The Crucial Ligaments

Diagnosis and Treatment of
Ligamentous Injuries
About the Knee

The
Crucial
Ligaments

Diagnosis and Treatment of
Ligamentous Injuries
About the Knee

Edited by

JOHN A. FEAGIN, JR., M.D.

Past President
The American Orthopaedic Society for Sports Medicine
Chicago, Illinois

Team Physician, 1968–1972
United States Military Academy
West Point, New York

Orthopaedic Surgeon
St. John's Hospital
Jackson, Wyoming

Churchill Livingstone
New York, Edinburgh, London, Melbourne   1988

Library of Congress Cataloging in Publication Data

The Crucial ligaments.

Includes bibliographies and index.
1. Cruciate ligaments—Wounds and injuries.   2. Knee—Wounds and injuries.   3. Knee—Surgery.   I. Feagin, John A., date. [DNLM: 1. Knee Injuries—diagnosis.   2. Knee Injuries—surgery.   3. Knee Prosthesis.   4. Ligaments, Articular—surgery. WE 870 C955]
RD561.C78   1988   617'.582   87-23920
ISBN 0-443-08549-8

Distributed in the United Kingdom by Churchill Livingstone, Robert Stevenson House, 1-3 Baxter's Place, Leith Walk, Edinburgh EH1 3AF, and by associated companies, branches, and representatives throughout the world.

Accurate indications, adverse reactions, and dosage schedules for drugs are provided in this book, but it is possible that they may change. The reader is urged to review the package information data of the manufacturers of the medications mentioned.

Acquisitions Editor: *Robert A. Hurley*
Copy Editor: *Margot Otway*
Production Designer: *Charlie Lebeda*
Production Supervisor: *Jane Grochowski*

Printed in the United States of America

First published in 1988

To my family
near and far, immediate and extended,
for understanding and support through all the years

Contributors

Paul J. Abbott, Jr., M.D.
Orthopaedic Surgeon, Virginia Beach Orthopaedics and Sports Medicine, Virginia Beach, Virginia

Harold Alexander, Ph.D.
Director, Department of Bioengineering, Hospital for Joint Diseases Orthopaedic Institute, New York, New York

James R. Andrews, M.D.
Clinical Professor, Department of Orthopaedics, Tulane University School of Medicine, New Orleans, Louisiana; Orthopaedic Surgeon, Alabama Sports Medicine and Orthopaedic Center, Birmingham, Alabama

Steven P. Arnoczky, D.V.M., Dipl. A.C.V.S.
Associate Professor, Department of Surgery, Cornell University Medical College; Director, Laboratory of Comparative Orthopaedics, The Hospital for Special Surgery, New York, New York

Inga Arvidsson, Dr. Med. Sc., R.P.T.
Lecturer, Department of Physical Therapy Education, Karolinska Institute, Stockholm, Sweden

Bernard R. Bach, Jr., M.D.
Assistant Professor, Department of Orthopaedic Surgery, Rush Medical College of Rush University; Director, Sports Medicine Section and Rush University Center for Sports Medicine and Athletic Injuries, Rush Presbyterian-St. Luke's Medical Center; Chicago, Illinois

James R. Bain, M.Sc.
Medical Products Division, W.L. Gore and Associates, Inc., Flagstaff, Arizona

Champ L. Baker, M.D.
Clinical Assistant Professor, Department of Orthopaedics, Tulane University School of Medicine, New Orleans, Louisiana; Director, Continuing Medical Education, Hughston Sports Medicine Hospital, Columbus, Georgia; Orthopaedic Consultant, University of Alabama School of Medicine, Tuscaloosa, Alabama

C. William Bolton, D.V.M.
Medical Products Division, W.L. Gore and Associates, Inc., Flagstaff, Arizona

William C. Bruchman, B.S.M.E.
Medical Products Division, W.L. Gore and Associates, Inc., Flagstaff, Arizona

J. Timothy Bryant, Ph.D., P.Eng.
Associate Professor, and Principle Investigator, Clinical Mechanics Group, Department of Mechanical Engineering, Queen's University Faculty of Applied Science, Kingston, Ontario, Canada

John J. Callaghan, M.D., M.A.J., M.C.
Assistant Professor, Department of Surgery, Uniformed Services University of the Health Sciences F. Edward Hébert School of Medicine, Bethesda, Maryland; Attending Surgeon, Orthopaedic Service, Walter Reed Army Medical Center, Washington, D.C.

Edmund Y. S. Chao, Ph.D.
Brooks-Hollern Professor of Bioengineering, Department of Orthopaedics, Mayo Medical School; Consultant, Section of Biomechanical Research, Department of Orthopaedics, Mayo Clinic and Mayo Foundation, Rochester, Minnesota

T. Derek V. Cooke, M.D., M.B., B.Chir., F.R.C.S.(C)
Professor of Surgery, and Chairman, Clinical Mechanics Group, Department of Surgery, Division of Orthopedics, Queen's University Faculty of Medicine, Kingston, Ontario, Canada

R. Raymond Cunningham, M.D.
Orthopaedic Surgeon, St. John's Hospital, Jackson, Wyoming

Walton W. Curl, M.D.
Orthopaedic Surgeon, Hughston Orthopaedic Clinic, Columbus, Georgia

Sandra Curwin, B.S.
Ph.D. Candidate, University of California, Los Angeles; Physical Therapist, UCLA Medical Center, Los Angeles, California

Dale M. Daniel, M.D.
Clinical Associate Professor, Department of Surgery, Division of Orthopaedics, University of California, San Diego, School of Medicine, La Jolla, California; Staff Physician, Department of Orthopedics, Kaiser-Permanente Medical Center, San Diego, California

Jesse C. DeLee, M.D.
Clinical Associate Professor, Department of Orthopaedics, University of Texas Medical School at San Antonio, San Antonio, Texas

Kenneth E. DeHaven, M.D.
Professor, and Head, Section of Athletic Medicine, Department of Orthopaedics, University of Rochester School of Medicine and Dentistry, Rochester, New York

Scott F. Dye, M.D.
Orthopaedic Surgeon, Ralph K. Davies Medical Center, San Francisco, California

Ejnar Eriksson, M.D.
Professor of Sportsmedicine (Traumatology), Karolinska Institute; Head, Division of Sports Medicine, Department of Orthopaedic Surgery, Karolinska Hospital, Stockholm, Sweden

John A. Feagin, Jr., M.D.
Past President, The American Orthopaedic Society for Sports Medicine, Chicago, Illinois; Team Physician, 1968–1972, United States Military Academy, West Point, New York; Orthopaedic Surgeon, St. John's Hospital, Jackson, Wyoming

Frank J. Frassica, M.D.
Senior Resident, Department of Orthopedics, Mayo Graduate School of Medicine, Rochester, Minnesota

James G. Garrick, M.D.
Director, Center for Sports Medicine, Saint Francis Memorial Hospital, San Francisco, California

Ramesh Gidumal, M.D.
Clinical Instructor, Department of Orthopedic Surgery, New York University School of Medicine; Orthopaedic Surgeon, Bellevue Hospital Center, New York, New York

Edward S. Grood, Ph.D.
Professor of Engineering Mechanics, and Director, Biomechanics Laboratories, Department of Aerospace Engineering and Engineering Mechanics, University of Cincinnati, Cincinnati, Ohio

Henry W. Hamilton, M.B., Ch.B., F.R.C.S.(Ed), F.R.C.S.(C)
Orthopaedic Surgeon, Port Arthur Clinic, Thunder Bay, Ontario, Canada

Charles E. Henning, M.D.
Clinical Assistant Professor, Department of Surgery, Division of Orthopaedics, University of Kansas Medical Center School of Medicine, Kansas City, Kansas; President, Mid-America Center for Sports Medicine, Wichita, Kansas

Robert W. Higgins, M.D.
Clinical Instructor, Department of Surgery, Division of Orthopedics, University of Mississippi School of Medicine; Orthopaedic Surgeon, Sports Medicine Section, Mississippi Sports Medicine and Orthopaedic Center, University of Mississippi Medical Center, Jackson, Mississippi

David V. Hoffman, M.D., F.R.C.S.(C)
Orthopaedic Surgeon, Port Arthur Clinic, Thunder Bay, Ontario, Canada

Peter A. Indelicato, M.D.
Associate Professor, and Director, Sports Medicine Section, Department of Orthopedic Surgery, University of Florida College of Medicine; Team Physician, University of Florida Athletic Association, Gainesville, Florida

Robert W. Jackson, M.D., F.R.C.S.(C)
Professor of Surgery, University of Toronto Faculty of Medicine; Chief of Staff/Chief of Surgery, Orthopaedic & Arthritic Hospital, Toronto, Ontario, Canada

Robert J. Johnson, M.D.
Professor of Orthopedic Surgery, and Head, Division of Sports Medicine, Department of Orthopedics and Rehabilitation, University of Vermont College of Medicine; Attending Physician, Medical Center Hospital of Vermont, Burlington, Vermont

Kenneth G. Jones, M.D.
Associate Clinical Professor, Department of Orthopaedic Surgery, University of Arkansas College of Medicine, Little Rock, Arkansas

Kenneth L. Lambert, M.D.
Orthopaedic Surgeon, St. John's Hospital, Jackson, Wyoming

Robert L. Larson, M.D.
Clinical Associate Professor, Department of Surgery, Division of Orthopedics, Oregon Health Sciences University School of Medicine, Portland, Oregon; Orthopedic Consultant, Athletic Department, University of Oregon, Eugene, Oregon

I. Martin Levy, M.D.
Attending Orthopaedic Surgeon, Jack D. Weiler Hospital of the Albert Einstein College of Medicine of Yeshiva University; Assistant Attending Orthopaedic Surgeon, Montefiore Medical Center; Assistant Attending Orthopaedic Surgeon, North Central Bronx Hospital and Bronx Municipal Hospital Center, New York, New York

Ronald E. Losee, M.D., D.Sc.
Private Practitioner, Ennis, Montana

Mary A. Lynch, M.D.
Mid-America Center for Sports Medicine, Wichita, Kansas

Kurt D. Merkel, M.D.
Senior Resident, Department of Orthopedics, Mayo Graduate School of Medicine, Rochester, Minnesota

Jeffrey S. Morris, M.D., M.B., B.Ch., F.R.C.S.(C)
Orthopaedic and Hand Surgeon, Joseph Brant Memorial Hospital, Burlington, Ontario, Canada

Werner Müller, M.D.
Privatdozent, Department of Orthopaedic Surgery, University of Basel, Basel, Switzerland; Head, Department of Orthopaedic Surgery, Kantonsspital Bruderholz, Bruderholz, Switzerland

Frank R. Noyes, M.D.
Director, Cincinnati Sportsmedicine and Orthopaedic Center; Clinical Professor, Department of Orthopedic Surgery, University of Cincinnati College of Medicine; Adjunct Professor, Department of Aerospace Engineering and Engineering Mechanics, University of Cincinnati, Cincinnati, Ohio

Bruce C. Ogilvie, Ph.D.
Professor Emeritus of Psychology, San Jose State University, San Jose, California

John R. Parsons, Ph.D.
Associate Professor, and Director, George L. Schultz Laboratories, Department of Surgery, Division of Orthopedic Surgery, University of Medicine and Dentistry of New Jersey-New Jersey Medical School, Newark, New Jersey

Lonnie E. Paulos, M.D.
Assistant Clinical Professor, Department of Surgery, Division of Orthopaedic Surgery, University of Utah School of Medicine; Director, Salt Lake City Knee and Sports Medicine, Salt Lake City, Utah

David W. Polly, Jr., M.D.
Instructor for Research, Department of Surgery, The Uniformed Services University of the Health Sciences F. Edward Hébert School of Medicine, Bethesda, Maryland; Orthopaedic Research Fellow, Division of Surgery, Walter Reed Army Institute of Research, Washington, D.C.

John S. Porter, M.D., F.R.C.S.(C)
Orthopaedic Surgeon, Port Arthur Clinic, Thunder Bay, Ontario, Canada

William G. Rodkey, D.V.M., Dipl. A.C.V.S.
Chief, Division of Military Trauma Research, Letterman Army Institute of Research, San Francisco, California

Thomas D. Rosenberg, M.D.
Assistant Clinical Professor, Department of Surgery, Division of Orthopedic Surgery, University of Utah School of Medicine; Director, Salt Lake City Knee and Sports Medicine, Salt Lake City, Utah

Franklin H. Sim, M.D.
Professor of Orthopedic Surgery, Department of Orthopedics, Mayo Medical School; Consultant, Department of Orthopedics, Mayo Clinic and Mayo Foundation, Rochester, Minnesota

George A. Snook, M.D.
Orthopaedic Surgeon, Cooley Dickinson Hospital, Northampton, Massachusetts; Consultant, University Health Service and Athletic Department, University of Massachusetts, Amherst, Massachusetts; Team Physician, University of Massachusetts Athletic Teams, Amherst, Massachusetts

William D. Stanish, M.D., F.R.C.S.(C), F.A.C.S.
Associate Professor, Department of Surgery, Dalhousie University Faculty of Medicine; Director, Orthopaedic and Sport Medicine Clinic of Nova Scotia, Halifax, Nova Scotia

J. Richard Steadman, M.D.
Assistant Clinical Professor, University of California, Davis, School of Medicine, Davis, California; Chairman, Medical Group, United States Ski Team, South Lake Tahoe, California

Mary Lou Stone, R.P.T.
Physical Therapist, Department of Orthopedics, Kaiser-Permanente Medical Center, San Diego, California

Robert A. Teitge, M.D.
Assistant Clinical Professor, Department of Orthopaedic Surgery, Wayne State University School of Medicine; Chairman, Department of Orthopedic Surgery, Hutzel Hospital, Detroit, Michigan

Russell F. Warren, M.D.
Associate Professor, Department of Surgery, Division of Orthopedics, Cornell University Medical College; Associate Attending Orthopaedic Surgeon, Chief, Sports Medicine Service, and Chief, Shoulder Service, The Hospital for Special Surgery; Team Physician, The New York Football Giants, New York, New York

Andrew B. Weiss, M.D.
Professor, Department of Surgery, and Chief, Section of Orthopaedic Surgery, University of Medicine and Dentistry of New Jersey-New Jersey Medical School, Newark, New Jersey

Preface

Over the centuries, the two central ligaments of the knee have been called the *genu-cruciata,* the *crucial ligaments,* and the *cruciate ligaments.* Galen referred to the genu-cruciata, and Robson, Hey-Groves, and Bosworth referred to the crucial ligaments, but all major references subsequent to 1936 refer to the cruciate ligaments.

The Crucial Ligaments was chosen as the title for this book. This title carries a double meaning—first, that it is the two crucial ligaments that form the central pivot of the knee, and second, that preservation or restoration of the ligamentous structures of the knee is crucial for optimal function and sports participation. Thus, my choice of title reflects the thrust of the book.

The Crucial Ligaments represents a summation of my clinical, laboratory, and team physician experiences. It also reflects thoughts and accomplishments of respected colleagues and mentors whose teachings I have known.

The Case Studies in Section 1, supported by the scientific and scholarly contributions in the other sections, provide a practical guide for the knee surgeon. This book emphasizes selectivity based on the principles of knee surgery. The resident may find a "ribbon match" that will help guide the management of a patient. The practitioner may seek a standard of practice. The mature craftsman will find examples and internal references to broaden his or her understanding of the principles of knee care, including physical examination, decision making, surgical care, and rehabilitation.

I have enjoyed preparing *The Crucial Ligaments* and deeply appreciate the colleagues who, through their knowledge and wisdom, have guided me. May this book fulfill its purpose so that you may teach those who follow.

Godspeed in your quest for science and skill in care of the knee.

John A. Feagin, Jr., M.D.

Acknowledgments

For Special Help in Preparing *The Crucial Ligaments*:

Lottie B. Applewhite, author's editor, Marsha J. Dohrmann, illustrator, and Venna Sparks, coordinator: They made a dream come true.

Drs. Larry VanGenderen and Bernard R. Cahill, for reviewing the case studies. Drs. Lowell M. Anderson, Robert A. Arciero, Kurt M. Chambless, Mark A. Broberg, and Charles D. VanMeter, for their critiques.

Our office staff: Rose, Dawn, Georgia, Kelly, Diane, Caroline, Annette, Juanita, Carri, Julie, Patricia, Brandy, and Lloyd.

The Churchill Livingstone staff, especially Robert A. Hurley and Margot Otway.

My partners, Drs. Kenneth L. Lambert and R. Raymond Cunningham, for spiritual and physical support as well as manuscript review.

Special Orthopaedic Mentors:

Drs. J. Leonard Goldner, Frank H. Bassett, Lloyd Taylor, Garnet F. Wynne, Ernest A. Brav, Walter Metz, George I. Baker, George E. Omer, Jr., David G. Paulsrud, Anthony Ballard, William E. Burkhalter, Marcus J. Stewart, William M. Deyerle, Augustus A. White, Jerry Sisler, Howard G. Abbott, Joseph R. Rokous, Douglas W. Jackson, the staff at Wrightington Hospital, Sterling B. Mutz, General George S. Woodard, Jr., Ralph Soto-Hall, Richard B. Welch, Robert L. Larson, F. James Funk, Jr., B. G. Weber, Werner Müller, Ejnar Eriksson, the ACL Study Group, and my colleagues in The American Orthopaedic Society for Sports Medicine

Exemplars:

Duke University and Dean Wilburt C. Davison, Sir John Charnley, the Past Presidents, and Board of Directors, of The American Orthopaedic Society for Sports Medicine

Special Friends:

Letterman Army Medical Center Staff, Fellows, and Residents

Jackson Orthopaedic Fellows and Residents

St. John's Hospital and Staff

Coach Tom Cahill, Ed Pillings, the Coaches and Trainers

The United States Military Academy, West Point: Staff, Faculty, Grads, and Cadets

Generals Andrew A. Goodpaster and William A. Knowlton

Drs. H. Edward Cabaud and William G. Rodkey

A. Graham Apley, F.R.C.S., M.B., M.R.C.S., and Dr. Stanley Hoppenfeld

My Patients

Thanks to each of you for your inspiration

*If I have been able to see further
it is because I have stood on the shoulders of giants.*
Sir Isaac Newton

Contents

SECTION 9
PROSTHETIC LIGAMENTS   493

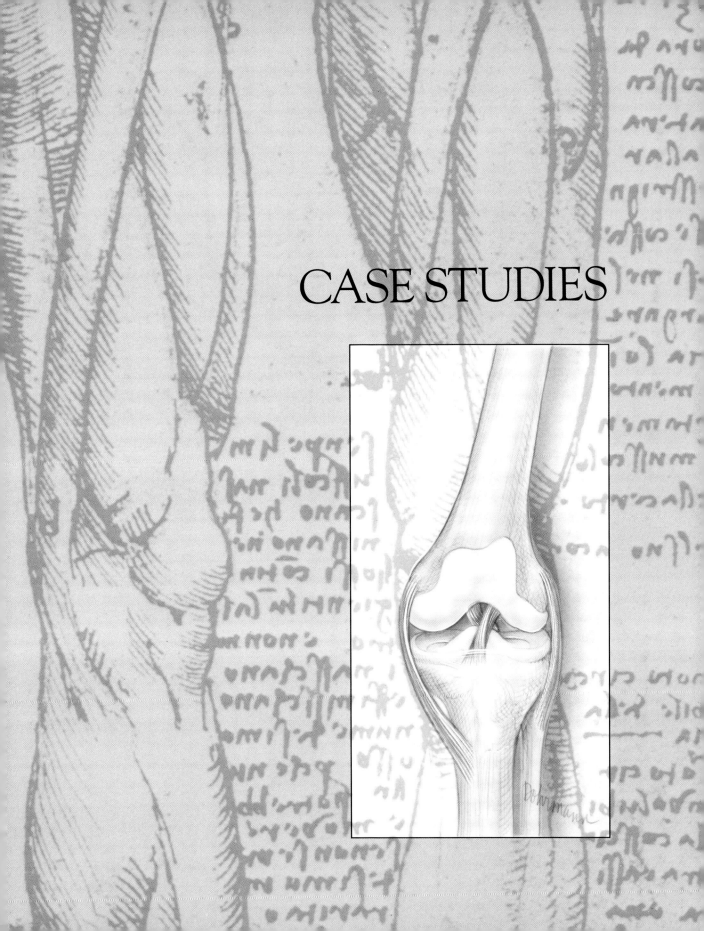

CASE STUDIES

Introduction: Principles of Diagnosis and Treatment

JOHN A. FEAGIN, JR.

Section 1 of *The Crucial Ligaments* is devoted to fifteen case studies of injured athletes. This introductory chapter presents the basic principles of diagnosis that I have found helpful and which are illustrated in the case studies. The case studies are organized in a consistent, algorithmic style. This style was chosen to stimulate the reader's thought processes and help him to refine, case by case, his knowledge of knee surgery.

The skills necessary for the diagnosis and treatment of knee ligament injuries are hard-earned and are the result of a never-ending quest for excellence. These skills are passed from generation to generation, perhaps more through our apprenticeships than our texts. These skills form the basis for good judgment, and become sources of unending pride.

One of the great teachers of orthopaedics had this to say:

> Accurate diagnosis, the essential preliminary to appropriate treatment, is difficult because the diagnostic pathway is beset by tripwires. A detailed history of the injury is seldom obtainable; the most complete ligamentous and capsular disruptions are often the least painful because the sensory nerve fibers also are torn, and sometimes they are the least swollen (because the torn capsule allows the effusion to leak away). Moreover, even an innocent radiograph can be misleading, because a ligament whose substance is torn is more difficult to repair than that which has avulsed its bony attachment. For all these reasons and because the initial physical assessment may determine the entire future athletic life of the patient, the initial examination must be both meticulous and systematic.
>
> A. Graham Apley, F.R.C.S., M.B., M.R.C.S, editor of the British issue of the Journal of Bone and Joint Surgery (personal communication, Jackson, Wyoming, May 1986).

It would be impossible to acknowledge all who, like Alan Apley, have guided me with their wisdom and philosophy. Some have been mentioned elsewhere; many the reader will get to know in Sections 2 through 9 of this book or the selected bibliography. The glossary is intended to standardize the semantics as they relate to our care of the knee. Drs. Grood and Noyes' concepts and terminology are used as the basis for a common language. The bibliography is a collection of readings from colleagues the world over whose contributions form the core of science and experience that are fundamental to the care of the knee.

I hope these case studies will help you to crystallize the principles of diagnosis and treatment of knee ligament injuries. The information and philosophy presented in this introduction should be kept in mind while reading the case studies. To facilitate integrating the introduction with the case studies, both are organized into sections on the history, physical examination, adjunct tests, rehabilitation, and decision-making.

HISTORY AND MECHANISM OF TRAUMA

In athletic trauma, the history is usually quite straightforward and the patient usually is aware of the details and circumstances. This is a luxury not always found in other fields of trauma. In obtaining the history, the physician should elicit from the patient the mechanism of injury, the swelling (immediate or delayed), the pain, the ability to continue participation, and previous injury or dysfunction.

Mechanism of Injury

The mechanism of injury alerts the physician to which ligaments were at risk in the knee. The most common mechanism of injury is a change of direction involving deceleration, with the foot fixed and with contact with another player. This classic injury of American football is the O'Donoghue triad—a tear of the anterior cruciate ligament (ACL), the medial collateral ligaments (MCL), and the medial meniscus (illustrated in Case Study 2).

As shoe/turf and ski/boot fixation devices have become more efficient, we now often see injuries caused by deceleration and change of direction that do not involve contact with another player. This type of injury is associated with a "pop," the inability to continue "play," and the onset over the next 24 hours of a relatively tense effusion. This mechanism was initially associated with the "isolated tear of the ACL" but, as has become clear with time and sophistication, there is seldom an isolated ligamentous injury to the knee. The knee is a harmonious symphony of ligaments, in which no ligament stands alone.

A recently identified mechanism, which occurs predominantly in the skier, is an abrupt contraction by the quadriceps to regain balance—similar to a powerful Lachman test—which pulls the tibia forward on the femur and tears the ACL. This injury may not even be associated with a fall.

Of course, there are other mechanisms of injury, but these three predominate and will serve the clinician well.

Pain

Many patients are able to walk off the field or ski down after a severe ligamentous injury. Pain is certainly a characteristic of these injuries, but perhaps the feeling of subluxation is more ominous and limiting to the patient. A tried and true dictum of ligament injury is that the more pain, the less severe the injury. It is probable that a complete tear so disrupts the nerve fibers that the pain is less severe. Certainly in a complete tear one can "open" the joint more readily with less discomfort to the patient.

The Pop

The pop is characteristic of a tear of the ACL. We know from Instron studies that the helicoid arrangement of the ACL allows it to store considerable energy before its elastic limit is reached. As a result, when the elastic limit is reached, the ligament bursts convulsively, and the patient defines this sensation as "a pop."

The pop is the part of the history that most reliably indicates ACL tear. Neither the MCL nor the capsuloligamentous structures tear with this pop, perhaps because they have broader origins and insertions and are generally flattened rather than helicoid. At any rate, the pop is characteristic of a tear of the ACL. It has been my experience that very few people will continue to play after sustaining an ACL injury. If they do continue, a more extensive injury may result, i.e., subluxation of the tibia on the femur, an event which is quite incompatible with sport and the cutting mechanism.

Onset of Swelling

Swelling, which can be appreciated by physical examination, is often delayed for 6 to 24 hours. The artery to the ACL, a branch of the posterior geniculate, is not substantial and is easily tamponaded. In the surgical care of acute cases, blood has been seen to "drip much like a leaky faucet." This explains the slow accumulation of the effusion. If the effusion is contained by the capsular mechanism, then it will reach maximum within 12 to 24 hours. If, however, a lesion of the capsule coexists with the ACL injury, the effusion may be slight because the fluid escapes through a rent in the capsuloligamentous structure.

If effusion develops immediately after injury, one should suspect an osteochondral fracture. Bleeding into the joint is more brisk with an osteochondral fracture than with a torn ACL; this distinction is a subtle diagnostic clue. The fluid is usually aspirated since its character and the presence or absence of fat are important diagnostic signs.

HISTORY OF PREVIOUS INJURY

Is the injury truly acute or was there a previous laxity or disability? Too often the athlete "forgets" that the knee was previously injured. Once reminded, the athlete can usually offer the details. These details take on added meaning when the x-ray films are reviewed as one seeks evidence of old injuries through osteophyte formation.

Simple as it is, the history can be a useful diagnostic tool. In fact, in my experience, deceleration, cutting injuries that are associated with a pop and with the gradual onset of effusion over the ensuing 24 hours will prove in 85 percent of cases to be ACL tears. Since ACL tear is seldom an isolated injury, the examiner's task is to verify the ACL tear and seek out associated injuries through the physical examination.

PHYSICAL EXAMINATION

The physical examination is an art and a science. The specific ligamentous injury is sought primarily by comparing the excursion of the tibia on the femur in the injured and uninjured knee. This is done by imparting stress through a range of motion. This sounds complex but in reality it can be quite precise, particularly if the clinician can get the patient to relax while he examines the well leg first. Using the well leg as a standard for comparison is a must.

The position of comfort for the patient is frequently the position in which he is found. I prefer to begin the examination with the patient in this position. The initial examination can be particularly revealing when it occurs before the onset of effusion

and muscle spasm. A single examination is seldom definitive. Re-examination is essential and appropriate. Sometimes a change in venue will help both physician and patient to relax and will result in a more productive physical examination. Ice is a useful adjunct to the physical examination as it decreases pain and promotes relaxation.

Inspection — Look!

The injured knee must be considered in the context of the entire patient. The patient's physiologic age, body fat, and muscle mass reflect his or her previous selection of activities. I consider these to be key observations during the physical examination. The brachioradialis and gastrocsoleus are excellent muscles to observe, since they are seldom developed by adult activity and thus reflect the activities of youth.

In addition to the knee, the leg as a whole should be inspected. Is the skin intact? Are there abrasions, old scars, or bruising? The state of the skin may give information about the direction, force, and mechanism of injury, and the past history. The shape of the joint and upper and lower limb segments, their general alignment, and any atrophy or swelling (localized or diffuse) should be noted. These observations lead to the laying on of the hands — palpation.

Palpation — Feel!

The hands of the skilled examiner are a wonderful arthrometer. The palpatory examination of the knee involves a subtle gradient of force application. The initial laying on of the hands is done on the normal side with only sufficient pressure to feel the subtleties of the knee's form. This complements the visual inspection. When the form is ascertained, more pressure is applied to distinguish induration — the hardness of the various tissue planes. Induration often is the clue to the severity as well as the site of injury. Gentle flexion of the knee, where possible without pain, is helpful during this search for induration because it may separate some of the anatomic structures and help to localize more precisely the sites of injury.

Finally, palpation is conducted with slightly more vigor to identify tenderness and/or gaps in the underlying soft tissues. This must be done with the patient's full knowledge and cooperation, and the patient must appreciate the precision with which this portion of the examination can be conducted. Gentleness is the key to this precision.

Problems left unattended within the knee do not become easier with the passage of time. Initial subtleties become blunted by induration, edema, and effusion which develop days after injury. One misses important details by not examining the knee-injured patient shortly after the injury occurs.

Movements — Move!

Should the examiner begin with active or passive movements? I prefer to ask the patient to move the well leg within the range of motion that is comfortable and possible for him. This gives a standard of comparison for the injured leg. Then I ask the patient to move the injured extremity within the bounds of comfort. This shows the range of motion available to position the leg for the ligamentous examinations.

Flexion/Extension
One of the goals of movement is to place the extremity in the best position for isolating and examining the different ligamentous structures (see Ch. 10). If hyperextension can be achieved, it is a good position to begin in. If the knee is stable in hyperextension, the medial and lateral capsuloligamentous structures and the posterior cruciate ligament (PCL) are intact. Thus, the maximum amount of information is gained quickly.

The collateral ligaments are best examined at hyperextension, neutral, and 30° flexion (Fig. 1). The technique that Smillie taught me still seems the most useful — the patient's foot is pinioned against the examiner's hip, so both hands are free to palpate the joint lines and ligamentous structures.

Varus/Valgus Angulation
Laxity in hyperextension to varus or valgus angulation are ominous signs that indicate disruption of key ligamentous structures. If in hyperextension the joint is lax to valgus angulation, the medial capsuloligamentous structures and the posterior cruciate ligament are probably interrupted. If in hyperex-

tension the knee is lax to varus angulation, the arcuate complex and posterior cruciate ligaments are probably disrupted. When varus and valgus angulation are applied with the knee at 0° flexion, the ACL and PCL are slackened sufficiently that these tests are diagnostic of medial or lateral capsular injuries. At 30° flexion the cruciates are in their most relaxed state and pathologic laxity palpated is capsular laxity (see definitions in Chs. 9 and 10).

Rotation
The appreciation of increased rotatory excursion requires careful attention to detail. With the hip and knee flexed 90°, internal and external rotation stress are applied first to the well and then to the injured leg (Fig. 2). This test can give quite meaningful information on the status of the cruciates, as well as the complementary medial lateral capsuloligamentous structures. I have found this test particularly useful.

AP Glide
The essence of the physical examination is an appreciation of pathologic excursion of the tibia with respect to the femur. AP glide is a particularly sensitive test, but may be misinterpreted if the relation of the tibia to the femur is not understood and the test is started in the wrong place. This misinterpretation most frequently occurs when the test is begun with the tibia inadvertently posteriorly subluxed on the femur. AP glide is best determined with the fingers measuring the translation of the tibia on the femur in an AP direction (Fig. 3). The fingers are quite accurate arthrometers though perhaps often undertrained.

Combined AP Glide and Rotation
By examining the medial and lateral compartments separately for AP glide, rotation can also be appreciated (Fig. 4). These combined movements are usually elicited in the pivot shift tests (see Adjunct Tests) and are eloquently described in Chapters 9 and 10.

Patellar Movements
The patella — which after all is the second joint of the knee — is not to be underestimated or underdiagnosed. The patella should be examined for ex-

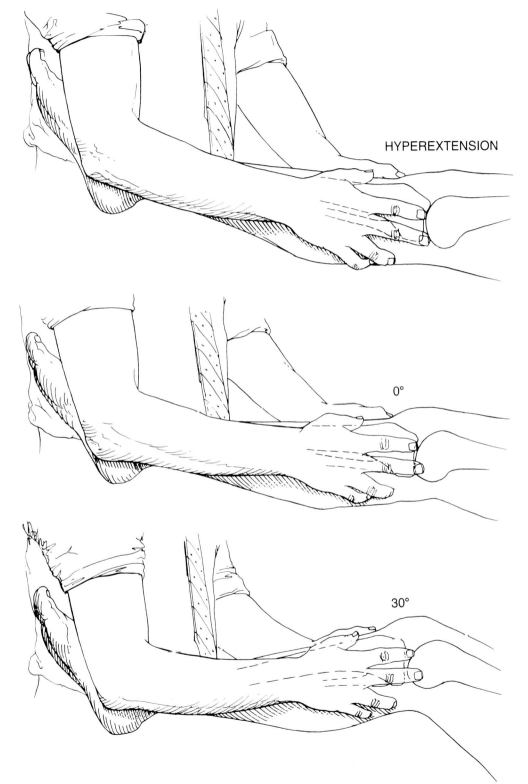

Fig. 1. The collateral ligaments are best examined at hyperextension, 0°, and 30° knee flexion. The technique was taught to me by Smillie.

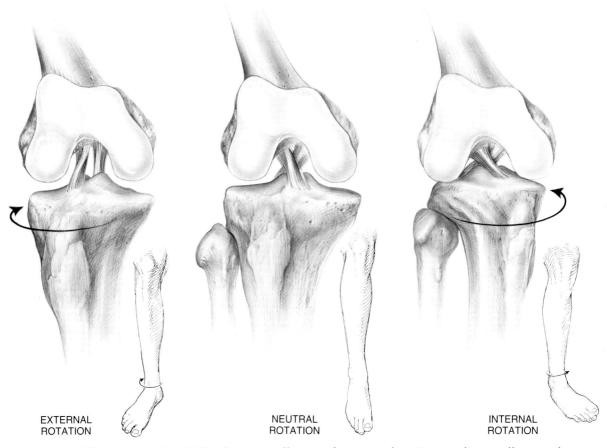

Fig. 2. Hip and knee flexed 90°; tibia externally rotated, in neutral position, and internally rotated. Note tightening of the cruciates with internal rotation.

EXTERNAL ROTATION

NEUTRAL ROTATION

INTERNAL ROTATION

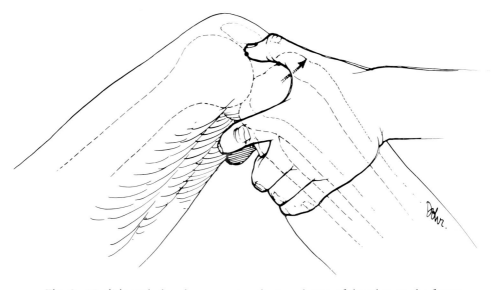

Fig. 3. AP glide with thumbs measuring the translation of the tibia on the femur.

Fig. 4. Combined AP glide and rotation. By examining the medial and lateral compartments separately a sense of rotation is appreciated.

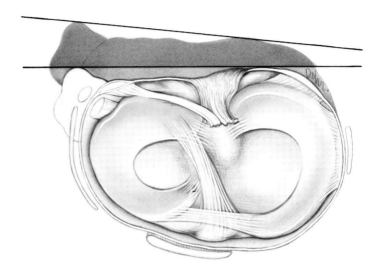

cursion, and the patient will indicate tenderness, pain, and apprehension (Fig. 5). This sometimes forgotten joint is too often the limiting factor after treatment. Thus, establishing its limits on the initial physical examination is especially appropriate.

ADJUNCT TESTS

An adjunct test is one that has become routine either because it is a specific test for a particular anatomic entity or because it has assumed significance

through a clinical meaning assigned by the founder. Such adjunct tests—physical and radiographic examinations—have proved reproducible in the hands of many.

The supine or sitting position seems to be the standard for examination. Too often we forget the other side of the joint, which is brought to view when the patient is prone. I have found the prone position to be particularly helpful when performing the Lachman and medial translation tests.

Besides the static examination, there is also a dynamic examination which requires assumption of

Fig. 5. The patella is examined for excursion, pain, and apprehension.

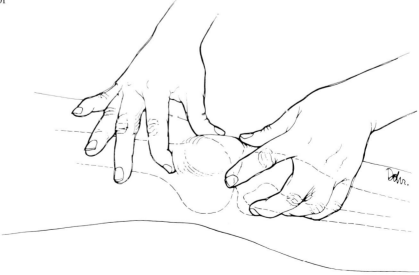

different positions. Standing, walking, or running give a keener appreciation of the limitation of function of the joint and the patient. In complex instabilities, it often is advantageous to record functional activities on videotape or film and to examine them in slow motion.

It is sometimes wise to perform the definitive physical examination elsewhere. The sideline is often not conducive to the meticulous attention to detail required of both patient and examiner. Sometimes merely a change in time and circumstances is advantageous; and should be so determined by the examiner. *Two tests, Lachman and pivot shift, are essential for every practitioner to master.*

Physical Examination Tests

Lachman Tests

With the knee flexed at 30° and the patient relaxed, the lower leg may be drawn forward on the upper leg by firmly stabilizing the femur and drawing the tibia forward on the femur (Fig. 6). Increased anterior excursion on this test is pathognomonic of a torn ACL. The end point should be graded as hard or soft. The end point is said to be hard when the ACL abruptly halts the forward motion of the tibia on the femur. The end point is soft when there is no ACL and the restraints are the more elastic secondary stabilizers. In this book the results of this test will be

described as mild (1+), moderate (2+) or severe (3+). Mild corresponds to 0 to 5 mm pathologic laxity, moderate to 6 to 10 mm, and severe to 11 to 15 mm of excursion greater than that of the uninvolved leg. The Lachman test is specific, reliable, and minimally painful to the patient, and should be mastered.

The only disadvantage of the Lachman test is that it is difficult to perform with small hands. This may be overcome by placing the patient prone (Fig. 7) and, with the knee in 30° flexion, accomplishing the same motion. Not only does gravity assist the examiner in this position, and the patient is usually more relaxed, but also the fingers may be free to palpate the femorotibial relationship. The test gives the same information whether the patient is supine or prone.

Another test I perform in the prone position is medial–lateral translation of the lower leg on the upper leg with the knee flexed 30°—a cruciate-deficient knee will manifest increased medial translation (see Ch. 8).

Pivot Shift Test

In its various forms, for example the MacIntosh test, the Losee test (Fig. 8), the Slocum test, the flexion-external rotation Drawer test (Noyes), and the Jerk test (Hughston), the pivot shift test helps the examiner to determine the abnormal translation and rota-

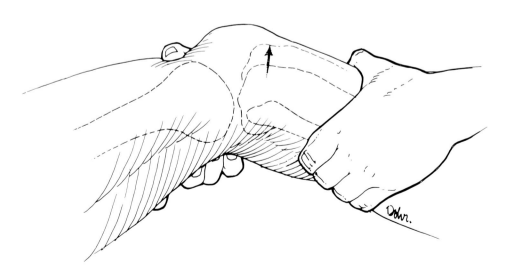

Fig. 6. The Lachman test.

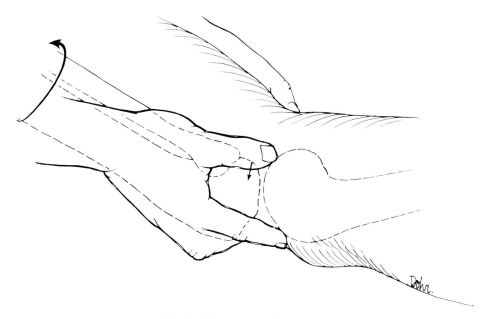

Fig. 7. The *prone* Lachman test.

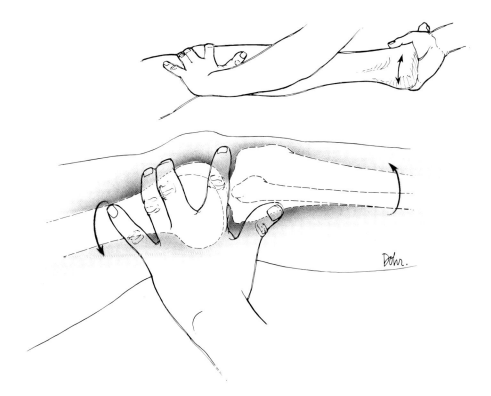

Fig. 8. The pivot shift test as described by Losee (Ch. 12).

tion of the medial and lateral compartments of the knee. Positive results in any of these tests depend, I believe, upon an incompetent ACL. If the MCL is disrupted, there may not be sufficient restraining force medially for the test to be meaningful. The test may be falsely negative because of muscle spasm. A false positive test is quite rare and would lead one to suspect either congenital laxity or congenital absence of the ACL (See Ch. 12).

Some wish to grade the results of the pivot shift test, as it is both a translatory and a rotatory phenomenon. This may be desirable since stretching of the secondary capsuloligamentous restraints increases the pathologic laxity in both translation and rotation.

The pivot shift test, in any of its presently recognized modifications, is sufficiently useful and specific to the examiner that he should *master* one or more of its variants.

Examination Under Anesthesia

The examination under anesthesia (EUA) should always be a concomitant of the arthroscopic examination. It is just as important during the EUA to examine the well leg first. With the muscles relaxed under anesthesia, subtle laxities may be apparent that were not fully appreciated in the office examination. It always gives a sense of satisfaction, however, when the examination under anesthesia yields the same findings as the office examination.

Radiographic Tests

What standard views and what special examinations should the examiner consider? What will be the role of computed tomography (CT) and magnetic resonance imaging (MRI)?

Fig. 9. The "tunnel" view.

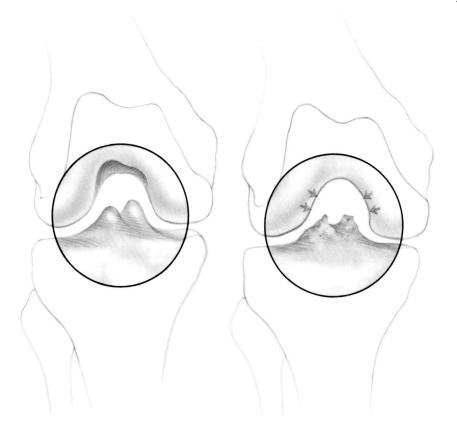

Standard Views

What standard radiographic views should the examiner request? The lateral view is accepted as standard by most physicians. The traditional AP view is under challenge from the tunnel view and the weightbearing tunnel view. In both tunnel views the knee is flexed and the beam is tangential to the tibia, so that the weightbearing surfaces of the femur on the tibia and the intercondylar notch (Fig. 9) are emphasized. I prefer either tunnel view to the AP view.

The patella view is likewise a part of the "standard" radiographic examination of the knee. Many views have been described and each has its proponents. I prefer the Merchant view because it is easier to standardize. It must be realized that all of these patellar views are static—the angles that can be measured from each are valuable but must be interpreted in light of the patient's pathology. It is doubtful that any of the views were intended to stand alone.

In our clinic is we routinely obtain a lateral view of the knee, a tunnel view with weightbearing where appropriate and practical, and a Merchant view of the patella.

Stress Radiographs and Arthrography

Stress radiographs, in both a varus/valgus and an AP plane, can be quite sophisticated and can give the physician valuable insight, although they have been used more for research than for clinical applications.

Arthrography has been developed into a refined science. It is a relatively noninvasive technique, usually performed by someone other than the surgeon. The anatomy is evaluated and recorded in situ before distension. Though indications for arthrography seem to decrease as skills in arthroscopy increase, I believe there will always be a place for a skillfully performed arthrogram.

Imaging

Technetium-99 scanning may be useful in the chronic knee to detect the increased cellular activity characteristic of degenerative arthritis (see Case Study 14). Computed axial tomography (CAT) has only begun to be used for the knee. CAT can be quite useful in the dynamic evaluation of the poste-

rior corners, where the arthroscope is often limited. The ACL and PCL can be visualized and their bulk and substance determined. The patella and its restraining ligaments, as well as adhesions and plicae, can be inspected. Cine-CT scanning adds yet another dimension which will help us in more effective care of patellar tracking problems. *Magnetic resonance imaging (MRI) promises to enhance our understanding of the soft tissues and their role in knee support and function.* This tool, though in its infancy, is already of diagnostic value (pp. 328–332).

The imaging modalities are useful in the diagnosis of knee disorders, but, helpful as they may be, they must not replace the manual skills.

Arthroscopy

The arthroscope is still young and yet already it has a proven place in the diagnosis and treatment of knee ligament injuries. Several generations of arthroscopes and tools have already appeared and vanished. The video record is yet another important adjunct to arthroscopy. The examination under anesthesia, a concomitant to arthroscopy, is likewise a benefit. The arthroscope has verified that ACL injuries are seldom isolated lesions and are frequently associated with medial or lateral meniscal tears. This certainly makes sense given our understanding of knee kinematics.

The arthroscope does not replace the manual examination; rather, it augments it and provides added validity and reliability. The clinician turned arthroscopist can focus with more certainty on the areas of pathology.

The arthroscope, used both diagnostically and therapeutically, has added a major new dimension to the art and science of knee surgery.

DECISION MAKING

Decision making is often a neglected art. Decision making is the logical conclusion of the diagnosis and selection of treatment. One of the joys of "decision making" is including the informed patient and/or his family in the process. Including them implies that they are interested in, have been educated about, and understand the implications of the problem. Involving the patient (and family) is the responsibility of the treating physician. Besides being given an outline of the necessary diagnostic tests required to arrive at the point of decision making, the patient or responsible party must understand the proposed therapy and its indications, limitations, and contraindications. These aspects are fundamental to "informed consent." The importance of rehabilitation, including its probable duration, as it relates to the proposed management must be outlined. Managing the rehabilitation of his patients is a special privilege of the knee surgeon, and a rightful part of our discipline. The patient must consider the necessary rehabilitation commitments before agreeing to the proposed treatment process.

REHABILITATION

In this section I originally intended to cover rehabilitation in two ways—first, a rather didactic cookbook of rehabilitation techniques, and second, the theory of rehabilitation as discussed in Section 8. However, in Chapter 25 Drs. Arvidsson and Eriksson provide a "cookbook recipe" for rehabilitation after anterior cruciate ligament surgery. Their regimen is nearly all-inclusive and obviates a presentation of the same material here. Their recipe incorporates the current biomechanical principles and the considerations of soft tissue care, and emphasizes early return to function. It is eminently practical. I endorse the program they outlined for postoperative rehabilitation. It may be applied to most of the case studies. The specifics of my personal program for postoperative rehabilitation after ACL surgery are well covered by the contributors in the rehabilitation section. I would feel comfortable applying appropriate portions of their programs to any of the patients outlined in the 15 case studies.

However, I will add the following comments:

A close relationship among the physical therapist, patient, and surgeon is necessary for the success of all rehabilitative plans.

The combination of an overzealous patient and an overzealous therapist can undo even the best work of the surgeon.

"Life after physical therapy," i.e., a self-motivated program, is imperative where endurance and agility are required.

Agility, proprioception, and balance are not adequately emphasized in our current programs. These skills can be enhanced by using existing local resources such as remedial dance, aerobic exercise programs, and personal fitness and conditioning courses.

Objective testing should be undertaken as a reward for the patient. This test should be performed at about the sixth to eighth month, using the Cybex or Orthotron (Cybex, Division of Lumex, Inc., Ronkonkoma, NY) or an equivalent instrument for testing the hamstrings and quadriceps. Hip abductors or abdominals are tested. Simple agility drills are included to ensure that agility has not been neglected. Use of a laxity arthrometer such as the KT-1000 (MEDmetric Corporation, San Diego, CA), Knee Laxity Tester, or Genucom system, when available, usually is also helpful.

COMMENT

The case studies that follow will help to crystallize these principles of diagnosis and treatment. New facets of diagnostic radiography give promise of procedures that will further confirm the findings of manual examination. Rehabilitation techniques, too, are becoming more scientific, so that we can monitor the patient more accurately and speed the patient's progress. Decision making, an art and science, can facilitate the treatment program because it elicits the patient's cooperation. However, all the technology [the techniques,] will not replace the hands-on physical examination by a skilled physician.

The glossary and annotated bibliography will prove to be useful resources. The case studies, with their timelines, may be considered singly or in sequence as the reader desires.

CASE STUDY 1

Isolated Anterior Cruciate Ligament Injury

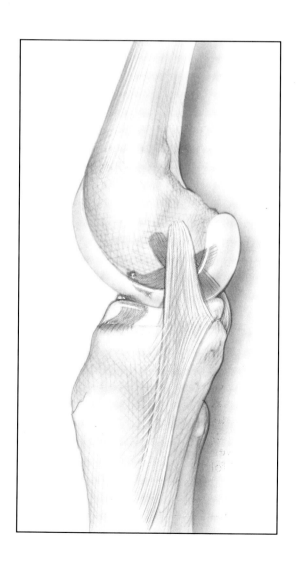

HISTORY

A 17-year-old secondary school athlete who lettered in football, basketball, and track sustained a noncontact deceleration injury to his right knee as he "cut" to the left in the second football game of his junior year. He felt a pop and was unable to continue play.

Knee Examination
(Physician On-Field)

Diagnostic Clues	Findings
Effusion	None
Tenderness	Diffuse/nonspecific
Lachman test	2 + positive*/soft end point
Drawer test	Uncertain
Pivot shift test	Not attempted
Varus/valgus	Stable
Patella apprehension	Negative
Range of motion	10 to 90°, mild discomfort
Gait	Walked with a limp
Neurovasculature	Intact
Other	None

  * 1+ means 0 to 5 mm pathologic laxity, i.e., abnormal tibial excursion on the femur; 2+ means 6 to 10 mm pathologic laxity; 3+ means 11 mm or more of pathologic laxity, i.e., increased excursion of the tibia on the femur on the injured leg when compared to the normal leg.

The knee injury occurred while the team was on the road, and the examining physician's treatment consisted of splinting and referring the patient to his home-town orthopaedic surgeon. The following day you the surgeon confirmed the history. The physical examination was difficult to duplicate, but revealed the following:

Diagnostic Clues	Findings
Effusion	+Moderate
Tenderness	Medial at jointline; lateral along iliotibial tract
Lachman test	2+ positive*/soft end point
Drawer test	1+ positive/soft end point
Pivot shift test	Could not be accomplished because of tense effusion and hamstring spasm
Varus/valgus	Stable
Patella apprehension	Negative
Gait	Antalgic
Neurovasculature	Intact
Radiographs	Negative except for effusion

* See Glossary.

The athlete and his parents were justifiably concerned. They desired diagnosis and counsel.

COMMENTS

This history was straightforward and suggested a tear of the ACL or subluxation of the patella. The patient was a dedicated, disciplined athlete, and was determined to continue recreational sports.

Persistence, patience, expertise, and a positive doctor/patient relationship will sometimes allow duplication of the initial physical findings, but, as in this case, swelling and spasm often mask critical features. It was explained to the patient and his family that the manual examination was not accurate enough to permit a decision, and that manual and arthroscopic examinations under anesthesia were indicated.

Although the joint could have been aspirated in the office to determine the presence or absence of fat, this would not have obviated the need for arthroscopic examination under anesthesia. Also, the possibility of more than an "isolated ACL" injury is such that a torn meniscus could be expected in approximately 70 percent of cases such as this.[4,9] In addition, arthroscopy may detect capsular rents or blushing of the capsule (indicative of tearing of secondary restraints).

The patient wanted his knee repaired as well as possible, and was willing to cooperate in the necessary rehabilitation if the ACL required repair. He was admitted to the hospital on the following day (day 3 after injury).

There certainly is not a consensus that operative care is either the best choice or the accepted standard for the "isolated ACL." This lack of unanimity, perhaps more than any other factor, was the impetus for this book — i.e., it was written in an attempt to understand better how and when the injured knee can be managed best by surgery.

COURSE OF ACTION

Physical Examination

The physical examination is critical in a case such as this. *The well leg must be examined first to provide a "baseline" standard of comparison.* Repeat physical examination can often be confirmatory, and *icing the knee* for 1 to 4 hours may be especially helpful. A change in venue sometimes is necessary to obtain a critical knee examination. Nevertheless, the physical examination should not be deferred; if possible, a firm, accurate diagnosis should be made within 24 hours of injury.

Problems in the knee that are left unattended do not get easier over time. Initial subtleties can become blunted by the induration, edema, and effusion that develop in the days after injury. One misses important patient feedback by not examining the patient early. Arthroscopic skill does not confer authority to neglect the manual physical examination. Not all pathology is intraarticular. The hands are a wonderful "arthrometer," and manual examination is a necessary precursor that complements the arthroscope.

The philosophy and technique of the physical examination were discussed in the Introduction. The principles I follow in the physical examination are as follows:

Examine the patient in the position of comfort. Examine the well leg before the injured leg.

Examine (feel) gently for induration and tenderness.

Examine for stability through a range of motion.

Examine the excursion of the medial and lateral compartments in response to both anteroposterior and rotatory testing through a range of flexion/extension.

Examine for stability as well as for pathologic laxity.

Diagnostic Studies

The following diagnostic studies should be performed in cases such as this:

Joint aspiration
Examination under anesthesia (EUA)
Diagnostic arthroscopy

Special Considerations

The age of this patient (17 years) is important, as it reflects his social responsibilities, lifestyle, rate of maturation, and intended use of his limb. Adolescents and young adults rarely tolerate alterations in their lifestyle as easily as some older patients. One may query the older patient about lifestyle modifications; even so, many are unwilling to alter their activity level. The young adult's wishes about surgery and restoration of function must be respected. Surgeons often ask at what age ACL reconstructive surgery should not be done. I have not found a cutoff, since I know people in their sixties who would be quite disabled by an unstable knee. Nevertheless, one must recognize that older patients are likely to suffer stiffness, adhesions, and poor healing, and the surgeon should modify both the operation and the postoperative care accordingly.

Body fat, muscle mass, and the distribution of muscle and fat reflect the patient's previous activities. I consider them to be key observations in the physical examination. The brachioradialis and gastrocsoleus are excellent muscles to check, since they are seldom developed in adulthood without specific attention and thus reflect the activities of youth.

As in the case under discussion, injuries do not always happen near the patient's home; however, it is important to maintain continuity of care. For example, an epidemic of ACL injuries is occurring at ski slopes. The place of injury may even be another country. Patients sometimes forcefully demand that the attending physician operate immediately. This should only be done when it is in the best interest of the patient and there is provision for continuity of care.

PLAN

What makes the practice of medicine unique is the infinite variability of "the plan." The subtle integration of all relevant factors—some obvious, some learned through experience, and some intuitive—in formulating the ideal treatment plan for a patient is the goal for which we all strive. Perfecting this art is an unending quest and is what keeps physicians vital through years of practice. Experience is important in formulating a treatment plan. Sometimes the surgeon is uncertain or underconfident. Sometimes the plan is "just not right." Usually I propose a tentative plan to the patient and then back off to allow response to the initial implications. I always let patients know that their input and insight are essential in formulating a plan for their care.

I often find that my time is equally divided between the physical examination and formulating the plan with the patient. Ultimately, however, the physician is responsible for the contract made with the patient. If the patient finds it difficult to establish a firm contractual relationship, he or she should seek a second opinion.

For this patient, the plan could have ranged from simple splinting to major reconstructive repair; there is no certain, single ACL injury treatment algorithm in our current state of knowledge. Philosophically, I would not have allowed this patient to ignore his lesion and "push on," as this would have jeopardized the secondary restraints. In my experience, active patients who have been allowed to test their secondary restraints after initial ACL injury have had disastrous results (J.A.F.). My choice for this type of injury is to complement the manual examination with an examination under anesthesia, diagnostic arthroscopy, and treatment of the injury under the same anesthesia. Results of ACL primary reconstruction are gratifying when the surgeon is able to restore *isometricity and revascularization* with a structure of adequate strength.

If this patient had declined surgery, I would have considered immobilizing the knee in 20° flexion for 4 to 6 weeks. This course at least would have allowed the secondary restraints to begin healing, and might have allowed the ACL to fall upon the PCL and gain a secondary source of attachment and blood supply (Fig. 10). I believe this is why the natural history of ACL injury was not quite so unsatisfactory in the past as today: immobilization after injury, formerly the usual recommendation, gave opportunity for the secondary restraints to heal, as well as for the ACL to join with the PCL, somewhat as described in the surgical repair of Wittek.[13]

Nonoperative care does not mean nondiagnostic care. One should not be tempted to make an incomplete diagnosis of a knee problem. Because the art of cruciate ligament repair is still imperfect, it is often tempting not to operate. Indeed, it is sometimes unwise to operate. Patient populations differ, and physicians too often fail to appreciate the idiosyncracies of their own patient populations. In this patient, I do not believe that nonoperative care would have been a good choice. The patient's current and future levels of activity were too high for a treatment regimen that did not restore the mechanics of the knee.

Primary repair of the interstitially torn ACL is seldom adequate, although the work of Marshall et al[8] presents some argument for interstitial repair. The interstitial nature of the torn helicoid structure, the scant blood supply, and the obtuse nature of the intercondylar notch all make it difficult to perform a primary repair that will restore isometricity, vascularity, and tensile strength. Augmentation grafting has been the procedure of choice in most hands. Prosthetics are not widely available at the time of this writing, but prosthetics, prosthetic research, and the potential for prosthetic repair will be discussed in Section 9.

Various procedures have been described for intraarticular reconstruction (see Ch. 20). Most of these procedures are applicable to both acute and chronic situations, but most are described, or applied, as chronic salvage procedures. This fact makes evaluation of results difficult, since in most of the cases for which they have been used, the ACL was not the only source of laxity. Most intraarticular procedures also reference the Jones operation,[6] and are described as modifications of the Jones procedure. This seems to be historically appropriate. Jones' current philosophic approach has been expressed elsewhere (see Ch. 20).

The central third of the patella tendon may well be more ligament than tendon in nature and function.[1] It is a sensible choice for a graft by today's standards.[3] One third of the structure usually confers adequate strength, and its harvest produces few complications. The question of vascularity is not yet resolved. Most surgeons prefer to make some attempt to provide vascularity, whether by maintaining the fat pad attachments, applying a synovial pedicle from the PCL, or routing the graft interstitially through the residual cruciate. Inadequate attachment of the graft and inaccurate placement that obviates isometricity have been

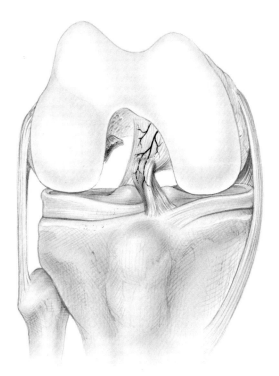

Fig. 10. The torn anterior cruciate ligament falls upon the posterior cruciate ligament and thus gains a secondary source of attachment and blood supply. This drawing illustrates the results of immobilization but is similar to the outcome of a surgical repair technique used by Wittek.[13]

major causes of failure. The surgical technique described in Ch. 21 will address these problems.

Thus, the first phase of the treatment plan for athletic patients with injuries such as this is a prompt, definitive diagnostic study, usually consisting of manual and arthroscopic examinations under anesthesia. Augmentation grafting of the ACL usually is accomplished under the same anesthesia.

Many ask, "Why arthroscopy if you are planning an arthrotomy in any event?" The arthroscope has reduced our need for wide surgical exposure, and provides more accurate diagnosis for the posterior parts of the knee than does the standard open joint exploration. Subtle meniscal and capsular tears, often not appreciated in open surgery, become apparent. Thus, at our clinic, we usually do an arthroscopic examination even when the pivot shift test is positive on the manual examination under anesthesia. Ultimately, I believe augmentation grafting will be accomplished through the arthroscope, which gives even more reason to gain expertise in this technique.

The procedure for this patient was as follows:

1. The knee was examined under anesthesia before the tourniquet was inflated. It was inspected, palpated, and checked for capsular induration. The competency of the central pivot was determined, as was the status of the secondary restraints.
2. The knee prepped, draped, and examined with arthroscope.
3. The knee was reprepped and draped.
4. The joint was exposed surgically through a single incision (which may be either straight medial, straight midline, or straight lateral).
5. The graft (center third of the patella tendon) was harvested.
6. Intercondylar notchplasty was performed.
7. Bone tunnels were placed central to the anatomic ACL origin and insertion.
8. The isometricity of the graft was checked.
9. The graft was fixed and tension adjusted.
10. Range of motion was checked and the elimination of pivot shift ensured.
11. The incision was closed.
12. A compression wound dressing was applied.

The operative procedure followed is described in more detail by Lambert and Cunningham in Ch. 21.

POSTOPERATIVE CARE AND REHABILITATION

Immediate

Ligaments that are isometrically placed, properly tensioned, and given a chance of nourishment through nearby vascularity can be amazingly resilient and can give gratifying results. Thus, a discussion of rehabilitation in this type of patient presupposes bone-to-bone internal fixation and isometric placement with a vascular leash that will not be jeopardized by early range of motion. There are three immediate postoperative goals:

Protection of the repair
Relief of pain
Prevention of adhesions

Continuous passive motion (CPM) has a function in achieving all three goals, and seems to be an effective adjunct to knee surgery (see Ch. 26). The CPM, cycling from 20° to 50° of flexion, is used frequently—usually beginning the day of the operation or the following day. Knowing that the joint can be moved comfortably so soon after the operation gives the patient confidence toward a home mobilization program. Marcaine (bupivacaine) 0.5 percent injected through the tissue layers at the time of closure seems to relieve some of the postoperative pain. Epidural analgesia through an indwelling catheter has proved effective in speeding recovery rehabilitation (see Ch. 25). Respiratory monitoring is essential if morphine is administered by indwelling catheter.

The usual hospital stay of this type of patient is 3 days. During that time, three types of exercises are emphasized:

Isometric exercise through an arc of 30° to 60° for the quadriceps and hamstrings
Vertical exercises for postural balance, such as toe rises and weight shift from right to left working toward single leg balance, as comfort allows

Exercise of the upper body and trunk muscles with a special emphasis on the abdominal and gluteus maximus muscles and on the opposite leg

The patient is taught to use crutches. We instruct the patient that the crutches are for balance, and to judge weightbearing by comfort. With proper internal fixation of the graft, the torque transmitted through the foot will not jeopardize a properly reconstituted ligament. Thus, we allow full weightbearing as soon as the patient can tolerate it. This approach has markedly enhanced our rehabilitation.

The firm compression dressing applied at the end of the operation is maintained for 7 to 10 days, until the first office visit. A light compressive dressing is then applied, often a thigh-length antiembolic hose. Care is taken not to impart venous constriction through elastic bandage about the knee. Phlebothrombosis is a paramount consideration even in young patients. Protection is afforded the ligaments by either a removable soft splint at 30° flexion, a 30° to 60° hinged cast, or one of the commercial hinged soft orthoses. For this patient, we chose to use a soft splint. This protection is maintained until the bone blocks of the augmentation graft are presumed to be healed at 6 weeks (see Timeline).

At each office visit, progress is reviewed, and the next stage of rehabilitation outlined. The stages are as follows:

Stage 1. Isometric stage — concentric tightening of the quadriceps and hamstrings so as not to impart quadriceps thrust which might jeopardize the graft (approximately 6 weeks)
Stage 2. Isotonic stage — emphasizes the strength through a range of motion with the hamstrings given preference over the quadriceps. The bicycle is particularly useful during this stage.
Stage 3. Restoration of endurance and agility through a functional rehabilitation program. This stage varies in length, depending on the ultimate functional requirements of the patient (which in this case were high)

Repeated manual examinations for ligamentous competency are not performed during these early office visits. However, a gentle Lachman test (20

lbs) can be reassuring. The patient sleeps without protection of the splint from the 6th week, and may wean himself from the daytime use of splint, 6 to 8 weeks postoperatively, as his judgment, strength, balance, activity level, and safety dictated.

Long Term

Long-term rehabilitation is, perhaps, the most neglected portion of patient management. Some of the structural and biomechanical abnormalities of the muscles, ligaments, and gait have been demonstrated objectively (see Ch. 25). A return to full function is the goal of the surgical procedure, but without rehabilitation it will not be attained. Sir John Charnley once said that a perfect operation requires little rehabilitation (personal communication, 1972, Wrightington, U.K.) I agree, but we are far from having a perfect knee operation. As we approach perfection, we will see a decrease in the demand for rehabilitation. Indeed, we have already seen an example of this trend, as arthroscopic meniscectomy replaced open meniscectomy.

Common to all long-term rehabilitation programs are the goals of *strength, endurance,* and *agility.* The SAID principle (specific adaption to individual demands)[12] is also applicable. These goals should be explained to the patient, and objective criteria for performance established. Practically speaking, this functional rehabilitation is difficult because it is beyond the purview of many physical therapists, and such goals are often too expensive for the patient. Rehabilitation facilities, health centers, and YMCAs can be participants by prescription, to the benefit of the patient and the facility. Unfortunately, most insurance companies have failed to appreciate this liaison in spite of its cost effectiveness.

Whenever possible, the patient should be encouraged to engage in bicycling, therapy pool walking, and level cross-country skiing if available, rather than in an impact-loading activity such as running.

Finally, there is return to competition. It is not necessarily national or even local competition — primarily it is self competition, the drive to turn the clock back to "do it again," with vigor and commitment and without pain or giving way. This is the ultimate goal. We should prepare athletic patients

CASE STUDY 1
Isolated ACL

Day of Injury	2	3	4	5	6	7	8	9	10	14	21	30	6	12	6	12
														WEEKS		MONTHS
			DAYS													

On Field Exam • Ice • Splint

Office exam • Ice • Splint

EUA • Arthroscopy • ACL augmentation graft • CPM 20°–50° • Removable soft splint • Discharge from hospital

Home PT program — 20 min 3 × daily

Office recheck • Isometrics • Toe rises • Trunk, upper body resistive exercises • D/C crutches when gait near normal • ROM 20°–50° • Weightbearing to comfort

Increase walking to tolerance • Begin strength training

Weightbearing to comfort • Isometrics

Bone blocks healed • D/C splint • Begin bicycle exercises if flexion 110° • ROM 20°–60° • No quad thrust • Skip rope with or without Endurance walking • Toe rises • Trunk, upper body resistive exercises • Isometrics

Endurance walking • Bicycle exercises (brace optional) • Swimming/water exercises simple agility patterns • Strengthen hamstrings and gluteals • Caution against jumping • Begin arthrometer rests

Sports participation when strength, endurance, and agility sufficient (brace optional) • Repeat strength and arthrometer rests
Return to all sports (brace optional)

such as the one described to work gradually toward this goal—the restoration of lifestyle for a lifetime of usage. A gratifying and unifying event for patient and surgeon is actual "return to competition."

PROBLEMS, COMPLICATIONS, FOLLOW-UP RESULTS

What can we expect of a patient who follows the regimen described—success, failure, satisfaction, disappointment, a shortened career? Evaluation techniques and recording methods are still too crude to answer this critical question.

Many will say the repair performed for this patient was philosophically and aesthetically acceptable, but what about back-up procedures? This was a primary case, and I have never felt obligated to back up a well-done, acute, "isolated" ACL augmentation. Certainly, back-up procedures can be justified, but the clinical results of primary surgical augmentation grafting of the reconstructed ACL both in the laboratory[2] and in our clinical experience[7] (see Ch. 21) are such that it seems disruptive to move other tissues, destroy further proprioception, and add to the rehabilitation time already surgically imposed. Back-up procedures and anatomic reconstruction of the corners is a necessary part of our armamentarium in chronic cases (see Ch. 23).

No adequate, standardized, universally accepted short-term or long-term form with which to compare our results has been developed—though many of us have tried.[5] The current arthrometers, at best, have given objective measurement of laxity, albeit only in a limited number of planes.

"Selectivity" is essential to determine which patients are candidates for knee surgery.[10,11] The practitioner must be cautious at this time, and must establish his standards in consultation and by comparison with others in the field.

SUMMARY

This case involved a 17-year-old outstanding athlete who sustained an "isolated ACL" during an athletic competition. In consultation, the patient elected an accurate diagnosis and surgical repair. The central third of the patella tendon was used for augmentation grafting. We were confident of the fixation and isometricity of the graft, and could closely supervise this dependable patient, so we permitted protected motion in the early postoperative period.

The long-term results for patients treated in this manner have been excellent. The operation has proved to be reproducible. Rehabilitation, both short-term and long-term, has been stressed until strength, endurance, and agility are restored. Bracing, return to competition, and complications will be discussed elsewhere.

REFERENCES

1. Apley AG: Letter to the Editor. J Bone Joint Surg 62A:487, 1980
2. Cabaud HE, Feagin JA, Rodkey WG: Acute anterior cruciate ligament injury and augmented repair. Experimental studies. Am J Sports Med 8:395–401, 1980
3. Clancy WG Jr, Narechania RG, Rosenberg TD et al: Anterior and posterior cruciate ligament reconstruction in rhesus monkeys. A histological, microangiographic, and biomechanical analysis. J Bone Joint Surg 53A:1270–1284, 1981
4. DeHaven KE: Diagnosis of acute knee injuries with hemarthrosis. Am J Sports Med 8:9–14, 1980
5. Feagin JA, Blake WP: Postoperative evaluation and result recording in the anterior cruciate ligament reconstructed knee. Clin Orthop 172:143–147, 1983
6. Jones KG: Reconstruction of the anterior cruciate ligament. A technique using the central one-third of the patellar ligament. J Bone Joint Surg 45A:925–932, 1963
7. Lambert KL: Vascularized patellar tendon graft with rigid internal fixation for anterior cruciate ligament insufficiency. Clin Orthop 172:85–89, 1983
8. Marshall JL, Warren RF, Wickiewicz TL: Primary surgical treatment of anterior cruciate ligament lesions. Am J Sports Med 10:103–107, 1982
9. Noyes FR, Bassett RW, Grood ES, Butler DL: Arthroscopy in acute traumatic hemarthrosis of the knee. Incidence of anterior cruciate tears and other injuries. J Bone Joint Surg 62A:687–695, 1980
10. Noyes FR, Matthews DS, Mooar PA, Grood ES: The symptomatic anterior cruciate-deficient knee. II. The results of rehabilitation, activity modification, and counseling on functional disability. J Bone Joint Surg 65A:163–174, 1983
11. Noyes FR, Mooar PA, Matthews DS, Butler DL: The

symptomatic anterior cruciate-deficient knee. I. The long-term functional disability in athletically active individuals. J Bone Joint Surg 65A:154–162, 1983

12. Wallis EL, Logan GA: Figure Improvement in Body Conditioning through Exercise. Prentice Hall, Englewood Cliffs, NJ, 1964

13. Wittek A: Zur Naht der Kreuzbandverletzung im Kniegelenk. Zentralbl Chir 54:1538–1541, 1927

RECOMMENDED READING

See also Chs. 12, 14, 17, this volume, and K.G. Jones in Ch. 20, this volume.

Dehne E: The spinal adaptation syndrome (a theory based on the study of sprains). Clin Orthop 5:211–219, 1955

Fairbank TJ: Knee joint changes after meniscectomy. J Bone Joint Surg 30B:664–670, 1948

Feagin JA, Cabaud HE, Curl WW: The anterior cruciate ligament. Radiographic and clinical signs of successful and unsuccessful repairs. Clin Orthop 164:54–58, 1982

Feagin JA, Curl WW: Isolated tear of the anterior cruciate ligament. 5-year follow-up study. Am J Sports Med 4:95–100, 1976

Galway HR, MacIntosh DL: The lateral pivot shift. A symptom and sign of anterior cruciate ligament insufficiency. Clin Orthop 147:45–50, 1980

Hunter LY, Funk FJ (eds): Rehabilitation of the Injured Knee. CV Mosby, St. Louis, 1984

Merchant AC, Mercer RL, Jacobsen RH, Cool CR: Roentgenographic analysis of patellofemoral congruence. J Bone Joint Surg 56A:1391–1396, 1974

Müller W: The Knee. Form, Function, and Ligament Reconstruction. Springer-Verlag, New York, 1983, pp. 8–13

Noyes FR: Flexion rotation Drawer test for anterior cruciate insufficiency. p. 924. In Edmonson AS, Crenshaw AH (eds): Campbell's Operative Orthopaedics, 6th Ed. CV Mosby, St Louis, 1980

Pavlov H: The radiographic diagnosis of the anterior cruciate ligament deficient knee. Clin Orthop 172:57–64, 1983

Slocum DB, James SL, Larsen RL, Singer KM: Clinical test for anterolateral instability of the knee. Clin Orthop 118:63–69, 1976

CASE STUDY 2

O'Donoghue's "Triad" — ACL Tear, Complete, MCL Tear, Complete, Peripheral Tear of the Medial Meniscus

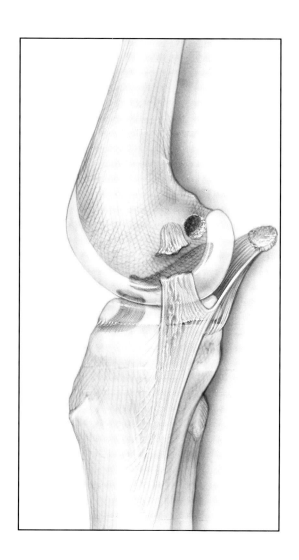

HISTORY

A 21-year-old college junior, a first-string running back, was struck on his planted right leg while advancing the ball. He experienced severe pain and did not attempt to rise from the turf. The on-field examination revealed gross laxity, and he was helped from the field with the leg splinted.

Knee Examination
(Team Orthopaedic Surgeon/Sideline)

Diagnostic Clues	Findings
Effusion	Mild
Tenderness	Medially
Lachman test	3+ positive*/soft end point
Drawer test	3+ positive/soft end point
Pivot shift test	Not attempted
Varus/valgus	3+ valgus opening in full extension, stable in full extension to varus testing
Patella apprehension	Patellofemoral joint stable
Range of motion	Too painful to elicit
Gait	Unable to bear weight
Neurovasculature	Intact
Radiographs	Not available
Other	Medial side is completely "blown out"

* See Glossary.

COMMENTS

This case represents the classic injury of American football as described by O'Donoghue.[12] This "triad" injury became more frequent through increased ef-

25

ficiency of the helmet and shoulder pad, contact below the waist (the "crack-back block"), and enhanced fixation of the shoe-turf interface. As both the speed of the game and the force of impact increased in the late 1950s, these injuries became all too common. Game films allow analysis of the disruptive forces that can be applied to the knee through this classic mechanism. Peterson (O'Donoghue Presentation at the American Orthopaedic Society for Sports Medicine meeting, Lake Tahoe, CA, 1981), through study of game films and the injury pattern, promulgated rule changes which have been responsible for a marked decrease in this devastating injury.

This patient had a chance at a professional sports future, and would be called an "elite" athlete. The next season was important to both player and coach. Because of this ominous history, it was important that planning proceed directly and expeditiously.

COURSE OF ACTION

Physical Examination

The on-field examination revealed that the injury was undoubtedly a surgical lesion by today's standards. It was merely a matter of when and how to perform the operation. A meniscal lesion was suspected on the basis of the mechanism of injury and the physical examination. The location of the meniscal disruption should be identified with intent to repair the torn portion and thus retain the meniscus. Given the gross valgus opening, the all-important posterior oblique portion of the medial collateral ligament was undoubtedly also torn.[6]

Even to the most experienced surgeon, the variety of MCL tears seems almost infinite (Fig. 11). Nevertheless, one should attempt to divide the medial capsuloligamentous complex into anatomic segments, search with diligence for tears of the individual parts, and recognize that many variations may be encountered. The direct portion of the medial ligament can be torn at either its meniscofemoral or its meniscotibial portions; the superficial portion of the ligament can be torn at either or both ends. The posterior oblique portion of the medial collateral ligament can be torn at either end or interstitially. All of the above can occur in combination.[7] The type

of lesion will frequently determine the best surgical exposure, and thus it is important to be alert to the nature of the tear so as to ensure the most direct entry into the joint for repair of the meniscus as well as to ensure complete repair of all torn medial capsuloligamentous structures.

Although a pivot shift may be helpful to determine the extent of injury, it would have been unnecessary to subject this patient to a subluxation test in the unanesthetized state. *Finding the knee stable to varus testing in extension confirmed the integrity of the lateral capsular ligaments and the posterior cruciate ligament.*

The patellofemoral mechanism can sometimes be disrupted in this injury, and when this occurs the lesion usually is at the attachment of the medial patellofemoral ligament to the linea aspera and medial intermuscular septum (Fig. 12).

Reexamination of injuries such as this in a stable, quiet milieu, away from the "heat of battle" and

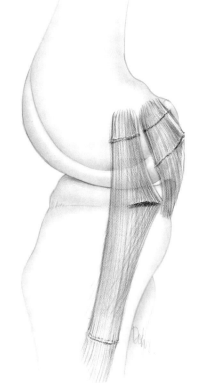

Fig. 11. The MCL is subject to an infinite variety of tears. The surgeon must divide the medial capsuloligamentous complex into anatomic segments and search for tears of the individual parts.

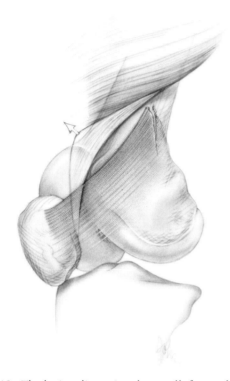

Fig. 12. The lesion disrupting the patellofemoral mechanism usually occurs at the attachment of the medial patellofemoral ligament to the linea aspera and medial intermuscular septum.

after the knee has been well iced, is important. Areas of maximum tenderness and induration are important clues. The gross laxity need not be reduplicated, but the subtle aspects of stability or laxity of the posteromedial and posterolateral corners will be important in the reexamination. Induration can be a clue to injuries in these areas and should be sought with gentle manual palpation. Two to six hours after injury is the best time for this reexamination. The "stable hinge" (i.e., residual intact ligamentous support), which usually remains even after a devastating injury of this nature, is as important in planning the operation as is the area of disruption.

Diagnostic Studies

The routine radiographs were carefully studied for bony evidence of capsular or ligamentous avulsion. Arthroscopy was not attempted because of the

danger of extravasation of the fluid through the disrupted medial compartment and possible compromise of the compartments of the lower leg. Furthermore, with a properly planned incision, it would be possible to open the knee widely and to explore visually even the posterior corners of both compartments.

Special Considerations

This patient obviously had exceptional physical ability, and our goal was to restore this ability so that he might attain his athletic potential. No qualified examiner could have missed the gross laxity with its surgical implications. It was clear that the operative repair should be done "at home" after the patient had been hydrated and mentally prepared for the operation and for his postoperative rehabilitation responsibilities. An operation of this type should be performed by a carefully chosen team. For an assistant I prefer an orthopaedic surgeon or highly trained surgical assistant who is experienced in knee surgery cases. The surgical technician and circulating nurse also must be well versed in the procedures. This type of operation is not the time for "on-the-job" training of an "on-call" operating room crew. It is important not to prolong tourniquet and surgical time needlessly.[3]

Rehabilitation should be closely supervised by the operating surgeon, and the patient should be given an estimate of how and when each activity level will be regained—such as range of motion, strength, agility, and return to his previous level of activity. In a patient of this type, these expectations are best covered preoperatively and reiterated at the appropriate time during the postoperative course, when the surgeon has the patient's full attention.

PLAN

As I prefer, the operation was planned for the morning following injury, after the patient had been counseled and hydrated. The knee was amply iced from the time of injury to the operation, to keep the disrupted tissues pristine and prevent the interstitial edema that complicates surgery. The "first team" was assembled, since obviously the first attempt at repair would offer the best chance of restoring the anatomic structures. A detailed preoperative examination under anesthesia should lead to the use of a single incision.

The repair in this type of case should be expeditious; tourniquet ischemia has been implicated as a cause for further muscular atrophy.[3] Securing isometric fixation of the medial ligaments with screw and washer (Fig. 13) allows early motion and the use of continuous passive motion in the postoperative period. All disrupted structures must be repaired. A diligent intraoperative physical examination at each stage of the repair will verify the restoration of stability and ensure that a ligamentous lesion has not been overlooked.

There is no place for nonoperative treatment in this type of lesion.

Examination under anesthesia is a part of the operative care. It is done immediately after induction of anesthesia, before the leg is prepped, and before the tourniquet is inflated. In addition to the obvious laxity, the surgeon searches particularly for induration at the posterior corners of the meniscoligamentous complexes and for excursion of the corners anteriorly and posteriorly. The stable hinge will dictate where the incision should be made. The incision should be made opposite this stability since it may be difficult to visualize both corners from either a medially or a laterally based incision. Both corners, however, can be reached from a straight midline incision.

In this patient, examination under anesthesia revealed a mild effusion (the remainder of the hemar-

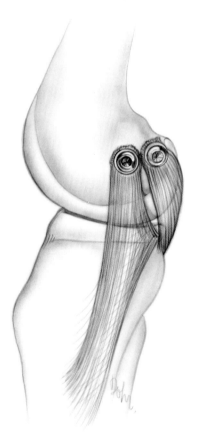

Fig. 13. The isometric fixation of the medial ligaments is secured with screw and washer so that continuous passive motion can begin in the immediate postoperative period, and subsequently the patient can begin early active motion.

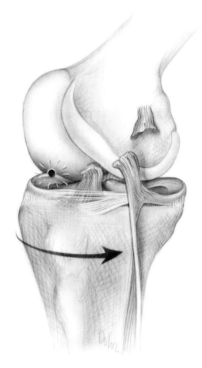

Fig. 14. The markedly positive Drawer test revealed that the tibia, with its conjoined menisci, could be brought quite anterior on the femur (the Finochietti sign). Both the posteromedial and posterolateral corners require careful evaluation for meniscocapsular disruption when this sign is identified.

throsis had leaked from the rent in the medial structures). The Lachman test showed a 3+ excursion with a soft end point, and the Drawer test was so markedly positive that the Finochietti sign[5] (Fig. 14) was identified. This confirmed that the tibia, with its conjoined menisci, could be brought quite anteriorly on the femur, which dictated a need for careful evaluation of both posteromedial and posterolateral corners for meniscocapsular disruption. The pivot shift was tested under anesthesia, and revealed that there was not only an anterior translation of the tibial plateau on the femoral condyles but also a gross rotatory subluxation.

The examination in this patient dictated that an incision adequate to visualize the pathology be made, either medial parapatellar or midline, extending from approximately 5 cm above the superior pole of the patella to the insertion of the superficial medial collateral ligament on the tibia (Fig. 15). The incision should be carried down to the plane of the prepatella bursa. This plane is used for dissection whenever possible. In dissecting the medial flap to reveal the medial pathology, great care must be taken to identify and preserve the nerve supply as well as possible (Fig. 16). In my experience, frequently it is not possible to preserve the infrapatellar branch of the saphenous nerve, but the saphenous nerve should be identified and protected. Its emergence from the fascia is quite variable.

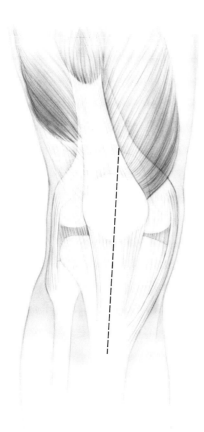

Fig. 15. A straight midline incision is adequate to visualize the pathology in the patient after the triad is diagnosed. The incision should extend from approximately 5 cm above the superior pole of the patella to the insertion of the superficial MCL on the tibia.

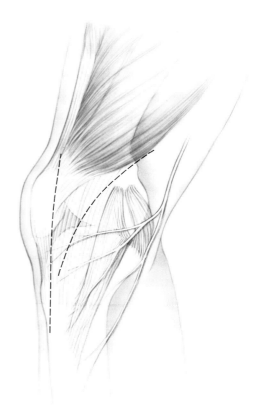

Fig. 16. The nerve supply must be identified and preserved as well as possible. The saphenous nerve, in particular, should be protected.

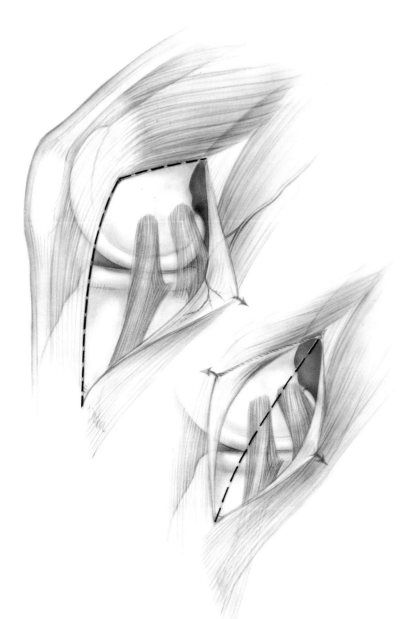

Fig. 17. The origin of the MCL in both its direct and oblique portions can be visualized by extending the medial retinacular incision obliquely along the vastus medialis obliquus and reflecting the fascia, or by incising the fascia along its parallel fibers overlying the tear of the deeper structures.

During the dissection medially, the capsular disruption should be sought to facilitate exposure of the deeper layers of the torn structures. Sometimes the rent extends through the fascia of the vastus medialis and this, of course, makes exposure easier since the lesion is essentially subcutaneous. More frequently, the medial fascia is intact, but the lesion can be palpated beneath this intact layer. I use one of two surgical alternatives: (1) to extend the medial retinacular incision obliquely along the vastus medialis obliquus (VMO) and reflect the fascia from superior to inferior, thus revealing the origin of the medial collateral ligament in both its direct and oblique portions, or (2) — the option chosen in this case — to incise the fascia along its parallel fibers overlying the tear of the deeper structures (Fig. 17).

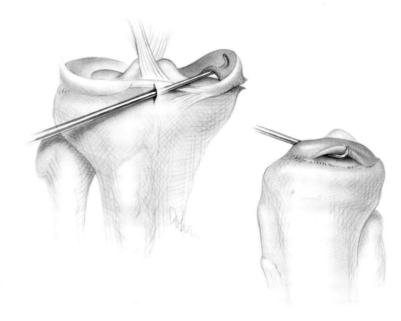

Fig. 18. The integrity of the meniscofemoral and meniscotibial ligaments is checked by visualizing the excursion of the probe along the superior and inferior surfaces of the meniscus.

Even when origin of the ligament is torn, there can still be tearing of surgical significance in its meniscotibial, meniscofemoral, and superficial components. After exposure of the conjoined origin of the superficial and direct heads of the medial collateral ligament, as well as of the posterior oblique portion of the ligament, the integrity of the meniscofemoral and meniscotibial ligaments is checked. This is accomplished by probing the meniscus along its superior and inferior surfaces while directly visualizing the excursion of the probe as well as the attachment of the meniscus to the tibial plateau (Fig. 18). Arnoczky,[1,2] Zlotsky (N. Zlotsky, West Point, NY, 1966, unpublished data), and others have verified that surgical repairs of the meniscus in this area are feasible, desirable, and reliable. If tears are demonstrated in this area, I usually use either the arthroscopic meniscal repair instruments or a 9D cutting needle and nonabsorbable size 0 suture to repair the meniscofemoral and meniscotibial ligaments. Sutures are passed but not tied.

The intercondylar notch is inspected next. *The ACL usually is torn interstitially* (Fig. 19).

The next step before repairing the ACL is visual exploration and probing of the posterolateral corner and the lateral meniscal attachments. This is facilitated by using a small, dull Hohmann-type retractor in the posterior tibial fossa at the site of attachment of the posterior cruciate ligament, thus levering the tibia forward on the femur (Fig. 20). This gives excellent visualization of the lateral meniscus in its posterior attachments. One should not forget, however, that the lateral meniscus attaches to the ligaments of Humphry and Wrisberg when

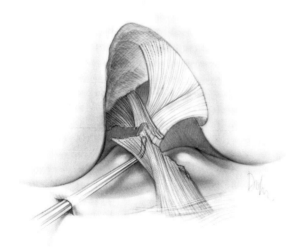

Fig. 19. In O'Donoghue's triad, the anterior cruciate ligament is usually torn interstitially.

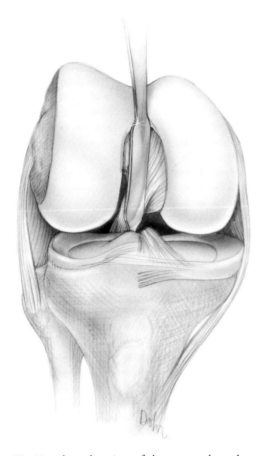

Fig. 20. Visual exploration of the posterolateral corner and the lateral meniscal attachments is facilitated by using a small, dull Hohmann-type retractor in the posterior tibial fossa at the site of the attachment of the posterior cruciate ligament. The tibia is levered forward by the retractor.

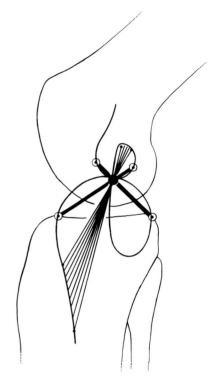

Fig. 21. The repair of the medial structures must be accomplished according to the theoretical course of the MCL and its position in relation to the Burmester curve. (Adapted from Müller W: The Knee. Form, Function, and Ligament Reconstruction. Springer-Verlag, New York, 1983.)

present and, rather than being firmly fixed to the tibial plateau, attaches to the femur superiorly. Again the probe is used to verify the integrity of the lateral meniscocapsular structures. If these structures are disrupted, they should be repaired. Repair can be accomplished through a counter-incision placed posterolaterally; the arthroscopic meniscal suture instruments are of great value in these situations.

In planning the repair of the ACL, the operating surgeon must decide whether to use semitendinosus tendon, patella tendon, allografts, or synthetic stent (augmentation). All have worked well

in the laboratory, but long-term clinical experience has yet to confirm the laboratory work on the value of allografts or synthetic stents.

One can then approach the repair of the MCL or the ACL in proper order, depending upon preference and choice of graft. The reconstructed ACL is not fixed under tension, however, until the MCL has been repaired. For the purpose of this discussion, we will assume that the medial collateral ligament is restored first. The surgeon must remember that sutures have already been placed for the meniscotibial and meniscofemoral portions of the tear. Attention is then directed to repairing the proximal and distal portions of the medial collateral and posterior oblique portions of the ligament. The medial patellofemoral ligament originating from the medial intermuscular septum will already have been visual-

Fig. 22. Tears of both medial collateral ligament and posterior oblique ligament. Repair with AO screws and spiked washers gives excellent fixation and allows early motion.

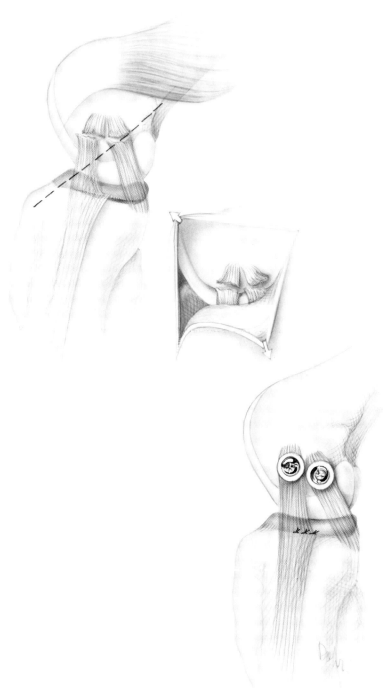

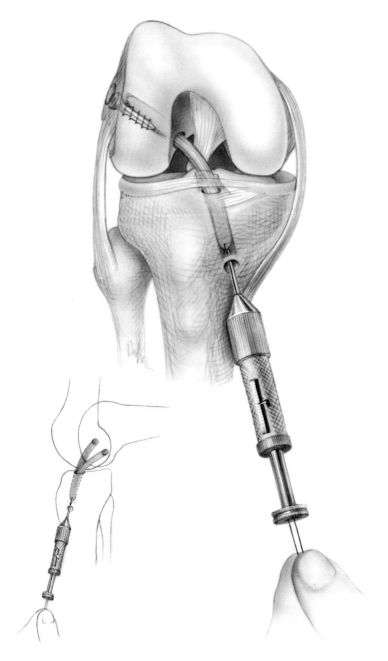

Fig. 23. After augmentation of the ACL, sutures should be placed in the tendon and the isometricity checked with a tensiometer through a range of motion.

ized beneath the vastus medialis obliquus, and, if disrupted, should be repaired.

The medial structures must be repaired according to Müller[11] (Fig. 21). To reattach the medial collateral ligament remote from its center of rotation is to guarantee limitation of motion and arthritic deterio-ration with "stretching out" of the repair. When both the origin and the oblique portions of the medial collateral are torn, I prefer to use a cancellous AO screw and spiked washer to repair each to their separate origins (Fig. 22). This technique has given excellent fixation and allowed for early motion. Lig-

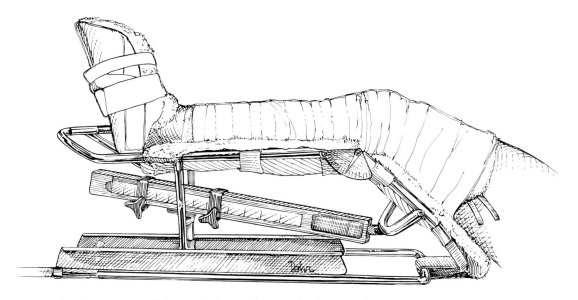

Fig. 24. The patient with leg in light supplemental splinting adjunctive to the cotton compressive dressing is returned to his hospital bed, and the continuous passive motion machine is adjusted to a range of 20° to 50° of motion.

ament reattachment studies have confirmed the efficacy of this approach. (D. M. Daniel, personal communication, San Diego, CA, 1987).

The superficial medial collateral ligament will often also be torn, and it too can be replaced near its insertion with a screw and washer.

Where interstitial tearing occurs, I try to use a Bunnell or Kessler type suture to approximate the ends, frequently alternating absorbable and nonabsorbable sutures of 0 and 1 size. On repair of the medial structures, there should be a range of motion from 0° to 90° with increasing stability to valgus testing so that the knee is stable in full extension and has no more than a 5 mm opening at 30° flexion. If this is not the case, then some portion of the tear of the medial collateral ligament has been overlooked and must be identified and reconstituted. The meniscus should be stable throughout this range of motion.

Most orthopaedic surgeons consider graft augmentation of the ACL to be essential. The techniques of Marshall[9] can be applied to the residual ligamentous stumps, but the interstitially torn ligament should be augmented or stented in some way,

to effect reliable repair. The patella tendon or doubled semitendinosus has worked well in my hands to restore cruciate stability in this situation.[8,10]

After the augmentation is completed, then the sutures for the ACL are placed under tension and its isometricity checked (using an Acufex or MEDmetric tensiometer; see also Chs. 21 and 22) (Fig. 23). Overtension exerts excessive pressure on the joint surfaces and the graft; grafts that have more than 4 mm excursion when cycled through a range of motion should be replaced. Bone-to-bone fixation after the manner of Lambert[8] has proven most effective in my hands.

After "tensioning" the ACL, the Lachman test may be trace-positive, but the pivot shift should have been eliminated. The surgical closure is straightforward; care is taken to restore each layer. Two drains are employed, one intraarticular and one subcutaneous. Subcutaneous closure should be meticulous, and intracuticular wire gives a most pleasing incisional healing.

The patient's *postoperative pain* is a major concern to the surgeon. It may be controlled by using gentle tissue techniques, minimizing dissection, injecting the incisional area with 0.5 percent bupivacaine (Marcaine), applying a firm compressive dressing, using continuous passive motion, and administering postoperative epidural analgesia. These details are important to the patient, the course of postoperative management, and the rehabilitation time (see Chs. 25, 26, and 28).

A compression bandage is applied firmly and the tourniquet is released. The amount of splinting inherent in the compression bandage will vary with the quality of repair and the philosophy of the surgeon. We frequently apply a removable supplemental splinting in addition to the cotton compressive dressing; this allows the patient to use the CPM machine on return to his hospital bed (Fig. 24).

The usual operative time is 1.5 hours. Tourniquet time may be decreased by releasing the tourniquet after the initial exposure is accomplished.

POSTOPERATIVE CARE AND REHABILITATION

The CPM is usually adjusted to a range of motion from 20° to 50°. The patient is expected to begin ambulation the day after surgery with weightbearing to comfort, and will use crutches for balance and an external splint for support over the compressive dressing when he is ambulatory. An isometric program involving the quadriceps and hamstrings through the 20° to 50° range of motion is instituted. A program of exercise for hip flexors, adductors and abductors, extensors, and trunk muscles is also initiated. Toe rises are also helpful to restimulate the gastrocsoleus complex as it spans the two joints. The well leg is emphasized as a "teacher" for the affected leg. Drains are removed 24 to 48 hours after operation. Effusion can be palpated through a properly tensioned Jones compression dressing. If significant effusion accumulates in the postoperative period it should be aspirated. The patient should not be discharged until he is afebrile. The hospital stay after operation at our institution averages 3 days. Before discharge the exercise program is reviewed with the patient by both physical therapist and surgeon, and written instructions for a home program are given to the patient (Ch. 25).

The patient is encouraged to record oral temperature daily, and should contact the surgeon's office if the temperature rises above 100.6°F (38.1°C).

The patient should be reevaluated 3 to 7 days postoperatively. At this visit, the compression bandage is changed and reapplied in the form of either a thigh-length antiembolism hose or a similar light elastic dressing that includes calf support. For a reliable patient, postoperative immobilization is maintained by an optional support, which is worn when the patient is ambulatory but may be left off when he is recumbent or performing the range of motion exercise program. A hinge cast or hinge orthosis is likewise effective. The patient is encouraged to continue to use the range of motion that he achieved on the CPM machine before hospital discharge (20° to 50°). This program is continued until the surgeon is satisfied that the ACL and ligamentous graft attachments are secure to bone. The first 6 weeks are called the *isometric phase* (phase 1), although weightbearing and early controlled range of motion were initiated immediately after the operation.

The patient is checked at intervals during the first 6 weeks, depending upon the need for observation and reinforcement of goals.

If a range of motion of 10° to 110° is not accomplished by the 12th week, the patient is counseled that his progress is not satisfactory, and the reason for the lack of progress is sought. Diagnostic arthroscopy may be necessary at this point to determine if there is low-grade infection, adhesions, inaccurate placement of the graft, or graft impingement.

The patient is usually bearing weight without crutch support throughout phase 2 (the *isotonic phase,* 6 to 12 weeks); he may use crutches for balance when he is at risk in either his social or work environment. Splint support is optional, but the knee should not be immobilized.

Phase 3 involves restoration of agility and endurance. This phase usually lasts as long as phases 1 and 2 together, and thus spans approximately the 12th to the 24th week after operation. The activities of this phase may be accomplished at the patient's local health club without supervision by a physical therapist, provided objective measurements of strength and range of motion are periodically available to the patient and surgeon. A bicycle, either indoors or outdoors, is advantageous during both phase 2 and phase 3. The Orthotron or Cybex are helpful in documenting progress at higher angular velocities during this phase. A simple clinical test to judge the end of phase 3 is when the patient can hop repeatedly with equal grace and agility on the affected and unaffected leg. The shoulders should not list during this maneuver, and thus the patient can self-test in front of a mirror (or observer) to determine his progress toward this goal.

PROBLEMS, COMPLICATIONS, FOLLOW-UP RESULTS

The most frequent complication is *stiffness*. Stiffness may be a result of inadequate restoration of the structures according to their anatomic origins, of adhesions of the suprapatellar pouch or lateral patellofemoral ligaments, of low-grade synovitis, or very rarely of infection. Loss of mobility of the patellofemoral joint is of special concern, and the patellofemoral joint should be mobilized daily in both superoinferior and mediolateral planes, by both the patient and the physical therapist. A full range of motion of the knee joint may be regained without regaining full excursion of the patellofemoral joint. In these cases patella compression is traded for excursion, which can lead to pain, chondromalacia, and arthrosis. Surgeon, physical therapist, and patient must be alert to this potential hazard, and early arthroscopy with lysis of adhesions and/or lateral release may be necessary.

Laxity may become progressive as a postoperative complication. This laxity usually results from one or more of the following three causes: (1) failure to identify at operation a tear of the capsuloligamentous lesion; (2) stretching of the repaired structures due to nonanatomic (and nonisometric) repair; and (3) reinjury, through the patient's negligence or bad luck.

A knee that shows increasing laxity during rehabilitation represents a serious complication, which must be discussed with the patient as soon as it is recognized. It is usually best to correct this laxity as soon as the patient's psyche and the tissues will allow.

A third complication is *sympathetic dystrophy,* particularly of the patellofemoral joint. The causes of this dystrophy are uncertain,[4] but I have often wondered if it sometimes results from excessive compression caused by a lack of freedom of the patellofemoral joint to assume its normal excursion during the postoperative rehabilitation. Radiographs can verify the sympathetic dystrophy, and sympathetic block is sometimes appropriate to disrupt the sequence of events associated with this diagnosis. Where patella compression or loss of excursion during the rehabilitation phase is identified, the anatomic source for this must be sought, and this must be corrected.

Last, there is a complication that I call *"failure to thrive."* This complication is manifested by muscle atrophy of the quadriceps and/or hamstrings, failure to gain range of motion, and a discoordinate gait. The patient and surgeon lose confidence in each other, and physical therapy seems ineffective. The cause of this failure to thrive must be sought. "Compensationitis," or lack of motivation on the patient's part, is often the cause of failure, and should be considered preoperatively. A direct approach to this problem by the supporting team, which may well include a representative of vocational rehabilitation, is appropriate. A Minnesota Multiphasic Personality Inventory or similar test will sometimes identify the cause of failure to progress and/or the need for psychologic or psychotherapeutic support.

Generally, the *long-term follow-up of the repaired and augmented ACL triad has been excellent.* Return to function within 1 year is to be expected; return of agility, endurance, and the cutting mechanism is usual when the principles outlined in this case study are followed. An accomplished athlete such as the patient described could expect to return to football. Bracing might be indicated, and a change of position for the ensuing season might be desirable. I would not allow him to participate in a contact fashion in spring practice, although he might run team drills with knee brace, shorts, shoulder pads, and helmet under the supervision of the coach and team physician. If an antalgic or protective gait, or effusion, ensued after return to his usual activities, he would have to halt those activities and return to supervised rehabilitation. The co-

CASE STUDY 2
O'Donoghue's Triad - ACL, MCL, Medial Meniscus

Day of Injury	2	3	4	5	6	7	8	9	10	14	21	30	6	12	6	12
													WEEKS		**MONTHS**	
			DAYS													

Admit to hospital • Ice • Hydrate

EUA • Repair MCL and meniscus • ACL augmentation graft

CPM 20–50° (optional) – Removable soft splints • Isometrics • Weightbearing to comfort

Remove drains

Discharge from hospital

Home PT program — Isometrics • Toe rises • ROM 20–50° • Trunk and upper body resistive exercises

Office recheck • Continue home PT program

D/C crutches when gait near normal • Increase ROM • Trunk, upper body resistive exercises

D/C splint • Begin bicycle exercises • Swimming/water exercises
Brisk walking • Bicycle exercises • Strength and gluteals • Skip rope • Increase
walking to tolerance • ROM 20–60° • No quad thrust • Increase ROM and endurance
Begin strength training • Strength and arthrometer tests

No contact sports • Continue agility drills (brace optional) • Strengthen
Contact sports • Repeat strength and arthrometer tests
Return to all sports (brace optional)

operation and coordination of the team physician, trainer, coach, and patient are important and must be agreed upon before he returns to team activities.

SUMMARY

This has been the case history of an elite college football player who sustained a triad in the classic fashion. Surgical repair was elected the day after the injury, and the ACL was repaired with an augmentation graft. The MCL was anatomically repaired, and early motion and early weightbearing initiated. The patient was protected over a period of at least 6 months after his injury until he had regained strength, endurance, and agility. Although "classic cases" such as this are not as common as they once were, they still represent a significant portion of orthopaedic practice and are a supreme challenge to our surgical expertise and rehabilitation skills.

REFERENCES

1. Arnoczky SP, Warren RF: Microvasculature of the human meniscus. Am J Sports Med 10:90–95, 1982
2. Arnoczky SP, Warren RF: The microvasculature of the meniscus and its response to injury. An experimental study in the dog. Am J Sports Med 11:131–141, 1983
3. Dobner JJ, Nitz AJ: Postmeniscectomy tourniquet palsy and functional sequelae. Am J Sports Med 10:211–214, 1982
4. Ficat RP, Hungerford DS: Disorders of the Patello-Femoral Joint. Williams & Wilkins, Baltimore, 1977
5. Finochietto R: Semilunar cartilages of the knee. The "jump sign." J Bone Joint Surg 17A:916–921, 1935
6. Hughston JC, Eilers AF: The role of the posterior oblique ligament in repairs of acute medial (collateral) ligament tears of the knee. J Bone Joint Surg 55A:923–940, 1973
7. Indelicato PA: Non-operative treatment of complete tears of the medial collateral ligament of the knee. J Bone Joint Surg 65A:323–329, 1983
8. Lambert KL: Vascularized patellar tendon graft with rigid internal fixation for anterior cruciate ligament insufficiency. Clin. Orthop 172:85–89, 1983
9. Marshall JL, Warren RF, Wickiewicz TL: Primary surgical treatment of anterior cruciate ligament lesions. Am J Sports Med 10:103–107, 1982
10. Mott HW: Semitendinosus anatomic reconstruction for cruciate ligament insufficiency. Clin Orthop 172:90–92, 1983
11. Müller W: The Knee. Form, Function and Ligament Reconstruction. Springer-Verlag, New York, 1983, pp. 81–84
12. O'Donoghue DH: Surgical treatment of fresh injuries to major ligaments of the knee. J Bone Joint Surg 32A:721–738, 1950

CASE STUDY 3

ACL Tear, Complete, with MCL Sprain, Incomplete

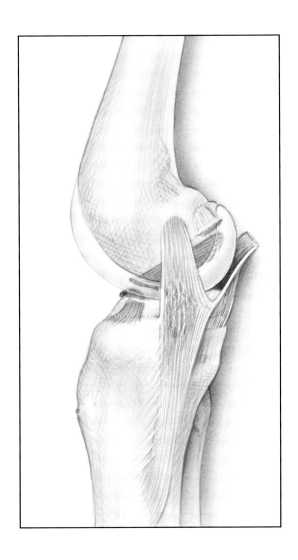

HISTORY

A 32-year-old woman, a novice skier, teacher, and mother of two small children, fell while skiing down a fairly steep slope. She experienced immediate knee pain. The mechanism of injury was unclear to the patient. She did not recall hearing a "pop." On attempting to bear weight, she experienced pain and a feeling of instability. The ski patrol was called to sled her down the slope.

Knee Examination
(Orthopaedic Surgeon/Ski Clinic; Within 30 Minutes of Injury)

Diagnostic Clues	Findings
Effusion	None
Tenderness	Above the joint line, at origin of medial collateral and posterior oblique capsular ligaments
Lachman test	1+ positive*/soft end point
Drawer test	1+ positive/soft end point
Pivot shift test	Could not be adequately performed because of pain
Varus/valgus	2+ opening at 30° flexion, 1+ opening at 0° flexion, stable to valgus testing at hyperextension
	No abnormal varus opening
Patella apprehension	Negative
Range of motion	20° to 50°
Gait	Toe touch with support
Neurovasculature	Intact
Radiographs	Normal except soft tissue swelling; consistent with MCL injury
Other	None

* See Glossary.

41

COMMENTS

Skiing has produced a virtual epidemic of ACL injuries (see Ch. 16). The biomechanics of knee injury in skiing are still imperfectly understood. The skier is often uncertain about the mechanism of injury. Many different mechanisms of ACL injury occur in skiing, but torsion in a weight-bearing mode is common in the novice. In such cases secondary restraints are at risk. The "pop" is not so reliably heard by skiers as by turf athletes. Nevertheless, when patients are relaxed and feeling confident, they may say they heard a "pop." The feeling of instability when bearing weight is probably due to a tibiofemoral subluxation. Few novice skiers attempt to ski down after such an injury.

Although this patient was obviously not a competitive athlete and held a sedentary job, one should not underestimate her desire for the active lifestyle. Body fat can be an important clue to previous lifestyle, as can a quick survey of such key muscle groups as the gastrocsoleus, postural muscles, and forearm muscles. It would be unwise to underestimate this patient's desire to excel.

Injury to knee ligaments seldom occurs at home. Since the early examination is likely to be much

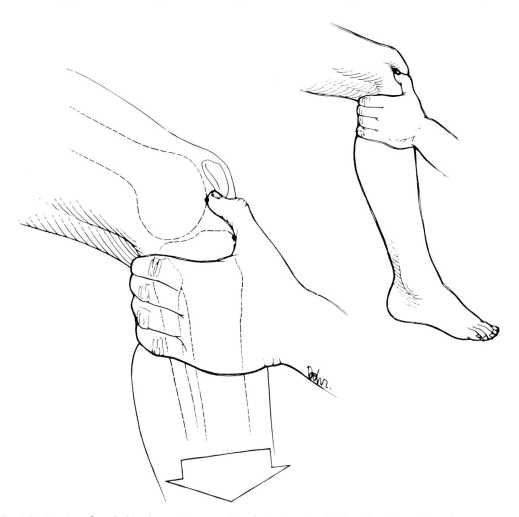

Fig. 25. Gravity often helps the patient to relax if he sits with his leg dangling while the examiner performs a gentle Drawer test. The result will frequently prove unequivocally positive and will serve as a diagnostic sign for the ACL tear.

more accurate than a later one, every effort must be made to be accurate in the initial examination and to transfer information to the patient's hometown orthopaedic surgeon.

The well leg must always be examined first. The Lachman test can certainly be 1+ (5 mm) in a normal leg, but there is a firm end point. It is useful to grade the quality of the Lachman and Drawer tests, although the end point is not always discernible because of hamstring spasm or associated injury. In this particular patient, the Lachman test had a firm end point on the well leg and was 1+ and soft on the injured leg. Often, too brisk an examination can cause pain that will mask the soft end point because of muscle spasm. When the Lachman test is equivocal or the end point uncertain, the Drawer test should be used. If the patient sits with the leg dangling, gravity often leads to relaxation, and a gentle drawer test will prove unequivocally positive (Fig. 25). This result is as diagnostic as a positive Lachman test. With medial laxity, the pivot shift test may not be accomplished or may be falsely negative. With MCL compromise, the Noyes test[4] would be the most gentle test for rotatory laxity.

The extent of the MCL complex tear must be accurately evaluated. In the normal leg, the valgus opening present at 30° flexion will usually diminish to complete stability in hyperextension. The injured leg should be examined in the same way. In this patient there was 2+ valgus opening at 30° flexion, 1+ opening at 0° flexion, and a stable knee in hyperextension. This result indicated some compromise of the medial collateral ligament but an intact posterior cruciate ligament. Tearing of the oblique portion of the MCL[2] is a common ski injury and may or may not occur with tearing of the ACL. Tears may be diagnosed manually and/or arthroscopically, but neither technique alone is absolutely certain. The combination of medial instability and cruciate laxity dictates a more aggressive course regardless of the patient's occupation.

A soft Lachman test, as in this patient, makes me suspect an ACL tear. I would not be confident that manual examination without examination under anesthesia (EUA) would define precisely the extent of medial collateral ligament tearing. Thus, I recommend arthroscopy to patients with this particular combination of signs.

COURSE OF ACTION

The patient returned home well splinted, with crutches, a well-documented examination, and x-ray films that were normal except for soft tissue swelling about the MCL. The office examination, a week after the injury supported the initial findings. To do nothing in this case would be to risk disaster. The patient may not want to ski again, but she will expect a stable knee. Manual examination would not give adequate information by which to treat this patient with confidence. Arthroscopy and EUA should be performed.

Physical Examination

The patient accepted the above reasoning and was admitted for EUA and arthroscopy. She also agreed to treatment as indicated by findings at that time.

Diagnostic Studies

It is important in cases such as this to join the information obtained from manual examination with that obtained from diagnostic arthroscopy. Arthroscopy can usually be performed, though care must be taken to avoid fluid extravasation. If this injury were an incomplete MCL tear without disruption of the posterior oblique ligament, it could be treated primarily as a cruciate ligament injury as long as more care was given to protecting the secondary restraints. However, if the case were underdiagnosed and the loss of integrity of the posteromedial capsuloligamentous complex were not appreciated, then nonoperative treatment would be associated with significant residual laxity.

Special Considerations

What percentage of patients with this type of injury are candidates for primary ACL reconstruction, given our current state of knowledge? A general answer to this question cannot and should not be given. All patients deserve a plan tailored to their goals and expectations. All of us desire a "happy" patient when the therapy is complete. It is the responsibility of the orthopaedic surgeon to elicit the patient's attitude. Although the patient can be told that one third of patients perform adequately without a cruciate, one third have a moderate disability, and one third do poorly, this information is of limited benefit to the patient since success or failure is 100 percent in his or her eyes.[5,6] Furthermore, the patient may not be able to appreciate the significance of the compromise of the posteromedial corner that may be demonstrated on the examination under anesthesia.

PLAN

The examination under anesthesia, conducted before applying the tourniquet, confirmed that the pivot shift in this patient was equally positive in internal and external rotation. Medially there was 2 + valgus opening at 30° flexion, 1 + opening at 0° flexion, and stability in hyperextension. The leg was then prepped and draped with the intent to do a limited arthroscopic examination and to proceed with definitive surgical repair as indicated and as consistent with the desires of the patient.

Routine medial and lateral arthroscopic portals are generally used to examine this type of case, but there is an important place for the superolateral or superomedial portal since these portals may allow (1) better visualization of the medial capsular structures at their origin, (2) visualization of the midportion of the ACL, and (3) excellent visualization of the lateral compartment, where compromise must always be suspected (Fig. 26).

Care must be taken on introducing the irrigation fluid that there is no leakage from the medial tear which might jeopardize the circulation of the lower leg. The assistant and the scrub nurse should be alerted to this possibility, although the surgeon has the ultimate responsibility.

I prefer to go straight to the pathology indicated by the physical examination so as to reduce the arthroscopy time and risk of fluid extravasation. I

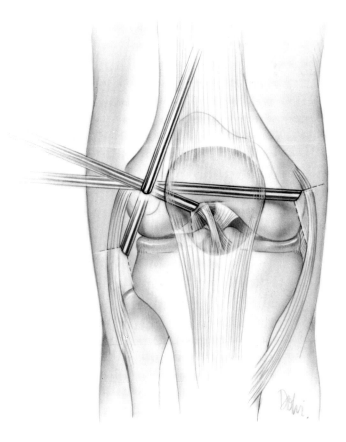

Fig. 26. The Patel superolateral portal provides better visualization of the medial capsular structures at their origin and of the midportion of the ACL. The lateral compartment can also be seen clearly from this portal.

frequently use a tourniquet in cases such as this because it also shortens the total arthroscopy time and thereby minimizes fluid extravasation. The probe is initially introduced through the lateral portal; with this approach one should be able to distinguish a complete from an incomplete cruciate tear. After defining the ACL tear (Fig. 27) the scope is directed to the medial compartment. The undersurface of the meniscus is probed to determine if there is disruption of the meniscotibial ligament or laxity of the meniscus. The superior portion of the meniscus is probed for evidence of capsular tear of either the posterior oblique ligament or the midportion of the MCL. Although the synovium may be intact, a hemorrhagic blush of the synovium may be diagnostic of a significant tear. An 18 gauge needle can be inserted opposite the blush and, by probing from externally, may further define the extent of a medial ligament tear. In this patient the medial capsuloligamentous complex was intact to arthroscopic examination, indicating an incomplete or extrasynovial MCL injury.

Upon completing the EUA and arthroscopy, the tourniquet should be released, the fluid expressed, and the lower leg carefully reexamined to ensure there has not been extravasation and compromise of

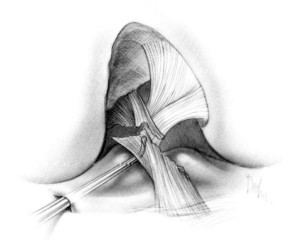

Fig. 27. After defining the ACL tear through the lateral portal, the arthroscope is directed to the medial compartment. The undersurface of the meniscus is probed to determine if there is either disruption of the meniscotibial ligament or laxity of the meniscus.

either the circulation or the compartments. Should fluid extravasation occur, surgery must be discontinued, compartment pressures monitored, and fasciotomy performed promptly if a compartment syndrome is detected.

Because the ACL lesion in this patient was complete and interstitial, it was necessary to decide whether augmentation grafting or a lateral isometric tenodesis would be best. Although I generally prefer augmentation grafting, in this case I used lateral tenodesis, since I think this too is an acceptable treatment for a patient of this activity level given our current state of expertise at reconstruction of the ACL. The choice of treatment was influenced by the patient's immediate needs as mother and teacher and the fact that she does not currently enjoy athletic pursuits that require cutting or abrupt change of direction.

The decision to do an isometric lateral tenodesis dictated lateral incision. Nevertheless, the fact that this operation may not be a permanent solution must be taken into consideration when incisions are chosen.

To perform this operation, first a 7.5 cm lateral incision is made overlying the posterior portion of the iliotibial band with the knee in 30° flexion (Fig. 28). An incision in the iliotibial band is made just anterior to the iliotibial tract. The iliotibial tract is defined and restored if there is a disruption. Then lateral isometric tenodesis is accomplished by securing a 2.5 to 4 cm strip from the tubercle of Gerdy to the isometric point on the lateral femoral condyle (Ch. 23).[1,3] This point may be difficult to identify precisely but usually is at the confluence of the lateral intermuscular septum with the anatomic tubercle for the lateral head of the gastrocnemius. The lateral tenodesis is then secured to the femur with the knee in 30° flexion, the lower leg in external rotation, and the tenodesis secured with a 6.5 mm cancellous screw. The pivot shift should be carefully checked, respecting the partially torn medial structures. Range of motion should give an indication that the lateral tenodesis is isometric. The Lachman test may remain trace-positive. The fascial layer is closed with absorbable sutures and the skin is closed with an intracuticular cosmetic closure.

The incision and tissue planes are infiltrated with 0.5 percent Marcaine (bupivacaine), a Jones-type

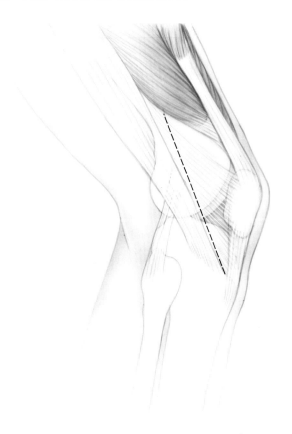

Fig. 28. A 7.5 cm lateral incision is made over the posterior portion of the iliotibial band with the knee in 30° flexion. An incision in the iliotibial band is made just anterior to the iliotibial tract. If there is a disruption of the tract it should be restored through this opening.

compression dressing is applied allowing flexion from 20° to 50°, and continuous passive motion (CPM) is initiated postoperatively in this range. This early motion decreases the patient's pain, gives the patient confidence in early motion, and enhances general rehabilitation.

POSTOPERATIVE CARE AND REHABILITATION

Postoperatively this patient was permitted to ambulate with crutches and bear weight to comfort. The CPM was continued at 30° to 50° of flexion as tolerated during the patient's hospitalization. A reinforced Jones compression dressing served as a splint. The usual isometric exercises and trunk rehabilitation program were instituted.

On discharge, the patient was instructed to continue the range of motion of 30° to 50° as accomplished on the CPM at least three times a day, and to bear weight using crutches for balance. The mechanics of tenodesis were explained to the patient so that she would not be concerned about the failure to obtain full extension immediately. The isometric tenodesis of the lateral aspect provided the patient with the opportunity to regain a full range of motion within 6 to 12 weeks.

During the office visit at approximately 10 days postoperatively, the Jones pressure dressing was replaced by a hinged cast allowing 30° to 50° flexion. Long antiembolic hose beneath this provided comfort and support. Localized constrictive devices such as elastic bandages about the knee can encourage edema of the lower leg and possible thromboembolic problems.

The patient continued the rehabilitation program — gradually increasing range of motion, increasing weightbearing, and following a hamstring exercise program through the sixth week (Ch. 27). At that time, an indoor bicycle was recommended. The patient was cautioned to avoid quadriceps thrust. Full extension and flexion past 110° would not be sought until after the 12th week.

After the 12 week, strength through range of motion was emphasized, with the hamstrings overriding the quadriceps, thus prohibiting quadriceps thrusts (Ch. 25). Great care was taken to evaluate the patellofemoral mobility throughout the rehabilitation period to ensure the patella was not bound by either adhesions or a lateral tenodesis. Binding of the patella retinaculum can cause undue patellofemoral pressure, limitation of excursion, and failure to progress as desired in the rehabilitation program (see Complications).

The final phase of rehabilitation was an agility program initiated at the 16th week. These exercises are simple but objective, and encourage proper body position, balance, and lateral directional stability.

The patient regained most of her agility by the 24th week and had full range of motion. Bracing would still be recommended, however, if she were to participate in active sports. Although such brac-

CASE STUDY 3
ACL (Complete), MCL (Incomplete)

Day of Injury	2	3	4	5	6	7	8	9	10	14	21	30	6	12	6	12
						DAYS							WEEKS		MONTHS	

Splint • Ice • Isometrics

Office exam by home physician • Crutches • Weightbearing to comfort

EUA • Arthroscopy • Lateral iliotibial band tenodesis

CPM 20°–50° • Removable soft splint • Isometrics • Weightbearing to comfort

Discharge from hospital

Home PT program

Office recheck — emphasize isometrics, toe rises • Trunk, upper body resistive exercises

D/C crutches when gait near normal

Increase walking to tolerance

Begin strength training • ROM 20°–50° • Weightbearing

Begin bicycle exercises • Trunk, upper body resistive exercises • Toe rises • Isometrics

Endurance walking • ROM 20°–60° • No quad thrust • Skip rope with or without splint

Begin simple agility patterns • Bicycle exercises • Endurance walking • No jumping

D/C splint • Strengthen hamstrings and gluteals • Caution against jumping

Sports participation when strength, endurance, and agility sufficient (brace optional) • Repeat strength and arthrometer tests

Return to all sports (brace optional)

Strength and arthrometer tests

ing may not stabilize the knee biomechanically, a sense of confidence is obtained from the proprioceptive support it provides and this seems to enhance patients' confidence in return to sport.

PROBLEMS, COMPLICATIONS, FOLLOW-UP RESULTS

There are a considerable number of potential pitfalls in the approach used on this patient. The *first pitfall* is to underestimate the MCL tear or the stability of the medial meniscus. The arthroscope is invaluable to avoid this pitfall.

The *second pitfall* is to miss a disruption of the iliotibial tract, thus allowing further anterolateral laxity. In this patient, surgical exposure precluded this complication. If an augmentation-type repair of the ACL had been selected, care would have been taken to ensure that the pivot shift was eliminated and anterolateral stability restored after graft augmentation. If this laxity is in doubt, then the iliotibial tract should be exposed and repaired.

The *third pitfall* is the possibility of creating a patella compressive syndrome either medially, laterally, or both. This pitfall must be guarded against during the surgical procedure and reevaluated throughout the rehabilitation process. If range of motion does not improve consistently between the sixth and twelfth weeks, and if a patient fails to progress under the therapeutic regimen described above, then consideration would be given to diagnostic arthroscopy, release of adhesions, and rebalancing of the patellar retinacula.

Each of the complications I have mentioned can be distressing, but it is the responsibility of the surgeon to be alert to the possibilities and to avoid them whenever possible.

Where the ACL has not been reconstructed, the results are uncertain. This is a disadvantage of the approach presented in this case, and the patient must understand the trade-off, the possible late complications, and the uncertainties. It perhaps takes more skill to accomplish an isometric extraarticular lateral reconstruction than to do an isometric augmentation grafting intraarticularly. Unfortu-nately, more surgeons feel comfortable with the lateral tenodesis, and thus it is covered in this case study. This patient presented a low-demand situation, and thus, if the surgical technique was reasonably accurate, the lateral tenodesis could be expected to hold up. If loosening had occurred, it would have been manifested by a reappearance of the pivot shift (particularly in external rotation) as the patient regained full extension. A patient's function, confidence, and ultimate satisfaction must be part of the final judgment. If increasing laxity does occur, it should not be ignored and should be dealt with through intraarticular augmentation if an optimal result is to be obtained.

SUMMARY

The case of a 32-year-old woman is presented—a teacher, mother, and novice skier who usually places limited demands on the knee. A thorough diagnostic study was accomplished, consisting of examination under anesthesia and diagnostic arthroscopy. A lateral isometric tenodesis was performed. Many feel this is the simplest approach to this type of anatomic deficit in patients with limited athletic usage. I personally prefer to do intraarticular augmentation, but respect the contributions and accomplishments of my colleagues through the years.

REFERENCES

1. Andrews JR, Sanders R: A "mini-reconstruction" technique in treatment of anterolateral rotatory instability (ALRI). Clin Orthop 172:93–96, 1983
2. Hughston JC, Eilers AF: The role of the posterior oblique ligament in repairs of acute medial (collateral) ligament tears of the knee. J Bone Joint Surg 55A:923–940, 1973
3. Krackow KA, Brooks RL: Optimization of knee ligament position for lateral extraarticular reconstruction. Am J Sports Med 11:293–302, 1983
4. Noyes FR: Flexion rotation drawer test for anterior cruciate insufficiency, p. 924. In Edmonson AS, Crenshaw

AH (eds): Campbell's Operative Orthopaedics. 6th edition. Mosby, St. Louis, 1980

5. Noyes FR, Mooar PA, Matthews DS, Butler DL: The symptomatic anterior cruciate-deficient knee. Part I. The long-term functional disability in athletically active individuals. J Bone Joint Surg 65A:154–162, 1983

6. Noyes FR, Matthews DS, Mooar PA, Grood ES: The sympotomatic anterior cruciate-deficient knee. Part II. The results of rehabilitation, activity modification, and counseling on functional disability. J Bone Joint Surg 65A:163–174, 1983

CASE STUDY 4

ACL Tear, Complete, with Lateral Capsular Avulsion Fracture (Segond's Sign)

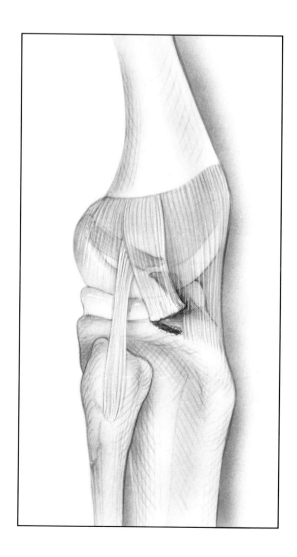

HISTORY

A 35-year-old affluent executive, an accomplished skier, was skiing fast, under ideal conditions, on a well-groomed slope. On the "last run," fatigued, he "stood up" and abruptly changed direction to avoid a slower skier. He caught an outside edge, fell over the downhill ski, and felt a "pop" and pain about the right knee. He was unable to ski down comfortably, but did manage to walk 250 meters to the aid station where the Ski Patrol suggested he "see a doctor."

Knee Examination
(Patient's Orthopaedic Surgeon At Home,
Approximately 48 Hours after Injury)

Diagnostic Clues	Findings
Effusion	Tense
Tenderness	Tender, anterolateral tibial joint line
Lachman test	2+ positive*/soft end point
Drawer test	2+ positive/soft end point
Pivot shift test	Too painful to elicit
Varus/valgus	Stable to valgus testing. Varus testing equivocal, caused pain, but suggested laxity at 30°
Patella apprehension	Negative
Range of motion	10° to 50°
Gait	Antalgic
Neurovasculature	Intact
Radiographs	Effusion, and a 5 mm lateral tibial metaphyseal avulsion fracture
Other	None

* See Glossary

51

COMMENTS

As mentioned in Case Study 3, ACL injury has become nearly epidemic (see Ch. 16). The absolute increase in the frequency of this injury represents more than just diagnostic recognition. The equipment and our current style of skiing, i.e., sitting back and using the tails of the skis to enhance the stiff, high boot, produces a "positive Lachman force" that jeopardizes the ACL (see Case Study 13). Groomed slope conditions allow higher speeds. The slopes are frequently crowded. Obstacles often require sudden deceleration or change in angular velocity of the knee joint. The binding never "sees" the injury, because bindings are generally designed to "recognize" forces as they relate to the tibial shaft and are "too slow" to respond to angular moments that jeopardize the ACL. When quadriceps fatigue occurs, the skier tends to stand up. This brings the ACL into the narrow portion of the femoral intercondylar notch, where it may be jeopardized by either the sharp intercondylar ridge (with hyperextension), or by being tented over the medial or lateral confines of the notch or the PCL (with rotation) (Fig. 29). Internal rotation is anatomically far less forgiving[1] (Fig. 30) (see Ch. 16).

Fig. 29. The ACL is at risk in hyperextension, where it may be jeopardized by the sharp intercondylar ridge. Also, it is at risk with rotation, where it may be tented over the medial or lateral confines of the notch, or the PCL.

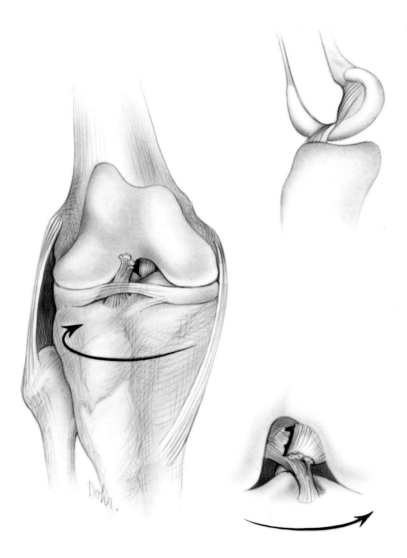

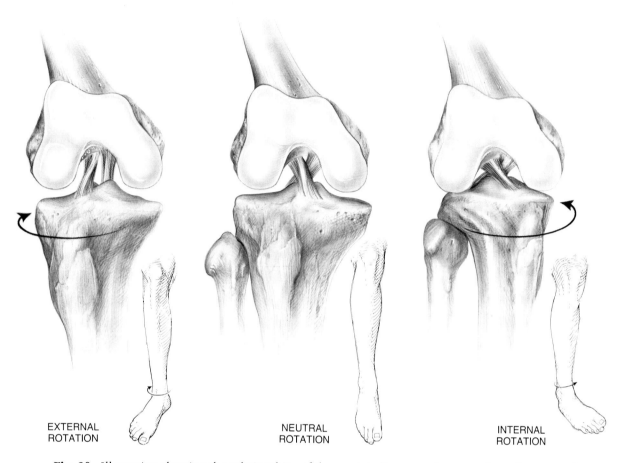

EXTERNAL
ROTATION

NEUTRAL
ROTATION

INTERNAL
ROTATION

Fig. 30. Illustration showing the relationships of the cruciate ligaments in external rotation, neutral position, and internal rotation. **(A)** External rotation unwinds the cruciate ligaments and allows the joint surfaces more freedom. **(B)** The anatomic (neutral) position. **(C)** Internal rotation entwines the cruciate ligaments and closes the joint space, thus restricting the freedom of motion between the surfaces.

After an ACL injury, the patient can seldom ski down but is usually able to "walk into the clinic." Effusion, just as in the turf injury, is slow to develop and usually requires 24 hours to reach its maximum. Segond's sign,[6] the lateral capsular avulsion fracture, (Fig. 31, radiograph) seems more common in skiing than in turf injuries, probably because of the frequency of internal rotation in skiing. Segond's sign is probably an indication of avulsion of the lateral capsular ligament and is usually associated with a tear of the ACL. The examining physician must be alert to the possibility of significant knee laxity when the Segond's sign is present.

COURSE OF ACTION

ACL laxity with a lateral capsular avulsion fracture may be a clue to total lateral capsular disruption. The lateral compartment must be examined meticulously for laxity to determine the extent of injury.

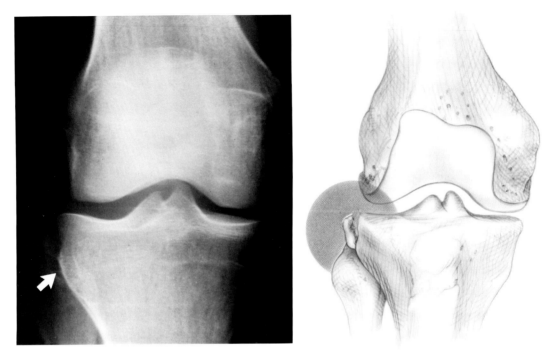

Fig. 31. The lateral capsular avulsion fracture (Segond's sign).

The Segond lesion cannot be ignored if a satisfactory functional result is to expected.

Physical Examination

A routine knee examination may be attempted, but when there is capsular disruption, pain frequently limits manual diagnostic testing in the office examination. Although varus laxity is tested exactly like valgus laxity, through a range of motion, the lateral laxity is frequently more difficult to appreciate. It is especially helpful to place the patient in the prone position for examination. The posterior portion of the joint can be better visualized and the lateral capsule better palpated (Fig. 32) than if the patient is supine. The Lachman test can be performed with ease in this position. Increased posterolateral laxity would suggest a tear of the arcuate complex.[4] For inexplicable reasons, sometimes a patient is more relaxed in the prone position, and the physician can evaluate the laxity more accurately.

Diagnostic Studies

Examination under anesthesia (EUA) and arthroscopy are nearly requisite in a patient with this history. As usual, the surgeon must be aware of the possibility of fluid extravasation through the lateral capsular injury, but the tense effusion found on physical examination suggests that the joint has sealed itself. An arthrogram would be of less value than EUA and arthroscopy.

Special Considerations

In contrast to the athlete, society seldom grants the executive the time to "get well." Thus the surgeon is often faced with the patient's desire to have the operation on Friday so he can be back in the office on Monday. This expects too much of most surgical procedures, of the healing process, and of the doctor-patient relationship.

The patient's age and activity level, as well as his body fat, are also considerations in decision mak-

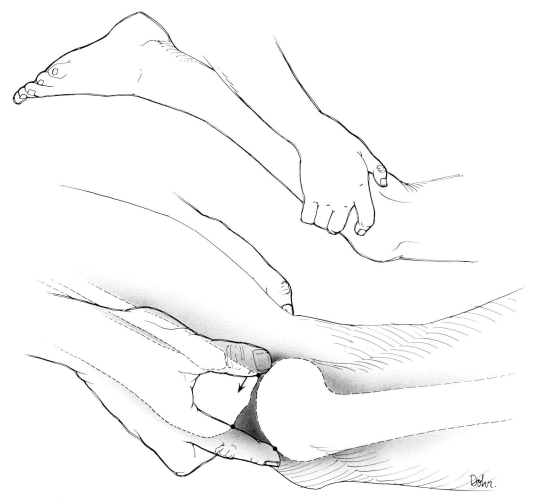

Fig. 32. The prone Lachman test. With the patient in the prone position, the posterior portion of the joint can be better visualized and the lateral capsule better palpated than if the patient is examined in the supine position.

ing. The "executive" may consider himself active, but a body fat of 30 percent would belie this opinion. It is helpful to know Cooper's aerobic point system[3] and apply it to the patient to determine how much exercise he takes. His exercise can then be further divided into straight-ahead and cutting activities. I know of many patients who do well on a jogging program without a cruciate ligament. They do not, however, engage in tennis, skiing, or sports requiring abrupt change of direction.

PLAN

The recommended plan for this patient starts with an examination under anesthesia and diagnostic arthroscopy. The patient and surgeon should decide before the anesthesia whether to proceed with reconstruction if the ACL is torn. Certainly, if the lateral capsule is responsible for pathologic laxity, it should be repaired.

If the patient deferred ACL reconstruction at this time, I would consider the Wittek alternative.[7] In this procedure, the surgeon repairs the residual stump of the proximally torn ACL to the PCL (Fig. 33).[7] This does not restore the four-bar linkage as described by Müller,[5] but it does decrease the Lachman and pivot shift signs. The procedure can be accomplished through a 5 cm incision subsequent to the arthroscopy and, in fact, with specialized tools it may even be accomplished arthroscopically. This procedure is not meant to be definitive. Rather, it provides an inexact restraint, applicable to the patient with open epiphyses or to the "older" patient.

Sometimes, however, the busy professional is the most successful of postoperative patients after a major ACL reconstruction. The self-discipline that has elevated him to his position of leadership will help him to rehabilitate rapidly. Undoubtedly, this executive's goal will be to return to as near normal function as the surgeon can grant. Herein is the essence of the art of including the patient in the decision making in orthopaedic surgery.

Though "nonoperative care" is often tempting in the "older" patient, caution must be advised. The 35-year-old may have 30 more years of sports enjoyment and will not appreciate being disabled early in his career by a surgeon insensitive to the demands he might place on his knee in his long future. Thus, I would not select nonoperative care for this patient.

Examination under anesthesia (EUA) and arthroscopy are recommended to patients of this type; reconstruction of the ACL should also be offered. The patient should be encouraged to seek a second opinion if he wants one. The operation is scheduled

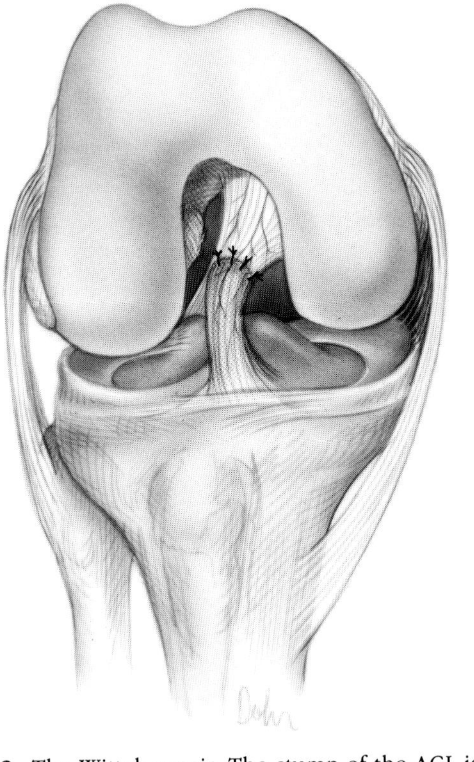

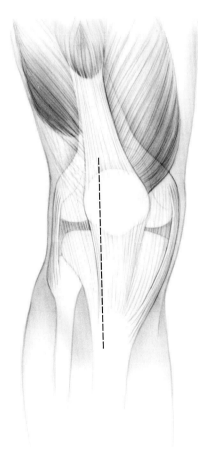

Fig. 33. The Wittek repair. The stump of the ACL is sutured to the intact PCL—a compromise that does not restore the four-bar linkage but affords some restraint.

Fig. 34. The surgical approach to an ACL tear with lateral capsular avulsion fracture through a straight incision 1 cm lateral to the infrapatella tendon.

Fig. 35. The Segond's lesion (avulsion fracture of the mid-third of the lateral capsule from the tibia) is repaired with AO screw and washer.

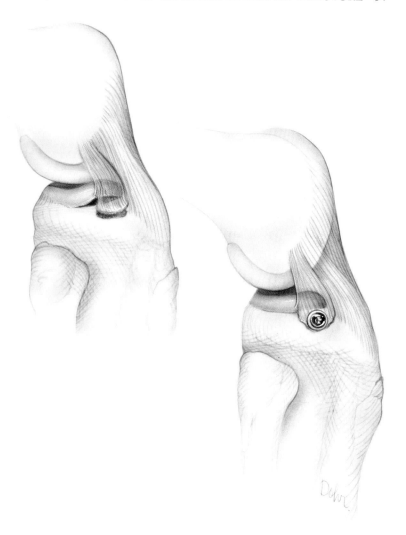

as soon as is practical since lateral capsular injuries are more difficult to repair as edema develops and the tissue planes become less well defined.

Examination under anesthesia is critical in determining the extent of the lateral capsular disruption. As usual, the well leg is examined carefully first before examining the injured leg. The injured leg is examined before inflating the tourniquet.

When this patient was examined under anesthesia, the surgeon found at 30° flexion an increased lateral opening to varus testing. This would connotate some tearing of the lateral capsule associated with the Segond's sign. In addition, there was a markedly positive Lachman test, Drawer test, and pivot shift test.

The EUA was followed by diagnostic arthroscopy. Care must be taken during this procedure to watch for extravasation of fluid from the lateral compartment. Both assistant and nurse should be alerted to this possibility and assist the surgeon in watching for it. At arthroscopy the interstitial tear of the ACL was confirmed, and the medial compartment was found to be intact, as was the patellofemoral compartment. There was mild chondromalacia of the patellofemoral joint, as is so frequently found in the athlete. In the lateral compartment the popliteus tendon was intact to probing. The lateral meniscus exuded hemorrhage from the portion anterior to the popliteus tendon when the probe elevated the meniscus. There was also blushing of the capsule adjacent and superior to the lateral meniscus anteriorly, compatible with a mid third lateral capsule tear. Thus, there was an interstitial tear of the ACL and disruption of the integrity of the lateral capsular mechanism; operative intervention was indicated if an excellent result was to be obtained.

The approach we use in this situation is a straight incision 1 cm lateral to the infrapatella tendon (Fig. 34). The iliotibial band is then opened in line with its fibers after the manner of Bruser,[2] parallel to the joint line. This reveals the extent of capsular disruption and allows for repair of the lateral capsular avulsion as well as the meniscal periphery. The

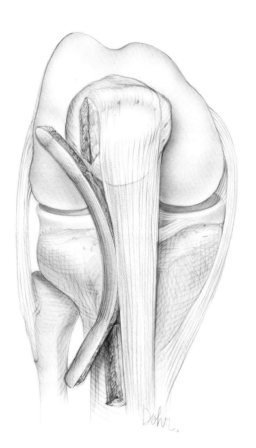

Fig. 36. The ACL lesion is repaired with a tendon graft from the lateral third of the patella tendon.

meniscal sutures are placed and tied at this time. The avulsion fracture of the mid-third of the lateral capsule from the tibia is replaced and held with an AO screw and washer (Fig. 35). Attention is directed to the interstitially torn ACL.

The ACL is treated with a lateral-third patella tendon graft since a lateral exposure has already been obtained (Fig. 36). The free graft is passed through the interstices of the residual ACL and is covered by the synovium of the PCL. The lateral third of the patella tendon is longer than either of the other thirds, and thus the bone plugs will not be flush with the femoral and tibial surfaces, respectively. More care is required here for chamfering, and it may even be desirable to fill the deficient tibial canal with locally obtained bone graft. The graft can then be secured with an AO screw external to the tibial canal (Fig. 37).

In closing the wound, a gap may be left compatible with the lateral retinacular release, but the stability of the lateral third of the capsule must not be compromised.

POSTOPERATIVE CARE AND REHABILITATION

Because of his age, the postoperative care of this patient was different than described in the preceding case studies: first, the knee was not immobilized; second, continuous passive motion (CPM) and range of motion were emphasized; and third, arthroscopy at 12 weeks would be recommended if motion were not increasing and there was evidence that adhesions were binding down the suprapatella pouch. Quadriceps thrust was definitely avoided later in the rehabilitation, not only to avoid straining the repaired structures, but also to respect the chondromalacia diagnosed at arthroscopy. Weightbearing to comfort was allowed. Toe rises were emphasized, and every effort was made to get the patient on a bicycle by 6 weeks. This type of patient will usually require the formal services of physical therapy because the experiences and demands of the rehabilitation process will be foreign to his usual daily discipline.

Fig. 37. The lateral third of the patella tendon is longer than the other parts of the tendon. The graft may be secured with an AO screw external to the tibial canal. Bone graft is added to the canal.

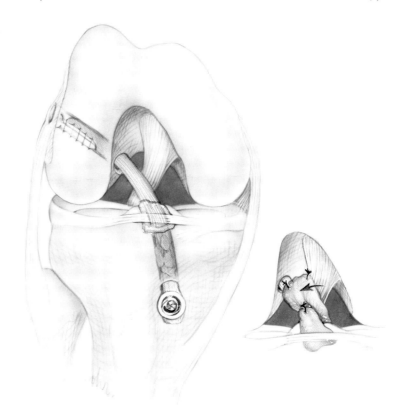

PROBLEMS, COMPLICATIONS, FOLLOW-UP RESULTS

The potential problems associated with surgery in a patient such as this are (1) failure on the part of the patient to put his therapy ahead of his demanding profession, (2) failure on the part of the surgeon to appreciate the extra time needed by a patient of this nature, and (3) failure to arrange for physical therapy supervision as well as continued guidance from the surgeon. Adhesions form all too quickly and patellofemoral compression is a major concern. Adhesions can usually be prevented by early range of motion. Sometimes early arthroscopic intervention and/or lateral retinacular release are indicated to release the patella compressive syndrome and adhesions of the suprapatella pouch.

The follow-up results have been good in patients of this type when the above cautions have been observed. A bad result, however, can be expected if a patient in his active mid-years is deprived of the "rightful" joy of continued athletic participation either because of knee instability or because of poor surgical results.

SUMMARY

Although this patient could have been managed either surgically or nonsurgically, given our current standards, the lateral capsular injury weighted the balance in favor of surgery, and the patient was handled in an aggressive postoperative manner so that he would gain 120° of flexion by the eighth week and thus was able to bicycle and work on his strength and range of motion without using quadriceps thrust or other patella-compressing exercises. A patient of this nature requires the utmost skills of our craft as regards both surgical technique and rehabilitative care to ensure success.

CASE STUDY 4
ACL (Complete), Positive Segond's Sign

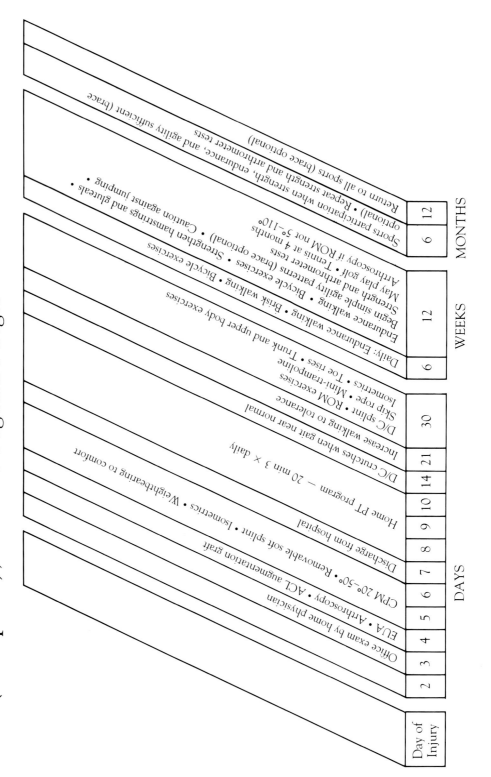

Day of Injury	2	3	4	5	6	7	8	9	10	14	21	30		6	12		6	12	

DAYS   WEEKS   MONTHS

Office exam by home physician

EUA • Arthroscopy • ACL augmentation graft

CPM 20–50° • Removable soft splint • Isometrics • Weightbearing to comfort

Discharge from hospital

Home PT program – 20 min 3 × daily

D/C crutches when gait near normal

Increase walking to tolerance

D/C splint • ROM exercises

Skip rope • Mini-trampoline

Isometrics • Toe rises • Trunk and upper body exercises

Daily: Endurance walking • Brisk walking • Bicycle exercises

Begin simple agility patterns (brace optional) • Strengthen hamstrings and gluteals

Endurance walking • Bicycle exercises • Caution against jumping

Strength and arthrometer tests

May play golf • Tennis at 4 months

Arthroscopy if ROM not 5°–110°

Sports participation when strength, endurance, and agility sufficient (brace optional) • Repeat strength and arthrometer tests

Return to all sports (brace optional)

REFERENCES

1. Bousquet G, Rhenter J-L, Bascoulergue G, Million J: L'illustré de Genou, Guy More, Le Coteau, France, 1982, p. 1030

2. Bruser DM: A direct lateral approach to the lateral compartment of the knee joint. J Bone Joint Surg 42B:348–351, 1960

3. Cooper K: The New Aerobics. M Evans, New York, 1970

4. Hughston JC, Norwood LA: The posterolateral Drawer test and external rotational recurvatum for posterolateral rotary instability of the knee. Clin Orthop 147:82–87, 1980

5. Müller W: The Knee. Form, Function, and Ligament Reconstruction. 1983, Springer-Verlas, New York, pp. 67–68, 8–13

6. Segond P, as cited by Losee RE: Orthop Clin North Am 16:97, 1985. Recherches cliniques et expérimentales sur les éspanchements, sanguins du genou par entorse. Progres Med (Paris) 7:297,319,340,400,419, 1897

7. Wittek A: Zur Naht der Kreuzbandverletzung im Kniegelenk. Zentralbl Chir 54:1538–1541, 1927

CASE STUDY 5

ACL Injury with Displaced Fracture of the Tibial Eminence

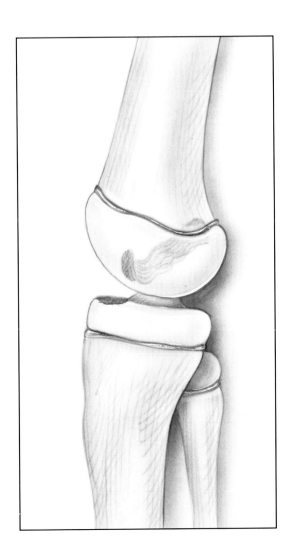

HISTORY

A 9-year-old boy was struck by a car and knocked aside. He was conscious, frightened, in obvious pain, and unwilling to bear weight on his right leg. The boy was taken to the emergency room. The knee was tensely effused, but the skin was intact. The child resisted a critical examination of the knee, but the Lachman test seemed positive with a soft end point.

Knee Examination
(Orthopaedic Surgeon/Emergency Room)

Diagnostic Clues	Findings
Effusion	Tense
Tenderness	Generalized
Lachman test	2+ positive*/soft end point
Drawer test	Could not be determined
Pivot shift test	Could not be determined
Varus/valgus	Stable
Patella apprehension	Negative
Range of motion	Resisted because of pain
Gait	Unwilling/unable to ambulate
Neurovasculature	Intact
Radiographs	6 mm upward displacement of tibial eminence, and significant effusion with fat
Other	None

* See Glossary.

COMMENTS

This mechanism of injury, "being knocked aside," is not so often appreciated in the child, although veterinarians deal with it frequently. Indeed, ACL laxity caused by this mechanism in the dog has a bad prognosis, particularly in the larger breeds. Degenerative arthrosis and lameness are the usual concomitants. To fail to identify this injury in this child would be to risk similarly poor long-term results. It is probably the whipping action of being knocked aside, rather than direct contact, that compromises the cruciate.

Where there is bony or chondral fracture, the onset of effusion is immediate. Effusion is tenser than in the interstitially torn ACL, and there will be gross fat in the aspirate. In contrast, with an interstitially torn ACL, fat droplets in the bloody aspirate are few.

The critical nature of this injury may be underestimated by the emergency physician, but should not be missed by the examining orthopaedic surgeon. The radiographs do not always reveal the obvious, and sometimes it requires a bright light and a high index of suspicion to appreciate fully the extent of the injury.

COURSE OF ACTION

Physical Examination

The well leg must be examined first, particularly as stability in the child is so variable. The increased excursion and soft end point, taken with the radiographic findings, are absolutely diagnostic of ACL incompetency associated with the fracture. The positive Lachman test can be elicited even with the effusion, but gentleness is necessary. The other tests are extremely difficult and usually require anesthesia.

Diagnostic Studies

A four-view x-ray study is usually sufficient in this type of case, although tomography is sometimes required. An arthrogram would be inappropriate. Arthroscopy will be discussed under Surgical Procedure.

Special Considerations

Even this patient's youth would not favor a good result if anatomic restoration were not the goal of treatment. The parents and child were made aware that the unstable knee would give a poor result and that the anatomy of the knee could and should be restored. Anesthesia and surgery are required to do this, and I prefer to operate promptly before the fracture fragments become softened or blunted.

PLAN

It was recommended to this patient and his family that examination under anesthesia (EUA) and diagnostic arthroscopy be followed by replacement of the tibial fracture fragment by either arthroscopic or open techniques, as appropriate.

Treatment

Although it has been reported that these fractures can be reduced in full extension,[2,5] often the fragment has extruded itself from beneath the intermeniscal ligament; although full extension may appear to reduce the fragment, actually it is not recessed beneath this ligament (Fig. 38). Arthroscopic intervention is therefore indicated to ensure that a stable anatomic configuration is restored and that there are no other intracapsular disruptions.

The EUA is usually critical—seldom can a complete examination of the medial and lateral capsular supporting structures be obtained in an outpatient setting in an injury of this nature. Again, the well leg must be examined carefully before the affected leg. The effusion is aspirated under anesthesia before the examination. The fluid was found to reflect gross fat with droplets too numerous to count. There was no induration of the capsular structures.

The Lachman test was indeed 3+ after aspiration under anesthesia, with a soft end point. The Drawer test was 3+. The pivot shift was actually positive bilaterally but with more translation in the affected knee. Children often have sufficient physiologic laxity that a positive pivot shift can be obtained under anesthesia in a normal leg.

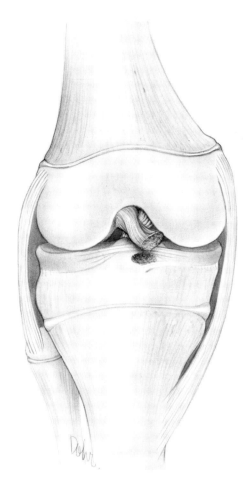

Fig. 38. With displaced fractures of the tibial eminence, the fragment often extrudes itself from beneath the intermeniscal ligament.

The knee was stable to varus/valgus testing and the patella could not be dislocated. A full range of motion was not attempted for fear of displacing the fragment further.

Standard medial and lateral arthroscopic portals are not always used initially in the evaluation of this injury. A superolateral portal, as described by Patel,[4] can be helpful in defining the anterior half of the joint, and particularly this injury. It will best show the relationship of the fracture fragment to the intermeniscal ligament. In my experience the fragment is usually above the ligament, and although the fragment can be approximately replaced using arthroscopic instruments, it is difficult to rearrange the fragment anatomically beneath the ligament in a stable fashion. Furthermore, the fracture fragment is often delicate and itself is frequently comminuted. Thus, after defining the fracture fragment arthroscopically, the joint is diligently searched for other intraarticular injuries. Frequently, however, this lesion is "isolated." In this patient the physical examination suggested that the lesion was isolated and, indeed, no other abnormality was noted at arthroscopy. The ACL was not interstitially torn, as evidenced by arthroscopic examination. The PCL was intact.

When this type of fracture cannot be replaced anatomically by arthroscopy, the limb is repripped and redraped and a small, straight medial, 3 cm incision is made which allows visualization of the intercondylar notch. The fat pad is carefully dissected laterally from the region of the intermeniscal ligament so that the latter can visualized. Sometimes it is necessary to divide and elevate the anterior horn of the medial meniscus and/or the intermeniscal ligament to reduce the fracture. The work of Cabaud et al[1] indicates that the anterior horn of the meniscus will heal quite well when repaired after surgical division. The exposure usually facilitates accurate reduction and fixation. After the fracture fragment or fragments are replaced in their bed and anatomic orientation is achieved, then two size 0 Kessler-type nonabsorbable sutures[3] are placed in the distal portion of the cruciate and through the fracture fragment (Fig. 39A). A 7 cm Keith needle can be inserted retrograde, through the physis, to receive the previously placed sutures (Fig. 39B). For strength and retention, two such sutures are placed, giving four-quadrant fixation to the fracture fragment. The fracture usually reduces as the knee is brought into full extension, and the sutures are tied with the knee in full extension (Fig. 39C). Thus, the epiphyseal plate is not violated, and secure internal fixation is obtained.

The intermeniscal ligament and/or horn of the medial meniscus is repaired, but with absorbable suture, and the medial extension of the fat pad replaced in its anatomic location. Radiographs should be taken in the operating room to verify fracture fragment relocation. The C-arm may be useful in the operating room for cases of this nature, particularly

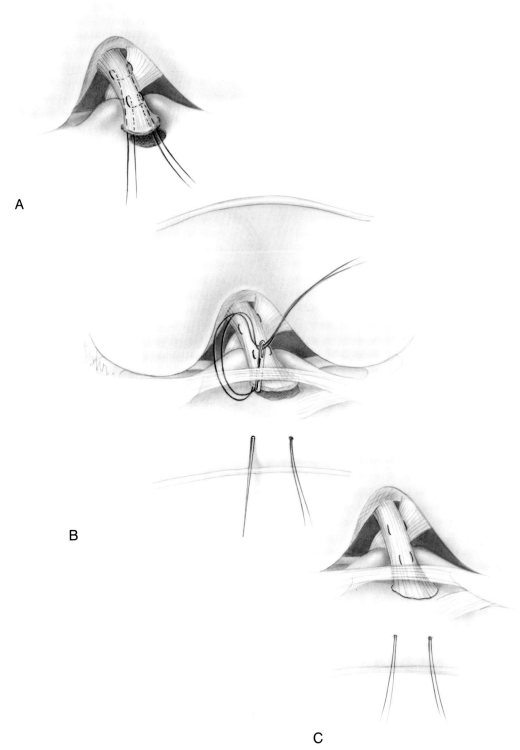

Fig. 39. After the fracture is reoriented anatomically, the ACL is repaired. **(A)** Two Kessler-type sutures are placed in the distal portion of the cruciate through the fracture fragment. **(B)** A 7-cm Keith needle is inserted retrograde through the physis to receive the previously placed sutures. **(C)** Sutures are tied with the knee in full extension.

CASE STUDY 5
ACL Injury, Tibial Eminence, Age 9

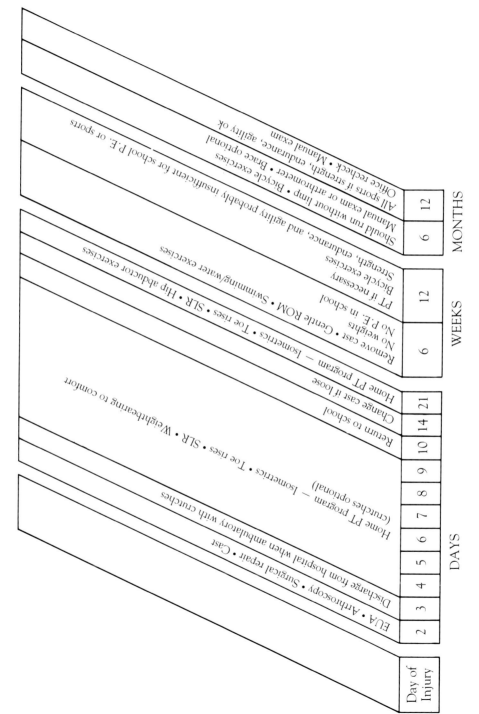

EUA • Arthroscopy • Surgical repair • Cast

Discharge from hospital when ambulatory with crutches

Home PT program — Isometrics • Toe rises • SLR • Weightbearing to comfort
(crutches optional)

Change cast if loose
Home PT program

Return to school

Remove cast • Isometrics • Toe rises • SLR • Hip abductor exercises
No weights
No P.E. in school
Bicycle exercises
PT if necessary
Gentle ROM • Swimming/water exercises
Strength, endurance, and agility probably insufficient for school P.E. or sports

Manual exam or arthrometer • Bicycle exercises
Should run without limp
Strength, endurance, agility ok
Office recheck • Manual exam • Brace optional
All sports if strength, endurance, agility ok

Day of Injury	2	3	4	5	6	7	8	9	10	14	21	6	12	6	12

DAYS   WEEKS   MONTHS

where one cannot visualize with the scope that the fracture is anatomically reduced and is stable in full extension. A drain is placed in the knee, and I usually apply a cylinder cast at this time, splitting it before departing from the operating room. Swelling is usually minimal, and the drain can be removed without disrupting the cast.

Stiffness and rehabilitation are, of course, a different problem in the child than in the adult, and healing of the fracture fragment in its anatomic location is paramount. The protection of the limb while the fracture heals dictates the postoperative care.

POSTOPERATIVE CARE AND REHABILITATION

Healing of a fracture fragment of this nature usually takes 6 weeks. The operative cast will not maintain control for this length of time, and usually must be changed at 10 to 14 days. The knee is immobilized in extension for 6 weeks in a properly fitting cylinder cast, and on removal of the cast, soft splints are applied with an Ace bandage to protect the child until his strength, confidence, and range of motion have returned. Crutches are appropriate in the immediate postoperative period for comfort, but most children dispense with them, and we have seen no harm in this practice.

Physical therapy is not instituted for fear of disrupting the healing fragment, and it is explained to the parents that it will probably be 12 to 16 weeks before the child walks without a limp. If atrophy is present after this period then therapy may be initiated. The surgeon must, however, be alert to the possibility that continued atrophy is caused by adhesions restricting the mobility of the patella. In practice, complications are few, physical therapy is seldom necessary, and a return to normal function and stability can be expected within 5 months of injury.

PROBLEMS, COMPLICATIONS, FOLLOW-UP RESULTS

Complications are usually the result of failing to treat the original injury in a timely fashion or failing to achieve anatomic restoration with secure internal fixation. It is essential to the management of this problem to realize that the intermeniscal ligament can obstruct reduction.

The follow-up results in terms of function, stability, and continued growth of the physis are usually excellent. The radiographs at 1 year often show some hypertrophy and/or calcification about the eminence, but this does not seem to interfere with knee function or affect the long-term excellent results.

SUMMARY

A 9-year-old child was "knocked aside" by an automobile. This mechanism of injury frequently produces a cruciate ligament injury in the child. A tense effusion usually occurs immediately, and aspiration will reveal gross fat. The Lachman test is usually elicited without anesthesia, with the soft end point being obvious to the physician and parents. The four-view radiographic study is essential and a bright light review of these films will usually reveal the extent of the fracture, thus obviating tomography. The arthroscope is invaluable to define the fragment and occasionally to obtain anatomic replacement. All too often, however, the intermeniscal ligament blocks arthroscopic reduction of the fracture, and open surgery is necessary. The operation can be accomplished through a small anteromedial incision. Division of either the anterior horn of the medial meniscus or the intermeniscal ligament is sometimes necessary to replace the fragment. This structure, when repaired, will heal.

Reduction should be confirmed radiographically in the operating room, and immobilization in extension is appropriate to protect the reduced fragments, since internal fixation techniques usually have limited strength. The long-term results of the anatomic restoration of these fractures are excellent in terms of function and stability, although x-ray films may show slight calcification and asymmetry of the tibial eminences.

REFERENCES

1. Cabaud HE, Rodkey W, Fitzwater JE: Medial meniscus repairs. An experimental and morphologic study. Am J Sports Med 9:129–134, 1981

2. Kennedy JC (ed): The Injured Adolescent Knee. Williams and Wilkins, Baltimore, 1979, pp. 141–156
3. Kessler I: The grasping technique for tendon repair. Hand 5:253–255, 1973
4. Patel D: Proximal approaches to arthroscopic surgery of the knee. Am J Sports Med 9:296–303, 1981
5. Roberts JM: Fractures and dislocations of the knee. pp 940–945. In Rockwood CA Jr, Wilkins KE, King RE (eds): Fractures in Children. Vol 3. JB Lippincott, Philadelphia, 1984

CASE STUDY 6

PCL Tear, Complete, Lateral Capsular Disruption, and Associated Diaphyseal Fracture of Femur

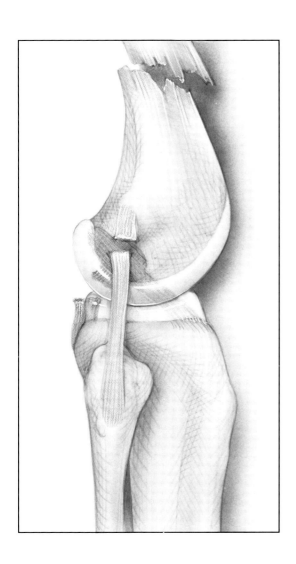

HISTORY

A 26-year-old passenger, seatbelted, in the right front seat of a motor vehicle, sustained a "dashboard" injury to his knee in a head-on collision. The patient was transported stable, neurologically intact, and well-splinted to the hospital. Initial evaluation revealed no evidence of increasing intracranial pressure and no visceral injuries. There was an obvious fracture of the right femur with hemarthrosis of the knee.

Knee Examination

Diagnostic Clues	Findings
Effusion	Moderate
Tenderness	Diffuse and difficult to localize
Lachman test	Difficult to quantitate, but questionable posterior sag of the tibia on the femur
Drawer test	Could not be attempted
Pivot shift test	Not attempted
Varus/valgus	Contraindicated because of fractured femur
Patella apprehension	Too painful to perform
Range of motion	Too painful to perform
Gait	Inappropriate to test
Neurovasculature	Intact
Radiographs	Confirmed a diaphyseal fracture of femur; no knee fractures although effusion obvious
Other	Knee aspirate/bloody with fat droplets too numerous to count

COMMENTS

The history of this patient injured in a head-on collision obviously reflects abrupt deceleration. The knee was most probably flexed at 90°. This position of the leg resulted in a fractured femur in addition to the "dashboard" injury to the knee, and could also have resulted in a dislocated hip. Although the vascular system appeared to be intact, the possibility of an intimal flap tear of the artery also had to be considered. An arteriogram is often indicated in such cases even when the distal pulses are intact. The fat aspirated from the knee could have been either intrarticular in origin or injected by the fractured femur perforating the suprapatella pouch. As for treatment, the fractured femur had obvious priority, assuming the vasculature was intact. The surgical team, having decided that the patient was in satisfactory condition for operation, scheduled an arteriogram and closed nailing of the femur as soon as possible.

COURSE OF ACTION

Physical Examination

The examination of the knee was of necessity limited because of the unstable femur. The appropriate primary concern was the vascular status, since normal pulses do not rule out a vascular injury. The physical examination included palpation for compartment swelling of the lower legs and a very careful documentation and monitoring of the neurovascular status.

The fracture required stabilization; this was handled as soon as the arterial status was resolved.

Although the tear of the PCL was obvious, it was important to quantitate the extent of disruption of the posterior capsule. Manual palpation can sometimes be helpful at this stage, as sometimes even parts of the gastrocnemius are torn from their origins by violent injuries of this type. Thus, the physical examination of this patient's knee, given the unstable femur, was not up to the standards we have illustrated in other case studies, and we were especially diligent in continuing to monitor the knee to gain progressive information that would bear on the treatment of this problem when the time came.

Diagnostic Studies

In this particular case, I would favor *an arteriogram to rule out vascular compromise before embarking on either stabilization of the femur or knee surgery.* Arthroscopy was contraindicated because of the possible gross disruption of the posterior capsule. After stabilization of the femur, stress radiographs of the knee were obtained and demonstrated varus laxity.

Special Considerations

The key to the management of this patient's injuries was the timing of the operation. It is the surgeon's choice whether to deal with the femur and the knee at the same surgical sitting or to delay the knee procedure. I personally prefer to stabilize the femur and wait approximately 10 days before embarking on the knee reconstruction, as was done in this patient. *Care must be taken from the beginning that a Steinmann pin is not inserted for traction in a manner that will ultimately compromise or delay reconstructive knee surgery because of an infected pin site.* The knee surgeon must guard this domain jealously if it is threatened by the fracture surgeon. Certainly, there is no problem if a pin is placed for traction during the closed nailing and removed after the procedure is finished.

Pulmonary embolus is a distinct possibility, and delaying the knee reconstruction does not guarantee that the risk of pulmonary embolus will be over. The swelling and tissue damage about the thigh caused by the femoral fracture may make it difficult to use a tourniquet for the knee surgery even at 10 days. Knee surgery can be accomplished without a tourniquet, but provisions for blood replacement should be made. The knee operation must be well planned and proceed expeditiously to avoid unnecessary blood loss and trauma.

Had this case involved a diaphyseal fracture of the tibia in association with a posterior cruciate ligament injury, I would have favored reconstruction of both bone and ligament in the same surgical sitting. The risk to the circulation is less with a tibial injury and, because a tourniquet can be used, blood loss and tissue damage pose less threat to life and limb. Although I prefer to stabilize the diaphyseal femoral fracture surgically, had internal injuries prevented my accomplishing this, we would have placed a femoral pin for traction in a position that would preclude connection with the knee joint. The femur would still take precedence over the knee as soon as the patient was medically stabilized. Although it is not a desirable course, I have deferred knee surgery for 3 to 4 weeks until the general condition of the patient was stabilized.

PLAN

Treatment

The treatment plan recommended for this 26-year-old patient was to examine the knee under anesthesia at the termination of femoral rodding and to ascertain the stability of the medial and lateral posterior capsules. This information might help in later planning to determine the extent and urgency of knee reconstruction. Certainly, an isolated posterior cruciate ligament tear might well be deferred, whereas complete capsular disruption should be treated surgically. In this patient, after a stable rodding of the femur, it was seen that the knee was unstable to varus testing in full extension, signifying a tear of the posterior cruciate as well as of the lateral capsule. Therefore, the patient was returned to surgery for knee reconstruction within 10 days of injury.

Although one can accept nonoperative care for the "isolated" rupture of the posterior cruciate ligament, *nonoperative care for PCL rupture with capsular disruption is untenable.*[6]

The surgical planning must include a discussion of the anterior versus posterior approach, and of what structure is to be used to augment the PCL. Arthroscopy is sometimes possible at 10 days when it would not have been judicious at the time of the initial injury. Nevertheless, at the slightest hint of posterior extravasation of the fluid, arthroscopy would have to be terminated.

In this particular case, I did not do arthroscopy because of the risks already cited. Instead, I made a long (15 cm) straight lateral parapatella skin incision and a medial patellar retinacular incision to allow lateral dislocation of the patella (Fig. 40).

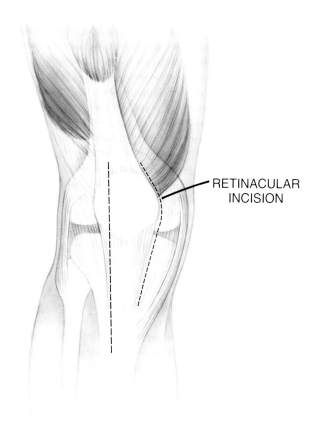

Fig. 40. The dotted lines indicate the straight lateral parapatellar skin incision and the medial patellar retinacular incision.

When repairing this type of injury, the type of graft to be used should be chosen before the operation—either a one-third patella tendon graft or a gracilis tendon free graft if the cruciate was interstitially torn. Both can be harvested from the incision described. In most cases of this nature, the lateral capsular tear is the more disruptive; hence rationale for the lateral skin incision, which allows the surgeon to dissect on this side.

With the patella dislocated, the tibia may be levered forward to the full extent of excursion of the ACL with a dull Hohmann retractor in the fossa of the PCL. The extent of capsular and posterior cruciate injury is best determined at 90° of flexion with the leg hanging and the popliteal fossa free (Fig. 41).

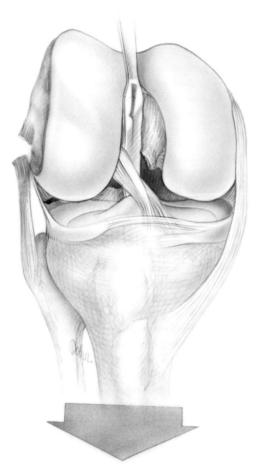

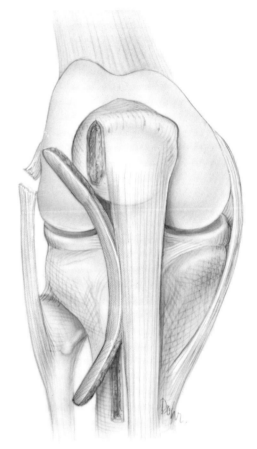

Fig. 42. A graft from the lateral third of the patella tendon is harvested with bone plugs at either end.

Fig. 41. The knee is in 90° flexion and the lower leg hangs for gravity distraction. Then the tibia is levered forward to the full extent of the ACL's excursion by using a dull Hohmann retractor in the fossa of the posterior collateral ligament. Now the extent of capsular and PCL injury can be determined.

It is not unusual to find a bony avulsion off the tibial attachment of the PCL, and this can be restored by using the techniques of O'Donoghue.[4,5]

In this 26-year-old patient, however, there was interstitial tearing of the PCL, and augmentation grafting was deemed essential for restoration. Since the ACL was intact, we decided to use the lateral third patella tendon graft harvested with bone plugs at either end (Fig. 42). The procedure is described in detail elsewhere (see Ch. 21). The drill guide is

essential for precision drilling, particularly of the tibial tunnel (Fig. 43). The tibial tunnel should be started quite inferiorly so as to minimize the angle through which the graft must pass at the tibial juncture. The femoral side is quite straightforward. It is slightly more difficult to bring the tibial bone plug into the posterior cruciate fossa because of limited ability to "turn the corner." This bone plug may be undersized (i.e., 6 mm) and shortened in length to facilitate passage. An interference fit is still sought by drilling a smaller hole and, as usual, care must be taken to chamfer the bony tunnels at their origin and insertion to avoid abrading the augmentation graft. The graft is pulled through the residual PCL stump to provide a vascular pedicle and ligamentous scaffolding. The graft is positioned at this stage but is not tensioned (Fig. 44).

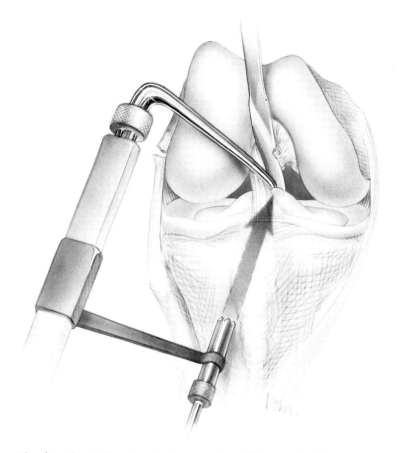

Fig. 43. The drill guide aids in precision drilling of the tibial tunnel.

The posterior medial capsule is usually not disrupted, and often the lateral capsular sutures can be placed intraarticularly by opening the knee widely in varus and bringing these sutures through drill holes in the tibia as described by O'Donoghue[4] (Fig. 45).

Dissection may still be required through the iliotibial band and beneath the lateral head of the gastrocnemius to ensure that there has been no disruption of the arcuate complex or fabella ligamentous system. This can usually be accomplished through the same skin incision by working "around the corner" and by mobilizing the lateral head of the gastrocnemius. In my experience, a single incision has healed better than double incisions while still giving adequate exposure. If the popliteus tendon is torn, it must be located and repaired. The popliteus

is a *key stabilizer* of the knee and an essential component of the lateral complex.[2,7,8] The meniscal suture set from the arthroscopic tray may be useful even in an open procedure to allow rapid placement of key sutures in the posterior aspect of the joint.

After the lateral capsular structures are repaired, the posterior cruciate ligament graft is tensioned (Fig. 46).

A helpful adjunct described by Müller[3] is "olecranization of the patella"—a technique that prevents posterior sag of the tibia on the femur which would stress the graft. A 4.5 mm Steinmann pin is placed through a prebored hole in the patella and driven into the tibia with the tibia and femur in appropriate alignment, and the graft is then tensioned (Fig. 47). The olecranization procedure limits the range of motion of the knee but protects the graft

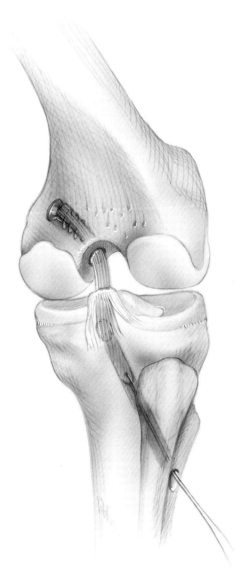

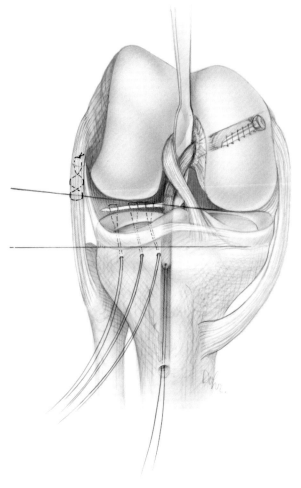

Fig. 45. The lateral capsular sutures are placed intraarticularly through drill holes in the tibia, as described by O'Donoghue.[4,5]

Fig. 44. The graft is pulled through the residual posterior cruciate ligament stump to provide a vascular pedicle and ligamentous scaffolding. The graft is positioned but not tensioned (posterior view).

from posterior sag during early healing. This pin may be removed between the fourth and sixth week.

Just as the circulation was checked before initiation of any surgical procedures, it must be checked carefully after this knee reconstruction.

POSTOPERATIVE CARE AND REHABILITATION

Although I have not had occasion to place a patient such as this on continuous passive motion (CPM), I believe I would consider doing so. The quality of fixation for the injuries described should be as good as for other injuries that benefit from CPM (provided the anatomy is equally well understood and the techniques of fixation equally applied). Certainly, even with "olecranization" of the patella to of flexion and extension. The patient would be instructed in isometric contractions of the quadriceps and hamstrings through this range of motion. Thus, the initial postoperative exercise program consists of early range of motion, early weightbearing, isometric exercises and, additionally, toe rises.

At the end of 4 to 6 weeks, the patella-tibial pin would be removed and range of motion would be increased. Thus, with bone-to-bone augmentation grafting of the PCL and restoration of the capsular anatomy, earlier rehabilitation can be initiated and adhesions, ankylosis, and prolonged convalescence minimized.

If range of motion failed to progress from the 6th to the 12th week, then arthroscopy would be indicated to ascertain and correct the cause.

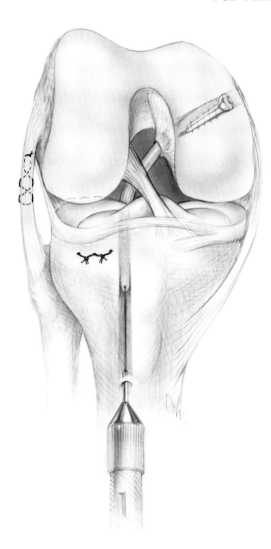

Fig. 46. The lateral capsule is repaired and the PCL is tensioned.

the tibia, CPM through a limited range would be advantageous. The intraarticular Steinmann pin, described by Godfrey,[1] might lead to further stiffening, and thus should be avoided in favor of olecranization and CPM.

The patient would be allowed to bear weight to comfort with a range of motion from 20° to 50°. Though I know of no brace that absolutely prevents subluxation, a hinge-type brace may well be considered to give the patient lateral support and control

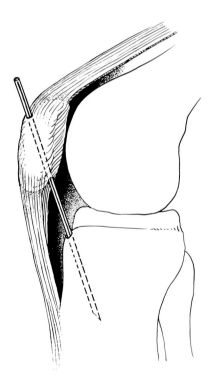

Fig. 47. To prevent posterior sag of the tibia on the femur, which would stress the graft, a 4.5 mm Steinmann pin is placed through a prebored hole in the patella and driven into the tibia with the tibia and femur in appropriate alignment. The graft is then tensioned. Müller (personal communication, 1984) called this "olecranization of the patella."

CASE STUDY 6
PCL (Complete), Lateral Capsule, Femoral Fracture

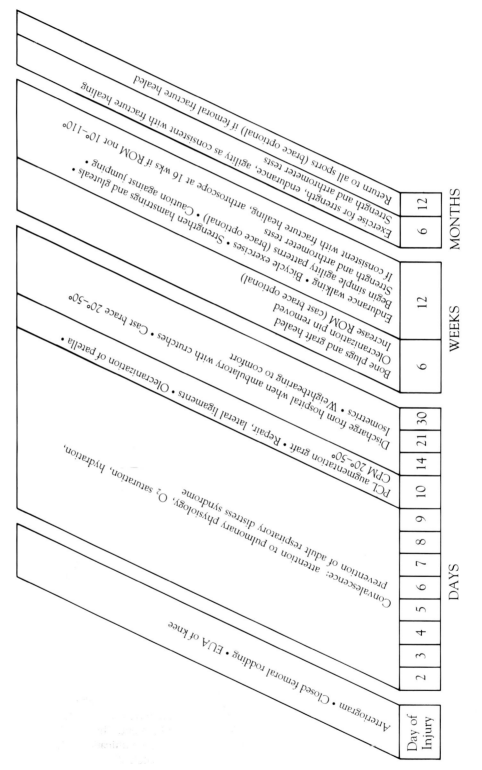

DAYS

Day of Injury	2	3	4	5	6	7	8	9	10	14	21	30

WEEKS

6	12

MONTHS

6	12

• Arteriogram • Closed femoral rodding • EUA of knee

Convalescence: attention to pulmonary physiology, O_2 saturation, hydration, prevention of adult respiratory distress syndrome

PCL augmentation graft • Repair, lateral ligaments • Olecranization of patella • CPM 20°–50°

Discharge from hospital when ambulatory with crutches • Weightbearing to comfort • Cast brace 20°–50°
• Isometrics

Bone plugs and graft healed
Olecranization pin removed
Increase ROM (cast brace optional)
Endurance walking • Bicycle exercises • Strengthen hamstrings and gluteals • Begin simple agility patterns (brace optional) • Caution against jumping
Strength and arthrometer tests if consistent with fracture healing

Exercise for strength, endurance, arthroscope at 16 wks if ROM not 10°–110°
Strength and arthrometer tests
Return to all sports (brace optional) if femoral fracture healed, agility as consistent with fracture healing

PROBLEMS, COMPLICATIONS, FOLLOW-UP RESULTS

Four major possible complications should be uppermost in the mind of the surgeon: (1) late arterial compromise, (2) infection as a result of the profound tissue damage in the limb and extensive prior surgery, (3) the inadvisability to use a tourniquet for the second procedure because of damage to the thigh, and (4) phlebothrombosis and/or compartment syndrome.

Ankylosis could ensue because of injury to the quadriceps mechanism as well as because of the major reconstruction about the knee. Residual posterior instability has always been a problem; however, with the advent of patella tendon grafting and olecranization of the patella-tibial joint, the results of this operation seem to have improved.

Patellofemoral arthrosis can ensue rapidly if there is an uncorrected posterior laxity. Once established, it is unrelenting in its progression, and reconstruction may be too late to prevent it. Complications are more likely in a patient such as this because of the complex nature of the injury, the inherent anatomic pitfalls, and the infrequency with which we are confronted with such an injury. The surgeon must be prepared not only for each individual complication, but for the occurrence of a combination of complications.

There are too few cases of this type to give specific follow-up results. Before aggressive internal fixation came to be used for femoral fractures, these cases were often treated by skeletal traction. Skeletal traction left residual deformity of the femur, and the disability caused by the femur deformity could not be distinguished from that due to the knee instability. My impression is that results for this type of knee injury have improved significantly since employment of early rigid skeletal fixation followed by anatomic repair, augmentation grafting, and early motion of the knee.

SUMMARY

This case was presented to show the relation between the instability of the associated fracture and the injured contiguous joint. The case further emphasizes the care of traumatized soft tissues above

and below, as well as at, the joint level. The femoral artery, because of its anatomic fixation, is a critical consideration in this case. Often, in our modern surgery, care of the fracture is the responsibility of one orthopaedic team and care of the soft tissue injuries about the knee the responsibility of another. This arrangement necessitates close cooperation and planning so that one team does not inadvertently place traction pins that might compromise the knee reconstruction by a later team. Timing and judgment related to the surgical procedures are obviously a delicate matter in such a case, but the patient's general well-being is of paramount importance, and separating the surgical procedures in time may decrease the risk of adult respiratory syndrome. Although the contributing factors are not absolute, these are complications of such magnitude that every opportunity must be taken to prevent them. A good result from repair of the posterior cruciate ligament can be expected when isometric reconstruction, augmentation grafting, and firm fixation are applied and the capsular injuries recognized and repaired.

REFERENCES

1. Godfrey JD: Ligamentous injuries of the knee. Curr Prac Orthop Surg 5:56–92, 1973
2. Müller W: The Knee. Form, Function, and Ligament Reconstruction. Springer-Verlag, New York, pp. 73–75
3. Müller W: Paper presented at the 2nd Meeting of the European Society for Knee Surgery and Arthroscopy, Basel, Switzerland, Oct 1–4, 1986
4. O'Donoghue DH: Reconstruction for medial instability of the knee. Technique and results in sixty cases. J Bone Joint Surg 55A:941–955, 1973
5. O'Donoghue DH: Treatment of Injuries to Athletes. 4th Ed. WB Saunders, Philadelphia, 1984, pp. 501–502
6. Parolie J, Bergfeld JA: Long-term results of nonoperative treatment of "isolated" posterior cruciate ligament injuries in the athlete. Am J Sports Med 14:35–38, 1986
7. Seebacher JR, Inglis AE, Marshall JL, Warren RF: The structure of the posterolateral aspect of the knee. J Bone Joint Surg 64A:536–541, 1982
8. Southmayd MW, Quigley TB: The forgotten popliteus muscle. Its usefulness in correction of anteromedial rotatory instability of the knee. A preliminary report. Clin Orthop 130:218–222, 1978

CASE STUDY 7

Knee Dislocation—ACL Tear, Complete, PCL Tear, Complete, and Medial or Lateral Capsular Disruption

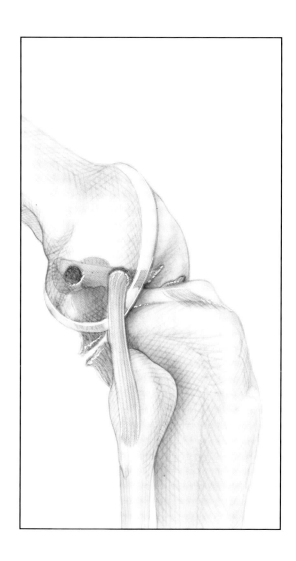

HISTORY

A 21-year-old college football punter (senior) was struck by an incoming player who had been blocked into him. The opposing player, airborne, landed heavily on the fixed leg of the punter just after the ball had left his other foot. The patient lay on the field writhing in pain, with obvious deformity of the knee.

Knee Examination
(Team Physician/On Field)

Gross deformity, with the skin tented over the prominent medial femoral condyle.

Extreme pain, and the writhing of the player, prevented the normal examination.

The neurovasculature, as best as could be determined, seemed to be intact.

The athletic trainer applied traction as the orthopaedic surgeon gently moved the knee into anatomic position. The relocation was attended by marked relief of pain so that the leg could be splinted and the player removed from the field.

COMMENTS

Knee dislocation is a true emergency, and an on-field dislocation strikes terror in the hearts of all concerned. Because most knee dislocations can be reduced early on with relative ease, I prefer to put the crowd and the referees aside and immediately try to relocate the knee manually in the direction that seems logical. This was accomplished, and the patient's pulses were intact and of good quality both before and after reduction. The knee could then be splinted in the position of comfort and a careful sideline examination accomplished.

COURSE OF ACTION

Knee Examination
(Orthopaedic Surgeon/Team Physician/On Sideline)

Diagnostic Clues	Findings
Effusion	Mild
Tenderness	Medial and lateral
Lachman test	Grossly positive/without end point
Drawer test	Positive anterior/with posterior sag
Pivot shift test	Too unstable to attempt
Varus/valgus	Valgus gross laxity at 30°, 1+* opening in full extension
	Varus gross laxity at 30°, 2+ opening in full extension
Patella apprehension	Equivocal
Range of motion	10° to 30° with laxity, tending toward re-dislocation with further motion
Gait	Not applicable
Neurovasculature	No decrease in pulses
Radiographs	Unobtainable on sideline
Other	On-field reduction gave pain relief sufficient to allow definitive sideline knee examination

* See Glossary.

Diagnostic Studies

The most important initial diagnostic study in this type of injury is *observation*. An intimal flap tear of the popliteal artery is an injury of major concern. The sideline situation is an excellent opportunity to ice the knee, immobilize it in slight flexion, and observe the circulation to the lower limb for 15 to 20 minutes before proceeding with further definitive care. *Arteriography is obligatory* in all complete knee dislocations, and should be scheduled immediately. Arthroscopy is contraindicated. Varus/valgus x-ray films might be considered under anesthesia, but are usually not necessary to support the manual examination. The routine x-ray films would be altered to consist of anteroposterior, lateral, and right and left obliques, as the patient would have difficulty in assuming the position required for patellar and tunnel views.

Special Considerations

The status of the arterial circulation overrides all other considerations in this type of case. It is nearly a universal standard to perform an arteriogram. It certainly grants the surgeon peace of mind, as he proceeds with the ligamentous repair, to know that an intimal flap tear is not waiting to displace itself and jeopardize the status of the lower limb. Thus, I would *not* pursue ligamentous repair until reassured by a normal arteriographic study.

PLAN

Although diagnosis and reduction of this type of injury are an emergency, I prefer to do surgery as an elective procedure. This serves two purposes. First, it ensures that no latent compromise of the artery, nerve, or anatomic compartments exists. Second, it allows for optimal surgical circumstances — operating room team support, family support, patient support.

The repair of this injury is an operation of such magnitude that it should be done by a trained team under optimal conditions. For this patient, the sideline examination was the best examination that would be available until the examination under anesthesia (EUA). Given that the neurovascular status was carefully ascertained well before surgery and was not in doubt, the next critical element of the physical examination was to determine if a "stable hinge" existed. Usually a portion of one corner remains intact, and since I prefer to do the operation through a single incision, it is important to make the incision opposite the stable hinge whenever possible. In this patient, the stable hinge appeared to be about the posteromedial corner at the insertion of the semimembranosus (1+ as compared to 2+ opening in full extension on physical examination). This is a common site of residual intact tissue. Thus, a long, straight incision would be used, either directly midline or approximately 5 cm lateral as in Case Study 6.

The retinacular incision would be along the medial aspect of the patella to allow lateral dislocation of the patella. The preoperative plan included provisions for grafting both the ACL and the PCL as well as inserting a Steinmann pin to olecranize the patella (see Case Study 6).

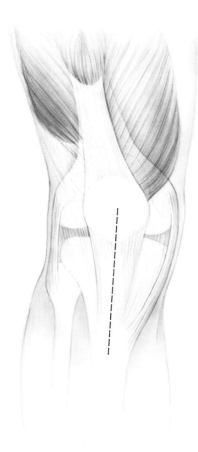

Fig. 48. A 24 cm straight midline skin incision and a medial retinacular incision allow dislocation of the patella and visualization of the interstitially disrupted cruciate ligaments.

Kennedy's review[2] of results following dislocation are well known. I do not believe, however, that in today's sporting society these results should dictate our treatment plan. I, therefore, do not recommend nonoperative care for a knee joint dislocation with complete tear of ACL and PCL and capsular disruption.

A long (24 cm), straight midline skin incision was made. A medial retinacular incision then allowed dislocation of the patella (Fig. 48). I seldom find a need for a posterior skin incision in these cases if dissection of the flaps is carefully accomplished medially and laterally. On dislocation of the patella, both cruciates were found to be interstitially disrupted. The posterior horns of both medial and lateral menisci were torn loose from their tibial attachments (Fig. 49A). The posteromedial corner was otherwise intact, but the medial collateral ligament was torn interstitially above the meniscus, and there was a complete tear of the entire lateral ligamentocapsular complex. The lateral collateral ligament and popliteus tendon were torn near their femoral insertions (Fig. 49B).

We repair injuries of this type according to the following procedure.

1. Peripheral capsular sutures can be placed by subluxing the joint through the leverage of a small Hohmann retractor placed into the tibial fossa of the posterior cruciate ligament. These capsular sutures can then be brought through holes in the tibia after the manner of O'Donoghue.[4] The meniscal repair kit from the arthroscopy kit is sometimes useful to place nonabsorbable sutures into the periphery, which are not tied at this stage of repair (Fig. 50).
2. Attention is then directed to the lateral capsule. The arcuate complex is identified and tagged with several sutures that will draw it to its origin on the tibia. The popliteus tendon is retrieved and will be brought into a tunnel in the femur or held with a Bunnell-type suture (Fig. 51).
3. Attention is then directed to the cruciate ligaments. Synthetic stent or allograft would be ideal for this case, but since these are not yet generally available or adequately tested, autogenous graft

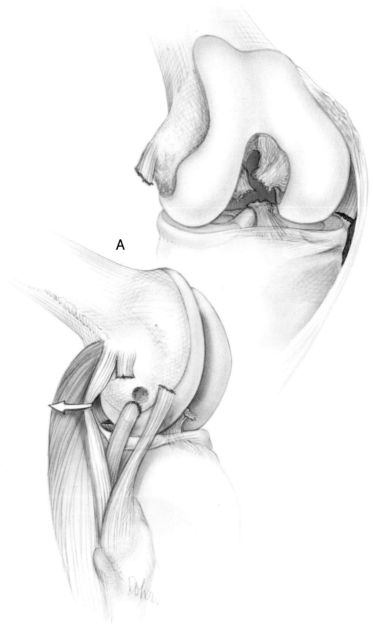

Fig. 49. (A) The posterior horns of both the medial and lateral menisci were torn loose from their tibial attachments and the MCL was torn interstitially above the meniscus. **(B)** The lateral collateral ligament and popliteus tendon were torn near their femoral insertions.

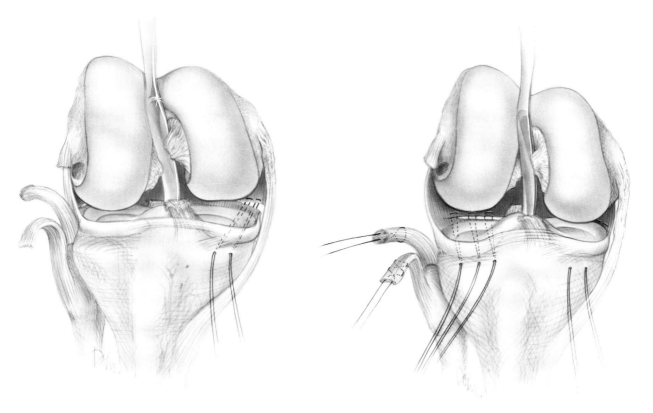

Fig. 50. Sutures are placed in the periphery but not tied.

Fig. 51. The arcuate complex is tagged with several sutures. The popliteus tendon will be brought into the tunnel in the femur.

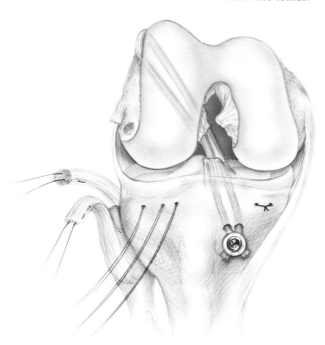

Fig. 52. The PCL will be augmented with the mid-third of the patella tendon, and the ACL has been augmented with a semitendinosus free tendon graft.

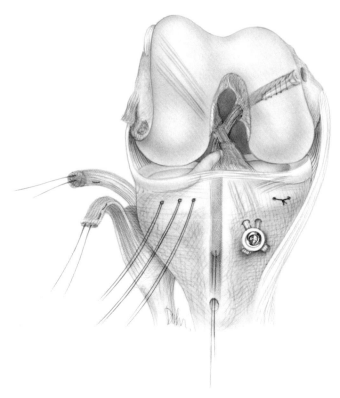

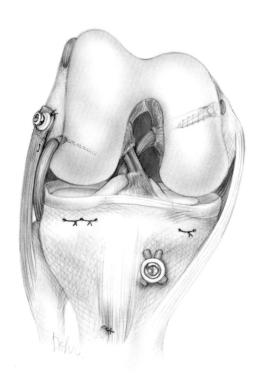

Fig. 53. The grafts are provisionally tensioned with the knee flexed 30°.

Fig. 54. Repair of the capsular structures is completed by using the screw and washer. They facilitate repair and accuracy of placement, and allow earlier motion of the joint because they enhance fixation.

was used. The mid-third patella tendon was used for the posterior cruciate and a semitendinosus free tendon graft for the ACL (Fig. 52).[3] Needless to say, harvesting these grafts involves additional surgical trauma and time. If satisfactory prosthetic or allograft material were available and proven, it certainly would be used in a case of this magnitude.

4. The posterior cruciate graft is placed in the manner described in Case Study 6. The anterior cruciate graft is positioned through the residual stump of the ACL as described by Mott.[3] One end of the cruciate grafts are fixed, and they are provisionally tensioned with the knee flexed 30° (Fig. 53). Care must be taken so that the tibia is not posteriorly subluxed on the femur during this tensioning. The meniscal sutures are tied and their anatomic position checked through a range of motion.

5. Attention is then directed to the capsular structures. Since in injuries of this type the arcuate complex is usually torn from its bony origin on the femur, this is an ideal place to use the AO screw and washer. As previously mentioned, using the screw and washer facilitates repair and accurate placement, enhancing fixation to allow earlier motion (Fig. 54).

6. Before the final tensioning of the two cruciate

ligaments, the femur must be accurately reduced on the tibia. Olecranization of the patella seems to be one of the best ways of accomplishing this (Case Study 6). Once this is accomplished, and with the knee in 30° flexion, the PCL is tensioned and secured, and then the ACL tensioned and secured. The Lachman sign is then tested, posterior sag is checked, varus/valgus stability ascertained, and range of motion determined. It is usually possible to change the tensioning of any of the major ligaments at this stage if the methods of fixation described have been used.

7. It is best to loosen the tourniquet after approximately 1 hour to prevent the atrophy that seems to occur with prolonged tourniquet time.[1] Two drains should be placed in a case of this magnitude. Closure time can be shortened by the use of skin staples. The compression dressing, as always, is critical.

The goal in this knee, after tensioning of the ligaments, would be to have a range of motion from 20° to 50° without undue tension on any of the components of the repair. This would allow use of continuous passive motion (CPM) and markedly reduce postoperative pain and the risk of ankylosis. Other methods for relief of postoperative pain and improvement in function are as described in Case Study 2 and Chapters 25 and 28.

POSTOPERATIVE CARE AND REHABILITATION

The immediate postoperative care was no different from that described in the preceding case studies. Patients of this type are more prone to lower leg swelling with a risk of phlebothrombosis, so anticoagulation might be considered, although it has not been the standard in my care and was not used in this case.

The patient was retained in the hospital under observation longer than for a routine two-ligament injury, to avoid dependent edema and its complica-

tions. A hinge cast or orthosis from 20° to 60° range of motion was used for support.

This is the type of case in which to consider arthroscopic reexamination at 8 weeks, if the range of motion has not progressed satisfactorily. This "relook" would be done when the patella pin was removed, which would allow for arthroscopic lysis of adhesions in the suprapatellar pouch and gentle manipulation under anesthesia using arthroscopic control. The surgeon may consider the possibility of lateral retinacular release either at the time of the original operation or at the time of this reexamination. Whether to perform this "relook" at 8 weeks is a difficult decision for both patient and surgeon. It is of little use to "discover" 12 to 16 weeks after repair that the patient has severely restricted motion that precludes further therapeutic exercise or progress toward normal gait and function. Adhesions are only more difficult to release at this later stage.

PROBLEMS, COMPLICATIONS, FOLLOW-UP RESULTS

As has been repeatedly mentioned, the most serious complication in this type of case is vascular compromise. Adequacy of the vascular status must always be uppermost in the mind of the surgeon. Vascular compromise may take the form of disruption of the artery at the time of injury, intimal flap tear, thrombotic occlusion of the artery, or compartment syndrome. Deep vein thrombosis is more common postoperatively in cases such as this than in less complex cases. Infection is a major concern because of the complexity of the operation.

Arthrofibrosis has been the most common postoperative problem, and this is why I believe that arthroscopic evaluation at 8 weeks, to lyse adhesions, can be justified.

No one has reported a large series of patients with knee joint dislocation and surgical repair. The availability of improved augmentation grafting materials will allow the operation to be accomplished with less trauma and more expeditiously. Follow-up results after such an operative procedure can be ex-

CASE STUDY 7
Knee Dislocation — On-Field Reduction

Day of Injury	2	3	4	5	6	7	8	9	10	14	21	30	6	12	6	12
DAYS													**WEEKS**		**MONTHS**	

- Ice • Splint • Arteriogram
- EUA • ACL/PCL augmentation grafts • Repair of capsuloligamentous complexes
- CPM 20°–50° • Removable splint • Isometrics • Weightbearing to comfort
- Discharge from hospital when ambulatory (cast brace 20°–50°)
- Home PT program — 20 min 3× daily
- Office recheck • Continue home PT program
- D/C crutches when gait near normal • Increase ROM resistive exercises
- D/C splint • Begin bicycle exercises • Trunk, upper body strength training • ROM 20°–60° • No quad thrust • Skip rope • Increase
- Brisk walking • Bicycle exercises • Swimming/water exercises • Increase ROM and endurance • Strength and gluteals • Strengthen hamstrings and gluteals • Strengthen
- No contact sports
- Continue agility drills (brace optional)
- Repeat strength and arthrometer tests
- Arthroscopy at 4 to 6 mo if ROM < 10°–110°
- Return to all sports (brace optional)

pected to be far better than nonoperative results, providing the ligament repairs have been isometric and complete.

SUMMARY

This case of knee joint dislocation with ligamentous disruption represents one of the most serious athletic injuries that can occur to the lower extremity. A dislocation of the knee is a major threat to the viability of the lower limb. The diagnosis, reduction, and vascular evaluation are an emergency that outweighs all other considerations. Surgery should be deferred until the arterial status has been determined accurately by both observation and arteriography. Reparative ligamentous surgery may be performed as an elective procedure, usually within 24 hours of the injury. The sequence of repair, as described in this case, is complex. It is necessary to repair both cruciate ligaments, and augmentation grafting of both is usually required. CPM is desirable in the immediate postoperative period. The postoperative management, however, is no different from that described, in the preceding case studies except that one is more cautious about allowing dependency and is especially observant for vascular complications.

Arthroscopic reevaluation may be performed between the 8th and 12th weeks if range of motion is not progressing. A satisfactory result from this type of injury can be expected if details are diligently attended to by the surgeon, the patient, and the other team members.

REFERENCES

1. Dobner JJ, Nitz AJ: Postmeniscectomy tourniquet palsy and functional sequelae. Am J Sports Med 10:211–214, 1982
2. Kennedy JC: Complete dislocation of the knee joint. J Bone Joint Surg 45A:889–904, 1963
3. Mott HW: Semitendinosus anatomic reconstruction for cruciate ligament insufficiency. Clin Orthop 172:90–92, 1983
4. O'Donoghue DH: Reconstruction of medial instability of the knee. Technique and results in sixty cases. J Bone Joint Surg 55:941–955, 1973

CASE STUDY 8

Isolated Posterior Cruciate Ligament Injury, Complete

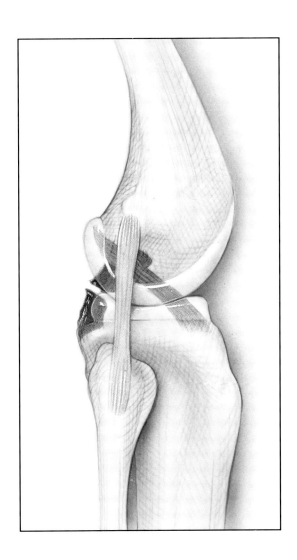

HISTORY

An 18-year-old helmeted motorcycle rider "broad-sided" a car crossing his path. The impact speed was approximately 25 km/hour. The motorcyclist's knee struck the handle bars as he was projected into the car. On-site examination suggested he was in-

Knee Examination
(Orthopaedic Surgeon/Emergency Room)
(1 Hour after Injury)

Diagnostic Clues	Findings
Effusion	Mild
Tenderness	Posteromedial and posterolateral capsules, and anterior tibial tuberosity
Lachman test	Equivocally positive
Drawer test	1+ positive posterior*/soft end point
Pivot shift test	Negative, but reverse pivot shift is questionably positive
Varus/valgus	Valgus: 2+ opening at 30° flexion; trace-positive opening at full extension.
	Varus: 2+ opening at 30° flexion; 2+ opening at full extension; 1+ opening in hyperextension
Patella apprehension	Negative
Range of motion	0° to 90°
Gait	Antalgic
Neurovasculature	Intact
Radiographs	Normal, except for joint effusion
Other	Tenderness of midpopliteal area with induration and fullness

* See Glossary.

91

tact neurologically but had sustained a knee injury. He was carried by ambulance to a tertiary trauma center where he arrived within 20 minutes of the accident. The skin was intact over the injured part. The knee examination demonstrated posterior laxity.

COMMENTS

A knee injury of this nature is only occasionally an "isolated" injury. The knee has not been dislocated and there is no evidence of vascular compromise, so the knee has low priority compared to a search for other injuries the patient may have sustained in the accident.

The speeds that produce a PCL injury are often deceptively slow. Such an injury may occur as a result of direct contact with astroturf, as a deceleration injury when a skier strikes a tree, upon contact with another player in a soccer game, upon striking an obstacle while riding a snowmobile, or in a myriad of other deceleration situations where the tibial tubercle is impacted. Although a PCL tear is not an emergency, if surgery is decided upon, early arthroscopy before edema develops facilitates diagnosis and repair.

COURSE OF ACTION

Physical Examination

The physical examination of the patient's knee suggested that the capsule was intact and that the PCL alone had been injured. The manual examination is critical in this type of injury. The reverse pivot shift[1] should be a part of the physical examination whenever rotatory laxity is suspected. In this case, the reverse pivot shift test was only trace positive, suggesting that the posterolateral capsule was intact. EUA and arthroscopy are usually required to verify the complete extent of the injury. The arcuate complex is particularly at risk, and unrecognized posterolateral laxity can be disabling.[2,4]

Diagnostic Studies

Routine four-view x-ray series are obtained for this type of injury and should be examined under bright light to search for avulsion fractures that may indicate the location of the PCL injury. A bone fleck would suggest avulsion and the possibility of primary surgical repair without grafting. Arthroscopy can usually be accomplished and can be extremely helpful. As always, extravasation of extracapsular fluid into the posterior compartment must not be allowed. Arthrography would not be a direct approach to the diagnosis. There was no need for an arteriogram in this patient, as the trauma appeared minimal—but had there been doubt, or significant swelling of the popliteal fossa, arteriography would have been wise.

Special Considerations

There is no uniformity of opinion about surgical reconstruction of the PCL when the lateral capsule is not also injured. Manual examination is not fully reliable in determining if the injury is limited to PCL tear alone. I recommend arthroscopic diagnosis to this type of patient. Although I prefer primary repair for isolated PCL injuries for much the same philosophy and reasons as outlined in Case Study 1, I recognize that this is not a uniform standard. The reason for primary repair is that posterior instability may lead to a progressive patellofemoral malacia and ultimately to degenerative arthritis—a significant complication for which there is no good treatment. *It is frustration with the patellofemoral consequences of posterior cruciate instability that leads me to recommend early repair.* Many surgeons will choose nonoperative care in the case of "isolated" PCL injury,[5] and they are not to be criticized, considering the current state of knowledge and techniques of cruciate surgery. The patient should be counseled that there is no definite standard treatment. In some states an 18-year-old patient such as this is still a minor and the parents should be included in the decision making. However, the patient's desires should prevail. If the patient elects nonoperative treatment, then I recommend placing the leg in a cylinder cast with the knee in 5° to 10° of flexion for

5 weeks. A lateral radiograph should be taken at appropriate intervals to be certain the knee is not subluxed posteriorly. It is quite acceptable to immobilize the knee in full extension. Some prefer 10° to 30° orthosis. A rehabilitation program would then be followed as diligently as though the patient had had reparative surgery, and would not differ from the latter in detail or goals.

If, however, as in this case, the patient and his family elect definitive care, he would be scheduled for examination under anesthesia (EUA) diagnostic arthroscopy, and reconstruction and/or repair as indicated.

PLAN

The EUA to determine the stability of the posteromedial and posterolateral capsule is an essential part of the plan for this type of case, with diagnostic arthroscopy to verify stability of the posterior horns of the menisci.

In this patient physical examination under anesthesia confirmed direct posterior instability without evidence of instability at either posteromedial or posterolateral corners. There was approximately 20° more extension on the injured than on the uninjured side, and the posterior sag was obvious. The reverse pivot shift was trace positive, but since the lateral capsule was intact, it was not grossly positive.[1] The fact that the arcuate complex stabilized the knee laterally as hyperextension was reached is favorable.

Arthroscopy showed that the menisci were stable posteriorly, the ACL intact, and the PCL intact at its femoral origin. It was difficult to ascertain whether the PCL tear was interstitial or occurred at its tibial fossa insertion. The knee was repatted and redraped for surgical reconstruction. We reconstructed the PCL according to the following procedure.

A medial parapatellar incision is made to allow subluxation of the patella (Fig. 55). Since in this case arthroscopy confirmed that there were no other posterior compartment injuries, the surgeon could proceed with reconstruction of the cruciate immediately. On exposing the intercondylar notch, the

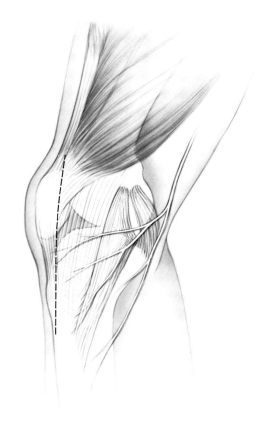

Fig. 55. A medial parapatellar incision allows subluxation of the patella, and the surgeon can proceed with reconstruction of the PCL.

cruciate injury is defined by using the probe and smooth forceps. It is more difficult to determine the nature of the PCL injury when the ACL is intact and complete subluxation of the tibia is not possible. Nevertheless, the Hohmann retractor placed posteriorly in the tibial fossa with the knee flexed 90° can assist in defining the tear (See Case Study 7). The PCL deserves augmentation grafting for the same reasons that this technique has been successful in treatment of ACL injuries. The semitendinosus, gracilis, and patella tendons have all been used with success in grafting the PCL. The selection appears to be the surgeon's choice. All are readily available through the incision and approach described.

The placement of the tibial drill hole is critical (See Case Study 6). The goal is to thread the graft through the interstices of the torn ligament and

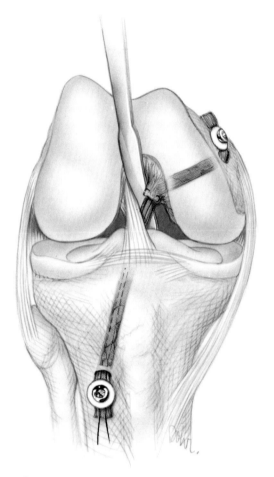

Fig. 56. The gracilis graft is threaded through the interstices of the torn ligament and through the anatomic insertion on the tibia. The graft may be held with an AO screw and washer at either end of the bony tunnel. Then the tunnels are packed with cancellous bone graft.

through the anatomic insertion on the tibia (Fig. 56). The insertion of the PCL in the tibial fossa is approximately 2 cm distal to the joint line. The insertion can be palpated through the notch and a drill guide carefully placed into this fossa. The holes should then be drilled with the knee at 90° flexion and the popliteal fossa freed from posterior pressure. A 3.2 mm hole is drilled using the drill guide with the hole placed at approximately a 30° angle in both the sagittal and horizontal planes to decrease the angle that the graft makes as it exits the tibia. The

3.2 mm hole, determined to be placed properly, is then overdrilled by using a 4.5 mm drill. This successive enlargement of the tunnel allows for more accuracy and lessens the chance of injury to the popliteal vessels.

Although I prefer to use mid-third patella tendon with bone plugs at either end, I will describe use of the gracilis tendon so as to contrast with Case Studies 6 and 7. The gracilis tendon is harvested from the pes anserinus under direct vision. A tendon stripper may facilitate harvesting, although it is possible to obtain the graft by an ancillary proximal incision. The doubled semitendinosus would be as acceptable as the gracilis. The 4.5 mm hole is then carefully chamfered by using the appropriate curette within the canal. The femoral hole is drilled with a drill guide and is quite accessible with the patella subluxed and the femoral origin of the posterior cruciate in direct view. A Kessler-type suture[3] is placed into the residual posterior cruciate ligament stump and the gracilis secured at either end by similar suture. The gracilis is then passed from the femoral canal through the interstices of the residual PCL stump. Passage is facilitated by expanding the stump with a Bunnell tendon grasper through the femoral canal before attempting to pass the gracilis tendon graft. An O'Donoghue-type suture passer is then placed through the tibial tunnel to the posterior portion of the joint where it can be grasped and brought forward into the joint so the sutures from the graft, as well as the residual stump, can be grasped. These are then brought through the tibial canal and out the anterolateral tibial metaphysis. The graft may be held with an AO screw and washer at either end of the bony tunnel, and the tunnels packed with cancellous bone graft (Fig. 56).

The tibial side is then tensioned. The graft usually can be placed isometrically with less difficulty than the ACL (because of the vertical nature of its fibers). I believe we often pull the graft too tight with the knee in flexion and posteriorly sublexed. Therefore, I prefer to set the tension with the knee in approximately 5° to 10° flexion with a bump placed beneath the tibia so as to provide a gentle anterior Drawer during tensioning of the PCL and graft. Olecranization can be considered with this procedure but is usually not necessary. After the PCL is tensioned in this position, the knee is cycled through a full range of motion to determine its isometricity and tension. Posterior sag of the tibia should be eliminated. Hyperextension of the knee is not allowed as this may prejudice the graft. A gentle posterior Drawer is accomplished. This Drawer may be trace positive, but the end point will be obvious. I prefer to immobilize such a knee in a cast in 5° to 10° flexion, although this practice perhaps varies from that of others. To me, it allows some semblance of bony stability and alignment without placing undue tension on the posterior capsule.

Continous passive motion (CPM) is not used because of concern about posterior subluxation of the femur on the tibia and stretching out of the graft. One difference between the ACL graft and the PCL graft is that gravity can easily pit the weight of the femoral portion of the limb against the graft, which may jeopardize the graft before it is healed.

Thus, the patient would leave the operating room immobilized in 10° flexion. This is not consistent with management outlined in previous ACL cases, but gravity weighs against the grafted PCL in the resting position, and further, the graft is usually somewhat more tenuous in strength than the original structure.

POSTOPERATIVE CARE AND REHABILITATION

The lower limb was maintained in a well-fitting cylinder cast for 6 weeks with the knee flexed 10°. Fortunately, because he is young, this patient may not have the residual stiffness older patients often develop from such immobilization. Perhaps if the patient were older and surgical repair were accomplished, then a 10° to 30° orthosis and/or olecranization of the patella would be considered to allow early motion.

Toe rises, isometric exercises, and weightbearing to comfort were allowed and encouraged.

After the cast is removed in cases such as this, patient-controlled range of motion would be in order from the 6th to the 12th week. A brace preventing hyperextension may be applied after removal of the cast for protection as the patient becomes more active. The goal would be to have sufficient flexion, i.e., 110°, by the 12th week to allow bicycling as a primary form of exercise. If this range of motion is not achieved by the 16th week, then the knee would be examined arthroscopically to determine if patella adhesions are present. The patient and physical therapist can practice patella mobilization throughout the rehabilitation, and in fact, the cast can be windowed to allow this during the period of immobilization.

Finally, at 12 weeks, resistive exercises are begun with the goal of restoring isotonic strength as well as endurance and agility.

PROBLEMS, COMPLICATIONS, FOLLOW-UP RESULTS

Recognition of the injury, counseling of the patient, and appropriate decision making are just as essential to success as accurate surgery. The augmentation graft is placed within approximately 1 cm of the critical vascular elements of the lower limb and must be placed with care. A failure to appreciate the effects of gravity and the mechanics of the PCL might lead to the blind application of a postoperative rehabilitation program similar to that for ACL injury. This would be a mistake and would jeopardize the integrity of the graft. The immature graft alone will not prevent posterior subluxation. It must be protected by either external or internal support.

Arthrofibrosis subsequent to immobilization can be a problem, and for this reason aggressive reexploration with the arthroscope is indicated if the patient fails to gain motion progressively so that bicycling can be accomplished by the 12th week.

As in ACL augmentation grafting, excellent results can be expected from PCL grafting, providing the graft has sufficient strength and is not stretched out by undue tension before the origin and insertion sites have healed. It is much easier to obtain isometricity in the PCL than the ACL because of its more vertical course. There are two major bands of the PCL, but compromise allows us to approximate them by a single graft. Some surgeons are tempted to treat the isolated PCL tear nonoperatively hoping that it will "reach" its tibial insertion. This and inap-

CASE STUDY 8
Isolated PCL

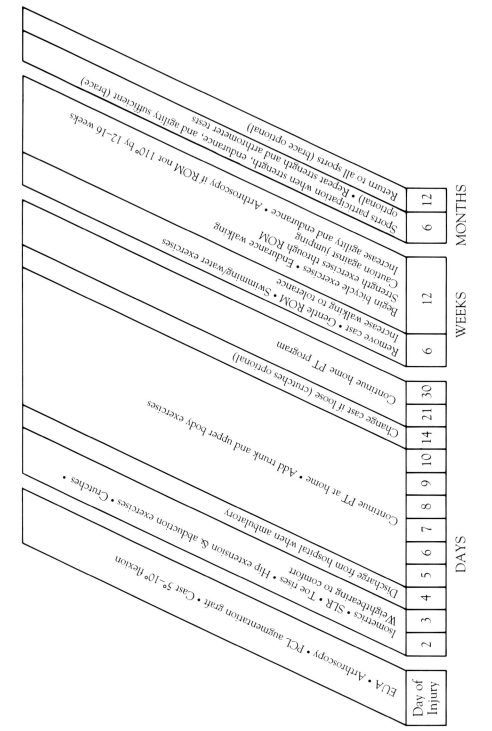

Day of Injury	2	3	4	5	6	7	8	9	10	14	21	30	6	12	6	12

DAYS — **WEEKS** — **MONTHS**

EUA • Arthroscopy • PCL augmentation graft • Cast 5°–100° flexion

Isometrics • SLR • Toe rises • Hip extension & abduction exercises • Crutches • Weightbearing to comfort

Discharge from hospital when ambulatory

Continue PT at home • Add trunk and upper body exercises

Change cast if loose (crutches optional)

Continue home PT program

Remove cast • Gentle ROM • Swimming/water exercises
Increase walking to tolerance
Begin bicycle exercises • Endurance walking
Strength exercises • Endurance walking
Caution against jumping ROM
Increase agility and endurance • Arthroscopy if ROM not 110° by 12–16 weeks

Sports participation when strength, endurance, and agility sufficient (brace)
(optional) • Repeat strength and arthrometer tests
Return to all sports (brace optional)

propriate therapy during the postoperative course are the usual causes of residual posterior laxity.

SUMMARY

Although in this case the patient was a motorcyclist, the mechanism of injury (deceleration) is common to other "sporting" activities. The injury is often unrecognized in the emergency room where the patient may not be seen by an orthopaedic surgeon. Late sequelae of this lesion may be "patella malacia" and degenerative arthritis. Thus, early identification of the injury may be important to a long-term result. Examination under anesthesia and arthroscopic evaluation are important to the management of this problem. Ample exposure for the posterior cruciate isolate can be obtained from the medial parapatella incision with the patella subluxed or dislocated. *Where interstitial tearing occurs, augmentation grafting is essential to obtain a satisfactory result.* The knee was immobilized postoperatively to minimize the stress of the weight of the limb against the graft. A good result can be expected in the operative care of this type of knee injury provided the details discussed in this commentary are taken into consideration.

REFERENCES

1. Jakob RP, Hassler H, Staeubli H-U: Observations on rotatory instability of the lateral compartment of the knee. Experimental studies on the functional anatomy and the pathomechanism of the true and the reversed pivot shift sign. Acta Orthop Scand 52(Suppl 191):1–32, 1981
2. Hughston JC, Jacobson KE: Chronic posterolateral rotatory instability of the knee. J Bone Joint Surg 67A:351–359, 1985
3. Kessler I: The grasping technique for tendon repair. Hand 5:253–255, 1973
4. Müller W: The Knee. Form, function, and ligament reconstruction. Springer-Verlag, New York, 1983, pp. 73–75
5. Parolie J, Bergfeld JA: Long term results of nonoperative treatment of "isolated" posterior cruciate ligament injuries in the athlete. Am J Sports Med 14:35–38, 1986

CASE STUDY 9

PCL Tear, Complete, and Arcuate Complex Tear, Partial

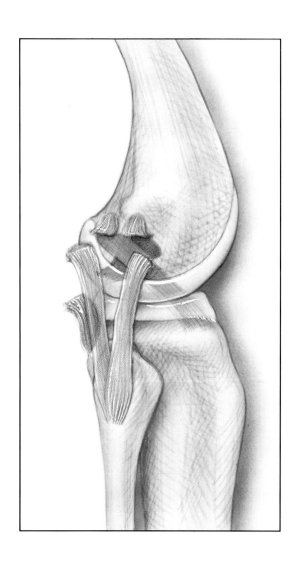

HISTORY

A 28-year-old competitive bicyclist was knocked off his bike by an oncoming car. The cyclist was wearing a helmet and was intact neurologically, and complained of a painful right knee. There were abrasions laterally, above, and below the joint line of the knee. The knee was unstable to varus stress at full extension.

Knee Examination
(Orthopaedic Surgeon/Emergency Room, 1 hour after injury)

Diagnostic Clues	Findings
Effusion	Trace
Tenderness	Posterolateral capsule proximal and distal to the joint line
Lachman test	Questionably positive
Drawer test	Posterior Drawer positive with soft end point
Pivot shift test	Positive reverse pivot shift
Varus/valgus	Valgus—trace opening in full extension, 1+* in 30° flexion Varus—3+ lateral opening at 30° flexion, 2+ lateral opening at 30°, 2+ lateral opening at hyperextension
Patella apprehension	Negative
Range of motion	0° to 70°
Gait	Antalgic
Neurovasculature	Intact
Radiographs	Negative
Other	Passive hyperextension of 20°

* See Glossary

COMMENTS

A deceleration injury such as this places at risk the PCL and posterolateral capsular ligaments. Major ligament laxity was detected on physical examination, and the presence of abrasions indicates that surgery should be performed early. Antibiotics should be injected/ingested immediately when surgery is contemplated in a case such as this.

COURSE OF ACTION

Physical Examination

One hour after injury is often too early for effusion and induration to be demonstrated fully. The history of injury and the physical examination in this case suggest significant posterior capsular injury. *Physical examination of this type of injury is more accurate if conducted in the supine, sitting, and prone positions.* The examination was initiated in the position in which the patient was found, i.e., supine. With the patient in this position the alert physician will check for posterolateral sag of the tibia—diagnostic of posterior cruciate and lateral capsule injury. In the prone position, several more tests are accomplished advantageously. The reverse Lachman test at 30° flexion can be performed and the posteromedial and posterolateral corners visualized while being palpated. In this type of injury one may feel a soft posterolateral corner during the reverse Lachman test (Fig. 57). The swelling and tenderness in the posterolateral aspect, even early after injury as in this case, can be better appreciated in the prone than the supine position. If the patient is asked to extend his hip, gravity sometimes will demonstrate the genu recurvatum.

If possible, the patient is then placed in the sitting position where the examining physician tests the knee again for the "soft" posterolateral Drawer test (Fig. 58). Testing internal and external rotation of the lower leg on the 30° and 90° flexed femur, in the sitting position, is helpful (Fig. 59). In a case such as this, where the posterolateral capsule is disrupted, there is increased external rotation on the injured side and decreased resistance to this test.

Diagnostic Studies

With this type of injury, four-plane radiographs should be carefully evaluated for flecks of bone that might indicate capsular injury. An arthrogram would not be of specific help. Examination under anesthesia (EUA) and arthroscopy are indicated as a part of the surgical repair. Arthroscopy, when it can be accomplished without extravasation, will verify the

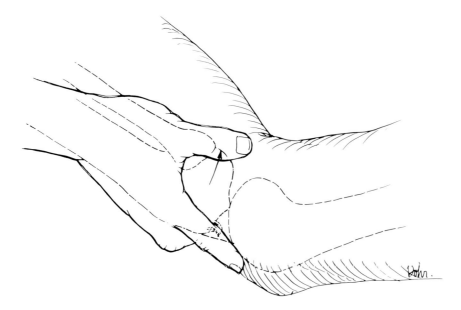

Fig. 57. The knee joint is tested with the patient in the prone position. The reverse Lachman test with the knee at 30° flexion can be performed. The posteromedial and posterolateral corners can be visualized while being palpated so that the examining physician can appreciate the swelling and the tenderness in the posterolateral aspect of the knee.

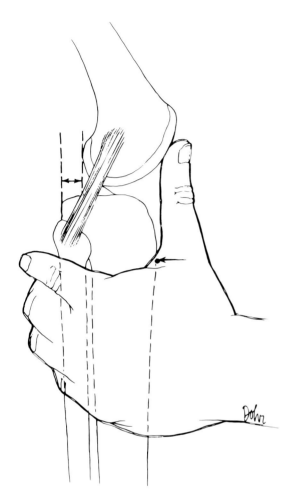

Fig. 58. With the patient in the sitting position, the examining physician can test the knee for the "soft" posterolateral Drawer.

intact status of the medial structures and assist in planning the exposure. The popliteus tendon can be evaluated arthroscopically.

Special Considerations

The special consideration in this case is the unsatisfactory natural history of the combination of PCL and posterolateral capsular laxity.[3] The late effects of this multiplanar laxity are particularly difficult to correct. Nonoperative care is not recommended, even for a relatively sedentary individual. Furthermore, the skin abrasions dictate that surgery should

be early, probably within 6 hours, rather than elective.

PLAN

The patient elected EUA, diagnostic arthroscopy, and surgical repair. Before surgery a review of the lateral anatomy is always beneficial.[1,2,4-6] I have found the book by Bousquet et al particularly graphic.[2]

Examination under anesthesia confirmed the lateral capsular laxity in hyperextension. This finding, plus the posterior Drawer test, confirmed the need for surgical repair.

The surgeon may attempt limited arthroscopy in a case such as this, realizing that extravasation has serious import. The arthroscopy must be accomplished rapidly, with limited manipulation and minimum fluid distension. In this patient, at arthroscopy, there was disruption of the posterolateral capsule above the level of the meniscus, the ACL and popliteus tendon were intact, and the PCL was interstitially torn. The medial compartment and patellofemoral joint were uninvolved.

Where to place the incision is a difficult decision in an injury to the PCL and posterior capsule. My preference is to use a single straight lateral incision long enough to allow dislocation of the patella laterally through a median parapatellar incision and to allow exposure of the posterolateral capsule through the iliotibial band incised in line with its fibers (see Case Study 6). That was the incision also used in this injured cyclist. The lateral head of the gastrocnemius is mobilized with the knee in flexion so that repair can take place along the line of the posterior capsule.

Sometimes, the status of the popliteus tendon cannot be ascertained with certainty with the arthroscope in an emergency situation. When this is so, I visually identify the popliteus tendon, not only to protect it but also to ensure its integrity.

I would not be critical of making two skin incisions in repairing this type of injury, although one is usually adequate. Good visualization of the posterolateral corner is critical. An accurate arthroscopic diagnosis is helpful in planning the surgical approach.

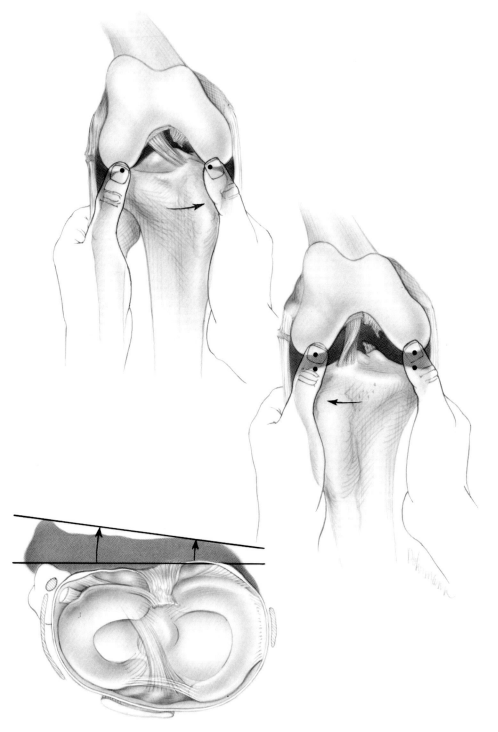

Fig. 59. With the patient in the sitting position (hip and knee flexed at 90°), the examining physician evaluates the internal and external rotation of the lower leg.

To perform the repair, first sutures are laid in the PCL and a lateral third patella tendon augmentation graft is harvested, somewhat as described in Case Study 6. The lateral third of the patella tendon is longer than the middle third and also allows for the beginning of the exposure of the lateral capsular structures. Closure is easier if the lateral third is used, and a lateral release is accomplished coincodent with the harvesting of the graft and the exposure of the lateral capsule.

The lateral capsule in this patient was torn interstitially (Fig. 60). The advantage of early surgery is that the torn structures can be accurately identified and anatomically restored. After these tissues have fused and obliterated the tissue planes, a surgical repair is less satisfactory. A thorough understanding of the anatomy, as emphasized in Ch. 20 and illus-

trated by Bousquet et al,[1,2] is helpful to understanding the complexity of the arcuate complex and its anatomic restoration.

An important intraoperative decision in this type of repair is determining how the repaired/augmented PCL and interstitially reapproximated lateral capsule will be supported and protected so that the weight of the lower limb segment will not jeopardize the repaired structures. Three approaches are possible, depending on the desire of the surgeon. The first is to place the knee in full extension and immobilize it in this position so that the joint geometry confers stability and anatomic alignment. The disadvantage of this procedure is that the joint must be held in a somewhat stiffened and straightened position for approximately 6 weeks.

The second method is to olecranize the patella. However, olecranization alone does not prevent the leg from rotating about the repaired posterolateral capsule, and may not afford this key structure sufficient protection. Nevertheless, provided this point is appreciated, the technique has significant advantages.

The third alternative is to hold the knee in approximately 45° flexion, which somewhat aligns the bony structures and takes the stress off the repaired structures. The disadvantage of this method is the strain it places on the patellofemoral joint and the difficulty of mobilizing the patellofemoral joint after immobilization for 4 to 6 weeks in this position.

My preference is to immobilize the knee 5° short of full extension; that was the option used for this patient.

POSTOPERATIVE CARE AND REHABILITATION

The postoperative care of this pernicious combination of ligamentous injuries is particularly difficult, and must not be underestimated. Stiffness, or ankylosis, is the most common complication. One must be quick and aggressive to resolve this problem if there is a failure to progress in the rehabilitation program. Accurate, objective records and regular office visits will help to avoid such complications. It is important to counsel the patient about the possi-

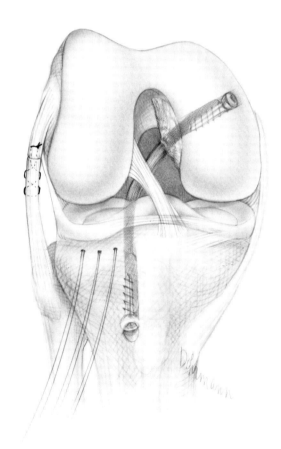

Fig. 60. Repaired arcuate complex and meniscocapsular ligaments. The PCL has been grafted.

CASE STUDY 9
PCL Tear, Arcuate Complex Tear, and Abrasions

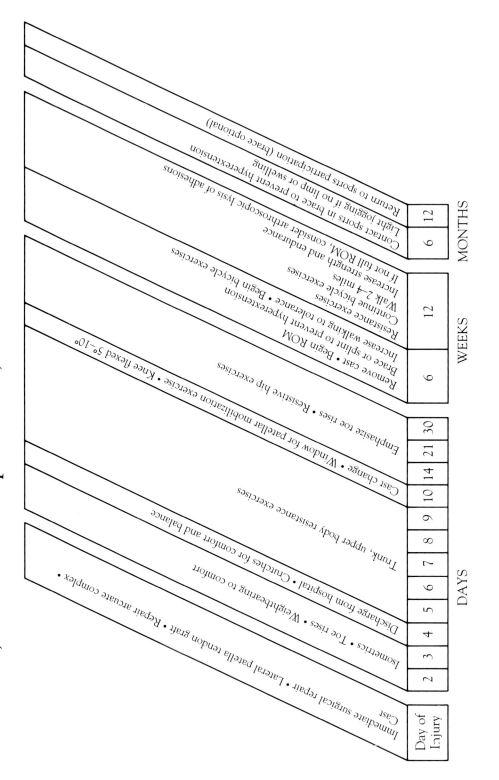

Day of Injury	2	3	4	5	6	7	8	9	10	14	21	30	6	12	6	12
					DAYS								WEEKS		MONTHS	

Cast

Immediate surgical repair • Lateral patella tendon graft • Repair arcuate complex

Isometrics • Toe rises

Discharge from hospital • Crutches for comfort and balance

Weightbearing to comfort

Trunk, upper body resistance exercises

Cast change • Window for patellar mobilization exercise • Knee flexed 5°–10°

Emphasize toe rises • Resistive hip exercises

Remove cast • Begin ROM
Brace or splint to prevent hyperextension
Increase walking to tolerance • Begin bicycle exercises
Continue bicycle exercises
Resistance exercises
Walk 2–4 miles
Increase strength and endurance

If not full ROM, consider arthroscopic lysis of adhesions
Contact sports in brace to prevent hyperextension
Light jogging if no limp or swelling
Return to sports participation (brace optional)

bility of unsatisfactory motion and the alternative courses of action that may become necessary.

The course of postoperative care differs somewhat depending on which of the three options for protecting the repair has been selected. With all three approaches, the leg is splinted for approximately 6 weeks to allow healing of both the graft and the interstitially torn posterolateral capsule. The foot is not immobilized since the ankle and foot should be left free to absorb rotatory torque regardless of whether the knee is held in extension or flexion.

Gravity is against the patient and surgeon in this injury. Weightbearing to comfort is allowed. Motion is regained slowly, with emphasis on toe rises, hip extension, hip abduction, and quadriceps strength — hamstring thrust is deferred. To rehabilitate a repair of this nature with too rapid motion and/or insensitivity to the effects of gravity probably would prejudice the quality of the repair. Olecranization of the patella may allow early motion, but the posterolateral capsule is still at risk from the rotatory pull of the biceps femoris.

Last, although bracing seems to be advantageous, it is difficult to line up the axis of the brace with the complex rolling and sliding motion of the knee in a manner that will protect the repair. Thus, bracing has not proved efficacious to protect the repaired structures during the immediate postoperative period.

PROBLEMS, COMPLICATIONS, FOLLOW-UP RESULTS

Complications are along four main lines: 1) missing the extent and implication of the posterolateral tear, 2) failure to understand at the time of surgical exposure the popliteus and posterolateral capsular anatomy, 3) inappropriate or inadequate postoperative immobilization, and 4) failure to restore range of motion in a timely fashion through inadequate postoperative care and supervision.

Each of these complications is a major concern, and any of them can lead to an unhappy result from the viewpoint of both the patient and the surgeon.

Follow-up results depend equally upon the quality of repair and the postoperative care. Both are

fraught with difficulty, and therefore the results with this injury have not been as satisfactory as with the injuries described in the preceding case studies. Perhaps with a better understanding of the physical examination and lateral capsular anatomy, our results in future years will be better.

SUMMARY

This case study describes a 28-year-old competitive cyclist who sustained a complete tear of the PCL and posterolateral capsule (arcuate complex), and discusses the treatment of this type of injury. The popliteus tendon remained intact. The surgery was done immediately because of abrasions. Limited arthroscopy confirmed that the popliteus tendon was intact. A single straight lateral incision was made, a lateral-third patella tendon graft was used to augment the interstitially torn PCL, and the posterolateral capsule was repaired by mobilizing the lateral head of the gastrocnemius through an incision in the iliotibial band.

The postoperative care of this type of injury requires careful support so the lower leg does not "sag" on the femur, thus jeopardizing through gravity the repaired structures. My preference for immobilizing the patient's leg is to place the knee 5° short of full extension to use the bony conformity to ensure alignment of the femur and tibia and to minimize the posterior sag effects of gravity on the tibial segment. This is one situation in which motion is delayed to ensure anatomic alignment.

The results of such acute repairs can be excellent, but require considerable attention to detail to restore the anatomy and protect the healing structures during the early postoperative period.

REFERENCES

1. Bousquet G, Millon J, Bascoulergue G, Rhenter J-L: Le refléction du ligament croisé antérieur par plastic activo-passive du pivot central et des points d'angle. [Reconstruction of the anterior cruciate ligament by active-passive surgery of the central pivot and angle points.] Rev Chir Orthop 66(Suppl 2):91–92, 1980

2. Bousquet G, Rhenter J-L, Bascoulergue G, Millon J: L'illustré du Genou. Guy Mure, Le Coteau, France, 1982

3. Hughston JC, Jacobson KE: Chronic posterolateral rotatory instability of the knee. J Bone Joint Surg 67A:351–359, 1985

4. Kaplan EB: The fabellofibular and short lateral ligaments of the knee joint. J Bone Joint Surg 43A:169–179, 1961

5. Müller W: The Knee. Form, Function, and Ligament Reconstruction. Springer-Verlag, New York, 1983

6. Seebacher JR, Inglis E, Marshall JL, Warren RF: The structure of the posterolateral aspect of the knee. J Bone Joint Surg 64A:536–541, 1982

CASE STUDY 10

Medial Collateral Ligament Injury, Complete

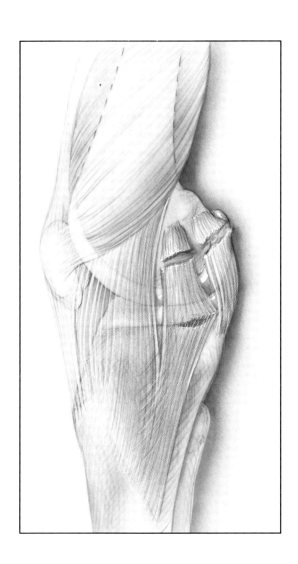

HISTORY

A 19-year-old professional hockey player was struck from the side as he was shooting. His foot was fixed, the skate did not give, and he sustained a severe valgus strain. He tried to continue skating but was ineffective because of pain and giving way. On the bench a physician examined the player's knee. There was 3 + valgus opening at 30° flexion and 1 + opening to valgus strain at 0° flexion. The morning after the injury the player was referred by his man-

**Knee Examination
(Orthopaedic Surgeon/Office)**

Diagnostic Clues	Findings
Effusion	Moderate
Tenderness	Tender, Origin medial collateral and posterior oblique capsular ligaments down to and including jointline
Lachman test	Trace positive*/firm end point
Drawer test	Trace positive/firm end point
Pivot shift test	Not attempted
Varus/valgus	Valgus 3+ opening at 30° flexion 1+ opening at 0° flexion Stable in hyperextension Stable to varus testing
Patella apprehension	Trace positive, without subluxation
Range of motion	0° to 30°
Neurovasculature	Intact
Radiographs	Medial soft tissue swelling
Other	None

* See Glossary.

agement to the orthopaedic surgeon for evaluation and care.

COMMENTS

The nature of the interface between the foot and the surface often determines the nature and extent of knee pathology. The difference between the ski/snow interface and the football shoe/turf interface was emphasized in Case Studies 3 and 4. The interface between skate and ice is more forgiving than that between shoe and turf. The skate may become trapped in a valgus sense, but without the rotatory deceleration of the lower limb segment so common in skiing. This results in a tear of the MCL rather than multiple ligament injuries. Thus, the skate/ice interface is unique, and the MCL tear is relatively common in hockey.

Tearing of the MCL is seldom accompanied by the audible "pop" so often associated with ACL injury. The linear rather than helicoid arrangement of the collagen fibers in the MCL possibly explains this difference. Depending on the application of force, the MCL may tear either from bone or interstitially. The MCL is a subtle gradation of ligaments (see Case Study 2) including the conjoined direct heads of the superficial and deep medial collateral, the posterior oblique portion of the medial collateral, the meniscofemoral, and the meniscotibial ligaments.

COURSE OF ACTION

Physical Examination

Injuries to the MCL result in a characteristic vaulting stiff-leg gait, which can be distinguished from the flexed-knee equinus gait of the effused knee usually associated with an ACL injury. In uniplanar instability, the quadriceps attempts to immobilize the acutely injured MCL. This is best accomplished in full extension. Thus, the patient walks by vaulting over the functionally lengthened injured leg. Left to his own devices, the patient will maintain this gait for many weeks. The functional results of this self-treatment are frequently quite satisfactory. In es-

sence, the patient fashions his own stabilizing brace.

As previously emphasized, it is important to know the limits of normality as defined by the "well" knee. The injured knee must be compared against this standard. Valgus opening of the injured knee in 0° extension signifies considerable disruption of the posteromedial capsule. It does not necessarily mean that the ACL or PCL is torn. Increased laxity in hyperextension, however, suggests not only a complete disruption of the posterior oblique capsular ligament but also a tear of the PCL. *This is the value of the hyperextension test.*

How often are these injuries associated with peripheral meniscal tears? The answer is not known with certainty because in most instances this injury is treated empirically without the benefit of diagnostic arthroscopy. Diagnostic arthroscopy, however, reveals a significant percentage of peripheral meniscal tears involving both the medial and the lateral menisci. The import of this finding is that these tears, when immobilized, must heal satisfactorily in a significant number of cases, since the complete MCL tear can be treated nonoperatively with relatively reliable results. Thus, tenderness and its anatomic location are key diagnostic findings in this type of injury.

A pivot shift with valgus strain should not be attempted with this type of injury since it depends upon an intact MCL, and further tearing of residual fibers and/or significant discomfort would be caused by an attempt to perform the pivot shift in this manner. *This is an ideal situation in which to use the flexion rotation Drawer test of Noyes.*[2] Emphasis can also be placed on subtle Lachman and Drawer tests. The Lachman test may be trace-positive or even 1+ positive with a disrupted MCL, but there should be a firm end point as distinguished from the soft end point when the ACL is involved. A Drawer test should confirm the findings of the Lachman test and seems to be even more helpful diagnostically. Physical examination can usually verify the integrity of the ACL.

It is seldom possible on physical examination of a complete MCL lesion to determine with certainty whether the meniscus is stable, torn at its periphery, or intact. On physical examination I cannot always determine exactly where the MCL is torn, but sometimes a critical palpatory examination will allow the defect in the ligament to be outlined. The defect usually correlates with the point of maximum tenderness previously found. *The most important aspect of the physical examination is to determine whether the laxity is uniplanar (MCL injury alone) or rotatory (cruciate involvement).* The latter (a two-ligament injury) should usually be repaired, whereas the former can be treated at the patient's and surgeon's discretion, and excellent results obtained from either operative or nonoperative care.[1]

Diagnostic Studies

A four-view x-ray series is routinely obtained for this type of injury. A stress ray film in 30° flexion and/or extension may be obtained, but it will not define whether or not a surgical procedure is indicated. I prefer to rely on manual and/or arthroscopic examination to determine the need for surgery, and I do not do stress radiographs unless they are needed for legal documentation. Arthrograms can be helpful to determine the integrity of the meniscus if there is a contraindication to arthroscopy. Arthroscopy, although it must be undertaken with care because of the capsular lesion, can be extremely helpful in deciding which cases are operative (i.e., involving an unstable meniscal lesion) and which are not.

Special Considerations

In this case, a special consideration was that the patient was a young professional athlete and there was a premium on his "return to function." "Management" has a right to encourage early return but not to risk unduly the player's future function. *Consultation with peers can ease the strain in such situations.*

The complete MCL tear can be treated nonoperatively; however, when the posterior oblique capsular ligament is involved, I prefer to examine the knee under anesthesia and perform diagnostic arthroscopy, particularly with an athlete at this skill level. Experience with high school and college players with complete MCL tears confirms that the natural history of the nonoperatively treated MCL

can be quite satisfactory when the posterior oblique capsular ligament is not disrupted. However, the knee does not always "tighten up" with time. One can expect the same laxity later that is found on the "sideline" examination. This residual laxity is surprisingly symptom-free provided it is uniplanar and there is no associated cruciate ligament injury. Radiographs do not show deterioration with time in the uniplanar injury.

A well-repaired complete MCL tear does not have to be immobilized completely. Certainly a range of motion of 30° to 60° can always be allowed, and sometimes even greater motion from 0° to 90° can be allowed. Thus, quadriceps atrophy is not always the concomitant of surgical care that it often is of nonoperative care. This fact, and the knowledge of the exact pathology, give me confidence in more prompt rehabilitation and return to function in the operatively treated knee. Limited exposure is implicit in this decision and thus arthroscopy is a helpful concomitant.

PLAN

Examination under anesthesia, diagnostic arthroscopy, and surgical repair were recommended to this patient. Most patients of this caliber understand the need for surgery and will follow the physician's recommendations.

Under anesthesia, the well leg is examined. The injured leg is then examined before applying the tourniquet. The *critical difference* between the knees is the laxity at varying degrees of flexion. With an MCL tear the knee should gain stability from 30° flexion to full extension. If the knee is stable in full extension, then the posterior oblique capsular ligament is intact, and I do not believe that surgical repair is advantageous. Arthroscopy is important in determining the stability of the meniscus and the integrity of its conjoined ligaments.

After careful physical examination under anesthesia, it was determined that this patient's knee was unstable to valgus testing in extension. This signifies that the posterior oblique capsular ligament was disrupted (Fig. 61). The ACL demonstrated a firm end point throughout a range of motion, as did the

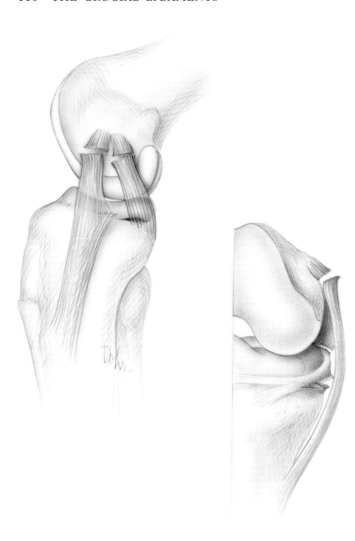

Fig. 61. Tear in the MCL and disruption in the posterior oblique capsular ligament. The disruption was identified by examination under anesthesia when it was determined that the knee was unstable to valgus testing in extension.

PCL. The stability of the patellofemoral mechanism was reaffirmed. The arthroscope was then introduced to determine the stability of the meniscus as well as to ensure that the manual examination for integrity of the ACL and PCL has been accurate.

Although I usually use the standard lateral portal for the arthroscope, with this type of injury I use a medial portal to define further the pathology of the medial compartment.

In this patient, the medial meniscus was seen to be slightly unstable and could be subluxed anteriorly with the probe in a manner that suggested that the meniscotibial ligament was torn. There was blushing of the posteromedial capsule superior to the meniscus. Even though the synovium was intact, blushing suggested a tear of the posterior oblique capsular ligament. The ACL in this patient was intact with good turgor of the anteromedial and posterolateral bands. Based on this information, it was decided to repair the complete MCL and posterior oblique capsular ligament tear.

To perform this repair, first the leg is reprepped and redraped, and a limited exposure of the MCL is accomplished. The patellofemoral mechanism must be carefully evaluated because the *same mechanism of injury that tears the MCL may also tear the* tibia. I usually look first for the meniscal pathology, trying to define it through the tear. The meniscotibial sutures may have already been placed arthroscopically, or may be placed at the time of open surgery. Both techniques can be satisfactory in anatomically stabilizing the meniscotibial ligament. Attention is then directed to the origin of the posterior oblique and conjoined superficial and deep portions of the medial collateral ligament (see Fig. 22 in Case Study 2). These are separate anatomic structures arising from separate anatomic tubercles. Individual repair of these two structures is usually accomplished using an AO screw and washer (Fig. 63). This serves as a good foundation for ligament repair.

Distally, the pes anserinus sometimes requires incision along the line of its fibers to inspect the insertion of the superficial portion of the MCL. This

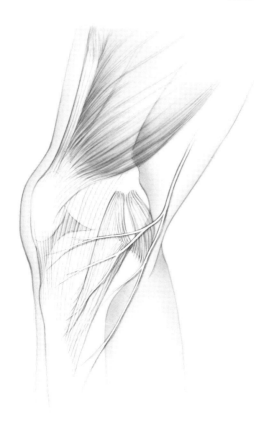

Fig. 62. A limited medial incision allows exposure of the MCL both proximally and distally.

patella ligamentous supporting structures at their origin from the intermuscular septum. These structures can be easily visualized at the time the origin of the MCL is visualized, and should also be repaired if they are torn.

After defining the MCL tear both manually and arthroscopically, I use a limited medial incision (Fig. 62). The incision must be somewhat extensile to allow for variations in the tear, and it must allow for exposure proximally and distally, since both origin and insertion of the MCL can be torn in the same case. The arthroscope allows me to know that I do not have to do further work in the interior of the joint. The usual incision extends from the origin of the posterior oblique portion of the medial collateral ligament on the femoral condyle to the midpoint of the insertion of the pes anserinus on the

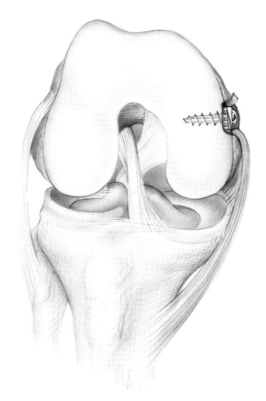

Fig. 63. The MCL and the posterior oblique ligament are individually repaired with AO screws and washers.

CASE STUDY 10
MCL Tear

DAYS

Day of Injury	2	3	4	5	6	7	8	9	10	14	21	30

- Ice • Splint
- Office exam
- EUA • Arthroscopy • MCL repair • Soft splint • CPM 20°–60° • ROM 60°–60° • Weightbearing to comfort
- Isometrics
- Discharge from hospital • Crutches for balance and comfort • Toe rises
- Home PT program • Trunk, upper body exercises
- Increase walking to tolerance
- Begin strength exercises 20°–60°
- Skip rope (soft splint optional)

WEEKS

6	12

- D/C soft splint • Endurance walking • Ok to begin limited skating
- Begin bicycle exercises if flexion 110° • Simple agility drills • 20 yard sprints
  (at 10 weeks)
- Noncontact, nonjumping sports (brace optional) • Bicycle exercises • Bicycle exercises (brace optional) • Caution against jumping • Strength
- Endurance walking • Strengthen hamstrings and gluteals

MONTHS

6	12

- Sports participation when strength, endurance, and agility sufficient (brace optional) • Repeat strength and arthrometer tests
- Return to sports (brace optional)
- Return to all sports (brace optional)

too is frequently torn in an injury of this magnitude, and defies restoration to its insertion. A mini-cancellous screw and washer work quite satisfactorily to hold the attenuated insertion of the MCL to its distalmost point on the bone. The stability can then be ascertained, and should be complete in full extension and allow no more than 1 + increased opening at 30° flexion. Closure is then accomplished in a routine fashion. I have never had to use substitute materials to augment repair of the MCL and have seldom been dissatisfied with the operative results of MCL and posterior oblique capsular ligament repairs.

POSTOPERATIVE CARE AND REHABILITATION

The quality of the repair is usually quite satisfying when anatomic principles are followed. The continuous passive motion (CPM) may be set from approximately 20° to 60° in the immediate postoperative period. In 2 to 3 days the patient is discharged from the hospital with instructions to continue this range of motion and to support the limb with an external soft splint when he is out of the house or subject to slipping or external trauma. Most patients prefer to use a splint intermittently for 4 to 6 weeks after injury. Full range of motion, however, may be slow to return because of the complexity of the ligamentous injury and may require the full 12 to 16 weeks. The patient may require protection during this time to prevent reinjury.

Rehabilitation in the face of operative repair can proceed rapidly since the pathology and the quality of repair are known. We work toward rapidly regaining strength through a functional range of motion, usually 10° to 90°. The patient ambulates with full weightbearing from the beginning. Valgus strain is, of course, guarded against, but significant rehabilitation can proceed within this limitation.

Rehabilitation in this manner will require relatively frequent meetings between patient, surgeon, and physical therapist.

PROBLEMS, COMPLICATIONS, FOLLOW-UP RESULTS

A most significant complication would be to overlook a tear of the ACL, which would result in rotatory laxity. Few complications or problems attend the operative or nonoperative care of the MCL, provided the patient diligently follows the rehabilitation regimen. Patients will have many questions regardless of the method of management and will need to be reassured at frequent intervals as definitive guidance is provided over the 12 to 16 weeks required for ligamentous healing.

Follow-up results for a complete MCL tear and posterior capsular ligament injury cared for surgically should be excellent. Uniplanar laxity is quite forgiving; thus one should not be concerned if there is 1 + laxity in the immediate follow-up period.

SUMMARY

This patient was an "elite" athlete, who for personal and professional reasons desired return to activity as soon as possible and for whom a good long-term functional result was obligatory. Given that the injury involved uniplanar laxity (i.e., the ACL was intact), excellent results could have been obtained either operatively or nonoperatively. Although I prefer operative management when the posterior oblique capsular ligament is torn, this is not necessarily the standard or obligatory treatment. The advantages of an aggressive approach are more certainty as to ligamentous repair, probably enhanced stability where the posterior oblique capsular ligament is involved, and earlier rehabilitation.

REFERENCES

1. Indelicato PA: Non-operative treatment of complete tears of the medial collateral ligament of the knee. J Bone Joint Surg 65A:323–329, 1983
2. Noyes FR: Flexion rotation Drawer test. p. 924, Fig. 9-53. In Edmonson AS, Crenshaw AA, (eds): Campbell's Operative Orthopaedics, 6th Ed. C.V. Mosby, St. Louis, 1980

CASE STUDY 11

Subluxation of Patella versus ACL Injury

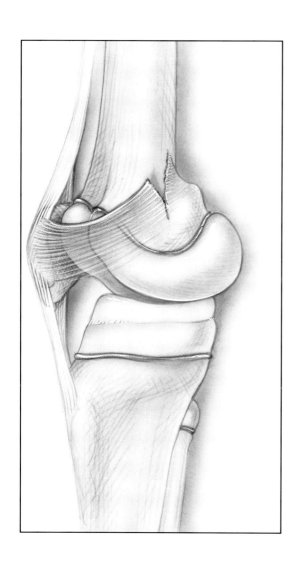

HISTORY

A 14-year-old elite gymnast dismounted the bar in practice, landed off balance, and felt a pop. Her knee buckled but she did not fall. She was unable to continue. Her gait was antalgic. There had been no previous episodes of similar injury.

Knee Examination
(Patient's Orthopaedic Surgeon/Emergency Room)

Diagnostic Clues	Findings
Effusion	Tense
Tenderness	"Medial parapatellar"
Lachman test	Equivocal
Drawer test	Negative
Pivot shift test	Could not be accomplished
Varus/valgus	Stability comparable through range of motion 10° to 30°
Patella apprehension	Positive
Range of motion	10° to 30°
Gait	Antalgic
Neurovasculature	Intact
Radiographic	Small "chips" medial to patella on Merchant view when examined under bright light
Other	None

COMMENTS

The ACL injury is as epidemic in gymnasts as in skiers. Nevertheless, the differential diagnosis between ACL disruption and patella subluxation with a chondral or osteochondral fracture is sometimes quite difficult. The mechanism of injury is often similar. Before arthroscopy was used diagnostically, 10 percent of knees opened as suspect of having ACL tears turned out to have patella subluxation with joint surface fracture.[1] Aspiration, of course, is helpful, but it does not obviate the decision of whether to perform diagnostic arthroscopy. The *onset of effusion* is more rapid with osteochondral fractures; the fat in the aspirated fluid is diagnostic of fracture. In this particular injury, there was a sense of urgency on the part of both the patient and her parents. Both ACL rupture and acutely subluxed patella may require surgical repair. The designation "elite gymnast" has a special connotation, but the orthopaedic surgeon must proceed on a course that is rational, logical, and one in which he and the patient ultimately feel comfortable.

COURSE OF ACTION

Physical Examination

Several clues as to whether an injury of this type is a patella subluxation or an MCL tear may be derived from the physical examination. Tenderness associated with subluxation of the patella is often found along the vastus medialis obliquus approximately 1 cm proximal to the origin of the MCL. It usually can be detected on physical examination and differentiated from the tenderness of the MCL which originates on the adductor tubercle. Patella subluxation is frequently associated with tenderness both medially and laterally along the patellar retinaculum, which is absent with ACL injury. The *patella apprehension test* should be performed in routine fashion (Fig. 64), but may be even more sensitive in the prone position. If possible I would also perform the patella apprehension test with the patient sitting and pressure applied laterally throughout the available range of motion. The physical examination suggested patella subluxation with an osteochondral fracture, and because there was no history of similar episodes, the injury was believed to be acute.

In a difficult case of this nature, I might ask the patient to return for reexamination the following day with the understanding that an examination under anesthesia (EUA) and/or diagnostic arthroscopy might be necessary to ascertain absolutely the pathology and implications of injury.

Diagnostic Studies

Careful attention to radiographic findings and examining the radiographs under the bright light are essential with this type of injury. As mentioned in the Introduction, I prefer the Merchant view, al-

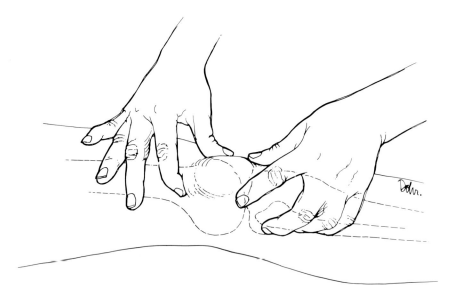

Fig. 64. The patella apprehension test should be performed in a routine fashion.

though other views can be quite satisfactory. Often, as in this patient, these tangential views will reveal parapatella fractures and/or loose bodies, and suggest whether the injury is acute or chronic. Arthrograms are not adequate to answer these questions and, therefore, are not usually recommended. In the future, MRI and CT may become valuable adjunct diagnostic tools. An EUA and arthroscopic examination are currently the most direct ways to proceed to precise diagnosis and the most appropriate treatment.

Special Considerations

This athlete undoubtedly desired to continue in competition, and it is doubtful that the orthopaedic surgeon could have effected a change in her chosen activities. To offer this suggestion as a remedy to such a patient might be inappropriate. The patient should know that there is difficulty with accurate diagnosis by manual examination. Some patellar retinacular tears must be repaired if stability is to be expected.[3] Thus I believe patella dislocation in an elite athlete, *if it is unstable to examination,* should be treated by surgical repair. Other clues about the integrity of the patella are the contour of the vastus medialis obliquus, an inadequate vastus medialis obliquus, and the Q-angle. In my experience, a Q-angle greater than 20°, particularly when associated with torsional malalignment, prejudices the stability of the patella.

PLAN

Diagnostic arthroscopy and repair as indicated were scheduled for this gymnast.

Although this patient could have been cared for nonoperatively, and such a course could not be criticized, I lean toward acute repair of the ligamentous disruption when it can be diagnosed with certainty.

Some criteria of laxity can be determined during EUA from the manual attempt to dislocate the patella in full extension and in varying degrees of flexion. If the patella is dislocatable through an arc from 0° to 30°, then I believe it is wise to repair the retinaculum if long-term stability is desired. When the patella cannot be dislocated and is quite similar

to the uninvolved side, I would not plan surgical repair unless findings at arthroscopy dictated further intervention. In this patient the patella was found to be dislocatable between 0° and 30°.

The arthroscope was introduced through a superolateral portal of the gymnast's knee ("Patel view"). This portal gives better visualization of the suprapatellar pouch as well as the medial and lateral femoral gutters, and more assurance of visualizing clearly a chondral or osteochondral fracture. This patient was found to have an osteochondral fracture of the lateral facet of the patella, approximately 1 cm in diameter, and blushing of the synovium of the medial gutter suggestive of a tear of the medial patellofemoral ligament.

An auxiliary anterolateral portal was made to obtain a more complete visualization of the posterior

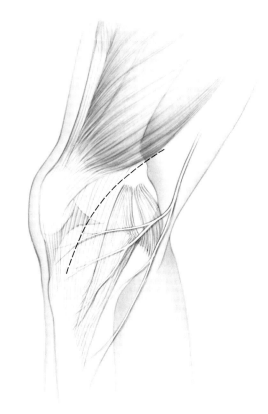

Fig. 65. A 7-cm incision made parallel to the vastus medialis obliquus. Beneath the reflected vastus medialis obliquus, an acute tear of the medial patellar ligament from the intermuscular septum can be seen.

horns of the menisci as well as of the contents of the intercondylar notch. They were normal.

The chondral defect of the patella was "verticalized" about its periphery, according to Shands' description.[5] The fragment was located and arthroscopically removed. Shands' work indicates that lesions under 1 cm do have the capacity to heal with fibrocartilage.

Since under anesthesia the patella was dislocatable between 0° and 30°, and a blush was seen in the medial retinaculum, a 7 cm incision was made distal and parallel to the vastus medialis obliquus (Fig. 65). The skin was mobilized, and the muscle was dissected off its underlying fascia. The underlying fascia was traced from the patella to the medial intermuscular septum. Here, beneath the reflected vastus medialis obliquus, an acute tear of the medial

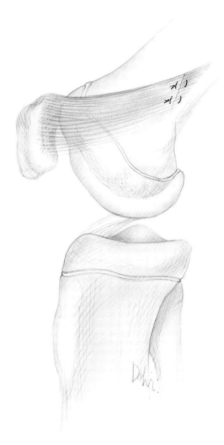

Fig. 66. When recognized acutely, the medial patellar ligament can be repaired.

patellar ligament from the intermuscular septum was found (see also Case Study 2). This ligament can be repaired when a tear is recognized acutely (Fig. 66).

Further medial reefing was not done, nor is it necessary in the face of an acute injury with repair. The question of whether to do a lateral retinacular release, particularly a limited one as described by Larson et al,[4] is up to the surgeon's preference. Many surgeons perform a retinacular release to ensure medial stability and try to prevent further lateral luxation. One must recognize the morbidity that may ensue if the lateral retinacular vessels bleed.

In this patient a lateral retinacular release was not done, as a good medial repair was obtained and the margins of the articular defect were verticalized. A defect of this size (<1 cm) would be expected to heal.

An intraarticular drain is usually placed at the end of this procedure, and a carefully applied Jones-type compression dressing is important to prevent hemarthrosis. Medial and lateral splints are used to limit motion. Patients are usually quite comfortable in this dressing and keep it in place for 10 days.

POSTOPERATIVE CARE AND REHABILITATION

After this procedure, the knee is retained in a snug Jones-type compressive dressing or splint support in full extension for approximately 6 weeks. Gradual mobilization is then allowed over the next 6 weeks. This patient's age was in favor of regaining a full range of motion without difficulty.

Sometimes a fiberglass cast is applied, as this allows swimming which can be beneficial during the initial stages of convalescence.

The isometric program and toe rises are important, and straight leg raising and abduction seem to stimulate the proximal end of the quadriceps. *Exercising both ends of the two-joint muscles is critical,* and the proximal end of the quadriceps is quite amenable to a vigorous isometric and isotonic exercise program.

The immobilization is removed 6 weeks after the operation, and the patient is allowed to regain motion over the next 4 to 6 weeks, at his or her own rate,

CASE STUDY 11
Subluxation of Patella versus ACL Injury

Day of Injury	2	3	4	5	6	7	8	9	10	14	21	30		6	12		6	12
						DAYS								WEEKS			MONTHS	

Injury • EUA • Arthroscopy • Debride chondral defect • Repair medial patellofemoral ligament • Splint or cast

Isometrics • Toe rises • SLR • Crutches • Weightbearing to comfort • Hip exercises

Discharge from hospital

Home PT program — 20 min 3 × daily

Return to school

Office recheck • Continue home PT

Isometrics • Toe rises • resistive exercises

Home PT program • Hip, trunk, and upper body resistive exercises • Toe rises • Add SLR • Weightbearing to comfort • Hip, trunk, and upper body

Cast off • Gentle ROM on own • Swimming/water exercises

No weights • No P.E. in school • Uphill walking • Jump rope

P.T. for strength through ROM • Bicycle exercises • Upstairs walking — careful downstairs

Sports participation when strength, endurance, and agility sufficient (brace optional) • Repeat strength and arthrometer tests

Return to all sports (brace optional)

without pressure from therapists, coach, or surgeon. At the end of 12 weeks, the patient should have flexion to 115°, which will allow bicycle riding. Bicycle riding is a desirable postoperative rehabilitation exercise. *The bicycle preferentially develops the vastus medialis obliquus as compared to other portions of the quadriceps.* The seat should be placed so that the knee flexes to 110°. A simple agility program is also a helpful adjunct to the cycling, walking, and skip-rope program. Although sometimes exasperatingly slow, the postoperative care is usually satisfactory to patient and physician. Patients are declared rehabilitated when they have a full range of motion on the operated side, hop equally well on either leg without trunk or shoulder shift, have right/left hamstring and quadriceps strength within 10 percent on the Orthotron or Cybex, and do not limp or reflect gait asymmetry with 40-yard interval sprints.

PROBLEMS, COMPLICATIONS, FOLLOW-UP RESULTS

There are few complications from primary repair of the medial patella supporting structures. The lateral release, when performed, is too frequently associated with hemarthrosis, hematoma, or synovial fistula. The lateral retinacular release also usually involves far more rehabilitation time; thus, one must be circumspect about the necessity for this procedure since adequate studies do not exist to document its efficacy.

Certainly, ankylosis and adhesions of the patellofemoral joint are not seen to the same extent after patellar ligament repair as after intraarticular cruciate ligament surgery.

The rehabilitation, although it requires no special techniques, can be difficult in this patient's age group. It sometimes may be agonizingly slow and patience is required. Nevertheless, restoration of the vastus medialis obliquus through isometric and short-arc quadriceps exercises is usually effective, and in patients such as this one the motivation to return to competition will usually predominate. Competition should not be allowed until the quad-

riceps and hamstring strength of the two legs are within 10 percent of each other.

The follow-up results of surgical repair of acute subluxation of the patella have been excellent. Chondral defects up to 1 cm do heal, and rearthroscopy has verified the work of Shands,[5] confirming a filling of the defect. Larger defects are, and can be, a significant problem. When this situation exists, the surgeon should refer to the work of Ficat and Hungerford.[2] Garrett reported his successful use of osteochondral allografts in the treatment of chondral defect of the femoral condyles (J.C. Garrett of Atlanta, Georgia, in presentation, Fifth Congress of the International Society of the Knee, Sydney, Australia, April 5–10, 1987.)

SUMMARY

A 14-year-old elite gymnast felt a pop from within the knee on dismount. Although frequently the pop indicates a disruption of the ACL, it can also indicate a lateral subluxation or dislocation of the patella. This patient suffered a lateral luxation of the patella with an osteochondral fracture and tearing of the medial retinacular supporting structures from the medial intermuscular septum deep to the vastus medialis obliquus. Physical examination under anesthesia was particularly helpful, showing that the affected patella was grossly unstable to manual stress. This patella excursion was in marked contrast to the opposite knee, particularly when tested from 0° to 30°.

Surgical repair was accomplished. It is necessary to reflect the vastus medialis obliquus to visualize the tear from the medial intermuscular septum. Medial reefing was not required, since there was no preexisting pathology. Lateral retinacular release can cause significant postoperative morbidity, and is not of certain benefit. The knee was immobilized for 6 weeks. Remobilization after this repair is usually not so difficult as with intraarticular reconstructions held for a similar period. Follow-up results of acute patella subluxation treated by surgical repair have been excellent, with return to competition and a low rate of reinjury or redislocation.

REFERENCES

1. Feagin JA: The syndrome of the torn anterior cruciate ligament. Orthop Clin North Am 10:81–90, 1979
2. Ficat RP, Hungerford DS: Disorders of the Patello-Femoral Joint. Williams and Wilkins, Baltimore, 1977
3. Kennedy JC: Ligamentous injuries in the adolescent. pp 161–204. In Kennedy JC (ed): The Injured Adolescent Knee. Williams and Wilkins, Baltimore, 1979
4. Larson RL, Cabaud HE, Slocum DB et al: The patellar compression syndrome. Surgical treatment by lateral retinacular release. Clin Orthop 134:158–167, 1978
5. Shands AR: The regeneration of hyaline cartilage in joints. Experimental study. Arch Surg 22:137–178, 1931

CASE STUDY 12

A Questionably Positive Pivot Shift

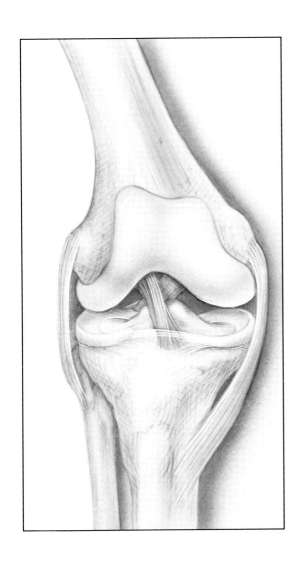

HISTORY

A 32-year-old professional ski instructor, skiing the moguls, caught an outside edge and vaulted forward. Her binding released, and she did a cartwheel into the next mogul. She felt immediate pain in the knee, but was able to ski down. Because she understood the importance of proper knee function in her work, she sought immediate medical attention. The unaffected knee was examined first, and it was noted that the patient was small of frame and generally demonstrated hyperextensile joints including laxity of the knees.

Knee Examination
(Orthopaedic Surgeon/Office)

Diagnostic Clues	Findings
Effusion	None
Tenderness	Over the medial and lateral ligamentous complexes
Lachman test	1 + positive*/firm end point
Drawer test	1 + positive/firm end point
Pivot shift test	Trace positive
Varus/valgus	Stable
Patella apprehension	Negative
Range of motion	0° to 90°
Gait	Apprehensive
Neurovasculature	Intact
Radiographs	Normal
Other	None

* See Glossary

COMMENTS

The accident described illustrates three mechanisms that place the ACL at risk:

1. The current style of skiing—that is, "sitting back" and using the stiff ski tails to unweight through avalement.[2] This can cause the force generated by the quadriceps contraction and the stiff boot to combine to create forward luxation of the tibia on the femur (an active anterior Drawer sign) sufficient to rupture the cruciate ligament without a fall.
2. Catching the outside edge, which usually causes internal rotation of the tibia on the femur, with "winding up" of the cruciates and a high risk of ACL rupture.
3. The deceleration of being thrown into the next mogul, whether the ski is attached or not.

This patient was a ski instructor, who was well-versed on knee injuries and was justifiably concerned that the injury might threaten her professional capacity and livelihood.

COURSE OF ACTION

Physical Examination

In the gracile, hyperextensile adult, as in the child, the tibia can often be luxated from the femur, mimicking the sensation of a pivot shift. The Losee test (see Ch. 12) done in internal and external rotation can discriminate between normality and abnormality, and this is also the time to use all the techniques of lateral compartment subluxation to discriminate subtle differences that might be present (see Ch. 10). *The most important yardstick for recognizing abnormality is the status of the well leg,* but sometimes the patient is unsure whether this leg might not have been injured also. The next check is then the firmness of the end point of both the Lachman and the Drawer tests. A second examination the following day allows further comparison of the stability and swelling between the two knees.

At the office examination on the day after injury, this patient showed no effusion in the knee, a range of motion of 0° to 110°, firm end points on the Lachman and Drawer tests, and mild induration and tenderness over the ligamentous structures of the medial and lateral capsules. The pivot shift was trace-positive in both knees.

Diagnostic Studies

The prime diagnostic study in this case was careful and repeated manual examination. Routine radiographs were helpful, showing no evidence of acute injury and no osteophytic spurring of the tubercles compatible with old injury. In cases of doubt the tunnel view can be obtained on both knees for comparison.

Special Considerations

This patient's livelihood (ski instructor), necessitating highly functional knees, is one important factor; another is the musculoskeletal anthropometry showing small bones and hyperextensile joints. These findings in this patient, as in the child, often mimic laxity similar to a tear of the ACL or PCL. Corroborating information may be obtained in objective fashion through arthrometer examination using devices such as the Genucom, KT-1000, or Stryker Ligament Tester. These devices, though new and expensive, are proving reliable for comparative examinations.

PLAN

Although one cannot have absolute confidence in the findings, there *must be a constant and diligent effort to refine and gain skill with the manual examination.* In this case, repeated manual examination assured the patient and physician that the injury was self-limiting. The radiographs showed no evidence of acute injury or osteoarthritis.

Observation and treatment of incomplete capsuloligamentous strains such as this are continued over 10 days to ensure there is no change in the physical signs, such as might occur with an ACL tear in which the synovium temporarily tamponaded the effusion.

In this patient the symptoms and apprehensive gait resolved in 5 days.

CASE STUDY 12
Questionably Positive Pivot Shift

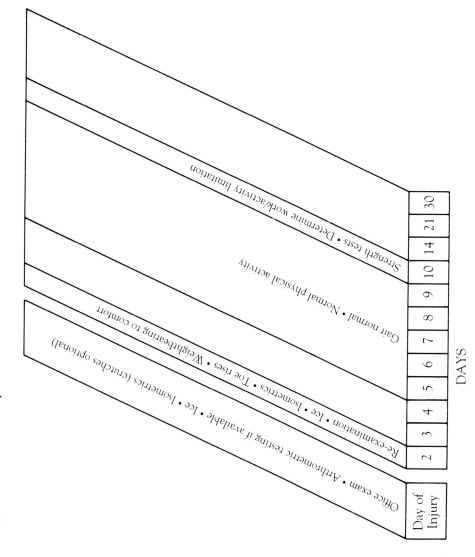

Day of Injury	2	3	4	5	6	7	8	9	10	14	21	30

DAYS

Office exam • Arthrometric testing if available • Ice • Isometrics (crutches optional)

Re-examination • Ice • Isometrics • Toe rises • Weightbearing to comfort

Gait normal • Normal physical activity

Strength tests • Determine work/activity limitation

REHABILITATION

No formal rehabilitation was necessary for this patient, but a comparative strength test (quadriceps/hamstrings and right leg versus left leg) were helpful to both patient and physician in timing the patient's return to work. A *strength difference* in the two legs of more than 10 percent would suggest that the injured knee was *vulnerable to reinjury*.[1] In my experience it is desirable for the quadriceps/hamstring strength ratio to be no less than 0.8 if reinjury is to be prevented and agility expected. These measurements can be accomplished with simple weights or through more sophisticated quantitative strength measurement equipment such as the Cybex or Orthotron.

PROBLEMS, COMPLICATIONS, FOLLOW-UP RESULTS

To overlook cruciate pathology and/or rotatory instability in a professional athlete can be disastrous. Sydnor and Andrews[3] have stated that the hyperextensile female may have a cruciate-dominant knee. The anthropometry cannot be ignored, nor can an ACL tear in an active person of this body habitus. Nevertheless, repeated physical examination can assure patient and physician that the structural integrity is sound.

SUMMARY

A professional athlete, a hyperextensile woman, presented with a knee injury and was justified in her concern that it might threaten her future function. She sought immediate attention and counsel, received supportive care and reassurance through the diagnostic process, and returned to full function. Physical examination and reliance on keenly honed manual skills are the answers to this type of problem.

REFERENCES

1. Abbott HG, Kress JB: Preconditioning in the prevention of knee injuries. Arch Phys Med Rehab 50:326–333, 1969
2. Joubert G: Teach Yourself to Ski. Trans. S. Thomas. Aspen Ski Masters, Aspen, Colorado. (French original: Pour Apprendre Soi-Même a Skier. Arthaud, France, 1970)
3. Sydnor RW, Andrews JR: Combined arthroscopy and "mini-reconstruction" techniques in the acutely torn anterior cruciate ligament. Orthop Clin North Am 16:171–179, 1985

CASE STUDY 13

ACL Tear, Incomplete, with Open Epiphyses

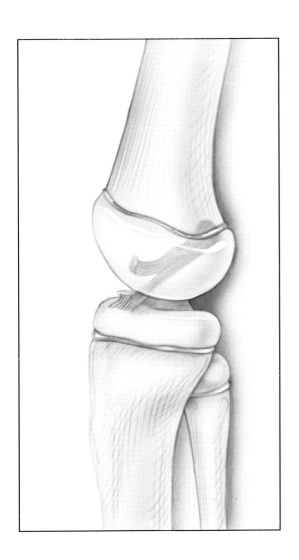

HISTORY

A 14-year-old soccer player was struck from the rear while in the act of shooting. The weighted leg was twisted, a pop was heard, and he was unable to continue to play. Radiographs revealed no acute injury. The epiphyses were "wide open."

Knee Examination
(Orthopaedic Surgeon/Office/2 Days after Injury)

Diagnostic Clues	Findings
Effusion	Moderate
Tenderness	Nonspecific
Lachman test	2+ positive*/firm end point
Drawer test	1+ positive/firm end point
Pivot shift test	Negative
Varus/valgus	Stable (20° to 70°)
Patella apprehension	Negative
Range of motion	20° to 70°
Gait	Antalgic
Neurovasculature	Intact
Radiographs	Normal adolescent
Other	None

* See Glossary.

COMMENTS

The mechanism of injury illustrated by this case places both the ACL and the epiphyses at risk. The negative pivot shift, in the face of the positive

127

Drawer and Lachman tests, suggests there was either an intact posterolateral band or inadequate relaxation.

The open epiphyses were a major factor, since they preclude some surgical procedures that require drilling through the epiphysis to implant an augmentation graft.

COURSE OF ACTION

Physical Examination

Repeat physical examination confirmed the negative pivot shift and 2+ positive Lachman test. An incomplete ACL tear was suspected, since integrity of the posterolateral bulk of the cruciate ligament is sufficient to negate the pivot shift. Approximately 10 percent of cruciate ligament tears are incomplete, and incomplete tears occur with nearly equal frequency in the anteromedial and posterolateral bands.[2] In this case the examining physician had confidence in his manual examination and knew the history, and therefore suspected a tear of the anteromedial band.

The pivot shift test requires only disruption of the posterolateral bulk of the ACL in order to be positive, and is quite specific for this structure. When the anteromedial band and secondary restraints are also torn or stretched, the pivot shift becomes "more positive" in both rotation and translation.

Diagnostic Studies

Routine roentgenograms were particularly important in this patient because at his age an osteochondral fragment, i.e., the insertion of the ACL, can be avulsed. The complexities of a partial ACL tear and the possibility of associated meniscal pathology are such that examination under anesthesia (EUA) and diagnostic arthroscopy were justified to ensure the best care for this young athlete.

Special Considerations

It was crucial in this patient to resolve the discrepancy between the positive Lachman and Drawer tests and the negative pivot shift. Since the natural history of partial tears of the ACL differs depending on whether the anteromedial or posterolateral band is torn, the discrepancy should be resolved to give appropriate guidance, care, and counsel. When the posterolateral band only is torn, there will be a positive pivot shift, and the knee is almost as much at risk as if there were a complete tear of the ACL. *The anteromedial band functioning alone will not protect the secondary restraints. The posterolateral band may protect them.*

A second consideration in this patient was the open epiphyses and the necessity of protecting them if operative intervention was elected. In addition to the disruptive effect of drilling on the epiphysis, it is possible that augmentation grafts can exert undue pressure on the epiphysis and result in growth disturbance. This has not yet been clinically documented.

PLAN

This athlete was young and would be "at risk" for many years; thus an EUA, diagnostic arthroscopy, and attention to the cruciate ligament problem were the method of choice to ensure a complete diagnosis and the best long-term results.

Before arthroscopy was used diagnostically, cases of this nature were normally managed by immobilizing the knee for 4 to 6 weeks. It is probable that the residual stump of the ACL frequently healed onto the synovium of the PCL. This fortuitously effects a repair after the manner of Wittek[3] (Fig. 67). Nevertheless, by today's standards, it is precarious to treat a patient in this manner, not knowing what one is treating, and unable to assure the patient of a reasonable outcome.

Treatment

The EUA confirmed the negative pivot shift and the 2+ positive Lachman test with a firm end point. The remainder of the examination remained unchanged.

Diagnostic arthroscopy showed the patellofemoral, medial, and lateral compartments to be intact. On probing, a tear of the anteromedial band was

Fig. 67. The ACL shows a partial tear.

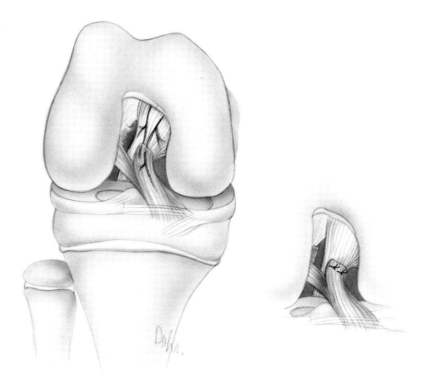

demonstrated. The posterolateral band was definitely intact and had good turgor.

The choice then, was between repairing the anteromedial band, reconstruction, and immobilization with the hope that the anteromedial band would heal.

Based on my experience, I chose to immobilize this patient's knee for 5 weeks at 30° flexion with the ankle and foot free. When partial tears involve only the anteromedial band, the residual laxity is minimal and subsequent injury infrequent (*provided the secondary restraints are protected* while they heal and the knee is rehabilitated). Immobilization not only promotes the cross-union previously described, but protects the residual ACL and secondary restraints as they regain structural integrity.

Reconstruction, as a primary procedure, was not indicated in this case. The results of treatment of anteromedial band tears by immobilization are usually satisfactory.

If the tear had involved the posterolateral bulk, the natural history would not be good, and failure of function with recurrent injury in the future could be expected.

POSTOPERATIVE CARE AND REHABILITATION

The postoperative care consisted of immobilization as described with emphasis on an isometric exercise program for the quadriceps and hamstrings. Active exercise of the gastrocsoleus and the muscles of hip, trunk, and upper extremities was encouraged. Weightbearing to comfort was allowed.

Isotonic and isokinetic rehabilitation, with regular objective follow-up examinations over a period of 2 years after the injury, is recommended for injuries of this type. Objective measurement of knee laxity with an arthrometer is helpful to document the stability and to ensure that there is no subtle stretching out of the residual cruciate ligament or secondary restraints.

CASE STUDY 13
ACL (Incomplete) Open Epiphyses

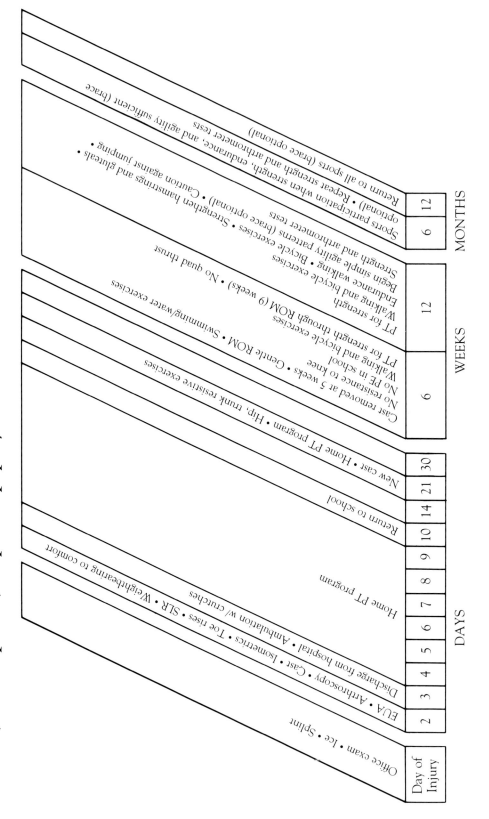

Day of Injury	2	3	4	5	6	7	8	9	10	14	21	30		6	12		6	12
														WEEKS			MONTHS	

DAYS

Office exam • Ice • Splint

EUA • Arthroscopy • Cast • Isometrics • Toe rises • SLR • Weightbearing to comfort
Discharge from hospital • Ambulation w/ crutches

Home PT program

Return to school

New cast • Home PT program • Hip, trunk resistive exercises

Cast removed at 5 weeks • Gentle ROM • Swimming/water exercises
No resistance to knee • No quad thrust
No PE in school
Walking and bicycle exercises
PT for strength through ROM (9 weeks)
PT for strength
Walking and bicycle exercises
Endurance walking • Bicycle exercises • Strengthen hamstrings and gluteals
Begin simple agility patterns (brace optional) • Caution against jumping
Strength and arthrometer tests
Sports participation when strength, endurance, and agility sufficient (brace optional) • Repeat strength and agility and arthrometer tests
Return to all sports (brace optional)

PROBLEMS, COMPLICATIONS, FOLLOW-UP RESULTS

This injury, incomplete tear of the ACL with open epiphyses, occurs in younger patients, so the immobilization is not attended by particular difficulties in rehabilitation caused by stiffness. This patient's youth also meant that his knee had to be protected from environmental pressures, and immobilization accomplished this.

When only the anteromedial band is involved, follow-up results are usually satisfactory. Sometimes it is difficult to distinguish the anteromedial band and the posterolateral bundle, since they are not discrete structures but form a continuum. The probe is as helpful in determining which of them is injured as the manual examination. When only the anteromedial band is involved the effusion is usually less, since the primary blood supply of the ACL originates from the posterosuperior corner of the posterolateral band.[1,2]

Infrequently with this type of injury, there is increasing laxity as well as increasing functional impairment. This increasing laxity usually indicates that the posterolateral band was involved more than had been originally appreciated. Perhaps the posterolateral band was correctly determined to be intact, but its elastic limit of deformation had been exceeded. Thus occasionally these knees become chronically unstable and must be treated by surgical means. Nevertheless, in spite of this, I have been pleased with the diagnostic examination and prognosis as described, and have found that the difference in the prognosis, depending on which band is involved, is quite predictable.

SUMMARY

This adolescent athlete had an incomplete tear of the ACL involving only the anteromedial band. This lesion, in contrast to tears of the posterolateral band, has a good prognosis without further surgical intervention. Postoperative care involved immobilization. This allowed healing of the torn portion of the ACL to its neighboring blood supply as well as healing within the residual ACL, which undoubtedly had undergone at least some degree of elastic deformation. The secondary restraints likewise needed to be protected to ensure their restitution.

The follow-up results in cases where only the anteromedial band is torn have been excellent. The same cannot be said for tears of the posterolateral band, and in fact these have a similar natural history to the "isolated" tear of the ACL as outlined in Case Study 1.

REFERENCES

1. Arnocsky SP, Rubin RM, Marshall JL: Microvasculature of the cruciate ligaments and its response to injury. An experimental study in dogs. J Bone Joint Surg 61A:1221–1229, 1979
2. Feagin JA: The syndrome of the torn anterior cruciate ligament. Orthop Clin North Am 10:81–90, 1979
3. Wittek, A: Zur Naht der Kreuzbandverletzung im Kniegelenk. Zentralbl Chir 54:1538–1541, 1927

CASE STUDY 14

ACL Insufficiency, Chronic, with Degenerative Arthritis

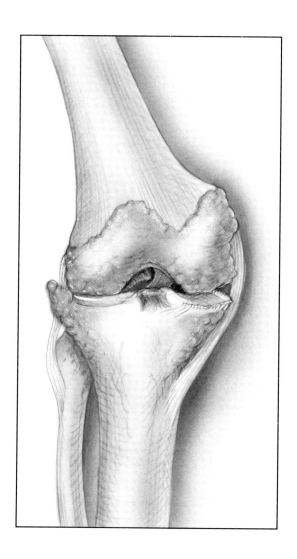

HISTORY

A 36-year-old self-employed electrician had symptoms of intermittent effusions, pain, and giving way in the knee. He had participated in college football

Knee Examination
(Orthopaedic Surgeon/Office)

Diagnostic Clues	Findings
Effusion	Mild
Tenderness	Not localized
Lachman test	2+ positive*/soft end point
Drawer test	1+ positive/soft end point
Pivot shift test	Trace positive
Varus/valgus	1+ valgus [opening instability] at 30°, stable at 0°
Patella apprehension	Crepitation with limitation of patella excursion medially and laterally
Range of motion	From 10° flexion to 10° lack of full flexion
Gait	Slight flexed knee, genu varum stance, with appreciable limp on fast walking
Neurovasculature	Intact, with 3 cm quadriceps atrophy
Radiographs	Fairbank's changes, grade II, with medial joint space narrowing. Spurring of the tubercular eminences, intercondylar notch stenosis. Mild degenerative arthrosis patella and significant periarticular osteophyte formation
Other	The patient is 5 ft 7 in tall and weighs 210 pounds. He has pes planus and significant callosities on the feet at the MP joint

* See Glossary.

133

for 1 year until a knee injury forced his "retirement" from football. Three years after his college knee injury, he had a medial meniscectomy. Now, 12 years later, he sought advise because the knee symptoms for the past year had stopped him from jogging and now inhibited recreational and vocational activities.

COMMENTS

The patient's history of injury and ensuing degenerative arthritis is a frequent sequela of American football. Perhaps a cruciate ligament injury was not detected at the time of injury or meniscectomy. The surgery of the 1950s and 1960s often did not deal with cruciate insufficiency, and "complete" meniscectomy was the dictum. Degenerative arthritis could be anticipated. In this case the patient was, in a very real sense, disabled at midlife, and was forced either to limit his activities significantly or change his occupation.

COURSE OF ACTION

Physical Examination

In a knee such as this patient's, the osteophytes "dampen" the pivot shift and decrease the excursion of the Lachman and Drawer tests. This is probably nature's "physiologic" method of restabilizing the knee in the face of cruciate laxity and/or loss of meniscal height. *A subtle sign is that the Lachman test is relatively more positive than is the Drawer test or pivot shift.* The osteophytes limit capsular excursion and seem to provide increasing stability as the joint approaches the extremes of flexion and extension. These are the motions first lost in this type of degeneration, and should be sought critically in the physical examination. The patient should be examined for this loss of motion in the supine position on a firm table with the limbs extended. He is asked to exert pressure on the examiner's hands placed beneath the patient's popliteal fossa (Fig. 68).

Loss of knee flexion is appreciated by measuring the heel-to-buttock distance with the patient supine and the hips in 120° flexion (Fig. 69). For goniometric measurement I prefer the prone position so that the hip is better stabilized and the angular knee motion can be measured accurately (Fig. 70).

Observation of the patient's normal and rapid gait should be a part of every knee examination; general alignment, subtle contractures, muscle weakness, and instability will often cause a limp not appreciated in the casual stance or walk. This patient had genu varum secondary to the loss of meniscal height and medial joint space.

Intermittent effusion, coupled with the loss of motion, is a prognostic indicator of increasing degenerative arthritis. The frequency and persistence of the effusions are clues to the patient's relative activity as well as to the extent of the arthrosis. Many patients will deny that activity causes the effusion, which occurs somewhat later. A daily exercise log

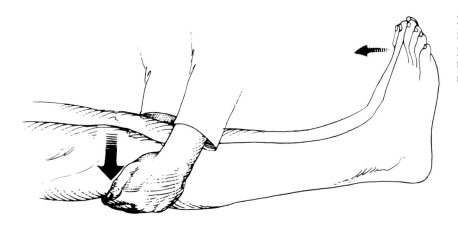

Fig. 68. The knee is tested for full extension. The examiner places his hands behind the patient's popliteal fossa and asks the patient to press against them.

Fig. 69. With the patient's hip in 120° flexion, the examiner measures the distance from the heel to buttocks. Compared with the opposite leg, the loss of flexion in the knee is obvious.

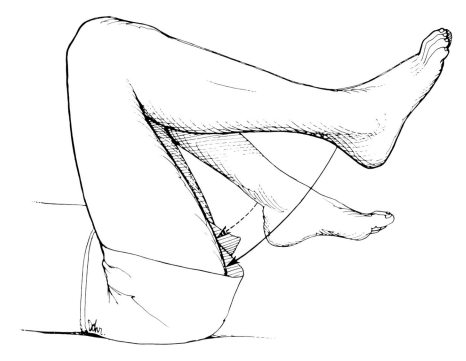

Fig. 70. The gonimetric measurements are more accurate with the patient prone so that the hip is stabilized.

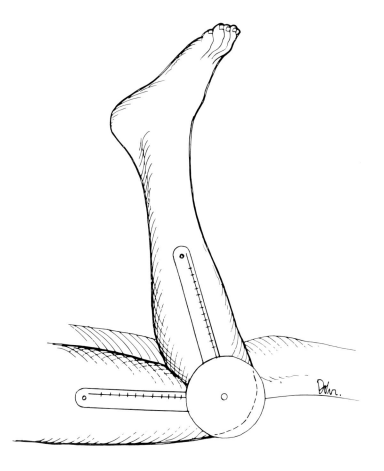

helps to sort out this matter in the minds of the surgeon and patient.

It is important to correlate the radiographic evidence with the physical examination, to gain some idea of whether the osteophytes that limit motion are in the patellofemoral joint or the knee joint. This analysis often helps to define the prognosis and will affect the operative choice.

Diagnostic Studies

An objective manual physical examination, with careful attention to documenting the objective findings in a reproducible fashion, are important in the long-term management of this type of patient.[1]

The routine four-view roentgenograms deserve careful scrutiny, and I would add to these views a comparison of right and left tunnel weightbearing views.[6] In the early stage of degeneration represented by this patient, Fairbank's signs can be separated from those of rotatory laxity by evaluating the medial and lateral compartments separately from the central compartment. *The central compartment reacts to rotatory laxity through early peaking of the tibial eminences and later through stenosis of the femoral intercondylar notch.*[2] (Fig. 71). Degenerative arthritis must be separated into its patellofemoral component and its tibiofemoral joint component. In chronic progressive disabling degenerative arthritis in a relatively young worker, I find it helpful to obtain a technetium 99m scan in addition to the routine radiographs. The technetium scan defines the cellular activity in each of the knee compartments. As the surgeon views the joint surfaces arthroscopically, it helps to know what is happening to the subchondral region. The ^{99m}Tc scan will often show that the disease is limited to one compartment, and this information, combined with a surface analysis through arthroscopy, will help to define the potential for osteotomy in this patient.

Fig. 71. The tunnel view, showing peaking of the tibial eminences ("Teton sign").

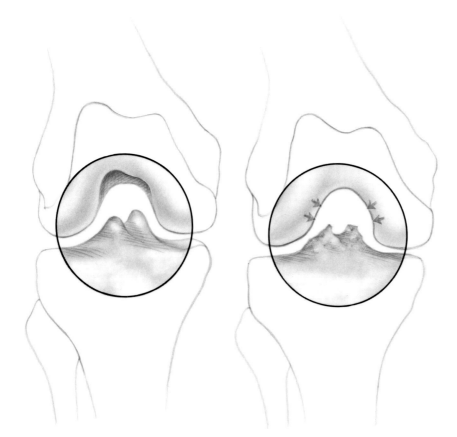

Also indicated are microscopic examination of the synovial fluid and sometimes percutaneous synovial biopsy.

Cybex or Orthotron strength and endurance curves for quadriceps and hamstring muscles are also helpful in the "data gathering" stage. Patellofemoral pain can result in a marked deterioration of the quadriceps strength curve with retention of hamstring strength.

Nowhere in knee surgery is it more important to interrelate all the diagnostic studies before formulating a plan than in a difficult case of this nature — old ACL injury, meniscal loss, plus deterioration through aging. The manual examination, radiographs, isokinetic and/or isotonic muscle studies, synovial fluid analysis, and ^{99m}Tc scan all give specialized information on the mechanics of the patellofemoral and knee joints that will help patient and surgeon in deciding on the course of treatment.

Special Considerations

This patient was self-employed. Thus, rehabilitation time and physical therapy were significant factors. The patient's lifestyle and ability to control his activity level, both recreationally and vocationally, were critical. The role of aspirin and other nonsteroidal antiinflammatory agents needed to be evaluated, as well as the possibility of gout, pseudogout, or other crystalline disease, or rheumatic arthropathy.

It is difficult to determine for a patient such as this what course of treatment will be best — a "conservative regimen," arthroscopic debridement, open debridement, realignment osteotomy, and/or ligamentous reconstruction. The surgeon is wise to move slowly until the full implications of the patient's symptoms and needs are appreciated.

PLAN

A patient such as this should be thoroughly counseled. He needs to understand that office evaluation will not yield the facts necessary to recommend a specific plan. In addition to routine radiographic examination, muscle power and strength measurements, ^{99m}Tc scan, and diagnostic arthroscopy may be useful, depending on the patient's desires and symptoms. After all the data are integrated, the operation is planned. In addition to arthroscopic examination and debridement, the surgeon should consider the possible usefulness of lateral retinacular release, facetectomy,[4] Pridie debridement,[5] ACL reconstruction, corner stability, and osteotomy. Needless to say, with this gamut of choices, every morsel of data is needed to assist in the decision-making process. The input of the patient and his family is a key to the proper timing for the proper operation, if surgery is the treatment of choice.

The nonoperative approach to this type of knee is perfectly acceptable, in that *there does not seem to be an identifiable "golden time" for intervention.* The patient should be apprised of this, and told that he can be followed objectively once the foundation of objective data has been established. The strength curves can be repeated at 6-month intervals. They are inexpensive and noninvasive. As objective data, they can be quite meaningful and usually are reproducible.

If nonoperative care is selected, then a regular exercise program with attention to weight control is essential and should be prescribed. The role of aspirin and nonsteroidal antiinflammatory agents will have to be deduced by trial and error and the patient's symptoms and desires. Occasionally this approach dramatically improves symptoms and results in patient satisfaction.

Should the knee be injected with corticosteroid? Repeated injection has been condemned — but a single diagnostic injection after an objective diagnostic evaluation can be quite helpful. Dramatic relief usually indicates that nonoperative care could work well. Cases in which corticosteroid gives no relief are usually those with more severe joint deterioration.

Patients for whom nonoperative care is chosen should be followed at regular intervals, such as quarterly during the first year after the diagnostic foundation is established.

Surgical Approach

Operative care in a patient of this age is usually based on minimal intervention with early return to function. Separation of the dysfunction of the patellofemoral joint from that of the knee joint and evaluation of the limitation of motion caused by the osteophytes are important.

In this patient, we decided that minimal intervention, i.e., arthroscopic debridement, would give us time to gather further objective data which would help in guiding the patient's course over the ensuing years. This patient did not feel that the loss of flexion particularly inhibited his activities, so restoration of full range of motion was not a goal of the surgery.

During arthroscopy it was determined that the medial meniscus was surgically absent and the lateral meniscus had a flap tear, the ACL was incompetent, and the cruciate notch was stenotic. The patellofemoral joint, as well as the medial compartment, displayed severe chondromalacia. The joint surfaces of the lateral compartment were relatively unaffected.

The flap tear of the lateral meniscus was debrided, the examination video-recorded, and arthroscopic lateral retinacular release was performed to decrease the lateral pressure syndrome[3] resulting from the osteophytosis (Fig. 72).

Alternative approaches are available to treat more severely disabled patients. In addition to arthroscopic debridement (which can be extensive), the surgeon can consider a more extensive lateral release and/or lateral facetectomy as described by O'Donoghue.[4] Often, the limitation of motion is a product of the tightening of the patellofemoral restraints and osteophytic overgrowth. Both problems can often be improved by the lateral facetectomy.[4]

If medial and lateral buttressing osteophytes are significant, they can be debrided either arthroscopically or as described by Pridie.[5] It has been my practice to also debride the osteophytes of the intercondylar notch because they often block full extension. This can be done arthroscopically without compromise of the existing soft tissue contained in the intercondylar notch.

Not many surgeons are willing to superimpose ACL reconstruction on an arthroscopic debridement, but our group has practiced this combination and is pleased with the outcome. If it is done, special attention must be given postoperative care to limit the possibility for arthrofibrosis. Also, harvesting the graft from the patella tendon must be considered carefully, in view of the status of the patellofemoral joint. Sometimes the lateral third of the infrapatellar tendon is a better choice, since harvesting it will accomplish lateral retinacular release and can be extended to lateral facetectomy without significantly extending the surgical trauma.

Finally, there is the role of osteotomy. Osteotomy is a key operation, necessary in the armamentarium of every knee surgeon. If chosen, it may be accomplished at the time of the other procedures. We have been quite satisfied with the results of combined

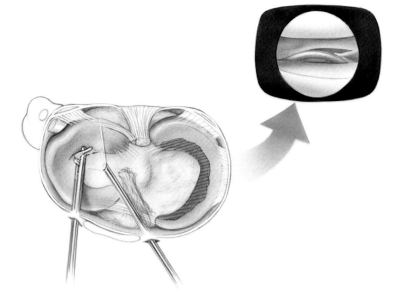

Fig. 72. A video record of the arthroscopic debridement of the lateral meniscus.

CASE STUDY 14
ACL, Chronic, with Degenerative Arthritis

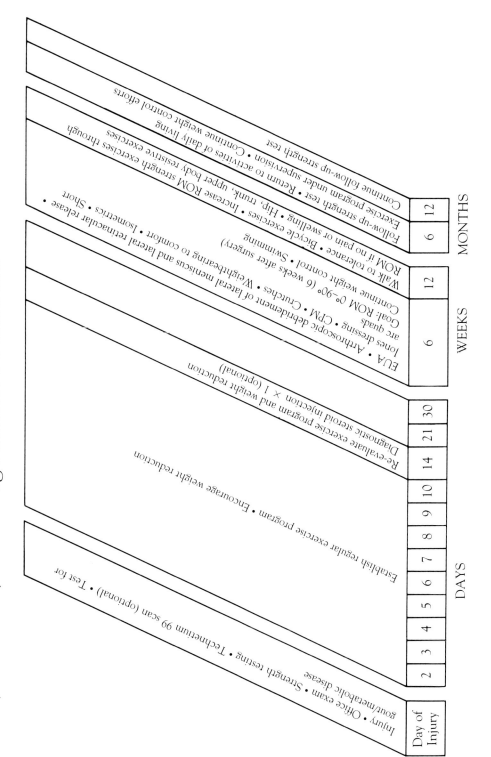

DAYS

| Day of Injury | 2 | 3 | 4 | 5 | 6 | 7 | 8 | 9 | 10 | 14 | 21 | 30 |

Injury • Office exam • Strength testing • Technetium 99 scan (optional) • Test for gout/metabolic disease

Establish regular exercise program • Encourage weight reduction

Re-evaluate exercise program and weight reduction • Diagnostic steroid injection × 1 (optional)

WEEKS

| 6 | 12 |

EUA • Arthroscopic debridement of lateral meniscus and lateral retinacular release • Short arc quads • Jones dressing • CPM • Crutches • Weightbearing to comfort • Isometrics • Continue weight control • Swimming

Goal: ROM 0°–90° (6 weeks after surgery)

Walk to tolerance • Bicycle exercises • Increase ROM if no pain or swelling • Continue weight control • Follow-up strength test • Return to activities of daily living • Continue weight control efforts

MONTHS

| 6 | 12 |

Increase ROM strength exercises through exercise program under supervision • Hip, trunk, upper body resistive exercises through Exercise program • Continue follow-up strength test

ACL reconstruction and osteotomy where fixation of the graft and osteotomy are secure. Range of motion may be initiated in the immediate postoperative period.

Total knee arthroplasty is obviously not a consideration at this time, at this level of our knowledge, but must be reserved for the "end-stage knee." The uncemented unicompartmental arthroplasty, however, may have application in carefully selected adults who are willing to reduce the demands on their knee in return for relief of pain and instability.

POSTOPERATIVE CARE AND EARLY REHABILITATION

The key to postoperative care is preventing swelling and adhesions (see Ch 25). Effective adjuncts have been (1) one or two large drains, (2) firmly applied Jones compression dressings, and (3) early range of motion through the continuous passive motion machine (see Fig. 24, Case Study 2). Epidural analgesia has helped in relieving pain and obtaining early motion in these patients with chronic ACL deficiency and degenerative arthritis. Even when the ACL reconstruction has been a part of the surgical procedure, a goal of motion from full extension to 90° flexion is sought as early as possible after the operation. If this range is not achieved by the 12th week, arthroscopic lysis of adhesions may be indicated. Postoperative care must be appropriately aggressive to match the pathology and the extent of the surgical intervention. A cast would not be appropriate even if ACL reconstruction and/or osteotomy were included in the treatment. Fixation of both ACL grafts and osteotomy must be secure enough to allow early active range of motion.

PROBLEMS, COMPLICATIONS, FOLLOW-UP RESULTS

Significant complications can develop from too much surgery, too soon. *One should attempt to match the surgical expectation to the patient's disability, desires, and pathology.* This is why extensive diagnostic studies are recommended so that the progress of the disease can be appreciated and matched to the patient's desires and disabilities.

The second complication is arthrofibrosis after surgical intervention. Usually this can be prevented through aggressive postoperative care including effective drainage, pressure dressings, continuous passive motion, and appropriate pain relief (see Ch. 28).

I seldom do manipulation under anesthesia. It is fraught with complications, does not reveal the underlying pathology, and is not nearly so effective and reliable as diagnostic arthroscopy with release of the offending structures.

Follow-up results have been gratifying to both patient and surgeon, but are difficult to quantitate because these are end-stage knees and the surgery is temporizing in nature. We do not know if the arthritic process can be altered or if its course is inexorable.

This patient was a relatively young self-employed electrician who needed reasonably functional knees in his work. He had already experienced significant limitation of recreational activities and was concerned about his vocational activities and endurance. It was explained to the patient that considerable diagnostic study was necessary before a decision could be made about surgical intervention. For this patient, minimal surgical intervention was recommended—arthroscopy and arthroscopic debridement. Nevertheless, I have described some alternative procedures which may be applied if indicated.

Significant postoperative risks are taken in performing too much surgery too soon on this type of knee. Pain, stiffness, limited motion, recurrent effusion, and pyogenic arthritis can all result in a knee that suffers a chronic state of siege from excessive external forces and deranged internal defenses. The potential problems can be reduced with care and concern for details by both the patient and physician during the preoperative and postoperative periods. The results of both limited and major surgical intervention can be gratifying if the patient selection is appropriate.

REFERENCES

1. Feagin JA, Blake WP: Postoperative evaluation and result recording in the anterior cruciate ligament reconstructed knee. Clin Orthop 172:143–147, 1983

2. Feagin JA, Cabaud HE, Curl WW: The anterior cruciate ligament. Radiographic and clinical signs of successful and unsuccessful repairs. Clin Orthop 164:54–58, 1982

3. Ficat RP, Hungerford DS: Disorders of the Patello-Femoral Joint. Williams and Wilkins, Baltimore, 1977

4. O'Donoghue DH: Facetectomy. South Med J 65:645–654, 1972

5. Pridie KH: Method of resurfacing osteoarthritis knee joints. (Abstract). J Bone Joint Surg 41B:618–619, 1959

6. Rosenberg TD, Coward DB, Scott SM: The flexion weight-bearing radiograph of the knee: Its anatomic basis and clinical significance. Clin Orthop (in press)

CASE STUDY 15

ACL-Deficient Knee, Multiply Operated, Global Laxity

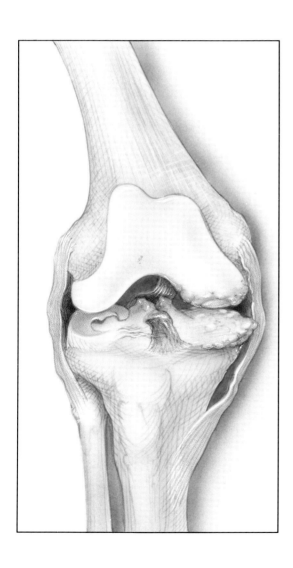

HISTORY

A 28-year-old national soccer player had multiple surgical procedures subsequent to an injury at age

Knee Examination
(Orthopaedic Surgeon/Office)

Diagnostic Clues	Findings
Effusion	Mild
Tenderness	Not localized
Lachman test	3+ positive*/soft end point
Drawer test	2+ anterior positive, trace positive posterior Anteromedial and lateral capsules soft to anterior Drawer testing at 30° and 90°. Posteromedial and posterolateral capsules soft to posterior testing in both 30° and 90° flexion.
Pivot shift test	Markedly positive in translation and rotation, in both internal and external rotation.
Varus/valgus	2+ varus and valgus opening (laxity) at 30°; 1+ varus and valgus opening (laxity) in full extension and hyperextension
Patella apprehension	Negative except for discomfort to palpation
ROM	Full
Gait	Abnormal, with lateral thrust
Neurovasculature	Intact, but with a 4 cm quadriceps atrophy
Radiographs	Grade II Fairbank's signs medially, tibial-eminence osteophytosis
Other	Multiple surgical incisions, well healed.

* See Glossary.

143

19. These operations, performed by reputable surgeons, consisted sequentially of medial meniscectomy and pes transfer at age 21, arthroscopic debridement of the lateral meniscus at age 23, and at age 26 combined intraarticular and extraarticular stabilization by using an iliotibial band "over the top" to substitute for the absent ACL and an extraarticular biceps transfer beneath the lateral collateral ligament. At presentation the patient complained of instability, pain, and inability to continue to play professional soccer. His symptoms were present even when he walked on the level during normal daily activities.

COMMENTS

Even for a high-performance athlete of relative youth, three surgical procedures to the knee over a 10-year span are significant, and in this patient have taken their toll physically and emotionally. The previous operations involved considerable tissue transfer and tissue loss. The possibility of neuropathy from repeated tourniquet ischemia, as well as inadequate or incomplete rehabilitation, must be evaluated. Finally, evaluating the patient's physical stamina and psyche in the face of possibly more surgical trauma are critical. The best intended surgery of its time (the 1970s) may not ultimately have proven best for this patient. The efficacy of the surgery of the 1970s has yet to be documented. Return to play, for such a patient, given his age and circumstances, should not be the primary goal. If surgery is undertaken, rehabilitation well may consume 2 years, and must be taken into consideration as the patient evaluates his long-term goals.

In addition to in-depth counseling with the patient, counseling with coach, family, and management would be appropriate to ensure that all realize the gravity of the situation, the limited playing potential, and the complexity of further surgery — with functional activities of daily living being the goal, not return to professional competition.

COURSE OF ACTION

Physical Examination

Physical examination revealed "global" laxity. Examination under anesthesia is usually not necessary in such cases. Nevertheless, the complexity of evaluation is such that manual examination may not be completed in one session. Often several repetitions of the manual examination, by several observers, are necessary to perceive accurately and record the "global" laxity.

The lateral thrusting gait exhibited by this patient is complex, for one never knows if it represents a loss of supporting tissue, a failure of rehabilitation, or a "learned gait" with implications of secondary gain. Videotape and/or high-speed gait photography are best for gait analysis in a patient with a multiply operated ACL-deficient knee and global laxity.

Diagnostic Studies

Routine radiographs with comparative weightbearing single-leg tunnel views should be obtained in patients with this type of injury to evaluate alignment and osteoarthritic change.[5] A computed axial tomography (CAT) scan is helpful in determining the patellofemoral joint alignment as well as the presence or absence of meniscal tissue in the posterior corners. This tissue needs to be preserved or repaired whenever possible. A gait laboratory examination with electromyographic recording is extremely helpful and serves as an objective standard by which to measure improvement. A ^{99m}Tc scan helps to determine the extent of progressing arthrosis.

Strength and power curves, as previously described for the quadriceps and hamstring muscles, would be valuable to determine if the knee has been maximally rehabilitated.

Psychological testing would be helpful to the patient and examiner to gain insight into the patient's psychological support systems (see Ch. 17).

Special Considerations

In this patient, the special considerations are the global laxity and the extent of the disability affecting his participation in sports as well as activities of daily living. Disability, not only from a functional aspect but also from a vocational rehabilitation aspect, must be considered. Help from the professional social services is too seldom made available to the "end-stage" athlete.

PLAN

The approach to a patient with complex anatomic laxity is perhaps nowhere better described than by Müller.[2] The fact that this is probably the last chance to obtain stability by surgical treatment, and the implications of a functional knee to the patient, must be appreciated. The diagnostic studies, although they may seem tedious and time consuming, will be essential in the final planning, timing of surgery, and nature of the procedure. Consultation between surgeons is essential to protect both patient and surgeon.

Nonoperative care may be appropriate until the patient's career is terminated. The timing and mutual goals are critical and will determine whether operative or nonoperative care is appropriate at the time of evaluation. Both patient and surgeon must understand that in some desperate cases fusion has been required for restoration of stability and function. It is unlikely that fusion would be acceptable to any of the persons involved, but sometimes the desperate nature of the situation can be better appreciated by realizing how limited the alternatives are in the knee with pain and severe "global" instability.

Operative care of this type of knee requires the highest order to skill and understanding of knee pathomechanics. The role of the central pivot, the definition of the residual stable hinge, knowledge of posterior capsular anatomy, and the availability and selection of graft material are all critical and part of preoperative planning. In my mind, *"dynamic substitution" no longer has a place.* Consideration must be given in a knee such as this to restoring some of the previous "dynamic transfers" to their anatomic points.

The posterior cruciate ligament was still possibly intact, although the physical examination suggested some attritional stretching. The ACL needed aug-

menting. An allograft or prosthetic graft would be preferable to tissue from the multiply operated knee. The iliotibial tract needed reconstructing. Tissue might have to be harvested from the well leg if the integrity of the iliotibial band was to be restored. The posteromedial and lateral capsules, as well as anteromedial and lateral capsules, will need "reefing." This must be planned carefully preoperatively to expedite teamwork, and to minimize surgical time. The ACL graft should be tensioned before evaluating the corners. The techniques of O'Donoghue[3,4] have merit in capsular plication. Undoubtedly, in this patient the arcuate complex would need advancing as described by Hughston and Jacobson.[1] There would be no dependence on dynamic substitution since this has failed the patient in the past.

The exact details of the operative procedure planned for this patient may be extracted from the writings of O'Donoghue,[3,4] Müller,[2] and Chapters 20 through 23. They are sufficiently complex that they defy adequate textbook description.

This patient elected to defer surgery, terminate his professional athletic career, and continue under the surgeon's care, but he wanted to know more about the postoperative requirements if surgery became necessary for him to continue functional activity.

POSTOPERATIVE CARE AND REHABILITATION

The proposed program included a long-term relationship with physical therapy. Objective goals and measurements would be reviewed periodically. The patient would be fitted with functional bracing to use in his activities of daily living. Patient, therapist, and surgeon must realize that if the patient elected surgery, the postoperative course and rehabilitation would require about 2 years of intense effort and dedication.

PROBLEMS, COMPLICATIONS, FOLLOW-UP RESULTS

The primary complication possibility is inadequate preoperative evaluation and too hasty dependence on the operation to restore the function to a goal that is not obtainable. Intraoperative use of the tourniquet can lead to muscle atrophy and possible sympathetic dystrophy. Furthermore, arthrofibrosis is a significant risk because of the four-quadrant nature of the surgery. A failure on the part of the patient's psyche, with the loss of will to rehabilitate himself, occurs frequently, and rejection of the patient by family, management, and the surgical team has occurred. These possibilities must be broached before embarking on a reconstructive procedure. Therapeutic and functional goals must be redefined and reinforced at frequent intervals.

Follow-up results after surgical procedures for "global" instability are largely disappointing. The vocational function desired is usually not obtainable. The patient's inability to regain elite sports skills or participate in athletic competition is frustrating. The psyche from previous surgery and disappointments is probably one of bitterness and hostility, with exasperation and despair. Sometimes the establishment of written goals and guidelines, almost in the form of a patient–surgeon contract, can be helpful so that each knows in advance the reasonable expectations.

SUMMARY

This patient was a 28-year-old nationally ranked soccer player whose only vocation was sport. Three previous knee operations had left him devastated physically and psychologically. Residual "global" instability after previous treatment in such a patient is threatening to the surgeon and demands the utmost caution, consideration, and consultation. The diagnostic studies necessary are complex and time consuming and will test the patient's endurance. Formal psychological testing can be an important adjunct. The timing of surgery is a primary consideration. Vocational rehabilitation must be considered preoperatively in exactly the same manner that provisions are made for physical rehabilitation.

Finally, if the patient and surgeon agree to surgical intervention again, this is "the last chance." All preparations must be accomplished in thorough detail so that there is no looking back by either patient or surgeon with regret about the timing of the surgery, the limited postoperative goals, and the lengthy rehabilitation.

It is appropriate that a case of this complexity should be the last in this section, for it is fraught with many pitfalls and requires knowledge extracted not only from the literature but also from the outstanding contributors of other sections of *The Crucial Ligaments*.

REFERENCES

1. Hughston JC, Jacobson KE: Chronic posterolateral rotatory instability of the knee. J Bone Joint Surg 67A:351–359, 1985
2. Müller W: The Knee. Form, Function, and Ligament Reconstruction. Springer-Verlag, New York, 1983, pp. 221–226
3. O'Donoghue DH: Reconstruction for medial instability of the knee. J Bone Joint Surg 55A:941–955, 1973
4. O'Donoghue DH: Treatment of Injuries of Athletes. 4th Ed. WB Saunders, Philadelphia, 1984, pp. 447–600
5. Rosenberg TD, Coward DB, Scott SM: The flexion weight-bearing radiograph of the knee. Its anatomic basis and clinical significance. Clin Orthop (in press)

Bibliography

Alm A, Gillquist J, Stromberg B: The medial third of the patellar ligament in reconstruction of the anterior cruciate ligament. A clinical and histologic study by means of arthroscopy or arthrotomy. Acta Chir Scand O(Suppl 445):5–14, 1974

The state of the art (circa 1974) on reconstruction of the anterior cruciate ligament.

Andrews JR, Carson WG Jr (eds): The Anterior Cruciate Ligament. Part I. (Symposium). Orthop Clin North Am 16:1–158, 1985

Andrews JR, Carson WG Jr (eds): The Anterior Cruciate Ligament. Part II (Symposium). Orthop Clin North Am 16:165–350, 1985

A two-part symposium authored by a host of world-class contributors who provide up-to-date knowledge on all aspects of knee injury diagnoses, surgery, and rehabilitation.

Andrews JR, Sanders R: A "mini-reconstruction" technique in treating anterolateral rotatory instability (ALRI). Clin Orthop 172:93–96, 1983

A detailed technical description of the extraarticular iliotibial band tenodesis.

Apley AG: Letter to the Editor. J Bone Joint Surg 62A:487, 1980

Is the structure that joins the patella to the tibial tubercle tendon or ligament? One of the world's greatest orthopaedic teachers addresses this subject.

Arms SW, Pope MH, Johnson RJ et al: The biomechanics of anterior cruciate ligament rehabilitation and reconstruction. Am J Sports Med 12:8–18, 1984

Arnoczky SP, Rubin RM, Marshall JL: Microvasculature of the cruciate ligaments and its response to injury. An experimental study in dogs. J Bone Joint Surg 61A:1221–1229, 1979

An important study of the vascular anatomy and its clinical applications.

Banks HH (ed): Major Sports Injuries: Tribute to Thomas B. Quigley, M.D. (Symposium). Clin Orthop 164:2–92, 1982

Bousquet G, Millon J, Bascoulergue G, Rhenter J-L: Le réflection du ligament croisé antérieur par plastic activo-passive du pivot central et des points d'angle. (Reconstruction of the anterior cruciate ligament by active-passive surgery of the central pivot and angle points.) Rev Chir Orthop 66(Suppl 2):91–92, 1980

Bousquet G, Rhenter J-L, Bascoulergue G, Millon J: L'illustré du Genou. Guy Mure, Le Coteau, France, 1982

A graphically illustrated book in French which reflects the immense experience and original thinking of the authors.

Brantigan OC, Voshell AF: The mechanics of the ligaments and menisci of the knee joint. J Bone Joint Surg 23A:44–66, 1941

The old original classic, perhaps outmoded but not to be forgotten. A scholarly piece of work which, for many years, was the cornerstone of our scientific body of knowledge on the anatomy and function of the knee.

Bruser DM: A direct lateral approach to the lateral compartment of the knee joint. J Bone Joint Surg 42B:348–351, 1960

Butler DL, Noyes FR, Grood ES: Ligamentous restraints to anterior-posterior Drawer in the human knee. A biomechanical study. J Bone Joint Surg 62A:259–270, 1980

Concept of secondary restraints about the knee and their interrelations with the ACL—a fundamental concept clearly presented.

Cabaud HE, Chatty A, Gildengorin V, Feltman RJ: Exercise effects on the strength of the rat anterior cruciate ligament. Am J Sports Med 8:79–86, 1980

Cabaud HE, Rodkey WG, Feagin JA: Experimental studies of acute anterior cruciate ligament injury and repair. Am J Sports Med 7:18–22, 1979

In an effort to resolve the failure of primary repair, experimental studies were conducted to evaluate augmented repair as a viable clinical alternative for acute as well as chronic ACL insufficiency.

Cabaud HE, Feagin JA, Rodkey WG: Acute anterior cruciate ligament injury and augmented repair. Experimental studies. Am J Sports Med 8:395–401, 1980

Cabaud HE, Rodkey WG, Fitzwater JE: Medial meniscus repairs. An experimental and morphologic study. Am J Sports Med 9:129–134, 1981

Cabaud HE, Slocum DB: The diagnosis of chronic anterolateral rotatory instability of the knee. Am J Sports Med 5:99–105, 1977

Campbell WC: Reconstruction of the ligaments of the knee. Am J Surg 43:473–480, 1939

Chen EH, Black J: Materials design analysis of the prosthetic anterior cruciate ligament. J Biomed Mater Res 14:567–586, 1980

Chick RR, Jackson DW: Tears of anterior cruciate ligaments in young athletes. J Bone Joint Surg 60A:970–973, 1978

Cho KO: Reconstruction of the anterior cruciate ligament by semitendinosus tenodesis. J Bone Joint Surg 57A:608–612, 1975

Clancy WG Jr, Narechania RG, Rosenberg TD et al: Anterior and posterior cruciate ligament reconstruction in rhesus monkeys. A histological, microangiographic, and biomechanical analysis. J Bone Joint Surg 63A:1270–1284, 1981

Clancy WG Jr, Nelson DA, Reider B, Narechania RG: Anterior cruciate ligament reconstruction using one-third of the patellar ligament, augmented by extra-articular tendon transfers. J Bone Joint Surg 64A:352–359, 1982

Presentation of the basis for the "Clancy Operation" which has become a standard for those who use patellar ligament augmentation surgery.

Clary BB, Couk DE: Experience with the MacIntosh knee prosthesis. South Med J 65:265–272, 1972

Cooper K: The New Aerobics. M Evans, New York, 1970

Collins HR, Hughston JC, DeHaven KE et al: The meniscus as a cruciate ligament substitute. Am J Sports Med 2:11–21, 1974

DeHaven KE, Collins HR: Diagnosis of internal derangements of the knee. The role of arthroscopy. J Bone Joint Surg 57A:802–810, 1975

DeHaven KE: Diagnosis of acute knee injuries with hemarthrosis. Am J Sport Med 8:9–14, 1980

Arthroscopy in the face of hemarthrosis is technically feasible and perhaps should be the standard of care for the high-demand athlete with an unresolved hemarthrosis. The article documents the evidence that the ACL is rarely an isolated lesion.

Dehne E: The spinal adaptation syndrome (a theory based on the study of sprains). Clin Orthop 5:211–219, 1955

Dobner JJ, Nitz AJ: Postmeniscectomy tourniquet palsy and functional sequelae. Am J Sports Med 10:211–214, 1982

Edmonson AS, Crenshaw AH (eds): Campbell's Operative Orthopaedics. 6th Ed. CV Mosby, St Louis, 1980

Eriksson E: Reconstruction of the anterior cruciate ligament. Orthop Clin North Am 7:167–179, 1976

Eriksson E, Häggmark T: Comparison of isometric muscle training and electrical stimulation supplementing isometric muscle training in the recovery after major knee ligament surgery. A preliminary report. Am J Sports Med 7:169–171, 1979

Fairbank TJ: Knee joint changes after meniscectomy. J Bone Joint Surg 30B:664–670, 1948

Feagin JA: The syndrome of the torn anterior cruciate ligament. Orthop Clin North Am 10:81–90, 1979

Summation of a clinician's experience (circa 1979) on

signs and symptoms often associated with instability of the knee.

Feagin JA Jr (ed): The Anterior Cruciate Ligament Deficient Knee (Symposium). Clin Orthop 172:2–163, 1983

Feagin JA, Abbott HG, Rokous JA: The isolated tear of the anterior cruciate ligament (Abstract). J Bone Joint Surg 54A:1340–1341, 1972

Feagin JA, Cabaud HE, Curl WW: The anterior cruciate ligament. Radiographic and clinical signs of successful and unsuccessful repairs. Clin Orthop 164:54–58, 1982

A description of tibial eminence spurring--the earliest radiographic sign of rotatory instability (the Teton sign).

Feagin JA, Curl WW: Isolated tear of the anterior cruciate ligament: 5-year follow-up study. Am J Sports Med 4:95–100, 1976

An acknowledgment that primary repairs of the ACL are not durable in the active patient even though repair is accomplished immediately following acute injury. Deterioration of the knee by reinjury, disruption of secondary restraints, and degenerative arthritis can be expected.

Feagin JA, Lambert KL: Mechanism of injury and pathology of anterior cruciate ligament injuries. Orthop Clin North Am 16:41–46, 1985

Fetto JW, Marshall JL: The natural history and diagnosis of the anterior cruciate ligament insufficiency. Clin Orthop 147:29–38, 1980

Ficat RP, Hungerford DS: Disorders of the Patello-Femoral Joint. Williams & Wilkins, Baltimore, 1977

Finerman G (ed): Symposium on Sports Medicine: the Knee. (Sponsored by the American Academy of Orthopaedic Surgeons, Denver, Colorado, April 1982). CV Mosby, St Louis, 1985

Finochietto R: Semilunar cartilages of the knee. The "jump sign." J Bone Joint Surg 17A:916–21, 1935

Funk JF (ed): Symposium on The Athlete's Knee. Surgical Repair and Reconstruction. (Sponsored by the American Academy of Orthopaedic Surgeons, Hilton Head, South Carolina, June 1978). CV Mosby, St Louis, 1980

Galway RD, Beaupré A, MacIntosh DL: Pivot shift: a clinical sign of symptomatic anterior cruciate insufficiency. (Abstract). J Bone Joint Surg 54B:763–764, 1972

A classic test which helps patient and physician better understand the functional event that was producing the disability.

Galway HR, MacIntosh DL: The lateral pivot shift: a symptom and sign of anterior cruciate ligament insufficiency. Clin Orthop 147:45–50, 1980

Gerber C, Matter P: Biomechanical analysis of the knee after rupture of the anterior cruciate ligament and its primary repair. An instant-centre analysis of function. J Bone Joint Surg 65B:391–399, 1983

Ginsburg JH, Whiteside LA, Piper TL: Nutrient pathways in transferred patellar tendon used for anterior cruciate ligament reconstruction. Am J Sports Med 8:15–18, 1980

Godfrey JD: Ligamentous injuries of the knee. Curr Prac Orthop Surg 5:56–92, 1973

Häggmark T: A study of morphological and enzymatic properties of the skeletal muscles after injuries and immobilization in man. (Doctoral thesis). Karolinska Institute, Stockholm, 1978

Häggmark T, Jansson E, Eriksson E: Time course of muscle metabolic changes during tourniquet ischemia in man. Int J Sport Med 2:50–53, 1981

Hauser ED: Total tendon transplant for slipping patella. A new operation for recurrent dislocation of the patella. Surg Gynecol Obstet 66:199–214, 1938

Hey Groves EW: The crucial ligaments of the knee-joint: their function, rupture, and the operative treatment of the same. Br J Surg 7:505–515, 1920

Hoppenfeld S: Physical Examination of the Spine and Extremities. New York: Appleton & Lange, East Norwalk, CT, 1976

A classic treatise for anyone interested in physical examination. Authored by a great teacher of orthopaedics--a friend and mentor.

Houston CS, Swischuk LE: Varus and valgus — no wonder they are confused. N Engl J Med 302:471–472, 1980

Hughston JC, Andrews JR, Cross MN, Moschi A: Classification of knee ligament instabilities. Part I. The medial compartment and cruciate ligaments. J Bone Joint Surg 58A:159–172, 1976
A two-part summary of a lifetime of experience evolving with a system designed to facilitate understanding and communication about knee instabilities.

Hughston JC, Andrews JR, Cross MJ, Moschi A: Classification of knee ligament instabilities. Part II. The lateral compartment. J Bone Joint Surg 58A:173–179, 1976

Hughston JC, Barrett GR: Acute anteromedial rotatory instability. Long-term results of surgical repair. J Bone Joint Surg 65A:145–152, 1983

Hughston JC, Eilers AF: The role of the posterior oblique ligament in repairs of acute medial (collateral) ligament tears of the knee. J Bone Joint Surg 55A:923–940, 1973
Description of the key role of a little appreciated knee stabilizer—the posterior oblique ligament.

Hughston JC, Jacobson KE: Chronic posterolateral rotatory instability of the knee. J Bone Joint Surg 67A:351–359, 1985

Hunter LY, Funk FJ (eds): Rehabilitation of the Injured Knee. CV Mosby, St Louis, 1984
A multiauthored, multifaceted reference that is valuable when one is designing a knee rehabilitation program.

Hunter GA (ed): Ligamentous Injuries of the Knee (Symposium). Clin Orthop 147:2–93, 1980

Indelicato PA: Non-operative treatment of complete tears of the medial collateral ligament of the knee. J Bone Joint Surg 65A:323–329, 1983

Insall JN (ed.): Surgery of the Knee. Churchill Livingstone, New York, 1984

Insall J, Joseph DM, Aglietti P, Campbell RD Jr: Bone-block iliotibial-band transfer for anterior cruciate ligament insufficiency. J Bone Joint Surg 63A:560–569, 1981

Jacobsen K: Osteoarthrosis following insufficiency in the cruciate ligaments in man. A clinical study. Acta Orthop Scand 48:520–526, 1977

Jacobsen K, Rosenkilde P: A clinical and stress radiographical follow-up investigation after Jones' operation for replacing the anterior cruciate ligament. Injury 8:221–226, 1977

Jakob RP, Hassler H, Staeubli H-U: Observations on rotatory instability of the lateral compartment of the knee. Experimental studies on the functional anatomy and pathomechanism of the true and the reversed pivot shift sign. Acta Orthop Scand 52(Suppl 191):1–32, 1981

James SL, Woods GW, Homsy CA et al: Cruciate ligament stents in reconstruction of the unstable knee. A preliminary report. Clin Orthop 143:90–96, 1979

Johnson RJ, Eriksson E, Häggmark T, Pope MH: Five- to ten-year follow-up evaluation after reconstruction of the anterior cruciate ligament. Clin Orthop 183:122–140, 1984
Probably the best follow-up study of ACL reconstructive surgery in the literature

Jones KG: Reconstruction of the anterior cruciate ligament. A technique using the central one-third of the patellar ligament. J Bone Joint Surg 45A:925–932, 1963
A landmark surgical description.

Jones KG: Reconstruction of the anterior cruciate ligament using the central one-third of the patellar ligament. A follow-up report. J Bone Joint Surg 52:1302–1308, 1970
Follow-up studies a decade later by the originator of the ACL patella tendon augmentation surgery.

Jones KG: Results of use of the central one-third of the patellar ligament to compensate for anterior cruciate ligament deficiency. Clin Orthop 147:39–44, 1980

Joubert G: Teach Yourself to Ski. Trans. S. Thomas. Aspen Ski Masters, Aspen, Colorado. (French original: Pour Apprendre Soi-Même a Skier. Arthaud, France, 1970)

Kaplan EB: The fabellofibular and short lateral ligaments of the knee joint. J Bone Joint Surg 43A:169–179, 1961

Kennedy JC: Complete dislocation of the knee joint. J Bone Joint Surg 45A:889–904, 1963

Kennedy JC (ed): The Injured Adolescent Knee. Williams & Wilkins, Baltimore, 1979

Kennedy JC, Roth JH, Mendenhall HV, Sanford JB: Intraarticular replacement in the anterior cruciate-deficient knee (Presidential address, American Orthopaedic Society for Sports Medicine, 1979). Am J Sports Med 8:1–8, 1980

Kettelkamp DB, Thompson C: Development of a knee scoring scale. Clin Orthop 107:93–99, 1975

Krackow KA, Brooks RL: Optimization of knee ligament position for lateral extraarticular reconstruction. Am J Sports Med 11:293–302, 1983

Lam SJS: Reconstruction of the anterior cruciate ligament using the Jones procedure and its Guy's Hospital modification. J Bone Joint Surg 50A:1213–1224, 1968

Lambert KL: Vascularized patellar tendon graft with rigid internal fixation for anterior cruciate ligament insufficiency. Clin Orthop 172:85–89, 1983
    A technique of fixation which allows early motion, weightbearing, and more vigorous rehabilitation through interference fit fixation of the bone-tendon-bone ACL graft.

Lambert KL: The syndrome of the torn anterior cruciate ligament (Review). Adv Orthop Surg 7:304–314, 1984

Laros GS, Tipton CM, Cooper RR: Influence of physical activity on ligament insertions in the knees of dogs. J Bone Joint Surg 53A:275–286, 1971

Larson RL: Rating sheet for knee function. In: Smillie IS: Diseases of the Knee Joint. Churchill Livingstone, New York 1974, pp 29–30

Larson RL: The knee — the physiological joint (Editorial). J Bone Joint Surg 65A:143–144, 1983

Larson RL, Cabaud HE, Slocum DB et al: The patella compression syndrome. Surgical treatment by lateral retinacular release. Clin Orthop 134:158–167, 1978

Lemaire M, Combelles F: Technique actuelle de plastic ligamentaire pour rupture ancienne du ligament croisé antérieur. (Plastic repair with fascia lata for old tears of the anterior cruciate ligament.) Rev Chir Orthop 66:523–525, 1980

Lipscomb AB, Johnston RK, Snyder RB et al: Evaluation of hamstring strength following use of semitendinosus and gracilis tendons to reconstruct the anterior cruciate ligament. Am J Sports Med 10:340–342, 1982

Losee RE, Johnson TR, Southwick WO: Anterior subluxation of the lateral tibial plateau. A diagnostic test and operative repair. J Bone Joint Surg 60A:1015–1030, 1978
    The best original description of the lateral compartment "event" and an extraarticular tenodesis to prevent the subluxation demonstrable on clinical examination of the knee.

Lynch MA, Henning CE, Glick KR Jr: Knee joint surface changes. Long-term follow-up meniscus tear treatment in stable anterior cruciate ligament reconstructions. Clin Orthop 172:148–153, 1983

Lysholm J, Gillquist J: Evaluation of knee ligament surgery results with special emphasis on use of a scoring scale. Am J Sports Med 10:150–154, 1982

Markolf KL, Mensch JS, Amstutz HC: Stiffness and laxity of the knee — the contributions of the supporting structures. A quantitative in vitro study. J Bone Joint Surg 58A:583–594, 1976

Marshall JL: Periarticular osteophtes. Initiation and formation of the knee of the dog. Clin Orthop 62:37–47, 1969

Marshall JL, Fetto JF, Botero PM: Knee ligament injuries. A standardized evaluation method. Clin Orthop 123:115–129, 1977
    John Marshall brought his veterinary experience and keen clinical and scientific mind to sports medicine. All of his works deserve review. This particular article established a common grading system. Dr. Marshall's death in a plane crash in 1979 was a tragic loss for the academic world of sports medicine.

Marshall JL, Girgis FG, Zelko RR: The biceps femoris tendon and its functional significance. J Bone Joint Surg 54A:1444–1450, 1972

Marshall JL, Warren RF, Wickiewicz TL, Reider B: The anterior cruciate ligament: A technique of repair and reconstruction. Clin Orthop 143:97–106, 1979

Marshall JL, Warren RF, Wickiewicz TL: Primary surgical treatment of anterior cruciate ligament lesions. Am J Sports Med 10:103–107, 1982

Merchant AC, Mercer RL, Jacobsen RH, Cool CR: Roentgenographic analysis of patellofemoral congruence. J Bone Joint Surg 56A:1391–1396, 1974

Mott HW: Semitendinosus anatomic reconstruction for cruciate ligament insufficiency. Clin Orthop 172:90–92, 1983

Müller W: The Knee. Form, Function, and Ligament Reconstruction. Springer-Verlag, New York, 1983
A classic example of clear thinking based on a superb knowledge of anatomy and a vast clinical experience. An essential reference text for any serious student of knee surgery.

Myers MH, McKeever FM: Fracture of the intercondylar eminence of the tibia. J Bone Joint Surg 41A:209–222, 1959

McConkey JP: Anterior cruciate ligament rupture in skiing. A new mechanism of injury. Am J Sports Med 14:160–164, 1986

McDaniel WJ Jr, Dameron TB Jr: Untreated ruptures of the anterior cruciate ligament. A follow-up study. J Bone Joint Surg 62A:696–705, 1980

McIntosh DL, Darby TA: Lateral subsitution reconstruction (Abstract). J Bone joint Surg 58B:142, 1976

MacIntosh DL, Tregonning RJA: A follow-up study and evaluation of "over-the-top" repair of acute tears of the anterior cruciate ligament (Abstract). J Bone Joint Surg 59B:511, 1977

McMaster JH, Weinert CR, Scranton P Jr: Diagnosis and management of isolated anterior cruciate ligament tears. A preliminary report on reconstruction with the gracilis tendon. J Trauma 14:230–235, 1974

Norwood LA, Cross MJ: Anterior cruciate ligament. Functional anatomy of its bundles in rotatory instabilities. Am J Sports Med 7:23–26, 1979

Norwood LA Jr, Cross MJ: The intercondylar shelf and the anterior cruciate ligament. Am J Sports Med 5:171–176, 1977

Noyes FR: Flexion rotation drawer test. As illustrated (Fig. 9-53, p. 924) in Edmonson AS, Crenshaw AA (eds.): Campbell's Operative Orthopaedics, 6th Ed. CV Mosby, St Louis, 1980

Noyes FR: Flexion rotation Drawer test for anterior cruciate insufficiency. As illustrated (Fig. 56-63, p. 2334) in Crenshaw AH (ed.): Campbell's Operative Orthopaedics, 7th Ed. Vol 3. St Louis: CV Mosby, St Louis, 1987

Noyes FR: Functional properties of knee ligaments and alterations induced by immobilization. A correlative biomechanical and histological study in primates. Clin Orthop 123:210–242, 1977

Noyes FR, Bassett RW, Grood ES, Butler DL: Arthroscopy in acute traumatic hemarthrosis of the knee. Incidence of anterior cruciate tears and other injuries. J Bone Joint Surg 62A:687–695, 1980
This article complements the article by DeHaven (1980) and verifies that ACL disruption seldom occurs as an isolated event.

Noyes FR, Butler DL, Grood ES et al: Biomechanical analysis of human ligament grafts used in knee-ligament repairs and reconstructions. J Bone Joint Surg 66A:344–352, 1984

Noyes FR, Butler DL, Paulos LE, Grood ES: Intra-articular cruciate reconstruction. I. Perspectives on graft strength, vascularization, and immediate motion after replacement. Clin Orthop 172:71–77, 1983

Noyes FR, DeLucas JL, Torvik PJ: Biomechanics of anterior cruciate ligament failure: an analysis of strain-rate sensitivity and mechanisms of failure in primates. J Bone Joint Surg 56A:236–253, 1974

Noyes FR, Grood ES: The strength of the anterior cruciate ligament in humans and rhesus monkeys. Age-related and species-related changes. J Bone Joint Surg 58A:1074–1082, 1976

Noyes FR, McGinniss GH, Mooar LA: Functional disability in insufficient knee syndrome. Sports Medicine 1:278–302, 1984

Noyes FR, Mooar PA, Matthews DS, Butler DL: The symptomatic anterior cruciate-deficient knee. Part I. The long-term functional disability in athletically active individuals. J Bone Joint Surg 65A:154–162, 1983

Noyes FR, Matthews DS, Mooar PA, Grood ES: The symptomatic anterior cruciate-deficient knee. Part II. The results of rehabilitation, activity modification, and counseling on functional disability. J Bone Joint Surg 65A:163–174, 1983

This two-part article is particularly useful to the practitioner attempting to understand the ACL syndrome and a rational approach to the nonoperative management of knee ligament injuries. Noyes' scientific contributions to the field of knee ligament surgery are internationally known and respected. All his works should be reviewed.

O'Donoghue DH. Surgical treatment of fresh injuries to the major ligaments of the knee. J Bone Joint Surg 32A:721–738, 1950

The American classic—the recognition of the "unhappy triad" and the plea for primary repair in preference to reconstruction.

O'Donoghue DH. Analysis of end results of surgical treatment of major injuries to the ligaments of the knee. J Bone Joint Surg 37A:1–13, 1955

O'Donoghue DH: Surgical treatment of injuries to ligaments of the knee. JAMA 169:1423–1431, 1959

O'Donoghue DH: A method for replacement of the anterior cruciate ligament of the knee. Report of twenty cases. J Bone Joint Surg 45A:905–924, 1963

O'Donoghue DH: Facetectomy. South Med J 65:645–654, 1972

O'Donoghue DH: Reconstruction for medial instability of the knee. Technique and results in sixty cases. J Bone Joint Surg 55A:941–955, 1973

O'Donoghue DH: Treatment of Injuries to Athletes. 4th Ed. WB Saunders, Philadelphia, 1984

Oretorp N, Gillquist J, Liljedahl S-O: Long term results of surgery for non-acute anteromedial rotatory instability of the knee. Acta Orthop Scand 50:329–336, 1979

Orr W: On the Contributions of Thomas, Jones, and Ridlon to Modern Orthopaedic Surgery. Charles C Thomas, Springfield, Illnois, 1949

Palmer I: On the injuries to the ligaments of the knee joint. A clinical study. Acta Chir Scand 81(Suppl 53):8–282, 1938

A historical classic which reflects the clinical syndrome, natural history, rationale, and results of the surgical approach. A superb work which will probably never be outdated.

Parolie J, Bergfeld JA: Long term results of nonoperative treatment of "isolated" posterior cruciate ligament injuries in the athlete. Am J Sports Med 14:35–38, 1986

Patel D: Proximal approaches to arthroscopic surgery of the knee. Am J Sports Med 9:296–303, 1981

Paulos LE, Butler DL, Noyes FR, Grood ES: Intra-articular cruciate reconstruction. II. Replacement with vascularized patellar tendon. Clin Orthop 172:78–84, 1983

Paulos LE, Noyes FR, Grood E, Butler DL: Knee rehabilitation after anterior cruciate ligament reconstruction and repair. Am J Sports Med 9:140–149, 1981

Pavlov H: The radiographic diagnosis of the anterior cruciate ligament deficient knee. Clin Orthop 172:57–64, 1983

Pridie KH: A method of resurfacing osteoarthritic knee joints (Abstract). J Bone Joint Surg 41B:618–619, 1959

Rockwood CA Jr, Wilkins KE, King RE (eds): Fractures in Children. Vol. 3. Lippincott, Philadelphia, 1984

Roberts JM: Fractures and dislocations of the knee. In Rockwood CA Jr, Wilkins KE, Kings RE (eds): Fractures in Children. Vol. 3. Lippincott, Philadelphia, 1984, pp 940–945

Rorabeck CH, Kennedy JC: Tourniquet-induced nerve ischemia complicating knee ligament surgery. Am J Sports Med 8:98–102, 1980

Rovere GD, Adair DM: Anterior cruciate-deficient knees: A review of the literature. Am J Sports Med 11:412–419, 1983

An excellent review of the literature, amply referenced.

Scapinelli R: Studies on the vasculature of the human knee joint. Acta Anat 70:305–331, 1968

Seebacher JR, Inglis AE, Marshall JL, Warren RF: The structure of the posterolateral aspect of the knee. J Bone Joint Surg 64A:536–541, 1982

Anatomic emphasis on the posterolateral corner of the knee.

Segond P: Recherches cliniques et expérimentales sur les épanchements sanguins du genou par entorse. Progres Med, Paris 7:379–381, 1879

Shands AR: The regeneration of hyaline cartilage in joints. Experimental study. Arch Surg 22:137–178, 1931

Slocum DB, James SL, Larson RL, Singer KM: Clinical test for anterolateral rotatory instability of the knee. Clin Orthop 118:63–69, 1976

Slocum DB, Larson RL: Rotatory instability of the knee. Its pathogenesis and a clinical test to demonstrate its presence. J Bone Joint Surg 50A:211–225, 1968

One of the first to bring to our attention the combined translation and rotation of the knee associated with ligamentous injury. A great contribution. Dr. Slocum was a distinguished gentleman and early leader in the diagnosis and treatment of knee instabilities.

Smillie IS: Diseases of the Knee Joint. Churchill Livingstone, New York, 1974

Southmayd W, Quigley TB: The forgotten popliteus muscle. Its usefulness in correction of anteromedial rotatory instability of the knee. A preliminary report. Clin Orthop 130:218–222, 1978

Steadman JR: Rehabilitation of acute injuries of the anterior cruciate ligament. Clin Orthop 172:129–132, 1983

Swearingen RL, Dehne E: A study of pathological muscle function following injury to a joint (Abstract). J Bone Joint Surg 46A:1364, 1964

Tegner Y, Lysholm J, Gillquist J: Rating systems in the evaluation of knee surgery (Abstract). Acta Orthop Scand 55:111, 1984

Tegner Y. Lysholm J, Nordin M et al: A test for evaluation of knee function (Abstract). Acta Orthop Scand 55:111–112, 1984

Tipton CM, Matthes RD, Maynard JA, Carey RA: The influence of physical activity on ligaments and tendons. Med Sci Sports 7:165–175, 1975

Torg JS, Conrad W, Kalen V: Clinical diagnosis of anterior cruciate ligament instability in the athlete. Am J Sports Med 4:84–93, 1976

Trent PS, Walker PS, Wolf B: Ligament length patterns, strength, and rotational axes of the knee joint. Clin Orthop 117:263–270, 1976

Turner DA, Prodromos CC, Petasnick JP, Clark JW: Acute injury of the ligaments of the knee: magnetic resonance evaluation. Radiology 154:717–722, 1985

Wallis EL, Logan GA: Figure Improvement in Body Conditioning through Exercise. Prentice-Hall, Englewood Cliffs, NJ, 1964

Wang JB, Rubin RM, Marshall JL: A mechanism of isolated anterior cruciate ligament rupture. Case report. J Bone Joint Surg 57A:411–413, 1975

Wang C-J, Walker PS: Rotatory laxity of the human knee joint. J Bone Joint Surg 56A:161–170, 1974

Warren RF: Primary repair of the anterior cruciate ligament. Clin Orthop 172:65–70, 1983

A more optimistic approach to primary repair and a follow-up report on the early work of Marshall.

Warren RF, Levy IM: Meniscal lesions associated with anterior cruciate ligament injury. Clin Orthop 172:32–37, 1983

Wittek A: Zur Naht der Kreuzbandverletzung im Kniegelenk. Zentralbl Chir 54:1538–1541, 1927

Wittek Von A: Kreuzbandersatz aus dem Lig. patellae (nach zur Verth). Schweiz Med Wochenschr 65:103–104, 1935

This surgeon obviously had a wealth of experience in treating knee injuries. We anticipate the day when the language barrier will no longer prevent the sharing of experiences and new techniques which advance the surgical sciences.

Woods GW, Homsy CA, Prewitt JM III, Tullos HS: A Proplast leader for use in cruciate ligament reconstruction. Am J Sports Med 7:314–320, 1979

Yerys P: Anterior cruciate reconstruction. Preliminary report of a new surgical technique. Orthop Rev 10:71–76, 1981

HISTORY
EVOLUTION
EPIDEMIOLOGY

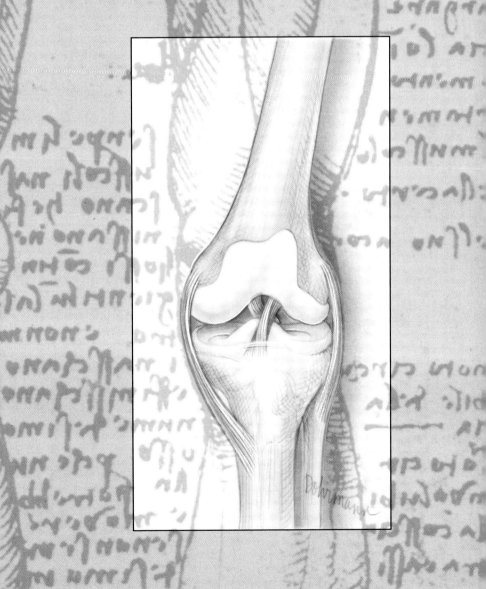

1
The ACL: A Historical Review

GEORGE A. SNOOK

One of the characteristics of modern surgical practice is the delusion that we are the first to present new concepts and treatments to our profession, only to discover upon closer examination that we have "reinvented the wheel." We sometimes forget that all of our accomplishments are only a few stones added to the massive wall of medical knowledge already built by our illustrious medical ancestors. This chapter will therefore serve as an introduction by acknowledging our debt to those practitioners who laid the foundations on which we build today.

Claudius Galen[12] of Pergamum and Rome must be given the credit for first describing the anatomy and nature of the anterior cruciate ligament (ACL). Before his writings, ligaments were thought to be part nerve and to have some sort of contractile power. Galen wrote that ligaments were the supporting structures of diarthrodial joints, serving as stabilizers of these joints and limiting abnormal motion. When discussing the knee he mentions the "genu cruciata."[12]

Interest in this structure lapsed for the next 1600 years as medical attention was drawn to infectious disease and major trauma. The injured ligament was mentioned only in connection with dislocations and severe sprains, and it could always be braced.

To Stark[19] in 1850 must go the distinction of first describing a rupture of the ACL. He treated two patients with casts and with apparent recovery, but he stated that they had slight residual disability.

Battle,[3] in 1900, published the first report of a repair of the ACL, performed 2 years earlier during treatment of a dislocated knee. Mayo Robson,[16] however, in 1903 reported an 8-year followup of a repair of the anterior and posterior cruciate ligaments in a miner injured in an earth fall 36 weeks earlier. His astonishing results revealed that the patient was working in the mine 8 hours a day and walking without a limp. His thigh circumferences were equal, he had full extension, and only slight limitation of flexion. There was no abnormal mobility and only a fine creaking on motion. We have been striving to equal these results ever since.[16]

In 1913 Goetjes[13] produced the first serious study of the ligament when he examined the mechanism of rupture on cadaver studies and accumulated 30 case studies including 7 of his own. He advocated repair of the acute rupture, replacement of the bony fragment rather than excision when avulsed from the tibia, and conservative management in the neglected case. He also recommended examination under anesthesia when the diagnosis was in doubt.[13]

In 1917 Hey Groves[14] published a short case report on the reconstruction of the ACL. He detached a strip of fascia lata from its insertion and routed it through a tibial tunnel. Two years later he presented 14 additional cases after modifying his procedure by detaching the graft from its origin rather than the insertion. This operation is the basis of the intraarticular reconstructions we use today.[15]

Alwyn Smith[1] in 1918 presented an overall review of the anatomy, biomechanics, mechanism of injury, diagnosis, and treatment of injuries to this ligament. He recommended reconstruction of neglected tears and modified Hey Groves's operation by bringing the end of the graft up to the medial femoral condyle to reinforce the medial collateral ligament. He advanced the sartorius insertion to provide extraarticular reinforcement and was the

157

first to attempt prosthetic reconstruction using a silk substitute. The latter operation failed at the 11th week.

The first use of the patellar tendon as a replacement for the ACL was described by Campbell[6,7] in 1936 and again in 1939. He directed the graft through holes in the tibia and the lateral femoral condyle, stating that this procedure was easier and produced less postoperative reaction than the Hey Groves procedure. He also called attention to the frequent association of tears of the ACL, medial collateral ligament, and medial meniscus.[6,7]

The first extraarticular reconstruction of the ACL was described by Bosworth and Bosworth[4] in 1936 using fascia lata grafts woven in a cruciate manner on the medial or lateral side of the knee.

Cubbins and his co-workers,[8] in 1937, summarized their work with a plea for immediate repair of these injuries and for reconstruction of the neglected tear. They also showed that there was a place for nonoperative therapy of dislocations using prolonged immobilization. They warned their readers that repair of this ligament took 1 year for complete recovery.[8]

In 1938, Ivar Palmer published his thesis "On the injuries to the ligaments of the knee joint."[18] In this detailed study of anatomy, biomechanics, pathology, and treatment, he reviewed the current state of the art. He also introduced several new thoughts such as the pathophysiology (biomechanics) of the subsequent changes in the knee joint, and anticipated several concepts in the future treatment of injuries of this ligament, as Eriksson[10] points out.

With the exception of Palmer's thesis, however, study of the ACL was still limited to case reports or descriptions of new surgical procedures. In 1941 this changed with the publication of Brantigan and Voshell's paper "The mechanics of the ligaments and menisci of the knee joint."[5] By thorough and detailed study of sections of different ligaments and analysis of the abnormal movements that resulted, the interaction between the several ligaments and menisci was demonstrated. This paper is usually quoted in any discussion of the biomechanics of the knee joint.[5]

The modern era may be said to begin with O'Donoghue[17] who in 1950 published his results on the treatment of injuries to the major ligaments of the knee in athletes. Although everything he said had already been stated, this paper was nevertheless unique. He presented 22 knee injuries treated by repair of the ligaments involved. In detailed descriptions of history, operative findings, method of repair, postoperative care, rehabilitation and analysis of success or failure, he clearly demonstrated the advantages of early diagnosis and treatment. More importantly, this paper dispelled the previously negative and hopeless attitude toward these injuries.[17] The reasons for this attitude are multiple. At the end of World War II there was a rise in the popularity of athletics. With the development of antibiotics, infectious disease ceased to be a major preoccupation of the medical profession and, at the same time, surgery became safer because of antibiotics and the improvements in anesthesia techniques. Undoubtedly the long successful winning streak of the Oklahoma University football teams also contributed: many of O'Donoghue's patients were from those teams.

Shortly after this, Augustine[2] initiated the concept of dynamic reconstruction of the ACL by transplanting the semitendinosus tendon through the back of the knee forwards into the tibia.

As progress was made in the diagnosis and treatment of injuries of the ACL, simultaneous advances were made in other fields of medicine that had a direct effect upon the study of the ligament. The first of these chronologically was the improvement of radiologic diagnosis, and especially arthrography.[11] In 1905, 10 years after Roentgen announced his discovery, Werndorff and Robinson performed the first arthrogram, a gas arthrogram of the knee. In 1908 Gocht described air contrast studies of the hip and, in 1930, Bricher and Oberholzer wrote of double-contrast arthrography. Lindblom in the late 1930s became the major proponent of arthrograms, but the popularity of the technique did not surge until the development of water-soluble media and the many technical developments in radiography in the late 1950s. While these advances are of extreme importance in the overall improvement in the diagnosis of joint lesions, their use in studies of the ACL is still limited.[11]

Another facet in the progress of treatment of these

injuries came from an entirely different field. Ivar Palmer had already stated that the results of investigations done in the laboratory, while invaluable, were not the final answer. The forces that act on the intact knee in the living human are not the same as those applied in the laboratory, and the cadaver knee is not the same as the living knee. Palmer emphasized that further research was necessary in the analysis of the actual injury at its occurrence. This was an impossibility, as no one could predict when an injury would occur in any particular individual. The problem remained unsolved until a few orthopaedic surgeons started working as physicians for American football teams. Coaches had been using films for scouting and teaching purposes since the early 1930s and, in this high-risk sport, the orthopaedic surgeon could also use them to analyze the mechanics of injury to the intact knee.

The other great advance had its inception in Japan when Professor Kenji Takagi first examined the inside of a knee with a cystoscope in 1918. Subsequent modifications finally resulted in 1931 in a practical arthroscope, and Takagi, Watanabe, Takeda, and Ikeuchi developed the techniques of single puncture and multiple puncture triangulation techniques. The first successful arthroscopic operation was in 1955 when Watanabe removed a benign tumor from a knee under arthroscopic control. With the development of fiberoptic transmission of light the use of arthroscopic surgical techniques increased rapidly and was spearheaded by pioneers such as Ward Casscells, Richard O'Connor, Robert Jackson, Lanny Johnson, Robert Metcalf, and many others.[20] Its importance in the treatment of ACL injuries lies in its use in early diagnosis. DeHaven[9] recommended the early use of the arthroscope in the acutely injured knee even in the presence of hemarthrosis. This procedure has led to early diagnosis and repair of these injuries, thus sparing the patient the more difficult reconstruction with its prolonged recovery.

Detailed studies of the cruciate ligaments have been performed to analyze the anatomy, function, biomechanics, and treatment. To list them all in this short introduction is impossible Descriptions of many of these studies can be found in other chapters in this book. The contributors to these chapters are leaders in current research on the cruciate ligaments.

REFERENCES

1. Alwyn Smith S; The diagnosis and treatment of injuries to the crucial ligaments. Br J Surg 6:176–189, 1918
2. Augustine RW: The unstable knee. Am J Surg 92:380–388, 1956
3. Battle WH: A case after open section of the knee joint for irreducible traumatic dislocation. Clin Soc London Trans 33:232–233, 1900
4. Bosworth DM, Bosworth BM: Use of fascia lata to stabilize the knee in cases of ruptured crucial ligaments. J Bone Joint Surg 18A:178–179, 1936
5. Brantigan OC, Voshell AF: The mechanics of the ligaments and menisci of the knee joint. J Bone Joint Surg 23:44–66, 1941
6. Campbell WC: Repair of the ligaments of the knee joint. Surg Gynecol Obstet 62:964–968, 1936
7. Campbell WC: Reconstruction of the ligaments of the knee. Am J Surg 43:473–480, 1939
8. Cubbins WR, Callahan JJ, Scuderi CS: Cruciate ligament injuries. Surg Gynecol Obstet 64:218–225, 1937
9. DeHaven KE: Diagnosis of acute knee injuries with hemarthrosis. Am J Sports Med 8:9–14, 1980
10. Eriksson E: Ivar Palmer. A great name in the history of cruciate ligament surgery. Clin Orthop 172:3–10, 1983
11. Freiberger RH, Kaye JJ, Spiller J: Arthrography. Appleton-Century-Crofts, New York, 1979
12. Galen C: On the Usefulness of the Parts of the Body. May MT (trans). Cornell University Press, Ithaca, New York, 1968
13. Goetjes H: Uber verletzungen der ligamenta cruciata des kniegelenks. Dtsch Z Chir 123:221-289, 1913
14. Hey Groves EW: Operation for the repair of the crucial ligaments. Lancet 2:674–675, 1917
15. Hey Groves EW: The crucial ligaments of the knee joint. Their function, rupture, and the operative treatment of the same. Br J Surg 7:505–515, 1919
16. Mayo Robson AW: Ruptured crucial ligaments and their repair by operation. Ann Surg 37:716–718, 1903
17. O'Donoghue DH: Surgical treatment of fresh injuries to the major ligaments of the knee. J Bone Joint Surg 32A:721–738, 1950

18. Palmer I: On the injuries to the ligaments of the knee joint. A clinical study. Acta Chir Scand 81(Suppl 53):2–282, 1938
19. Stark J: Two cases of ruptured crucial ligaments of the knee-joint. Edinburgh Med Surg 74:267–271, 1850
20. Watanabe M, Bechtol RC, Nottage WM: pp. 1–6. In Shahriaree H (ed): O'Connor's Textbook of Arthroscopic Surgery. JB Lippincott, Philadelphia, 1984

2

An Evolutionary Perspective

SCOTT F. DYE

As orthopaedic surgeons, we are of necessity students of human anatomy. The knee, being the largest and most intricate of human joints, presents perhaps the greatest challenge to our ability to comprehend articular structure and function. In the human knee one finds an extremely complex biomechanical system with many asymmetries of design.

A biomechanical system as complex as the human knee may be easier to understand if it is compared to the homologous structure of other animals. Sterling Bunnell[3] studied the evolution and comparative anatomy of the upper extremity and believed that the knowledge gained from an understanding of functional morphology would benefit his clinical practice of hand surgery. Perhaps, following Bunnell's example, knee surgeons could benefit from studies in comparative anatomy and evolution of the knee. Not only could we gain an aesthetic appreciation of the complex biomechanics of the knee, but also the findings might have a practical impact on our clinical approaches to knee problems. It would be helpful to discover more adequate animal models for our studies of the knee and its mechanisms. If comparative morphologic studies can help us to determine the commonality and significance of various structures of the knee, we may be able to gain insights that could be translated into better ligamentous reconstructions and total knee prosthesis designs applicable to our clinical practice.

Although several orthopaedic surgeons[2,5,9] have attempted to examine the evolution and comparative morphology of the knee joint, the best works on this topic have been produced by paleontologists and anatomists,[4,7,8,17,18] not orthopaedists. Some of the finest work was accomplished by Haines,[8] an English anatomist who described comparative knee transections of various species. However, he did not emphasize collateral ligament placement or functional morphology. Information from the current orthopaedic, paleontologic, and zoologic literature on knee function has not been synthesized.

This chapter attempts to provide an overview of the main evolutionary developments of the knee and, through the presentation of comparative functional morphologic data, to put these developments into perspective with the modern human joint.[6a]

APPROACHES TO PHYLOGENETIC STUDIES OF THE KNEE

When scientists attempt to discover answers to questions about phylogenetics and evolution of the knee, two basic approaches to the topic are often used. One approach involves examination of fossil femora, tibiae, fibulae, and footprints of extinct species, and the other involves examination of the knee structure and function of extant species.

Fossil femora, tibiae, and fibulae of representative extinct species were examined in conjunction with the vertebrate paleontology departments of the American Museum of Natural History, New York; the Museum of Comparative Zoology, at Harvard;

This paper was presented in part at the Fourth Congress of the International Society of the Knee, Salzburg, Austria, May 12–17, 1985.

and the California Academy of Sciences, San Francisco. Together with colleagues, I dissected the knees of representative extant tetrapod species, in conjunction with the California Academy of Sciences and the School of Veterinary Medicine, Auburn University, Auburn, Alabama (1983 to 1986).

How similar in design and function is the human knee to that of the first proximal joint of the hind limb of other species? At first glance it may appear that the knees of some animals differ markedly in structure and function from the human knee. For example, it is a common impression that the "knees" of birds flex backwards, that is, with the apex oriented posterior to the line of progression (Fig. 2-1). One may assume therefore, that the "knees" of birds are as different morphologically from the analogous human structure as the feet of birds are different from human feet. In fact, this assumption is not accurate, for in many respects human and the true avian knee are similar in both structure and function. The avian joint that looks like a "backwards knee" is in reality the ankle joint, with the actual knee (oriented apex anterior) usually well hidden under the wings (Fig. 2-1).

The knee of a chicken (*Gallus domesticus*), for example, has several striking similarities to the human joint, including a bicondylar cam-shaped distal femur, relatively flat tibial plateaus, the presence of a patella, intraarticular cruciate ligaments and menisci, a broad, flat medial collateral ligament, and a pencil-shaped lateral collateral ligament (Fig. 2-2). There are also morphologic differences; for example, the chicken knee has a femorofibular articulation and extensor digitorum longus originating on the lateral femoral condyle.

The commonality of anatomic characteristics between avian and human knees, while seemingly little else in their morphology is similar, raises many questions. Are these shared characteristics indicative of a common ancestor in the remote past, or were they derived independently? If humans and birds did share a common ancestor with similar characteristics, how long ago did such an animal exist? How similar in structure and function are the knees of humans and birds compared to other animals with hind limbs? If structural and functional similarities can be established between the knees of different orders of tetrapods, and in light of the often distant phylogenetic relationships and widely varying biomechanical demands, why should this be? The answers to these questions may provide some insight into the antiquity and adaptability of design of this unique joint.

PALEONTOLOGY

Based on examinations and other paleontologic evidence,[1,6,7,10,12,14,16-18] a summary of the major osseous developments of the knee is provided, as well as an overview of the phylogenetic relationships of extant tetrapod orders.

The osteology of the hind limb of all extant tetrapods can be traced back to analogous structures of the pelvic fins of extinct sarcopterygian lobe-finned fishes of the early Devonian period, approximately 370 million years ago (Fig. 2-3). Recent analysis of fossil data indicates that perhaps ancient dipnoans, ancestors of modern Australian lungfish, were the actual progenitors of all living tetrapods.[19]

The earliest evidence for ambulation with limbs comes not from fossil femora or tibiae but from the fossilized footprints left in mud by an early tetrapod.[14] The earliest osseous evidence of weightbearing hind limbs comes from the extinct amphibian

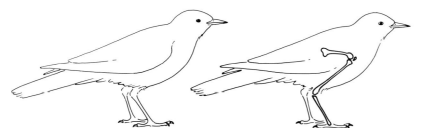

Fig. 2-1. Schematic representation of avian morphology demonstrates the knee well hidden under the wings and oriented with the apex anterior. (Dye SF: An evolutionary perspective of the knee. J Bone Joint Surg (A), in press, 1987.)

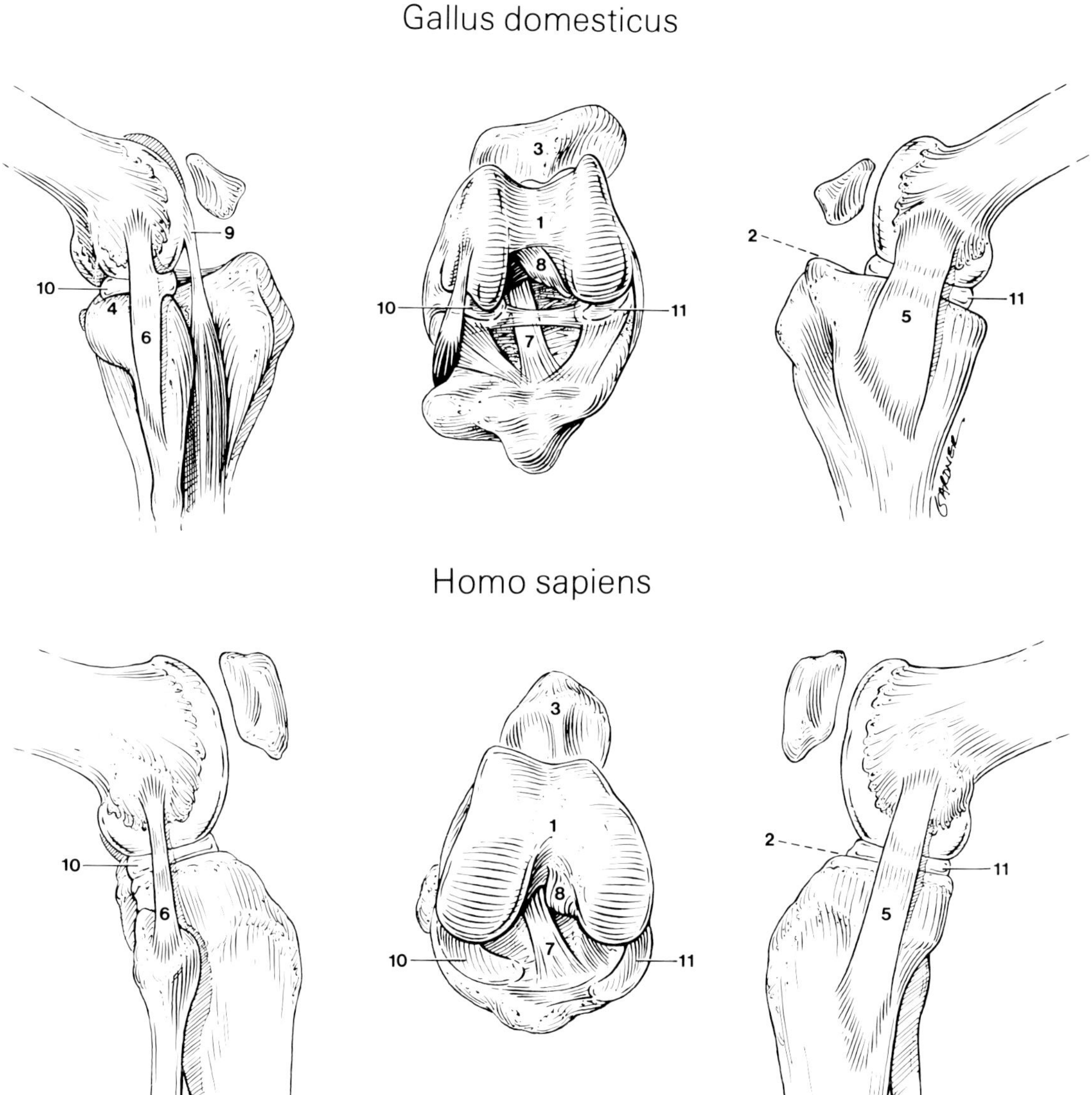

Fig. 2-2. Comparative knee morphology of *Gallus domesticus* and *Homo sapiens*. *1*, Bicondylar cam-shaped distal femur; *2*, flat tibial plateaus; *3*, osseous patella; *4*, fibular articulation with lateral femoral condyle; *5*, flat medial collateral ligament with distal tibial insertion; *6*, cord-shaped lateral collateral ligament; *7*, anterior cruciate ligament; *8*, posterior cruciate ligament; *9*, origin of extensor digitorum longus from lateral femoral condyle; *10*, lateral meniscus; *11*, medial meniscus. (Dye SF: An evolutionary perspective of the knee. J Bone Joint Surg (A), in press, 1987.)

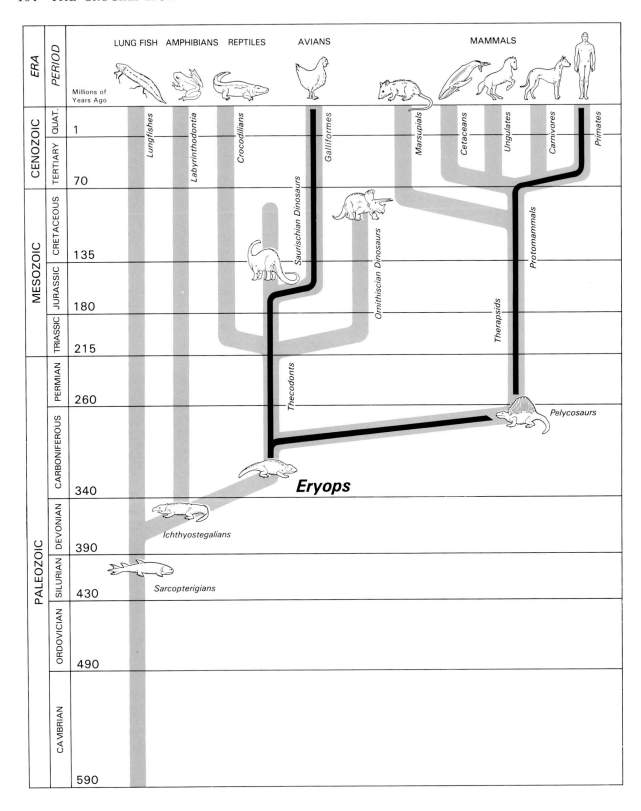

Eryops

Ichthyostega.[11] Even at this extremely early date in tetrapod evolution, approximately 360 million years ago, not only are femur, tibia, and fibula present and distinct, but the distal end of the femur already exhibited a bicondylar shape (Fig. 2-4). The proximal tibia was relatively flat and articulated with both condyles of the femur. The postaxial condyle of the femur (lateral femoral condyle analogue) also articulated with the proximal fibula. This fibular articulation with the femur is retained in the knees of reptiles, birds, and some primitive mammals. Apparently the femora of these ancient amphibians extended nearly perpendicular from the body, and thus *Ichthyostega* had the sprawling gait with flexed knees characteristic of the early land forms.

Approximately 350 million years ago the ichthyostegalians evolved into two main lineages: one (the labyrinthodonts) leading to modern amphibians such as the frog, and the other leading to the development of an amphibian species, *Eryops*. The lines leading to modern mammals and amphibians is presumably a genetic separation for at least 350 million years.

Eryops is considered of great importance by vertebrate paleontologists, since it is believed to represent the common ancestor of all living reptiles, birds, and mammals.[8,14,18] This species had a well-developed bicondylar distal femur with an increasing radius of curvature, a relatively flat tibia, and the primitive characteristic of fibular articulation with the femur. In his classic article on the evolution of the tetrapod limb, Haines[8] provides an elaborate reconstruction of the ligaments of *Eryops'* knee, including the presence of cruciate ligaments, asymmetrical collateral ligaments, and menisci (Fig. 2-5). Although the actual fossil evidence for this reconstruction is tenuous, the commonality of shared characteristics in the knees of most living tetrapods supports this conclusion.

By the early Mesozoic era, 215 million years ago, the lineages ancestral to living frogs (labyrintho-

donts), alligators and birds (thecodonts), and mammals (therapsids) were separate. The line leading to mammals branched off from that leading to reptiles and birds approximately 320 million years ago. Thus humans and chickens are separated by no less than 320 million years (Fig. 2-3).

Three major osteologic developments occurred about the knee during the Mesozoic (215 to 70 million years ago). By the Jurassic period (180 million years ago) most major orders of tetrapods had evolved a medial offset of the femoral head and internal rotation of the femur, which allowed the knee to be oriented with the apex anterior. This development resulted in a more efficient gait by bringing the limbs closer to the midline.

During the later Mesozoic, the fibular head of most protomammals ancestral to modern eutherian mammals receded to a point distal to the joint line, and thus the knees of most extant mammals (except some marsupials) do not exhibit the primitive characteristic of fibular articulation with the femur. The last major osteologic development of the knee was the independent development of an osseous patella in birds, some reptiles (lizards), and mammals, which apparently occurred approximately 65 to 70 million years ago.

COMPARATIVE ANATOMY

Paleontologists and zoologists consider modern amphibians degenerate in many aspects of their anatomy. Therefore, their knee morphology probably is not representative of the earliest amphibians. However, the knee of a frog (*Rana tigerinus*) does exhibit many similarities to the human knee. The femorotibial articulation has both internal and external ligamentous connections. In larger species, medial and lateral menisci are present. The single broad intraarticular ligament may represent the initial form of the protocruciate ligaments of extinct

Fig. 2-3. Schematic representation of the phylogenetic relationships of the major classes of tetrapods demonstrating *Eryops* as a common ancestor to living reptiles, birds, and mammals. (Dye SF: An evolutionary perspective of the knee. J Bone Joint Surg (A), in press, 1987. Adapted from Mossman DJ, Sarjeant WA: The footprints of extinct animals. Sci Am 250:75–85, 1983. Copyright © 1983 by Scientific American, Inc. All rights reserved.)

Ichthyostega

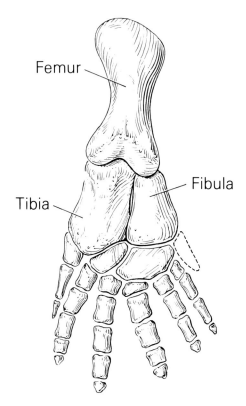

Fig. 2-4. Anterior view of the left knee of *Ichthyostega*—the oldest known knee from the fossil record—demonstrating a bicondylar distal femur and femorofibular articulation. (Dye SF: An evolutionary perspective of the knee. J Bone Joint Surg (A), in press, 1987. Adapted from Jarvik E: Basic Structure and Evolution of Vertebrates. Academic Press, Orlando, FL, 1980–81.)

amphibians. The medial collateral ligament is relatively broad and inserts distally on the proximal tibia, with the lateral collateral analogue being more rounded in cross-section and inserting on the proximal lateral tibia (the fibula having merged with the tibia through evolution). There is an analogous pes anserinus expansion, with insertion distally on the medial aspect of the proximal tibia anterior to the medial collateral ligament, that has a remarkable similarity to the human structure.

What is striking about the frog's knee (Fig. 2-6A), and indeed all the knees we have dissected to date (Fig. 2-6B – F), is that the *functional* dynamics appear similar. These knees have a complex rolling and gliding motion of the femur on the tibia, with the point of contact of the femur moving posteriorly on the tibia with flexion similar to a four-bar linkage system, as described by Müller (Fig. 2-7).[15]

The knee of a living reptile, the alligator, has closer similarity to the human knee than that of the frog. This species has a bicondylar distal femur, relatively flat tibial plateaus, asymmetrical medial and lateral collateral ligaments, and well-formed menisci.

The knee of the modern alligator (*Alligator mississippiensis*) also has three cruciate ligaments: an anterior and posterior cruciate ligament with origins and insertions similar to those in the human knee, and a smaller anterior cruciate ligament situated medial to the posterior cruciate. This tripartite division of cruciate ligaments, which is thought to be associated with the need for rotatory stability, may represent a developmental stage beyond the single broad intraarticular ligament of amphibians. The familiar morphology of two cruciate ligaments seen in birds and mammals thus may have been derived independently during the Mesozoic by regression of the smaller medial anterior cruciate.

The medial collateral ligament of the alligator is flat, broad, and inserts distally on the proximal tibia, as in the human knee. The lateral collateral ligament is round in cross-section and pencil-shaped; it inserts on the head of the fibula, which articulates with the lateral femoral condyle. There is a distinct analogue to the ligament of Wrisberg arising from the posterior horn of the lateral meniscus. This structure is also seen in turtles. In addition, the extensor digitorum longus has its origin on the lateral femoral condyle; this ancient characteristic is retained in the knees of most living tetrapods, including most mammals. The functional morphology (Fig. 2-6B) appears to follow closely the complex rolling and gliding motion of a four-bar linkage as described by Müller.[15]

The morphology of the chicken's knee (*Gallus domesticus*), which initially stimulated our interest in this topic, revealed all the similar characteristics found in the alligator except that it has two cruciate ligaments and no analogue to the ligament of Wrisberg. The functional dynamics of the chicken knee

Fig. 2-5. Soft tissue construction of the right knee of *Eryops,* an extinct amphibian ancestral to living reptiles, birds, and mammals. (Dye SF: An evolutionary perspective of the knee. J Bone Joint Surg (A), in press, 1987. Adapted from Haines RW: The tetrapod knee joint. J Anat 76:270–301, 1942. Cambridge University Press. © Anatomical Society of Great Britain and Ireland. Reprinted with the permission of Cambridge University Press.)

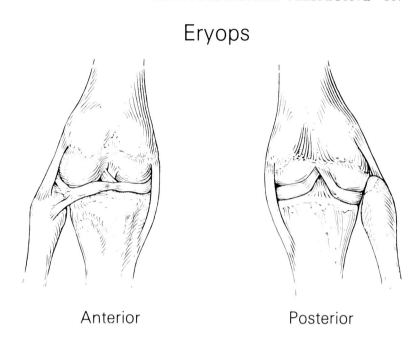

Eryops

Anterior   Posterior

follow the same pattern of a four-bar linkage system, with the femorotibial contact point moving posteriorly in flexion (Fig. 2-6C). In addition, the chicken has a combined motion of internal rotation of the tibia on the femur with flexion, a characteristic also found to some degree in the alligator and well developed in most mammals.

The overall design of most mammalian knees can be classified into three broad categories based on the form of the pes:[20] unguligrade (*ungulus,* Latin for hoof), digitigrade, and plantigrade (Fig. 2-8). The unguligrade knee (e.g., pig, horse, sheep) lacks full extension in the human sense and, therefore, is permanently loaded in flexion. Such knees have separate patellofemoral and femorotibial articulations. The digitigrade knee (e.g., carnivores such as the dog and cat) can be nearly fully extended but is functionally loaded most frequently in flexion and has a narrow confluence of the trochlea with the femoral condyles. The plantigrade knee (e.g., human, bear) is functionally loaded in full extension during portions of the gait cycle and in stance. This type of knee has a broad confluence of the trochlea with the femoral condyles.

The sheep (*Ovis aries*) is an excellent example of typical ungulate knee morphology (Fig. 2-6D). This

knee (which can be easily obtained within a "leg of lamb" from a butcher) has all the soft tissue components with which we are familiar in the human knee, including well-developed cruciate ligaments and menisci, asymmetrical collateral ligaments, and the insertion of the popliteus on the lateral femoral condyle. A significant anatomic difference is the origin of the common extensor on the lateral femoral condyle with the tendon crossing the knee. The functional morphology is similar to that of the human knee: there is a differentially greater roll-back of the femorotibial contact point of the lateral compartment (including the posterior translation of a highly mobile lateral meniscus) compared to that of the relatively stable medial compartment. The automatic internal rotation of the tibia on the femur in flexion is a manifestation of this differential motion.

A typical example of digitigrade knee morphology is found in the dog (*Canis familiaris*). The knee structure has all the soft tissue components found in ungulates including origin of the long extensor on the lateral femoral condyle. The functional morphology differs from ungulates (and humans) in that there is nearly equal roll-back of the femur on the tibia in both lateral and medial compartments

Frog

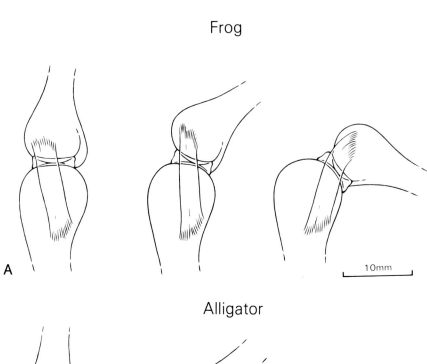

A

10mm

Alligator

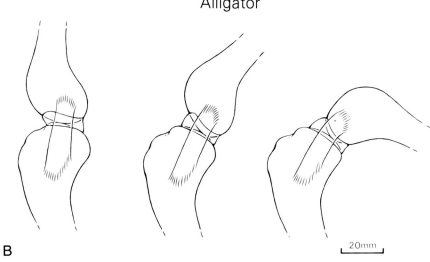

B

20mm

Chicken

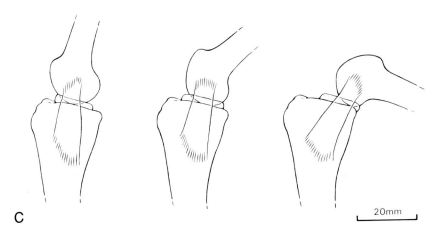

C

20mm

Fig. 2-6. Medial projections of the right knee of representative tetrapods demonstrating similarity of static anatomy and posterior rolling–gliding motion of the femur on the tibia. Illustrations are based on original dissections and video studies. **(A)** Frog *(Rana tigerinus)*. **(B)** Alligator *(Alligator mississippiensis)*. **(C)** Chicken *(Gallus domesticus)*. *(Figure continues.)*

Fig. 2-6 *(Continued).* **(D)** Sheep *(Ovis aries).* **(E)** Dog *(Canis familiaris).* **(F)** Human *(Homo sapiens).* (A, D, F from Dye SF: An evolutionary perspective of the knee. J Bone Joint Surg (A), in press, 1987.)

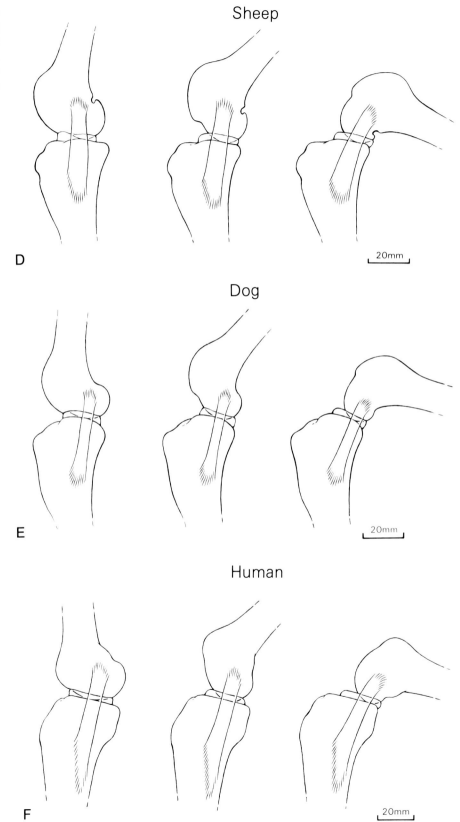

Sheep

D

20mm

Dog

E

20mm

Human

F

20mm

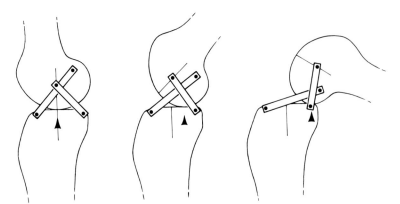

Fig. 2-7. Schematic representation of the knee as a four-bar linkage system demonstrating posterior displacement of the femorotibial contact point with flexion (Dye SF: An evolutionary perspective of the knee. J Bone Joint Surg (A), in press, 1987. Adapted from Müller W: The knee: Form, Function, and Ligament Reconstruction. Springer-Verlag, New York, 1983.)

(Fig. 2-6E). The posterior aspect of the medial tibial plateau slopes inferiorly almost as much as the lateral tibial plateau and thus allows a significant posterior displacement of the medial meniscus in flexion. This aspect of the functional morphology of the canine knee should be considered when one is using such an animal model.

The human knee (*Homo sapiens*) is an example of plantigrade morphology. The extensor digitorum longus does not cross the knee joint but has its origin off the proximal tibia. There are well-formed menisci and cruciate ligaments, as well as asymmetrical collateral ligaments. The functional morphology of the medial as compared with the lateral compartment exhibits a differentially greater roll-back laterally than in the ungulates.

COMMENTS

As shown in Table 2-1, one can compare the similarity of knee characteristics among the major categories of living tetrapods. If the commonality of characteristics from diverse orders of animals is accepted, what can be said from an evolutionary perspective regarding the development and significance of the knee joint?

It seems certain that the complex set of attributes we associate with "kneeness"—bicondylar distal femur, intraarticular cruciate ligaments, menisci, asymmetrical collateral ligaments, and other components—has an extremely ancient origin. The major osteologic and soft tissue components of the knee were probably well-developed by the time of *Eryops* (320 million years ago), a species representing the ancestor of reptiles, birds, and mammals. The *functional* morphology manifested by these sets of shared anatomic characteristics appears to approximate a four-bar linkage system as elucidated by Müller (Fig. 2-7).[15]

The general structural and functional similarity of the knees of diverse orders of animals implies that the knee is a special and profoundly adaptive biomechanical system unique among tetrapod joints. This observation has more impact when one real-

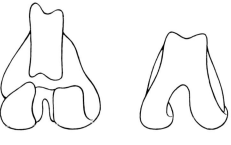
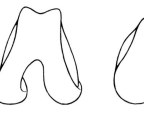
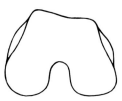

Unguligrade   Digitigrade   Plantigrade

Fig. 2-8. Representations of the distal femoral articular surfaces of unguligrade, digitigrade, and plantigrade mammals. (Dye SF: An evolutionary perspective of the knee. J Bone Joint Surg (A), in press, 1987. Adapted from Tardieu C: Morpho-functional analysis of the articular surfaces of the knee-joint in primates. In Chiarelli G (ed): Primate Evolutionary Biology. Springer-Verlag, New York, 1981.)

Table 2-1. Interspecies Comparison of Knee Characteristics

	Amphibians (frog)	Reptiles (alligator)	Avians (chicken)	Mammals Unguligrade (sheep)	Digitigrade (dog)	Plantigrade (humans)
Osseous Characteristics						
Bicondylar distal femur	Yes	Yes	Yes	Yes	Yes	Yes
Tibial plateaus	Yes	Yes	Yes	Yes	Yes	Yes
Femorofibular articulation	N/A	Yes	Yes	No	No	No
Osseous patella	No	Only in lizards	Yes	Yes	Yes	Yes
Soft Tissue Characteristics						
Flat MCL with distal insertion on the tibia	Yes	Yes	Yes	Yes	Yes	Yes
Cord-shaped LCL	Yes	Yes	Yes	Yes	Yes	Yes
Pes anserinus insertion on proximal tibia anterior to MCL	Yes	Yes	Yes	Yes	Yes	Yes
Menisci	Yes	Yes	Yes	Yes	Yes	Yes
Intraarticular ligaments	Yes	Yes	Yes	Yes	Yes	Yes
Ligament of Wrisberg analogue	No	Yes	No	Yes	Yes	Yes
Origin of long extensor off the lateral femoral condyle	Yes	Yes	Yes	Yes	Yes	No
Popliteus insertion on the lateral femoral condyle	No	No	No	Yes	Yes	Yes
Functional Characteristics						
Posterior femorotibial contact with flexion	Yes	Yes	Yes	Yes	Yes	Yes
Internal rotation of tibia with flexion	No	Yes	Yes	Yes	Yes	Yes

izes that it has taken less than 50 million years for cetaceans to lose almost all remnants of the hind limbs of their terrestrial ancestors.

ORTHOPAEDIC IMPLICATIONS

What are the implications of these data for orthopaedic surgeons, beyond an enhanced aesthetic appreciation of the knee? Despite the overall similarity of tetrapod knee design, differences exist between the human knee and those of commonly used animal models. For instance, dogs are digitigrade with a functional quadruped gait, and their knees are habitually loaded in flexion. Humans belong to the only known species that is both plantigrade (knees habitually loaded in extension) and functionally bipedal. We should be cognizant of such inherent dissimilarities in interpreting data from animal model studies. There is probably no ideal animal model for the human knee, but it seems possible that with

further comparative morphologic research an animal may be discovered (perhaps a small ursine species?) that will prove to be a functional morphologic improvement over currently used species.

The commonality of retained morphologic characteristics of the knee over eons implies that each anatomic component of this complex biomechanical system is needed for proper functioning of the whole system. (Parts that are not functional are not retained; e.g., whales have almost no remnants of hind limbs). Robert Larson,[13] in characterizing the knee as "The physiological joint," has described this concept exquisitely. Therefore, as orthopaedists we may not be able, with impunity, to modify surgically (through ligamentous reconstructions) or substitute (with total knee replacements) for knee morphology and expect our work to result in normal or near-normal function.

Through examination of the functional morphology of nonhuman knees, one realizes that a differential roll-back of the femur on the tibia greater in the lateral compartment than in the medial compartment is a common characteristic. This is also a well-established characteristic of the human knee, yet no external bracing system exists to incorporate this concept. Bracing systems with the same hinge design both medially and laterally are not capable of following the complex motion of the human knee. It seems clear that future improvements in knee brace design should include a differential medial and lateral hinge to allow for the normal asymmetrical physiological motion of the knee without undue stress on the ligaments. Taking into account such functional characteristics of normal knee morphology may also be of value in the future design of improved total knee replacement systems.

CONCLUSIONS

The human knee is the result of nearly 400 million years of tetrapod evolution. In this articulation we share a common musculoskeletal heritage with most living orders of terrestrial vertebrates. From an evolutionary perspective, we are beginning to appreciate the significance of the complex components of this unique joint.

Many questions regarding the knee remain unanswered. For example, what are the particular characteristics of a four-bar linkage system that have proven so advantageous to knee design? To what extent can these characteristics be modified and still result in acceptable function? Future investigations in this area will provide insights into functional knee morphology that may have a positive impact on the treatment of knee conditions.

REFERENCES

1. Barnett CH, Napier JR: The rotatory mobility of the fibula in eutherian mammals. J Anat 87:11–21, 1953
2. Brantigan OC, Voshell AF: The relationship of the ligament of Humphry to the ligament of Wrisberg. J Bone Joint Surg 28A:66–67, 1946
3. Bunnell S: Surgery of the Hand. JB Lippincott, Philadelphia, 1944
4. Craycraft J: The functional morphology of the hind limb of the domestic pigeon, *Columba livia*. Bull Am Mus Nat Hist: 144:173–268, 1971
5. DePalma AF: Diseases of the Knee. JB Lippincott, Philadelphia, 1955
6. Fox RC, Bowman MC: Osteology in relationships of *Captorhinus aguti* (Cope) (Reptilia: Captorhinomorpha). Vertebrata: 1–79, 1966
6a. Dye SF: An evolutionary perspective of the knee. J Bone Joint Surg (A), in press, 1987
7. Goodrich ES: Studies on the Structure and Development of the Vertebrates, Vol I and II. Dover Publications, New York, 1958
8. Haines RW: The tetrapod knee joint. J Anat 76:270–301, 1942
9. Herzmark MH: The evolution of the knee joint. J Bone Joint Surg 20:77–84, 1938
10. Howell AB: Speed in Animals. Hafner Publications, New York, 1942
11. Jarvik E: Basic Structure and Evolution of Vertebrates. Academic Press, Orlando, FL, 1980–81
12. Kemp TS: Mammal-Like Reptiles and the Origin of Mammals. Academic Press, London, 1982
13. Larson R: The knee—The physiological joint. Editorial. J Bone Joint Surg 65A:143–144, 1983
14. Mossman DJ, Sargeant WA: The footprints of extinct animals. Sci Am 250:75–85, 1983
15. Müller W: The Knee. Form, Function, and Ligament Reconstruction. Springer-Verlag, New York, 1983
16. Romer AS: Osteology of the Reptiles. University of Chicago Press, Chicago, 1956
17. Romer AS: The Vertebrate Body. WB Saunders, Philadelphia, 1963
18. Romer AS: The Procession of Life. Universe Books, New York, 1968
19. Rosen DE, Forey PL, Patterson C: Lungfishes, tetrapods, paleontology, and plesiomorphy. Bull Am Anat Hist 167:156–276, 1981
20. Tardieu C: Morpho-functional analysis of the articular surfaces of the knee-joint in primates. In Chiarelli G (ed): Primate Evolutionary Biology. Springer-Verlag, Berlin, 1981

3
Epidemiology of the ACL

JAMES G. GARRICK

Epidemiology is generally used in sports medicine as a means of identifying and describing the circumstances surrounding an injury. Although interesting from an esoteric perspective, the ultimate goal of such a study method is the manipulation of those circumstances to provide a greater degree of safety. The role of epidemiology is equally important in describing the conditions associated with reinjury. Because the primary goal of any treatment is the prevention of reinjuries, epidemiologic techniques are the means by which we evaluate the efficacy of treatment.

In theory, the investigation of diseases — injuries, in this instance — should be relatively straightforward in the athletic environment. Athletes enter the sport milieu healthy. Their level of fitness and the residuals of other injuries are measured and recorded. Their athletic activities are often carefully monitored, sometimes even filmed. A sophisticated level of medical care, offering the potential of providing early, precise diagnoses, is frequently readily available. Why then, is there such a paucity of epidemiologic information on anterior cruciate ligament (ACL) injuries? Perhaps more important, why is the treatment of this injury so controversial?

Part of the answer is quite simple: we have virtually no idea of the frequency of ACL injury. Without this basic information it is impossible to characterize a "natural history" of the injury, and without knowledge of the outcome of an untreated injury there is nothing with which to compare the results of treatment.

The major deterrent to establishing a natural history is the unreported injury. Cases are "lost" (unreported) at many points in the chain of events between the occurrence and treatment of the injury. Each time a case is lost, the remaining group of "found" cases becomes less representative of all ACL injuries. Given the fact that one chooses a regimen of management based on the results of a particular treatment in a group of patients, it is important to know what that group represents or who is in the group. Understanding the biases associated with the creation of the group allows one to place the results in proper perspective.

PERCEPTION OF THE INJURY

For an injury to be counted in an epidemiologic sense, the occurrence must be perceived as an injury, first by the patient and later by the physician.

Although virtually all athletes experiencing ACL injury realize that "something happened to the knee," its significance is perceived in a variety of ways. In a recent chart review of ACL sprains in skiers, we found that nearly half had skied off the slope under their own power without aid or notification of the ski patrol. Those who presented to us for medical care did so from 6 hours to 6 months after the injury. Although competent medical care was readily available, in many instances the injury was perceived as being not serious enough to require assistance.

Those skiers, all with clinical evidence of anterior instability, represent two obviously distinct groups: those who perceived themselves as being immediately disabled and required assistance getting off the slope, and those who lacked this perception until sometime later. Unfortunately, in an epidemiologic sense, a third group exists: those with the same injury who have not perceived themselves as being injured.

The severity of the injury plays a major role in how it is perceived. Generally injuries involving more than one structure are considered more severe. Thus injuries involving tears of the menisci or other ligaments are more likely to receive immediate care. Injuries involving multiple structures are also more likely to arise in certain sports, often involving different mechanisms of injury. For example, in the Hughston-Barrett series,[4] most ACL injuries with associated anteromedial instability were the result of "contact."

Thus, a study of a group of patients presenting for treatment immediately after injury may be biased toward involvement of multiple structures, and this group in turn may be biased toward contact injuries.

The duration of symptoms and the presence of recurrent injuries also push the patient toward seeking medical assistance. A patient with symptoms that interfere with the activities of daily living probably will seek assistance. Even these individuals do not seek care immediately (as evidenced by the study of patients with an acute hemarthroses). Fifty percent of these patients waited for over 48 hours after their injuries to seek treatment,[6] and within this group, 18 percent successfully ignored their disability for over a week.[6]

In the absence of symptoms associated with the activities of daily living, the patient's activity level is the major determinant of the perception of disability. If the injured athlete attempts to return to a demanding sport, the disability may become immediately apparent. Thus, those athletes injured during "the season" are more likely to seek care. This point is illustrated by the preponderance of ACL injuries occurring in athletes participating in team sports.

The situation differs significantly for recreational athletes. People often ski or play tennis only intermittently. The injured skier or tennis player may not have occasion to "test" the knee for some time, perhaps until the next ski season or vacation, and thus the injury may remain unreported.

These activity-related biases encourage the inclusion in series of patients participating in organized team sports, which are activities usually associated with younger athletes. Older athletes participating in intermittent recreational activities are less likely

to be seen and counted. This fact is documented in virtually every report listing the origins of ACL injury.

In an epidemiologic sense, activity-related biases are particularly troublesome. An ACL sprain is classically a noncontact injury, and yet contact sports (football, basketball, and soccer) lead the list of activities "causing" the problem.[5,6] One must be aware of the fact that it is not football, basketball, or soccer that "causes" the injury but rather specific acts undertaken by athletes participating in these sports. These acts — decelerating, twisting, cutting, and jumping — are common to many other activities. However, other activities are scarcely represented in lists of sports associated with ACL injuries. Many of them, such as tennis, ballet, and softball, involve thousands of participants undergoing the same types of maneuvers.

Perhaps football, and to a lesser extent basketball, involves another biasing variable: outside assistance in the perception of injury. Medical care is readily available to football players, so any injury is more likely to be recognized and reported. The football player usually does not have a chance to "wait and see if the injury is severe." This decision is made for him, a situation in stark contrast to that of the injured recreational athlete who must make the decision independently.

The loss of cases does not stop with the patient's perception of injury. Equally important is the ability of the medical professional to perceive the injury. Characterization of the classic history by Feagin and Curl,[2] description of the Lachman test by Torg et al.,[8] and the recent popularization of arthroscopy as a diagnostic procedure have provided the means by which injuries of the ACL can be diagnosed with considerable accuracy. Nonetheless, series continue to be reported.[3,5] Wherein this diagnosis is missed in the majority of initial encounters with medical professionals.[3,7] Many of these patients were ultimately identified only because they sought consultation for reinjuries. Therefore, to the growing list of biasing variables we must now add the ability of the treating physician to make the diagnosis. This last influences all of the other biases.

Circumstances that encourage the reporting of the injury, for example, team sports, the presence of other injuries, and ready availability of medical care also tend to lead the injured person to a medical professional capable of making the diagnosis. Conversely, when those who initially ignored the injury do get around to seeking care, they may seek it at the hands of someone unable to make the diagnosis. Thus, the injury is "unreported."

The passage of time after the injury does not always result in continued disability or recurrent injuries. With time, the functional manifestations of the injury disappear in some athletes. Aside from the theoretical considerations regarding the reporting or nonreporting of the initial injury, substantial clinical evidence shows that an appreciable number of ACL injuries fail to produce problems of a magnitude that require medical care.

DIFFERENCES BETWEEN ACUTE AND CHRONIC INJURY PATTERNS

If one assumes that the course after ACL injury is one of worsening problems, as time passes we will see evidence of increasing damage to the knee. This worsening pathology takes the form of increased numbers of meniscus tears and degenerative changes of the joint. These tears and changes are evident if we compare the pathology associated with fresh ACL injuries with the pathology in knees of patients with "chronic" problems.

DeHaven[1] and Noyes et al.,[6] in their studies of patients with acute hemarthroses, have defined the injuries associated with acute sprains of the ACL. They report, respectively, a 65 and 62 percent overall frequency of meniscal pathology with the lateral meniscus involved in 51 and 41 percent of all cases and the medial meniscus in 31 and 25 percent. The results of the two studies suggest that they present an accurate appraisal of the situation.

Feagin and Curl[2] observed meniscal pathology in patients who had sustained their initial injury more than 5 years previously; McDaniel and Dameron[5] studied injuries sustained an average of 35 months previously. They reported lateral meniscal pathology in 3 and 19 percent of the cases and medial meniscal pathology in 31 and 62 percent, respectively. The two groups of patients differed significantly; one group[2] had an earlier attempt at primary repair of the torn ACL, and the other group[5] presented for treatment because of symptoms presumably associated with an earlier ACL injury. In spite of these differences, both groups demonstrated a reversal in the ratio of lateral and medial meniscal involvement.

McDaniel and Dameron's work[5] further supports the thesis that lateral (rather than medial) meniscal pathology is more frequently associated with acute ACL injuries. The average time from injury to the initial operation was 5.1 months for those patients with isolated lateral meniscal tears, and 48 months for those demonstrating medial meniscal tears.

It is impossible to reconcile these differences in the frequency of meniscal pathology by assuming that, with time, more medial menisci become torn and that too many lateral meniscus tears are not counted. Two possibilities remain: (1) that most lateral meniscus tears associated with ACL injuries heal to such an extent that they are not apparent at the time of later operations; or (2) those patients with continued problems following an injury to the ACL represent an appreciably smaller subgroup of those who initially sustained the injury. If we assume the latter, at least half of those diagnosed as having an injured ACL will disappear from the orthopaedic care system, presumably because they do not perceive whatever problems they might have as meriting medical assistance. They become, in a sense, another group of patients with unreported injuries.

EPIDEMIOLOGIC SIGNIFICANCE

We are a considerable distance from specifically preventing ACL injuries. Not only are we failing to identify all who have sustained the injury, but also the diversity of description of the mechanism of injury suggests that we know little about exactly how the injury occurs. Given this lack of information it is difficult to alter these (undefined) circumstances. This latter situation will not change until mechanisms of injury can be defined more precisely than as "deceleration," "twisting," "cutting," or "jumping."

Epidemiology may play a role in injury prevention, and it may play an even larger role in the cruciate ligament "controversy" by determining how to assess accurately the results of treatment. The true "natural history" of this injury must be documented. In order to do this, a population wherein all of the anterior cruciate injuries are identified must be evaluated. Given the biases associated with the perception of injury and the bias associated with initial diagnosis, we cannot currently identify this entire population. As long as this deficiency of information exists we will never know whether the results associated with a particular treatment are the result of that treatment or merely a function of the inadvertent selection of patients who would have done well regardless of the management.

REFERENCES

1. DeHaven KE: Diagnosis of acute knee injuries with hemarthrosis. Am J Sports Med 8:9–14, 1980
2. Feagin JA, Curl WW: Isolated tear of the anterior cruciate ligament: 5-year follow-up study. Am J Sports Med 4:95–100, 1976
3. Fowler PJ, Regan W: The patient with symptomatic chronic anterior cruciate ligament insuffiency of the knee. Conservative management. Presented at the AOSSM annual meeting, Nashville, TN; July, 1985
4. Hughston JC, Barrett GR: Acute anteromedial rotatory instability: long term results of surgical repair. J Bone Joint Surg 65A:145–153, 1983
5. McDaniel WJ, Jr, Dameron TB, Jr: Untreated ruptures of the anterior cruciate ligaments. J Bone Joint Surg 62A:696–705, 1980
6. Noyes FR, Bassett RW, Grood ES, Butler DL: Arthroscopy in acute traumatic hemarthrosis of the knee: incidence of anterior cruciate tears and other injuries. J Bone Joint Surg 62A:687–695, 1980
7. Noyes FR, Mooar RA, Matthews BS, Butler DL: The symptomatic anterior cruciate-deficient knee. J Bone Joint Surg 65A:154–162, 1983
8. Torg JS, Conrad W, Kalen V: Clinical diagnosis of anterior cruciate ligament instability in the athlete. Am J Sports Med 4:84–93, 1976

ANATOMY
KINEMATICS

4

Anatomy of the Cruciate Ligaments

STEVEN P. ARNOCZKY
RUSSELL F. WARREN

Understanding the anatomy of the knee is crucial to understanding its function; this is especially true of the cruciate ligaments. The anatomy of the anterior (ACL) and posterior (PCL) cruciate ligaments is directly related to the function of these structures in constraining joint motion.[5,12,13,15,21,24,30,32,37] Likewise, the vascular anatomy of the cruciate ligaments plays a critical role in the ability of these structures to be repaired or reconstructed. Knowing this anatomy is a prerequisite for any discussion of cruciate ligament function, injury, or repair.

DEVELOPMENTAL ANATOMY

The development of the knee joint and its component structures has been the topic of many elegant and detailed embryologic investigations in both humans[2,11,14,16,28] and animals.[10] Studies have shown that the knee joint develops as a cleft between the mesenchymal rudiments of the femur and tibia in about the eighth week of development.[14,16,28] As the mesenchyme in the region of the future knee joint condenses to form the precartilage of the joint and the joint capsule, some vascular mesenchyme becomes isolated within the joint.[14] This tissue is the precursor to the intraarticular structures of the knee (cruciate ligaments and menisci).[14]

Early investigators considered the intraarticular structures of the knee to be derived from extraarticular muscles and ligaments, which they thought to be "drawn" into the joint during its embryonic evolution.[36] Subsequent studies, however, have demonstrated that the cruciate ligaments develop in situ, presumably in response to some genetic factor, and are not merely secondary capsular or muscular derivatives.[14,16]

The cruciate ligaments of the human knee joint first appear as condensations of vascular synovial mesenchyme at about 7 to 8 weeks of development.[14,16] By 9 weeks the cruciate ligaments are composed of numerous immature fibroblasts having scanty cytoplasm and fusiform nuclei, the long axes of which are parallel to the course of the ligaments.[14,16]

At 10 weeks the ACL and PCL are separate from each other and are easily distinguished from one another by the direction of their parallel fibers (Fig. 4-1). While no blood vessels are seen in the cruciate ligaments at this time, capillaries are noted in the blastema adjacent to the ligaments (Fig. 4-2).[14,16]

Over the next 4 weeks the cruciate ligaments become better differentiated from the adjacent tissues and the attachment sites appear to become more specialized. Blood vessels are also seen in the loose tissue surrounding the cruciate ligaments at this time.[14,16]

By 18 weeks the cruciate ligaments stand almost alone, and a few vascular elements are to be found within their substance. During the following weeks the chief changes, in addition to growth, are the increase in vascularity and the appearance of definite fat cells in the mass of connective tissue anterior to the cruciate ligaments and inferior to the

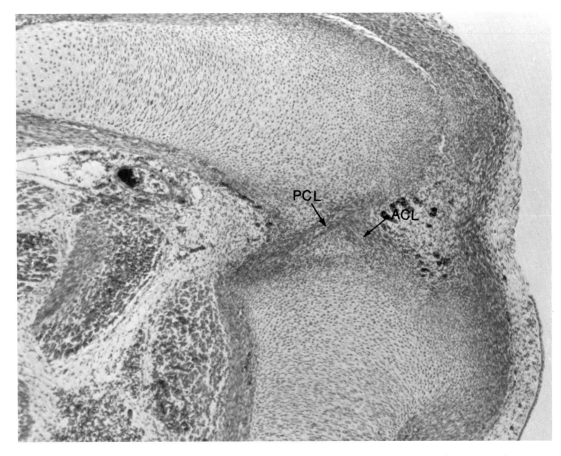

Fig. 4-1. Photomicrograph of sagittal section of an embryonic knee joint. The condensation of mesenchymal tissue forming the ACL and PCL is clearly visible. (H & E, original magnification × 10.)

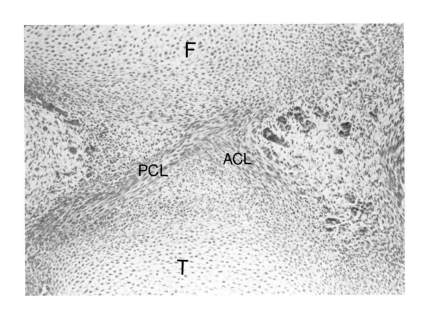

Fig. 4-2. Photomicrograph of sagittal section of an embryonic knee joint illustrating the ACL and PCL and the adjacent vascular tissue. *F*, femur; *T*, tibia. (H & E, original magnification × 100.)

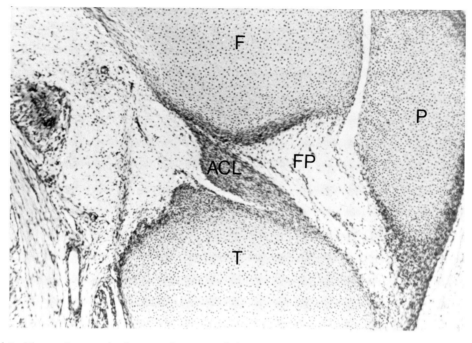

Fig. 4-3. Photomicrograph of a sagittal section of a human knee joint in approximately the 20th week of development. The anterior cruciate ligament *(ACL)*, infrapatellar fat pad *(FP)*, and patella *(P)* are clearly visible. *F,* femur; *T,* tibia. (H & E, original magnification × 40.)

Fig. 4-4. Photograph of a human knee joint at approximately the 20th week of development. Note that the cruciate ligaments and menisci are fully formed at this time.

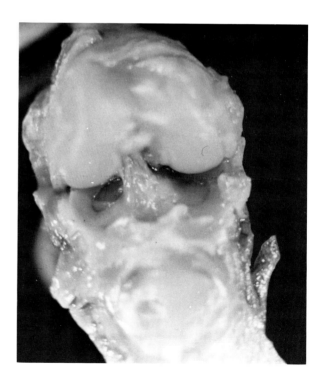

patella; thus the infrapatellar fat pad comes into being at this time (Fig. 4-3).[14,16]

By 20 weeks the cruciate ligaments resemble those of the adult, and their remaining development consists of marked growth with little change in form (Fig. 4-4).[14,16]

GROSS ANATOMY

The cruciate ligaments are bands of regularly oriented, dense connective tissue that connect the femur and tibia. They are surrounded by a mensentery-like fold of synovium that originates from the posterior intercondylar area of the knee and completely envelops the ligaments. Thus while the cruciate ligaments are intraarticular they are also extrasynovial. Several sources state that the PCL is the shorter and stronger of the two ligaments.[5,32] However, a study that examined the dimensions of the anterior and posterior cruciate ligaments in 24 adult cadaver knees revealed that the ACL had a mean length of 3.5 cm (±1 cm) and a mean midportion width of 1.1 cm (±0.1 cm).[15] The PCL in these specimens had a mean length of 3.8 cm (±0.4 cm) and a mean midportion width of 1.3 cm (±0.1 cm).[15] In a study evaluating the ultimate failure strengths of human cruciate ligaments, the PCL was found to be significantly stronger than the ACL.[23]

Femoral Attachment

The ACL is attached to a fossa on the posterior aspect of the medial surface of the lateral femoral condyle. The femoral attachment is in the form of a segment of a circle, with the anterior border straight and the posterior border convex. The long axis of the femoral attachment is tilted slightly forward from the vertical, and the posterior convexity is parallel to the posterior articular margin of the lateral femoral condyle (Fig. 4-5).[3,15,17]

The PCL is attached to the posterior aspect of the lateral surface of the medial condyle. As with the ACL, the attachment is in the form of a segment of a circle. However, in the PCL the long axis of the attachment is more horizontal. The upper boundary of the attachment is horizontal, and the lower

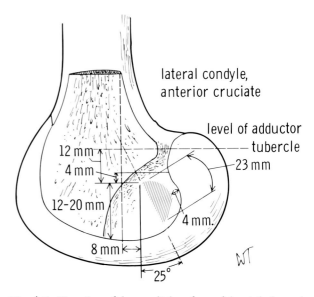

Fig. 4-5. Drawing of the medial surface of the right lateral femoral condyle showing the average measurements and body relations of the femoral attachment of the ACL. (Arnoczky SP: Anatomy of the anterior cruciate ligament. Clin Orthop 172:19–25, 1983.)

boundary is convex and parallel to the lower articular margin of the femoral condyle (Fig. 4-6).[7,15,17]

Tibial Attachment

The ACL is attached to a fossa in front of and lateral to the anterior tibial spine (Fig. 4-7). At this attachment the ACL passes beneath the transverse meniscal ligament, and a few fascicles of the ACL may blend with the anterior attachment of the lateral meniscus. In some instances fascicles from the posterior aspect of the tibial attachment of the ACL may extend to, and blend with, the posterior attachment of the lateral meniscus. The tibial attachment of the ACL is somewhat wider and stronger than the femoral attachment.[3,15,17]

The PCL attaches to the tibia in a depression just posterior to the articular surface of the tibia (Fig. 4-7). While this tibial attachment extends for several millimeters on the posterior surface of the tibia, the functional attachment of the ligament is proximal, the more distal attachment being quite thin. Immediately above the tibial attachment of the PCL a few

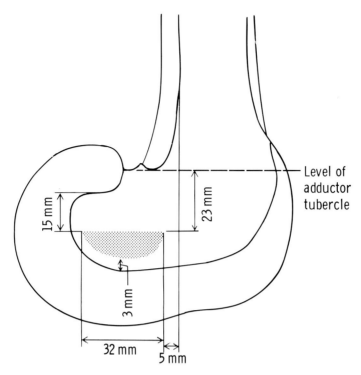

Fig. 4-6. Drawing of the lateral surface of the medial condyle of the femur showing the average measurements and bony relations of the femoral attachment of the PCL. (Girgis FG, Marshall JL, Monajem ARS: The cruciate ligaments of the knee joint; anatomical, functional, and experimental analysis. Clin Orthop 106:216–231, 1975.)

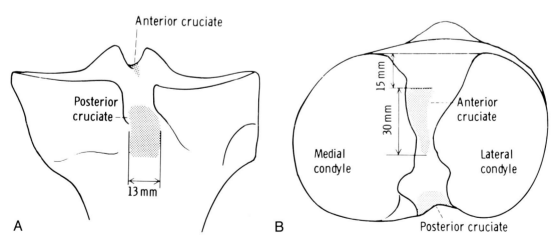

Fig. 4-7. Drawing of **(A)** the posterior surface of the tibia and **(B)** the upper surface of the tibial plateau to show average measurements and relations of the tibial attachments of the ACL and PCL. (Girgis FG, Marshall JL, Monajem ARS: The cruciate ligaments of the knee joint; anatomical, functional, and experimental analysis. Clin Orthop 106:216–231, 1975.)

fibers of the ligament can be seen extending laterally, where they blend with the posterior horn attachment of the lateral meniscus.[7,15,17]

SPATIAL ORIENTATION
ACL and PCL

The cruciate ligaments, as their name signifies, *cross* each other as they pass from the femur to the tibia. This spatial orientation is critical to the function of the cruciate ligaments as constraints of joint motion.[5,13,15,29,32]

The ACL courses anteriorly, medially, and distally across the joint as it passes from the femur to the tibia (Fig. 4-8). It also turns on itself in a slight outward (lateral) spiral. This is due to the orientation of its bony attachments.[3,5,15,24]

The PCL passes posteriorly, laterally, and distally across the joint as it courses from the femur to the tibia. It is narrowest at its midportion, fanning out

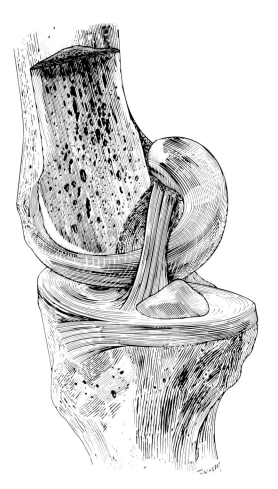

Fig. 4-8. Drawing of the ACL with the knee in extension showing the course of the ligament as it passes from the femur to the tibia. (Girgis FG, Marshall JL, Monajem ARS: The cruciate ligaments of the knee joint; anatomical, functional, and experimental analysis. Clin Orthop 106:216–231, 1975.)

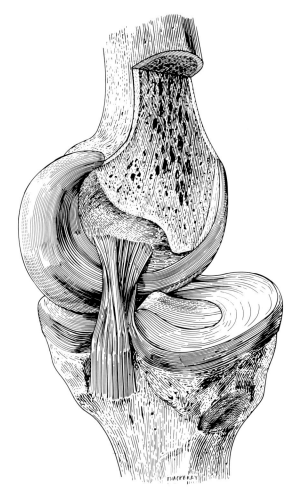

Fig. 4-9. Drawing of the PCL with the knee in extension showing the course of the ligament as it passes from the femur to the tibia. (Girgis FG, Marshall JL, Monajem ARS: The cruciate ligaments of the knee joint; anatomical, functional, and experimental analysis. Clin Orthop 106:216–231, 1975.)

Fig. 4-10. The femoral attachment of the ACL, demonstrating its broad attachment area and its multifascicular structure.

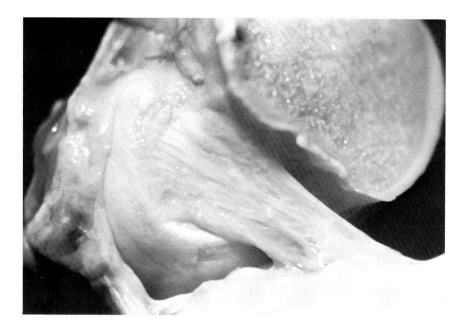

proximally on the femur and to a lesser degree on the tibia[7,15,22] (Fig. 4-9).

The orientation of the femoral attachments of the cruciate ligaments, because of its joint position (flexion/extension), is responsible for the relative tension of the ligament throughout the range of motion.[13,15] The cruciate ligaments are attached to the femur and tibia, not as a singular cord but as a collection of individual fascicles that fan out over a broad flattened area (Fig. 4-10).[3,30,37] In both the anterior and posterior cruciate ligaments these fascicles have been summarily divided into two groups.[13,15] In the ACL these include the anteromedial band (AMB) — those fascicles originating at the proximal aspect of the femoral attachment and inserting at the anteromedial aspect of the tibial attachment — and the posterolateral bulk (PLB) — the remaining bulk of fascicles that are inserted at the posterolateral aspect of the tibial attachment.[13,15] When the knee is extended the PLB is tight whereas the AMB is moderately lax. However, as the knee is flexed, the femoral attachment of the ACL assumes a more horizontal orientation, causing the AMB to tighten and the PLB to loosen (Figs. 4-11, 4-12).[13,15]

In the PCL the fascicles are divided into an anterior portion, which forms the bulk of the ligament,

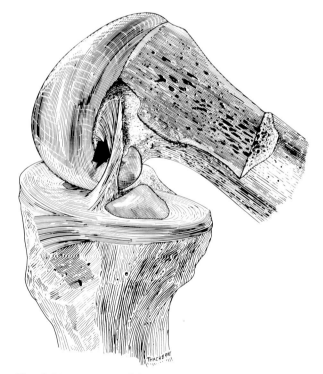

Fig. 4-11. Drawing of the ACL with the knee in flexion. Note the presence of an anteromedial band *(arrow)*. (Girgis FG, Marshall JL, Monajem ARS: The cruciate ligaments of the knee joint; anatomical, functional, and experimental analysis. Clin Orthop 106:216–231, 1975.)

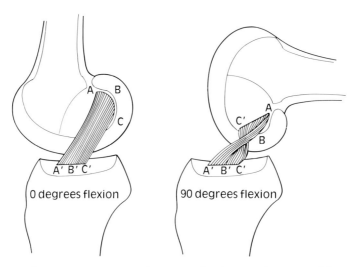

0 degrees flexion   90 degrees flexion

Fig. 4-12. Schematic drawing representing changes in the shape and tension of the ACL components in flexion and extension. In flexion, there is lengthening of the anteromedial band ($A-A'$) and shortening of the posterolateral aspect of the ligament ($C-C'$). Also present, however, is an intermediate component ($B-B'$), which represents the transition between the anteromedial band and posterolateral bulk, with fascicles in varying degress of tension. (After Girgis FG, Marshall JL, Monajem ARS: The cruciate ligaments of the knee joint; anatomical, functional, and experimental analysis. Clin Orthop 106:216–231, 1975.)

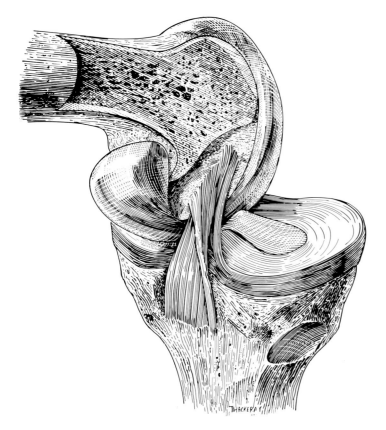

Fig. 4-13. Drawing of the PCL with the knee in flexion. Note that most of the ligament is taut while a small posterior band of fibers becomes loose. (Girgis FG, Marshall JL, Monajem ARS: The cruciate ligaments of the knee joint; anatomical, functional, and experimental analysis. Clin Orthop 106:216–231, 1975.)

Fig. 4-14. Schematic drawing representing the change in shape and tension of the PCL components in extension and flexion. In flexion there is lengthening of the bulk of the ligament ($B-B'$) and shortening of a small band ($A-A'$). $C-C'$ is the anterior meniscofemoral ligament (ligament of Humphry) attached to the lateral meniscus. (Girgis FG, Marshall JL, Monajem ARS: The cruciate ligaments of the knee joint; anatomical, functional, and experimental analysis. Clin Orthop 106:216–231, 1975.)

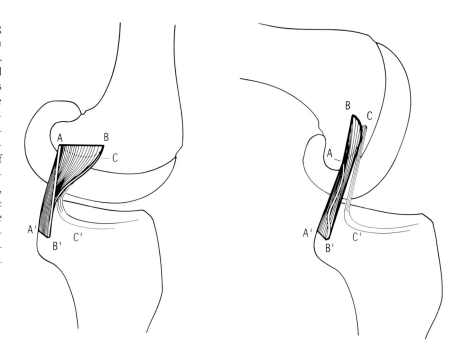

and a posterior segment, which is much smaller and courses obliquely across the joint (Fig. 4-9).[15] As with the ACL, flexion and extension of the joint alter the relative tautness of these segments. The anterior component, which arises from the convex portion of the femoral attachment, is robust and tightens in flexion while the smaller posterior portion tightens in extension (Figs. 4-13, 4-14).[15]

While this two-part designation provides a general idea of the dynamics of the cruciate ligaments through the range of motion, it is an oversimplification. The ligaments are actually a continuum of fascicles, different portions of which are taut throughout the range of motion.

Meniscofemoral Ligaments (Ligaments of Wrisberg and Humphry)

The meniscofemoral ligament is an accessory ligament of the knee that extends from the posterior horn of the lateral meniscus to the lateral aspect of the medial femoral condyle, close to the attachment of the PCL.[6,7,18,20,26] Once described as the "third cruciate ligament,"[33] this structure is intimately as-

sociated with the PCL and may divide to pass anteriorly and/or posteriorly to it. These divisions are respectively termed the anterior and posterior meniscofemoral ligaments[6,7,18,20,26] (Fig. 4-15).

The anterior meniscofemoral ligament (ligament of Humphry) is a fibrous fasciculus that originates from the posterior aspect of the lateral meniscus, extends obliquely medially and proximally in front of the PCL, and inserts into the medial condyle of the femur.[18-20,26] The ligament of Humphry, when present, can vary considerably in size and may be up to one third the size of the PCL or larger[18,26] (Fig. 4-16).

The posterior meniscofemoral ligament (ligament of Wrisberg) lies behind the PCL and extends from the posterior aspect of the lateral meniscus to the medial condyle of the femur.[18,20,26] The ligament of Wrisberg varies in size and in some specimens is half the diameter of the PCL[18] (Fig. 4-17).

The presence of these structures within the knee is quite variable. In one study, one or the other of these ligament bands was present, with equal incidence, in 71 percent of 140 knees examined.[18] In only eight of these knee were both the anterior and posterior meniscofemoral ligaments present together.[18]

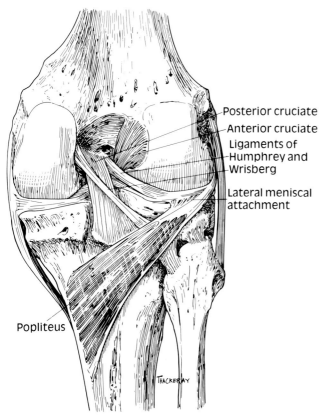

Fig. 4-15. Drawing of the posterior aspect of the knee joint showing the relationship of the anterior (Humphry) and posterior (Wrisberg) meniscofemoral ligaments to the posterior cruciate ligament. (Reproduced by permission from Warren RF, Arnoczky SP, Wickiewicz TL: Anatomy of the knee. In Nicholas JA (ed): The Lower Extremity and Spine in Sports Medicine. St. Louis, 1985, The C.V. Mosby Co.)

Because of the variability in the presence and size of the meniscofemoral ligament, its function is somewhat questionable. During flexion of the knee, the meniscofemoral ligament pulls the posterior horn of the lateral meniscus anteriorly, increasing the congruity between the meniscotibial socket and the lateral femoral condyle.[18]

MICROANATOMY

Ligaments

The cruciate ligaments are made up of multiple fascicles, the basic unit of which is collagen.[9] Nonparallel interlacing networks of these collagen fibrils (150 to 250 nm in diameter) are grouped into fibers (1 to 20 μm in diameter) that, in turn, make up a subfascicular unit (100 to 250 μm in diameter). These subfascicular units are surrounded by a loose band of connective tissue known as the endotenon. Three to twenty subfasciculi, bound together, form a fasciculus, which may be from 250 μm to several millimeters in diameter. These are surrounded by an epitenon. This interfascicular connective tissue also supports the neurovascular elements of the ligament.[1] These individual fascicles either are oriented in a spiral fashion around the long axis of the ligament or pass directly from the femur to the tibial attachment (Fig. 4-18). The entire continuum of fascicles, forming the ligament, is surrounded by the paratenon, a connective tissue covering similar to but much thicker than the epitenon.[9]

Ligament – Bone Attachment

The cruciate ligaments attach to the femur and tibia via the interdigitation of collagen fibers of the ligament with those of the adjacent bone.[8] The abrupt change from flexible ligamentous tissue to rigid bone is mediated by a transitional zone of fibrocartilage and mineralized fibrocartilage (Figs. 4-19, 4-20).[1,8] This alteration in microstructure from ligament to bone allows for a graduated change in stiffness and prevents stress concentration at the attachment site.[1,31] This zone may also impose a barrier to endosteal vessels entering the ligament at these attachment sites.

VASCULAR ANATOMY

The major blood supply to the anterior and posterior cruciate ligaments arises from the ligamentous branches of the middle genicular artery as well as some terminal branches of the medial and lateral inferior genicular arteries.[3,4,27,34,38]

The cruciate ligaments are covered by a synovial fold that originates at the posterior inlet of the intercondylar notch and extends to the anterior tibial insertion of the ligament, where it joins with the synovial tissue of the joint capsule distal to the infrapatellar fat pad. This synovial membrane, which forms an envelope about the ligament, is richly endowed with vessels that originate predominantly from the ligamentous branches of the middle geni-

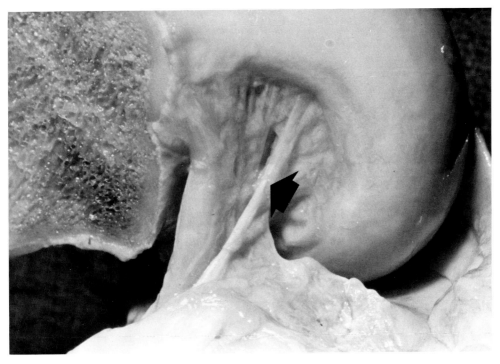

Fig. 4-16. Photograph of a knee joint specimen showing the presence of an anterior meniscofemoral ligament (ligament of Humphry) *(arrow)* and its relationship to the PCL.

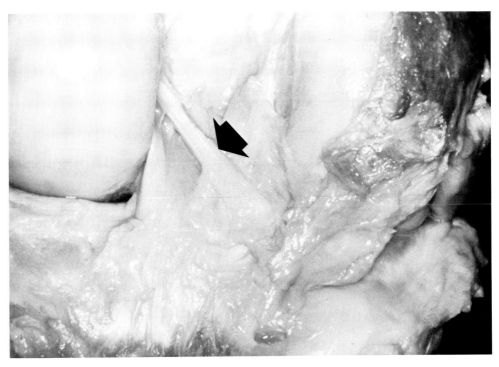

Fig. 4-17. Photograph of a knee joint specimen showing the presence of a posterior meniscofemoral ligament (ligament of Wrisberg) *(arrow)* and its relationship to the PCL.

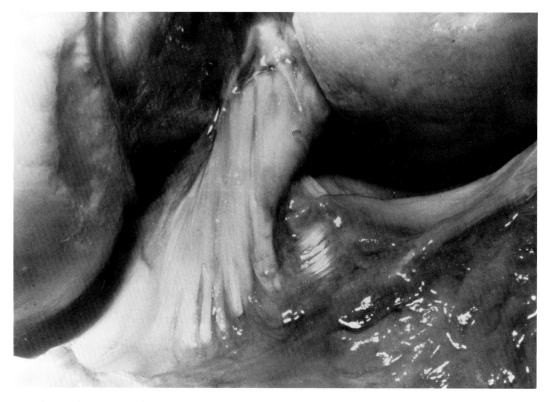

Fig. 4-18. Photograph of the ACL demonstrating the spiral and multifascicular nature of its structure. (Arnoczky SP: Anatomy of the anterior cruciate ligament. Clin Orthop 172:19–25, 1983.)

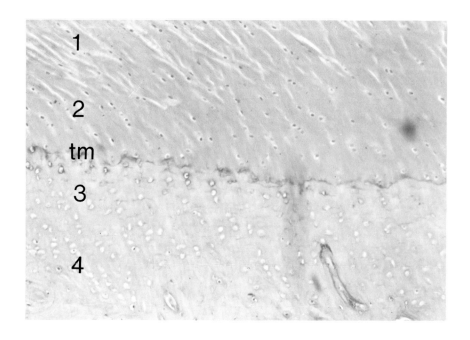

Fig. 4-19. Photomicrograph of the tibial insertion of an ACL illustrating the transition zone: *(1)* ligament, *(2)* fibrocartilage, *(tm)* tide mark, *(3)* mineralized fibrocartilage, *(4)* bone. (H & E, original magnification × 100.)

Fig. 4-20. Photomicrograph of the specimen in Fig. 4-19 as viewed under polarized light. Note how the collagen fibers of the ligament interdigitate with the collagen of the bone. (H & E, original magnification × 100.)

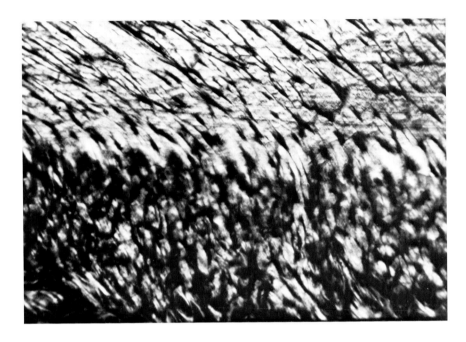

cular artery (Fig. 4-21).[3,4,27,34] A few smaller terminal branches of the lateral and medial inferior genicular arteries also contribute some vessels to this synovial plexus through its connection with the infrapatellar fat pad. The synovial vessels arborize to form a web-like network of periligamentous vessels that en-

sheath the entire ligament (Fig. 4-22). These periligamentous vessels then give rise to smaller connecting branches that penetrate the ligament transversely and anastomose with a network of endoligamentous vessels (Fig. 4-23).[3,4,27] These vessels, along with their supporting connective tissues,

Fig. 4-21. Sagittal 5 mm thick section of a human knee (Spalteholz technique) showing the branches of the middle genicular artery that supply the distal femoral epiphysis *(large white arrow),* the proximal tibial epiphysis *(large open arrow),* and the cruciate ligaments *(small white arrowheads). (F,* femur; *T,* tibia; *FP,* fat pad; *P,* popliteal artery.) (Arnoczky SP: Blood supply to the anterior cruciate ligament and supporting structures. Orthop Clin North Am 16:15 – 28, 1985.)

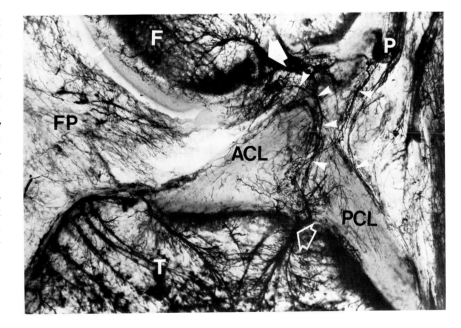

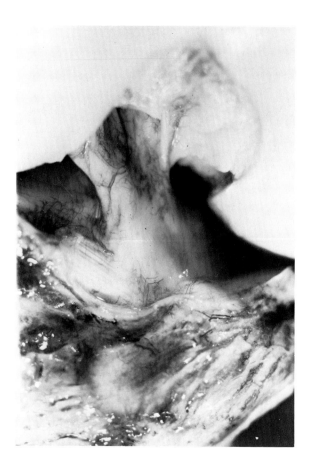

Fig. 4-22. Photograph of a human knee specimen injected with India ink demonstrating the synovial (periligamentous) vasculature on the surface of the ACL. (Note that the infrapatellar fat pad has been removed for better visualization). (Arnoczky SP: Blood supply to the anterior cruciate ligament and supporting structures. Orthop Clin North Am 16:15–28, 1985.)

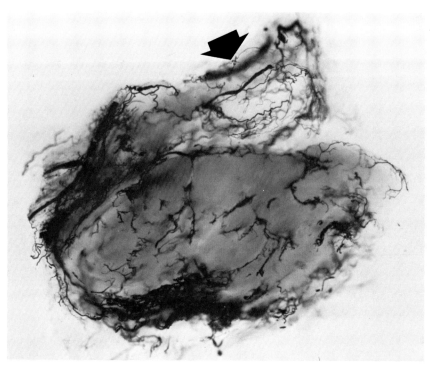

Fig. 4-23. Cross-section of a human ACL (Spalteholz technique) demonstrating the periligamentous as well as endoligamentous vasculature. The fold of synovial membrane *(arrow)* can be seen supplying vessels to the synovial covering of the ligament. (Arnoczky SP: Anatomy of the anterior cruciate ligament. Clin· Orthop 172:19–25, 1983.)

Fig. 4-24. Sagittal 5 mm thick section of a human knee joint (Spalteholz technique) showing the periligamentous vasculature of the ACL and PCL *(closed arrows)*. Note the absence of vessels crossing the ligamentous–osseous attachment of the ACL *(open arrows)*. (Arnoczky SP: Blood supply to the anterior cruciate ligament and supporting structures. Orthop Clin North Am 16:15–28, 1985.)

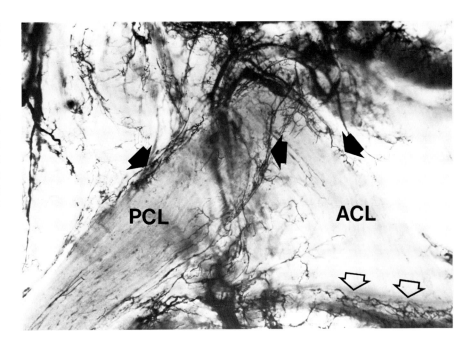

are oriented in a longitudinal direction and lie parallel to the collagen bundles within the ligament.[3,4,27]

The anterior and posterior cruciate ligaments are supplied with blood predominantly from soft tissue origins. While the middle genicular artery gives off additional branches to the distal femoral epiphysis and proximal tibial epiphysis, the ligamentous–osseous junctions of the cruciate ligaments do not contribute significantly to the vascular scheme of the ligaments themselves (Fig. 4-24).[3,4,27]

Although the location of the PCL places it in inti-

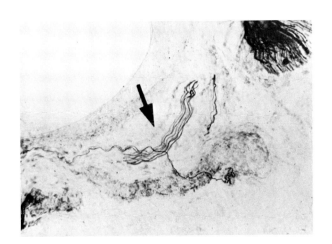

Fig. 4-25. Photomicrograph of an ACL showing nerve fibers in the synovium investing the ligament. (Kennedy JC, Alexander IJ, Hayes KC: Nerve supply of the human knee and its functional importance. Am J Sports Med 10:329–335, 1982.)

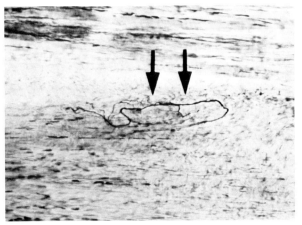

Fig. 4-26. Photomicrograph of a PCL showing the presence of a Golgi-like tension receptor within the ligament. (Kennedy JC, Alexander IJ, Hayes KC: Nerve supply of the human knee and its functional importance. Am J Sports Med 10:329–335, 1982.)

mate contact with the ligamentous branches of the middle genicular artery and the vascular synovial tissue of the posterior joint capsule, there is no evidence that the PCL has a better vascular supply than the ACL.

NERVE SUPPLY

The cruciate ligaments receive nerve fibers from branches of the tibial nerve (posterior articular branch of the posterior tibial nerve).[25] These fibers penetrate the joint capsule posteriorly and course along with the synovial and periligamentous vessels surrounding the ligaments to reach as far anterior as the infrapatellar fat pad.[25] Smaller nerve fibers have also been observed throughout the substance of the ligaments.[25,35] While most fibers are associated with the endoligamentous vasculature and appear to have a vasomotor function, some fibers have been observed to lie alone among the fascicles of the ligament.[25,35] These latter neural elements are located primarily within multiple clefts in the tibial origin of the ACL and in its richly vascularized synovial coverings (Fig. 4-25).[25,35] Golgi-like tension receptors have been identified near the origins of the ligaments as well as at the surface of the ligament beneath the synovial membrane (Fig. 4-26).[25,35] These mechanoreceptors are suggestive of some type of proprioceptive function and may provide the afferent arc for postural changes of the knee through deformations within the ligament.[25,35]

REFERENCES

1. Akeson WH, Woo SL-Y, Amiel D, Frank CB: The chemical basis of tissue repair: ligament biology. p. 93. In: Hunter LY, Funk FJ Jr (eds); Rehabilitation of the Injured Knee. CV Mosby, St. Louis, 1984
2. Anderson H: Histochemical studies on the histogenesis of the knee joint and superior tibio-fibular joint in human foetuses. Acta Anat 46:279–303, 1961
3. Arnoczky SP: Anatomy of the anterior cruciate ligament. Clin Orthop 172:19–25, 1983
4. Arnoczky SP: Blood supply to the anterior cruciate ligament and supporting structures. Orthop Clin North Am 16:15–28, 1985
5. Brantigan OC, Voshell AF: The mechanics of the ligaments and menisci of the knee joint. J Bone Joint Surg 23A:44–66, 1941
6. Brantigan OC, Voshell AF: Ligaments of the knee joint. The relationship of the ligament of Humphry to the ligament of Wrisberg. J Bone Joint Surg 28A:66–67, 1946
7. Clancy WG Jr, Shelbourne KD, Zoellner GB et al: Treatment of knee joint instability secondary to rupture of the posterior cruciate ligament. J Bone Joint Surg 65A:310–322, 1983
8. Cooper RR, Misol S: Tendon and ligament insertion. A light and electron microscopic study. J Bone Joint Surg 52A:1–20, 1970
9. Danylchuk KD, Finlay JB, Krcek JP: Microstructural organization of human and bovine cruciate ligaments. Clin Orthop 131:294–298, 1978
10. DePalma AF: Diseases of the Knee. JB Lippincott, Philadelphia, 1954
11. Ellison AE, Berg EE: Embryology, anatomy, and function of the anterior cruciate ligament. Orthop Clin North Am, 16:3–14, 1985
12. Fowler PJ: Functional anatomy of the knee. p. 11. In Hunter LY, Funk FJ Jr (eds): Rehabilitation of the Injured Knee. CV Mosby, St. Louis, 1984
13. Furman W, Marshall JL, Girgis FG: The anterior cruciate ligament. A functional analysis based on postmortem studies. J Bone Joint Surg 58A:179–185, 1976
14. Gardner E, O'Rahilly R: The early development of the knee joint in staged human embryos. J Anat 102:289–299, 1968
15. Girgis FG, Marshall JL, Monajem ARS: The cruciate ligaments of the knee joint. Anatomical, functional, and experimental analysis. Clin Orthop 106:216–231, 1975
16. Gray DJ, Gardner E: Prenatal development of the human knee and superior tibiofibular joints. Am J Anat 86:235–288, 1950
17. Gray H: Anatomy of the Human Body, 29th edition, Goss CM (ed). Lea & Febiger, Philadelphia, 1975
18. Heller L, Langman J: The menisco-femoral ligaments of the human knee. J Bone Joint Surg 46B:307–313, 1964
19. Humphry GM: Treatise on the Human Skeleton (Including the Joints). Macmillan, Cambridge, 1858
20. Kaplan EB: The lateral meniscofemoral ligament of the knee joint. Bull Hosp Joint Dis 17:176–181, 1956
21. Kaplan EB: Some aspects of functional anatomy of the human knee joint. Clin Orthop 23:18–29, 1962
22. Kennedy JC, Granger RW: The posterior cruciate ligament. J Trauma 7:367–377, 1967

23. Kennedy JC, Hawkins RJ, Willis RB, Danylchuk KD: Tension studies of human knee ligaments. Yield point, ultimate failure, and disruption of the cruciate and tibial collateral ligaments. J Bone Joint Surg 58A:350–355, 1976

24. Kennedy JC, Weinberg HW, Wilson AS: The anatomy and function of the anterior cruciate ligament as determined by clinical and morphological studies. J Bone Joint Surg 56A:223–235, 1974

25. Kennedy JC, Alexander IJ, Hayes KC: Nerve supply of the human knee and its functional importance. Am J Sports Med 10:329–335, 1982

26. Last RJ: Some anatomical details of the knee joint. J Bone Joint Surg 30B:683–688, 1948

27. Marshall JL, Arnoczky SP, Rubin RM, Wickiewicz TL: Microvasculature of the cruciate ligaments. Phys Sports Med 7:87–91, 1979

28. McDermott LJ: Development of the human knee joint. Arch Surg 46:705–719, 1943

29. Müller W: The Knee: Form, Function, and Ligamentous Reconstruction. Spinger-Verlag, New York, 1983

30. Norwood LA, Cross MJ: Anterior cruciate ligament: Functional anatomy of its bundles in rotatory instabilities. Am J Sports Med 7:23–26, 1979

31. Noyes FR, DeLucas JL, Torvik PJ: Biomechanics of anterior cruciate ligament failure. An analysis of strain-rate sensitivity and mechanics of failure in primates. J Bone Joint Surg 56A:236–253, 1974

32. Palmer I: On the injuries to the ligaments of the knee joint. A clinical study. Acta Chir Scand 81(Suppl 53):2–282, 1938

33. Poirier P, Charpy A: Traité d'Anatomie Humaine, Tome 1. Masson, Paris, 1899

34. Scapinelli R: Studies on the vasculature of the human knee joint. Acta Anat 70:305–331, 1968

35. Schultz RA, Miller DC, Kerr CS, Micheli L: Mechanoreceptors in human cruciate ligaments. A histological study. J Bone Joint Surg 66A:1072–1076, 1984

36. Sutton JB: Ligaments: Their Nature and Morphology. P. Blakiston and Son, Philadelphia, 1887

37. Welsh RP: Knee joint structure and function. Clin Orthop 147:7–14, 1980

38. Wladmirow B: Arterial sources of blood supply of the knee joint in man. Acta Med 47:1–10, 1968

5

Injury to the Medial Capsuloligamentous Complex

PETER A. INDELICATO

The tibial (medial) collateral ligament and adjacent posterior oblique ligament contribute to the confusion that surrounds the nomenclature and function of the ligaments of the knee, although they are not as controversial as the cruciate ligaments.

This chapter reviews the function, surgical anatomy, mechanism of injury, physical findings, and various approaches to treatment of injuries to the medial capsuloligamentous complex of the knee (Fig. 5-1).

FUNCTIONAL ANATOMY

Two basic theories are proposed about primary medial support against valgus stress to the knee. One theory was discussed by Hughston and Eilers[3] in 1973, and the other by Warren and associates[9] in 1974. Hughston and Eilers[3] stressed the importance of the posteromedial capsule and associated attachments of the semimembranosus. They called this structure the posterior oblique ligament. Warren and associates[9] concluded that the prime stabilizer on the medial side of the knee, to resist both valgus stress and external rotation with the knee in flexion, is not the posterior oblique ligament but the long anteriormost fibers of the tibial collateral ligament.

Hughston and Eilers' Theory

The authors[3] described the posterior oblique ligament as a distinct thickening or condensation of the posteromedial capsule that is firmly attached to the medial meniscus. The ligament is functionally inde-pendent of the medial (tibial) collateral ligament. The latter is anterior to this and superficial to the capsular ligament of the knee. The posterior oblique ligament, although somewhat lax as the knee goes into flexion, is "dynamized" by the muscular attachments of the semimembranosus tendon. In this fashion, the posterior oblique ligament has a significant influence on stability throughout the first 60° of flexion. Specifically, they pointed out that this important structure is "not a posterior area of the more superficial tibial collateral ligament." According to them, repairing the oblique ligament is the "keystone" to restoring function not only in the medial ligaments, but also in the anterior cruciate ligament (ACL).

> Following reapproximation of the torn ends of the posterior oblique ligament, light abduction stress should be applied to the tibia to test the adequacy of this part of the repair. If the repair is adequate, the medial joint space will not open during testing. . . . We do not repair the anterior cruciate ligament when it has a "mop-end" type tear. . . . Under these circumstances it is resected." Once the posterior oblique ligament and the remaining ligaments of the medial compartment are repaired, . . . "the positive anterior drawer sign is corrected."[3]

More recently, Hughston and Barrett[4] reviewed 154 patients with acute repairs performed on knees with anteromedial rotatory instability. The follow-up ranged from 2 to 21 years. They stated:

> We have approximated the middle third of the capsular and tibial collateral ligaments without per-

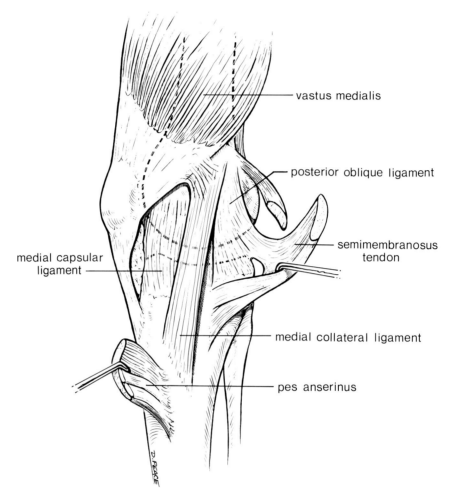

Fig. 5-1. Medial capsuloligamentous complex.

forming immediate repair on the posterior oblique ligament, and have demonstrated continued instability. On the other hand, we have repaired the posterior oblique ligament first, without repairing the middle third of the capsular and tibial collateral ligaments, and at 30 degrees of flexion have demonstrated stability to abduction stress. . . . Repair of the posterior oblique ligament is the key to medial instability at the moment of static fixation.[4]

Müller[7] also believes that the "semimembranosus corner" or posterior oblique ligament is paramount in abolishing any valgus laxity in the extended knee, even before the tibial collateral ligament or ACL is repaired. He claims that even though the posterior oblique ligament and tibial collateral ligament are functionally independent, they are both "dynamized," the former by the semimembranosus tendon, the latter by the vastus medialis (Fig. 5-2). The connections between the vastus medialis and tibial collateral ligament occur in the superficial layer near the femoral attachment site of the ligament. They are extremely important and should be preserved whenever possible because they serve as transmitters of neuromuscular impulses to the ligament when placed under tension and therefore are protective in nature. They also may help decrease the functional laxity secondary to applying tension on the longitudinal fibers of this ligament.

Müller[7] also claims that the tibial collateral ligament has some function in preventing external rota-

Fig. 5-2. According to Müller, the MCL is "dynamized" by the connecting fibers of the vastus medialis, and the posterior oblique ligament is "dynamized" by the semimembranosus.

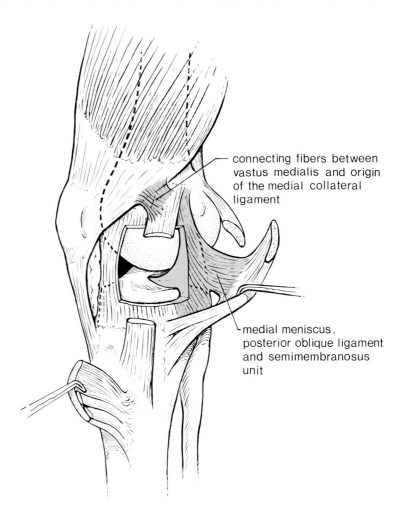

connecting fibers between vastus medialis and origin of the medial collateral ligament

medial meniscus, posterior oblique ligament and semimembranosus unit

tion of the tibia on the femur with the knee flexed (Fig. 5-3). However, the main deterrent to external tibial rotation is the posterior oblique ligament.

Warren and Associates' Theory

In contrast to both Hughston and Müller, Warren and associates,[9] after examining 32 fresh human knees at necropsy, concluded that the prime static stabilizer on the medial side of the knee is the long anteriormost fibers of the tibial collateral ligament.[8] These authors remarked that demonstrable medial opening to valgus stress with the knees in 45° flexion is indicative of damage at least to the anterior long fibers of the tibial collateral ligament. They indicted a rupture of the medial capsular ligament and posterior oblique ligament when "gross" instability is present to valgus stress testing.[9] They pointed out, however, that parallel fibers of the tibial collateral ligament within 5 mm of its anteriormost edge slacken as the knee goes into flexion and therefore are not as crucial to stability as the anterior edge of this same ligament. Thus, they seem to classify the tibial collateral ligament into three functional components:

1. The anteriormost long fibers of the superficial (tibial) collateral ligament are most important in preventing medial joint opening or abnormal external rotation of the tibia on the femur with the knee in flexion.

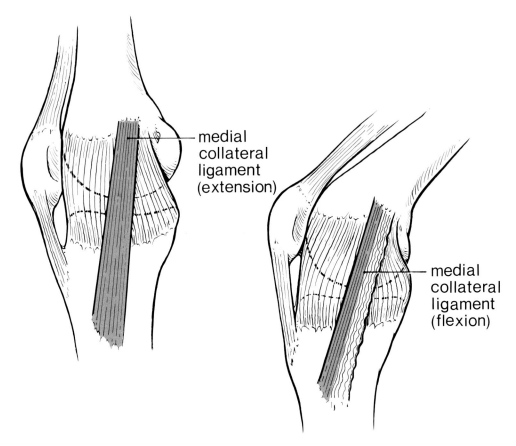

Fig. 5-3. The theory of Warren and associates: the anterior 5 mm of the MCL remains tight in flexion, and thus resists valgus stress and external rotation in this position.

2. The posterior (approximately) two-thirds of the superficial (tibial) collateral ligament are, according to the authors, slightly lax with the knee in flexion and therefore serve as "back-up" restraints against valgus and external rotary forces.
3. The oblique or posterior aspect of the superficial (tibial) collateral ligament Hughston has labeled the posterior oblique ligament. This is a thickening of the posteromedial capsule of the knee and is firmly attached and continuous with the medial meniscus in this location.

Other Observations

In general, any peripheral tear of the medial meniscus in the posteromedial corner would include a tear of the posterior oblique ligament. This is an important point that will be discussed in greater detail under Management.

As far as restraining external rotation is concerned, Warren et al.[9] again point out that only after sectioning the anteriormost long fibers of the tibial collateral ligament does one elicit a demonstrable increase in external rotation with the knee in flexion. If one were to section the deep medial capsular ligament and posterior oblique ligament, leaving the long fibers of the tibial collateral ligament intact, "a remarkable resistance to external rotation of the tibia was retained." On the other hand, a "permissible" amount of external tibial rotation was demonstrated once these long fibers were sectioned.[9] My own observation is that the amount of abnormal external rotation occurring with damage to the deep medial capsular ligament, the tibial collateral ligament, the posterior oblique ligament, or any combination of these ligaments is not the dramatic, classic "anteromedial rotatory instability" of the knee that one encounters with structural damage to the ACL.

As stated previously, Müller,[7] in contrast, claims that the main deterrent against external rotation of the tibia on the femur with the knee in flexion is not the tibial collateral ligament or any component of it but the posterior oblique ligament. In this aspect he is in total agreement with Hughston. In his recent book, Müller[7] points out that due to the direction of the ligament alignment, the tibial collateral ligament is tight in full extension. As the knee flexes, however, the tibia rotates internally (15°), allowing the ligament to slacken somewhat and thus increasing the amount of rotation that can and should normally occur between the tibia and femur. He claims that tears of the posterior oblique ligament alone will result in some abnormal external rotatory instability, and that classic anteromedial rotatory instability of the knee is only amplified with additional damage to the tibial collateral ligament and/or the ACL.[7]

Still another viewpoint was presented by Kennedy and Fowler[6] in 1971. They identified the deep medial capsular ligament as the primary restraint against external rotatory instability (Fig. 5-4), rather than the tibial collateral ligament (Warren et al.) or the posterior oblique ligament (Müller, Hughston). Kennedy and Fowler[6] clinically evaluated 42 knees by routine physical examination and also by a stress machine. They concluded that external rotatory instability is "caused by a tear of the medial capsular ligament with or without a partial or complete tear of the tibial collateral ligament."

Finally, in 1981, Grood et al[2] published an extensive study of the biomechanical restraints of cadaver knees. In general, they agreed with previously published data[9] and concluded the following:

The long parallel-oriented fibers of the tibial collateral ligament are the prime medial static stabilizer of the knee that resist medial opening to valgus stress.

Although this ligament contributes to medial support with the knee close to full extension (5° flexion), as the knee flexes (25° flexion) its im-

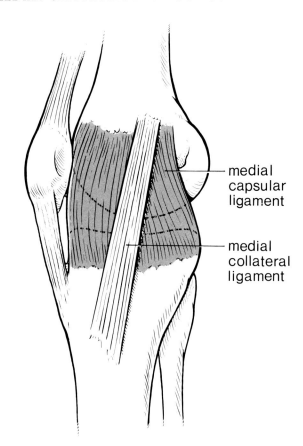

Fig. 5-4. The primary restraint against abnormal external tibial rotation, according to Kennedy and Fowler,[6] is the medial capsular ligament.

portance increases from providing 57 percent of the restraining force to providing 78 percent of the restraining force. This is due to the relaxation or laxity that develops in flexion to the other contributing structures, mainly the posteromedial capsule.

The deep midmedial capsular ligament, although important in that it provides a firm attachment site for the medial meniscus, does not serve as a primary restraint against straight medial opening.[2]

Some controversy still exists over which specific structures prevents abnormal medial opening and abnormal external rotation of the tibia on the femur. Although the posterior oblique ligament is the primary restraint according to some authorities (Müller, Hughston), the tibial collateral ligament appears to be the primary restraint against abnormal medial opening (Warren, Grood) and against abnormal external tibial rotation (Warren).[2,3,7,9]

SURGICAL ANATOMY

Fortunately, in contrast to the controversy that surrounds the function of the medial and posteromedial capsuloligamentous complex, generally, authorities agree on the relative anatomic location of the stabilizing structures. Müller has done an excellent job of classifying the medial capsuloligamentous complex into various layers. The importance of having a thorough understanding of these layers is more than academic; without it appropriate surgical exposures are most difficult, often confusing the relatively inexperienced surgeon and frustrating attempts to obtain a secure repair under proper tension.

Müller[7] and Warren and Marshall[8] have classified the medial capsuloligamentous complex into three separate layers. Layer I, the most superficial, includes the deep fascia from the patella tendon anteriorly to the popliteal fossa posteriorly. This layer also envelopes the medial hamstring tendons. Layer II is composed basically of one distinct structure, the tibial collateral ligament. Anterior to the tibial collateral ligament layer I joins the periosteum of the tibia, whereas posteriorly it joins the posteromedial capsule and posterior oblique ligament of the knee. As the fibers forming the tibial collateral ligament are followed from anterior to posterior, they become more obliquely and posteriorly oriented. As these fibers approach the "semimembranosus corner" they join the deep capsular ligament (layer III) and, combined, are referred to as the posterior oblique ligament of the knee. Extensions of the semimembranosus tendon sheath also appear to reinforce and "dynamize" this important posteromedial corner of the knee. The normal mechanics of the knee demands that the tibial collateral ligament have approximately 1.5 cm anterior–posterior excursion as the knee goes from full extension to full flexion.[7]

I have observed repeatedly at primary repair that a hematoma has dissected itself between the various layers, superficial and deep to the tibial collateral ligament, thus helping the surgeon to differentiate more easily the various layers for proper exposure.

Layer III is the deep capsular ligament and true "capsule" of the knee joint to whose inner surface is attached the synovium. The capsular ligament is easily identified as a separate layer through its anterior two thirds but becomes indistinguishable from the overlying oblique extensions of the tibial collateral ligament in its remaining posterior third. As stated previously, this condensation of these two structures, (the deep capsular ligament and oblique posterior extension of the tibial collateral ligament) is what Hughston and Eilers,[3] as well as Müller,[7] refer to as the posterior oblique ligament. The meniscus is firmly attached to this structure throughout its entirety, the attachment being firmest at this posteromedial corner. The capsule has more recently been popularly classified into meniscofemoral and meniscotibial portions to highlight its important attachment to the meniscus. However, other than serving as an anchor for the meniscus, the structural significance of the anterior and midthird region of this deep medial capsular ligament is relatively slight, as mentioned previously by Grood et al.[2]

MECHANISM OF INJURY

Whereas a "noncontact" mechanism of injury is frequently associated with so-called "isolated" tears of the ACL, most of the major injuries to the medial capsuloligamentous complex are the result of some blow or contact to the lateral aspect of the lower thigh or upper leg. Hughston and Barrett[4] claimed that 86 percent of the knees treated for acute anteromedial rotatory instability had sustained the damage as a result of contact. In our prospective evaluation of the treatment of complete tears of the medial capsuloligamentous complex, we evaluated the mechanism of injury in 51 patients diagnosed as having complete tears of the tibial collateral ligament and found that 47 (92 percent) sustained a blow to the lateral aspect of the lower thigh or upper leg.[5] Müller[7] speculates that a pure valgus injury to the knee without any rotatory component will damage the tibial collateral ligament with or without damage to the posterior oblique ligament. If valgus and rotation are combined simultaneously, however, tears mainly occur first to the posterior oblique ligament (semimembranosus corner) and possibly the ACL before the tibial collateral ligament is torn.

PHYSICAL FINDINGS

After a careful history is obtained, including as detailed an account as possible of the mechanism of injury, a thorough physical examination is essential to help clarify the extent of injury. Although this can occasionally be done adequately in an emergency room or office, thigh muscle relaxation is absolutely essential for adequate assessment of the static structures needed for stability of the knee. Even to the most experienced knee surgeon, an examination with the patient under spinal or general anesthesia may be required to obtain adequate muscle relaxation. Valgus stress testing with the knee in extension and 30° of flexion is still the single most important test to perform to evaluate the extent of damage to the medial capsuloligamentous complex. The degree of medial opening compared to the contralateral knee is a direct measure of damage to this complex.

Medial opening that occurs when valgus stress is applied to a knee in full extension is indicative of damage to at least the deep capsular ligament, the tibial collateral ligament, and the posterior oblique ligament. If there is gross opening, damage to the cruciates should also be strongly suspected. If the knee is stable in full extention, Müller[7] states that one can assume that there is probably no significant structural damage to the "semimembranosus corner." With the knee in 30° of flexion, the posterior capsule and a portion of the posterior oblique ligament relax. Medial opening now under valgus stress is indicative of damage to the tibial collateral ligament, the underlying midthird portion of the deep medial capsular ligament, and possibly to anterior fibers of the posterior oblique ligament. Grood et al.[2] recently showed that even a 5 to 8 mm increase in laxity is indicative of major tibial collateral ligament damage. The importance of develop-

ing a sensitivity for the "quality" of the "end-point" *where one should normally feel an "end-point"* cannot be overemphasized in this physical exam. In complete (grade III) tears of the medial capsuloligamentous complex, no firm end-point is encountered until an intact ACL is sufficiently loaded, which is quite beyond the point of medial opening seen in the contralateral knee.

Another point to keep in mind when performing a stress test on an injured knee is the fact that a component of axial rotation occurs along the long axis of the extremity during valgus testing. This rotatory motion seen can be misinterpreted as abnormal medial opening.[2] To minimize the risk of this happening, Müller[7] recommends that valgus stress testing done with the knee in 30° of flexion must be performed with the tibia slightly externally rotated. As mentioned earlier, he claims that the tibial collateral ligament is tight in external rotation and extension. As the knee flexes and internally rotates its mandatory amount (approximately 15°) this ligament slackens somewhat, allowing rotation to increase. The normal rotation that occurs when valgus stress is applied—neutral or internal rotation changing to external rotation—may be incorrectly interpreted as abnormal medial opening.[7]

However, as mentioned above, the abnormal external rotation that may be present following complete tears of the deep capsular ligament, the tibial collateral ligament, and even the posterior oblique ligament is not as significant as the classic anteromedial rotatory instability of the knee associated with tears of the ACL. The functional significance of the latter condition carries a much worse prognosis when compared to those medial injuries seen in conjunction with a normal ACL.

Finally, one does not usually find a massive hemarthrosis when injury is limited to only the medial capsuloligamentous complex, although soft tissue swelling is consistently present and easily detectable on examination. A massive hemarthrosis is, however, frequently encountered when structural damage to the ACL is present. One must keep in mind that when the "unhappy" triad of O'Donohue is present, the hemarthrosis may be minimal due to extravasation of blood through the tear of the medial capsule.

MANAGEMENT

The degree of suspected damage ascertained on physical examination determines the course of treatment best suited to secure a good result.

In mild (grade I) sprains to the medial capsuloligamentous complex, ice, compression, elevation, and some form of protection (crutches) may be used for a short period of time. Once the pain diminishes, mobilization of the knee is begun, followed by aggressive supervised rehabilitation aimed at restoring strength, power, and endurance to the injured extremity.

In moderate (grade II) sprains, the treatment is the same except that the period of protection is extended and the temporary application of a knee splint may be required for the patient's comfort. Usually within 7 to 10 days the pain is diminished to the point where the rehabilitation program can be easily commenced with little or no problem. While the splint is in place the patient is encouraged to do isometric quadriceps sets and straight leg raises against resistance. Usually, the patient has no difficulty in obtaining full knee extension even during the first week after the injury. Bergfeld has described an excellent rehabilitation program for the functional treatment of these moderate sprains.[1]

Primary Repair of Grade III Sprains

In severe (grade III) sprains to the medial capsuloliamentous complex, most authorities believe a primary surgical repair should be undertaken as soon as possible to secure the best possible functional results, especially if there is associated damage to the cruciate ligaments and/or meniscus.

Hughston and Barrett[4] recommend the primary repair of "all torn capsular ligaments, retinacula, and tibial collateral ligaments."[4] They believe that primary repair of the posterior oblique ligament, "semimembranosus corner," and medial meniscus whenever possible is the key to stability and a good result. In the long-term evaluation, they reported 73 percent satisfactory objective results, 89 percent satisfactory subjective results, and 89 percent satisfactory functional results using their rating system.

Müller[7] is very explicit about the treatment of complete (grade III) tears of the medial capsuloligamentous complex. "In third-degree injuries, or complete ruptures, the situation is definite. There is no chance that the torn ends will spontaneously reappose and form adequate scar, and only surgical repair can ensure a complete functional recovery."[7] He properly emphasizes the importance of using not only approximating sutures but also tension sutures in an attempt to reapproximate the torn structures as closely as possible. Their isometric position must be carefully checked during the procedure by repeatedly flexing and extending the knee. If they are too lax, tension needs to be increased; if too tight, they will cut through the soft tissue and therefore their tension needs to be reduced. The judicious use of a screw-toothed washer method of fixation is helpful when the rupture occurs near or at the site of insertion.

Normal anatomic connections that exist between the vastus medialis–tibial collateral ligament as well as between the semimembranosus–posterior oblique ligament should be left undisturbed whenever possible due to the important effect these muscles have in "dynamizing" these two ligaments. Both Hughston and Müller stress the importance of repairing the posterior oblique ligament to the medial meniscus; once accomplished, this repair dramatically reduces the amount of medial opening and anteromedial rotatory instability present.

It has been my observation that the associated meniscal tears seen in knees with damage only to the medial capsuloligamentous complex are, strictly speaking, "capsular" tears rather than "substance" tears of the meniscus. These tears are usually, if not always, through a plane that is relatively vascular and amenable to healing. On the contrary, so-called "isolated" tears of the ACL are also commonly associated with meniscal tears. Although these are also amenable to repair, they are probably more true peripheral "substance" tears of the meniscus, unlike the "capsular" tears associated with major lesions of the medial capsuloligamentous complex in which the ACL is not damaged.

The surgical technique of reattaching the meniscus to the capsule is usually straightforward. Simple interrupted 2-0 nonabsorbable suture is used. Frequently there is enough capsular tissue available to secure a stable repair without the need to drill holes. Direct visualization of the quality of the meniscal repair is determined prior to repair of the overlying tibial collateral ligament by moving the knee through a complete range of motion and observing whether "kinking" of the free edge of the meniscus occurs.

One must keep in mind the "layer" approach to the various levels discussed earlier to obtain the most suitable exposure. The surgeon should take advantage of the exposure afforded by the tears of the various ligaments and minimize the need to transect normal structures.

The rehabilitation program following primary repair of the medial capsuloligamentous complex has changed somewhat over the past 5 years. Whereas a 6-week course of rigid cast immobilization was routinely recommended, recently the concept of early "protected mobilization" has become more and more popular. *Allowing as much motion as possible without placing stress on the repair site is an extremely valuable determination that is best made in the operating room prior to skin closure.* The use of a long-legged hinged orthosis postoperatively is excellent for permitting a predetermined range of motion to take place. Strengthening exercises should begin while the device is in place. One must keep in mind the importance of strengthening major muscle groups both proximal (hip) and distal (ankle) to the knee early in the rehabilitation period even while the long leg orthosis is being worn.

Nonoperative Treatment of Complete (Grade III) Tears of the Tibial Collateral Ligament

It has been my contention that most complete (grade III) tears of the tibial collateral ligament of the knee can be successfully treated nonoperatively, provided certain criteria are met. A study was initiated in January 1979, to evaluate the effectiveness of this approach. The protocol consists of the following elements.

1. All patients undergo valgus stress testing under general and/or spinal anesthesia to determine the degree (I to III) of medial laxity present. As stated earlier, even a 5 to 8 mm increase in laxity compared to the opposite knee indicates major tibial collateral ligament damage.[2] In the study, a

10 mm increase in laxity or greater was required. As stated previously, the quality of the end-point when performing the valgus stress test is an extremely important physical sign to determine the "completeness" of the tear. In addition, the Lachman, anterior Drawer, and pivot shift tests were also done to evaluate the integrity of the ACL. Any patient suspected of having any structural damage to the ACL based on this clinical laxity test under anesthesia was eliminated from the study.

2. All patients undergo a thorough arthroscopic examination through both anterolateral and posteromedial portals to rule out any structural damage to the ACL and/or meniscus. If any exists, these patients also are eliminated from the study. (Patients eliminated from the study for damage to the ACL undergo primary repair with augmentation to correct the ACL damage, as well as a primary repair of the medial capsuloligamentous damage. Every effort is made to preserve the menisci.)

3. Those patients included in the study are then placed in a groin-to-toe cast while still under anesthesia. The knee is held in slight varus and 30° of flexion while the cast is applied. At the end of 2 weeks a hinged-cast or, more recently, a long-leg orthosis is applied to allow a range of motion from 30° to 80°. Weight-bearing with crutches is encouraged. Four weeks later the cast or orthosis is removed and aggressive therapy is initiated.

All of the patients included in our study are evaluated within 1 week following the initial injury; therefore, we have no experience treating medial injuries initially seen beyond this period of time.

The importance of appropriate, supervised physical therapy is as paramount in these patients as in those undergoing primary repair. The goal of the program was to restore strength, power, and endurance to the hip, thigh, and leg muscles by means of isometric, isotonic, and isokinetic forms of exercise. Agility training was also encouraged and supervised when possible.

Over the past 6 years we have treated over 50 patients in the manner described in the preceding paragraphs. The results to date are encouraging. Over half of the patients included in this study are varsity intercollegiate football players. All but one were able to return to the team with few or no complaints an average of 2 months following injury.

It is our belief that complete tears of the medial capsuloligamentous complex have a high potential for healing independent of primary repair, provided there is no structural damage to the ACL at the time of initial injury.

REFERENCES

1. Bergfeld J: Symposium: functional rehabilitation of isolated medial collateral ligament sprains. First-, second-, and third-degree sprains. Am J Sports Med 3:207–209, 1979
2. Grood ES, Noyes FR, Butler DL, Suntay WT: Ligamentous and capsular restraints preventing straight medial and lateral laxity in intact human cadaver knees. J Bone Joint Surg 63A:1257–1269, 1981
3. Hughston JC, Eilers AF: The role of the posterior oblique ligament in repairs of acute medial (collateral) ligament tears of the knee. J Bone Joint Surg 55A:923–940, 1973
4. Hughston JC, Barrett GR: Acute anteromedial rotary instability: long-term results of surgical repair. J Bone Joint Surg 65A:145–153, 1983
5. Indelicato PA: Non-operative treatment of complete tears of the medial collateral ligament of the knee. J Bone Joint Surg 65A:323–329, 1983
6. Kennedy JC, Fowler PJ: Medial and anterior instability of the knee. An anatomical and clinical study using stress machines. J Bone Joint Surg 53A:1257–1260, 1971
7. Müller W: The Knee — Form, Function, and Ligament Reconstruction. Springer-Verlag, New York, 1983
8. Warren LF, Marshall JL: The supporting structures and layers on the medial side of the knee — an anatomical analysis. J Bone Joint Surg 61A:56–62, 1979
9. Warren LF, Marshall JL, Girgis F: The prime static stabilizer of the medial side of the knee. J Bone Joint Surg 56A:665–674, 1974

6
Posterior Meniscal Capsuloligamentous Complexes of the Knee

I. MARTIN LEVY

The normal, complex motion of the knee is dependent on the successful interaction of muscle motors, capsular restraints, meniscal cartilages, and bony architecture.[38] Aberrations in any of these members can allow pathologic motions, inappropriate force transmission, apparent instability, and ultimately the destruction of the joint's gliding surfaces. Although the primary control of passive instability of the knee is accomplished by the knee's primary ligamentous restraints, contributions to this control, and ultimately the subtle differences in a given knee's stability, are dependent upon the secondary contributions of capsular restraints and the meniscal cartilages.[15,29] This chapter reviews the contributions of the knee's menisci and posterior capsule to the normal function of the knee and discusses the interplay between the anterior cruciate ligament (ACL) and the peripheral meniscoligamentous complexes.

ANATOMY

Menisci

The medial meniscus is a crescent-shaped fibrocartilage that covers the medial two thirds of the medial tibial plateau.[14,20] It is roughly triangular in cross-section. The peripheral margin is thickened whereas the central free edge is remarkably thin. The anterior extremity of the medial meniscus is narrower than the posterior extremity. The anterior limit or horn of the medial meniscus is firmly fixed by bands of fibrous tissue to the anterior intercondylar fossa of the tibia in front of the ACL.[20] A fibrous band (the transverse ligament of the knee) extends from the anterior horn of the medial meniscus to the anterior convex margin of the lateral meniscus.[14,20] The posterior limit of the medial meniscus is firmly anchored by a tough expansion of fibers from the periphery of the meniscus to a deep recess behind the medial spine of the tibia and anterior to the tibial attachment site of the posterior cruciate ligament (Fig. 6-1).[11] The peripheral border of the meniscus is attached to the fibrous capsule of the knee. Fibers from the femur and tibia extend into the cartilaginous peripheral third of the meniscus.[32] The meniscotibial fibers that firmly link the medial meniscus to the tibial border are known as the coronary ligament.

The lateral meniscus is more nearly circular than the medial meniscus and covers a greater percentage of the lateral tibial plateau than its medial counterpart.[14,20] It too is triangular in cross-section, but its width is constant over most of its length. Its anterior attachment is in front of the intercondylar eminence of the tibia just anterior to the attachment site of the ACL. The posterior horn is fixed to the intercondylar eminence of the tibia, in front of the attachment site of the posterior horn of the medial meniscus. Variably, fibrous bands (the ligaments of

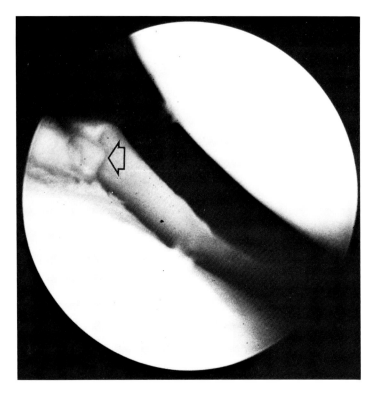

Fig. 6-1. Arthroscopic view of the posterior horn of the medial meniscus where it anchors into a deep recess anterior to the tibial attachment site of the PCL *(open arrow)*.

Humphry and Wrisberg) emanating from the peripheral margin of the posterior third of the lateral meniscus surround the posterior cruciate ligament (PCL) as the latter makes its way to the femur.[3,20,25] When present, the ligament of Humphry courses to the femur anterior toward the PCL, whereas the ligament of Wrisberg courses toward the femur posterior to the PCL. The capsular attachments of the lateral meniscus are not as firm as those of the medial meniscus, and in the posterolateral aspect are interrupted by the popliteus tendon as it travels toward its insertion on the tibia.[9,21] The defect created in the capsular attachment by the popliteus is not complete. As the tendon courses by the superior edge of the lateral meniscus, the superior capsular attachment (the superior fascicle) of the meniscus is interrupted but the inferior attachment (inferior fascicle) remains intact.[21] Further posteriorly, the inferior fascicle is breached but the superior fascicle is reestablished.

Using polarized light microscopy, Bullough et al.[4] examined the orientation of the collagen fibers of the knee's menisci. They determined that most of collagen fibers are arranged circumferentially. Radially oriented fibers are present to a lesser extent in the midzone of the meniscus. In addition, radially oriented fibers are present on the surfaces of the meniscus, predominantly the tibial surfaces. Electron microscopic evaluations of the collagen architecture of the knee's menisci by Inoue et al.[19] indicated that a regular interwoven network of collagen fiber bundles was present on the meniscus surface. Similar studies by Cameron and McNab[5] indicated that the ridges and grooves on the surface of the meniscus were predominantly in the longitudinal direction. This arrangement was common to both medial and lateral menisci.

Electron micrographs of the fiber orientation in the body of the meniscus supported the findings of polarized light microscopy. It appears that this longitudinal arrangement of fibers resists the tensile forces commonly experienced by the meniscus.[4,5] In addition, it is postulated that the radial fibers act to prevent crack propagation along the collagen bundles and thereby resist longitudinal splits of the meniscus.[4,5]

Arnoczky and Warren[1] have evaluated the vascular supply of the medial and lateral meniscus. The predominant supply is contributed by the inferior and superior, medial and lateral genicular arteries. These vessels give rise to a perimeniscal capillary plexus that branches extensively into vessels that supply the peripheral border of the menisci along their capsular attachments (Fig. 6-2). These perimeniscal vessels are oriented circumferentially with branches that project from them into the body of the meniscus.[1,2] The radial capillary projections course into the body of the medial meniscus between 10 and 30 percent of its width. Projections into the lateral meniscus extend only to 25 percent of its width. The usual perimeniscal plexus contributions are altered in the lateral meniscus in that portion adjacent to the popliteus tendon.[1,2] In this region a synovial pedicle extends to the lateral wall of the meniscus supplying the wall but not penetrating the body of the meniscus. This creates an avascular area adjacent to the popliteus tendon. The anterior and posterior horn attachment sites are supplied by the synovium covering the horns. The synovium in these areas is perfused by vessels contributed by the middle genicular artery and terminal branches of the medial and lateral genicular artery.

Posteromedial and Posterolateral Architecture of the Knee

Warren and Marshall[40] have described the architectural arrangement of the ligamentous structures of the medial side of the knee in terms of three consistent layers (Fig. 6-3). This method of description is particularly useful when one is considering those structures posterior to the longitudinal fibers of the superficial medial ligament.

After incising the skin and subcutaneous tissue on the medial side of the knee, the crural fascia (layer 1) is the first fascial plane encountered.[14,40] It invests the sartorius muscle and is continuous with the fascia that overlies the gastrocnemius and the posterior neurovascular structures. The superficial medial ligament lies deep to layer 1 and defines layer 2.[40] It is composed of two bundles of fibers, one vertical and one oblique. The vertical group originates from the femoral epicondyle and inserts posterior to the pes anserinus tendons on the proximal tibia. The fibers of the oblique bundle lie posterior to the longitudinal group of fibers. The oblique

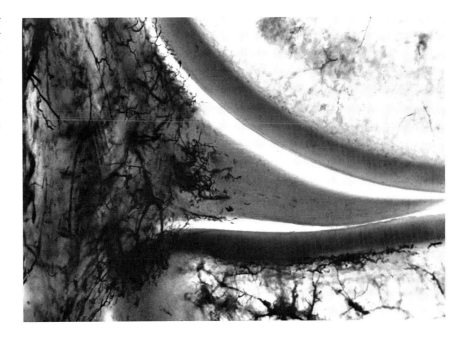

Fig. 6-2. Frontal section of the medial compartment of the knee demonstrating the branching radial vessels from the perimeniscal capillary plexus. (Arnoczky SP, Warren RF: Microvasculature of the human meniscus. Am J Sports Med 10:90–95, 1982. © 1982, American Orthopaedic Society for Sports Medicine.)

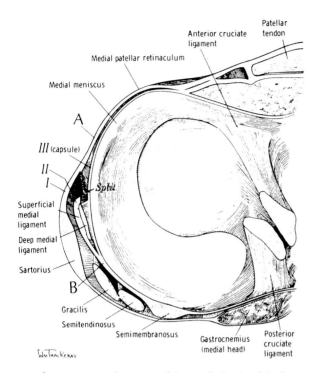

Fig. 6-3. Transaxial section of the medial side of the knee at the joint line. Three distinct layers are readily appreciated: crural fascia (layer 1, *I*), superficial medial ligament (layer 2, *II*), and capsule (layer 3, *III*)). Posteromedially layers 2 and 3 merge to form the posteromedial capsule. (Warren LF, Marshall JL: The supporting structures and layers on the medial side of the knee: an anatomical analysis. J Bone Joint Surg 61A:56–62, 1979.)

bundle also originates from the epicondyle, and ultimately inserts into the posteromedial aspect of the tibia just inferior to the articular surface. Alternatively, Hughston and Eilers[18] have designated the oblique fibers the posterior oblique ligament. They stated that the posterior oblique ligament is a thickening of the capsular ligament and is distinct from the fibers of the superficial medial ligament. Its proximal attachment is to the adductor tubercle of the femur. The ligament inserts by way of three distinct arms. Fibers of the superior arm coalesce with fibers of the oblique popliteal ligament as the latter extends laterally across the posterior capsule. The central arm inserts into the tibia just proximal to the groove created by the semimembranosus. Fibers from the inferior arm of the ligament pass from the adductor tubercle over the direct insertion of the

semimembranosus tendon and insert into the tibia posterior and inferior to that tendon. The posterior oblique ligament differs from the superficial medial ligament in that the former is firmly attached to the medial meniscus in the posteromedial aspect of the knee, whereas the latter has no attachments to the meniscus.[32]

The capsule of the knee joint, layer 3, inserts into the articular margins of the femur and tibia.[40] The more superficial capsular fibers course from the articular margin of the femur to the tibia. Deeper capsular fibers extend from the femur to the meniscus and from the meniscus to the tibia. The meniscotibial fibers are also known as the coronary ligaments.[32,40] The medial capsule is thin anteriorly, but deep to the superficial medial ligament the capsule of the knee thickens into a short band of vertically oriented fibers and is designated the deep medial ligament. Posterior to the deep medial ligament, the oblique fibers of the superficial medial ligament unite with capsular fibers of layer 3 to form the posteromedial capsule of the knee.[40] The posteromedial aspect of the knee is strengthened by fibrous extensions of the semimembranosus tendon sheath.[18,40] Fiber tracts from the semimembranosus tendon sheath coalesce and extend laterally and superiorly across the posterior capsule of the knee and form the oblique popliteal ligament. Part of the tendon of the semimembranosus muscle inserts directly into bone posterior to the verticle fibers of the superficial medial ligament. A second portion of the tendon courses more anteriorly and inserts deep to the superficial medial ligament on the proximal tibia.

Seebacher et al.[34] have used a layered approach to describe the architecture of the ligamentous supports of the lateral side of the knee (Fig. 6-4).[34] The most superficial layer (layer 1) is formed by the iliotibial tract anteriorly and the superficial portion of the biceps tendon and its expansion posteriorly. The iliotibial tract is firmly attached to both the lateral supracondylar tubercle of the femur and the lateral tibial tubercle (the tubercle of Gerdy) but remains independent of the deep capsule as it crosses the joint.[23] Fibers from the posterior edge of the iliotibial tract merge with fibers from the fascia overlying the biceps tendon.[23,34]

The anterior aspect of layer 2 of the lateral side is formed by the retinaculum of the quadriceps mus-

Fig. 6-4. Cross-section of the lateral side of the knee at the joint line. Layer 3, the capsule of the joint, divides postero-laterally into a superficial and deep lamina. (Seebacher JR, Inglis AE, Marshall JL: The structure of the posterolateral aspect of the knee. J Bone Joint Surg 64A:536–541, 1982.)

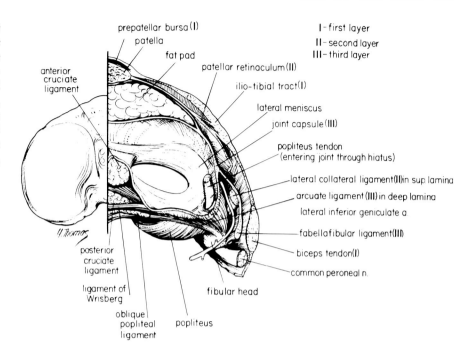

cle group. The proximal and distal patellofemoral ligaments contribute to the posterior aspect of layer 2. The patellomeniscal ligament courses from the lateral border of the patella to the margin of the lateral meniscus and on to the tubercle of Gerdy in this same layer.[34]

The lateral joint capsule, layer 3, attaches to the articular margins of the femur and tibia.[34] It divides into a superficial and deep lamina posterior to the overlying iliotibial tract.[34] The lateral collateral ligament lies between the two laminae of the joint capsule and extends from the lateral condylar tubercle of the femur to the lateral surface of the head of the fibula. The superficial lamina of the joint capsule continues posteriorly and terminates in the fabellofibular ligament.[34] Kaplan[24] found that when a fabella is present, a strong fabellofibular ligament (originating from the lateral gastrocnemius fabella and inserting on the apex of the fibula) was present. In the absence of the fabella the fabellofibular ligament was either completely absent or attenuated.[24,34] The deep lamina of the joint capsule is continuous with the lateral meniscus and forms the coronary ligament for that structure.[34] In addition, the deep lamina forms the popliteus hiatus and ultimately terminates as the lateral arch of the arcuate ligament.[24] The lateral arch extends from the fibular

styloid and crosses over the tendon of the popliteus.[24,34] The medial arch of the arcuate ligament is formed by fibers contributed by the oblique popliteal ligament as it arches over the popliteus muscle.[24] Last[27] has indicated that no less than half of the popliteus muscle is attached by the quadrilateral aponeurosis to the posterior peripheral margin of the lateral meniscus. The aponeurosis continues superiorly to blend with the deep capsule. The popliteus passes through an oval opening in the deep capsular lamina and into a plane between the deep lamina and the synovium lining the joint. The tendon of the popliteus is firmly adherent to the overlying arcuate ligament.

BIOMECHANICS: ROLE OF THE MENISCI AND POSTEROMEDIAL AND POSTEROLATERAL STRUCTURES IN STABILIZING THE KNEE

Menisci

Although speculation about the function of the knee's menisci had been made, the in vivo trials of King[26] suggested that the menisci protected the hyaline cartilage of the knee. The radiologic study of Fairbank[8] again suggested that the menisci prevented overloading of the articular cartilage. Cox and his colleagues[6,7] reaffirmed these conclusions. They examined the knee joints of dogs following partial or complete meniscectomies and showed that the degree of degenerative change present in the knee was directly related to the amount of fibrocartilage no longer present.

Methyl methacrylate forms were used by Walker and Erkman[37] to determine the area of contact between the tibia and femur under conditions of varying load. They determined that the tibiofemoral contact area of each compartment decreased by two thirds following meniscectomy from 6 cm² to 2 cm².[36,37] Using an arthrographic technique, Maquet et al.[31] found that tibiofemoral contact areas decreased significantly under conditions of physiologic load and were reduced again after dual meniscectomy. They concluded that the menisci formed a large portion of the weight-bearing surface independent of the angle of knee flexion. Fukubayashi et al.[10] used pressure-sensitive film to determine that in full extension and at 100 N load the contact area of the knee was 11.5×10^2 mm² with both menisci present and 5.2×10^2 mm² after dual meniscectomy. They determined that the menisci occupied 70 percent of the contact area.

Clinical observation of knee motion suggests that the passive stability of the knee is subject to change depending on the presence and competence of the menisci.[17,22] Huckel[17] suggested that loss of meniscal mass could be responsible for the relative looseness of a knee. Johnson et al.,[22] in reviewing 99 patients at 17 years following meniscectomy, found that 37 of their patients had demonstrable anteromedial rotational instability while only 24 had valgus rotational or anterior instability. This suggested that the menisci participated in the control of rotational stability.

Wang and Walker[38] evaluated the rotation of the tibia on the femur along a single axis at 25° of knee flexion. Cyclic rotational torques were applied and the degree of internal and external rotation was recorded. Following dual meniscectomy, half of the examined specimens demonstrated increases in rotational motion of 14 percent with an applied torque of 5 kg-cm. They concluded that the menisci of the knee contributed to the passive restraint of internal

and external rotation of the tibia on the femur. Hsieh and Walker[16] evaluated the effect of dual meniscectomy on total anterior–posterior motion of the knee at 0 and 30° of knee flexion under conditions of load and no load. They determined that the excision of both menisci had little effect on induced anterior or posterior translation, whether a load was applied or not. However, in one knee, when dual meniscectomy followed cutting of the anterior and posterior cruciate ligaments, the total anterior–posterior translation of the tibia on the femur was increased over that already produced by sectioning the cruciates.

Seale et al.[33] evaluated the effect of meniscectomy on internal–external and valgus–varus rotational stability of the knee in vitro. The knees were tested at multiple flexion angles and with an axial load of 50 pounds compressing the joint. They determined that medial meniscectomy allowed increased internal rotation of the knee, particularly at 20° of knee flexion. Lateral meniscectomy allowed increases in internal and external rotation of the knee. Medial meniscectomy allowed increased valgus rotation, which increased with the degree of flexion. Lateral meniscectomy resulted in increases in varus rotation and even greater increases in valgus rotation.

In vitro tests by Markolf et al.[30] indicated that the removal of the menisci from ligamentously intact knees had no significant effect on anterior–posterior tibial translation or internal–external rotation in unloaded or loaded specimens. However varus–valgus rotation increased after dual meniscectomy at both full extension and at 20° of knee flexion.

Levy et al.,[28] using an in vitro knee testing apparatus, demonstrated that isolated resection of the medial meniscus had no significant effect on induced anterior–posterior knee motion (Fig. 6-5). However, after section of the anterior cruciate ligament, medial meniscectomy resulted in increases in anterior displacement larger than those already increased by isolated section of the ACL. This increase in excursion was greatest at 90° of knee flexion with smaller but still statistically significant increases occurring at 30 and 60° of knee flexion. It seemed likely that after section of the ACL, the medial meniscus acted as a wedge between the tibial plateau

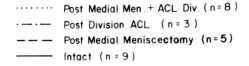

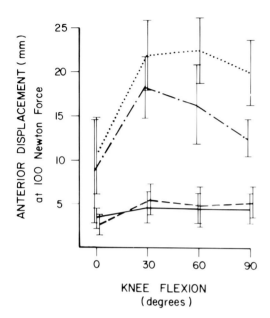

Fig. 6-5. Anterior displacement resulting from a 100 N anteriorly directed force as a function of the angle of knee flexion. (Levy IM, Torzilli PA, Warren RF: The effect of medial meniscectomy on anterior-posterior motion of the knee. J Bone Joint Surg 64A:883–888, 1982.)

and the femoral condyle, thereby restraining the tibia from further anterior displacement (Fig. 6-6).[28] For the posterior wedge to be effective, it was postulated that compressive forces across the joint were developed by the tightening of the medial supporting structures. Sullivan et al.,[35] in a follow-up study, supported this hypothesis. They demonstrated that sectioning the medial supporting ligaments resulted in significant increases in anterior displacement only after the ACL was cut. Gould et al.,[13] using a similar in-vitro knee testing apparatus, found that isolated lateral meniscectomy had no effect on forced anterior–posterior translation of the tibia (Fig. 6-7). In knees lacking both an ACL and a lateral meniscus, mean anterior displacement resulting from an applied anteriorly directed force did not differ significantly from the mean displacement

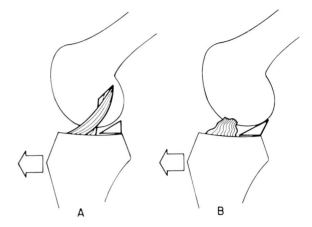

Fig. 6-6. (A) With an intact ACL, forward translation of the tibia stops before contact with the medial meniscus. (B) However, with disruption of the ACL, the posterior horn contacts the femoral condyle and acts as a wedge that resists further anterior tibial translation. (Levy IM, Torzilli PA, Warren RF: The effect of medial meniscectomy on anterior–posterior motion of the knee. J Bone Joint Surg 64A:883–888, 1982.)

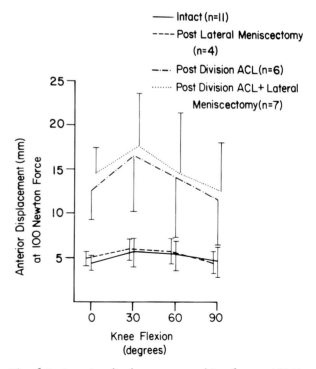

Fig. 6-7. Anterior displacement resulting from a 100 N anteriorly directed force as a function of the angle of knee flexion.

occurring after isolated section of the ACL. These results suggested that the lateral meniscus did not act as a significant block to anterior translation of the tibia after sectioning of the ACL. It is likely that these results reflect the greater mobility of the lateral meniscus. The ability of the lateral meniscus to move anteriorly and posteriorly during flexion and extension prevents it from contributing substantially to the restraint of the tibia.[13]

Posteromedial and Posterolateral Structures

The prime static restraint to valgus rotation of the knee is the superficial medial ligament.[15,39] Warren et al.[39] demonstrated in vitro that only after section of the long fibers of the superficial medial ligament was there a significant increase in the valgus rotation resulting from an applied force at 0, 30, and 45° of knee flexion.[39] After sectioning of the deep medial ligament, the posterior oblique fibers, or posterior capsule, the response of the knee to valgus torques did not significantly differ from the response of the intact knee.[39] Only after cutting the superficial medial ligament did the external rotation resulting from an applied external rotational torque increase significantly. Sectioning of the deep medial, posterior oblique, or posterior capsular ligaments did not significantly change the response of the knee to an applied external rotation torque at 0, 30, 45, or 90° of knee flexion.[39]

Grood et al.[15] examined the contribution of the collateral and capsular ligaments to the restraint of valgus and varus rotation in cadaveric knees. At 5° and 25° of knee flexion, the collateral ligaments were the primary static restraints to varus and valgus rotation. At 5° of knee flexion the medial posterior capsule contributed 17.5 percent of the restraining force resisting valgus rotation, compared to 57.4 percent contributed by the superficial medial ligament. At 25° of knee flexion the medial posterior capsule contributed only 3.6 percent to the restraint of valgus rotation compared to 78.2 percent contributed by the superficial medial ligament. At 5° of knee flexion the lateral collateral ligament contributed 54.8 percent of the restraining force to varus rotation. The lateral posterior capsule contributed 13.2 percent while the iliotibial tract, popliteus, and

biceps tendon contributed 5.0 percent of the restraint in vitro. At 25° of knee flexion the lateral collateral ligament contributed 69.2 percent of the restraint to varus rotation while the lateral posterior capsule contributed only 5.1 percent.

Sullivan et al,[35] using an in vitro knee testing apparatus, evaluated the contribution of the posteromedial structures to the restraint of anterior translation of the tibia on the femur before and after sectioning the ACL (Fig. 6-8).[35] Tests were performed at seven flexion angles between 0° and 90°. Progressive cuts of the medial side structures (the superficial medial ligament, the deep medial ligament, the oblique fibers of the superficial medial ligament, and the posteromedial part of the capsule) had no effect on anterior or posterior translation of the tibia when the ACL was intact. When sectioning of the ACL was followed by cutting the posteromedial part of the capsule, the oblique fibers of the superficial medial ligament or both, the anterior translation recorded was no greater than that seen after isolated sectioning of the ACL ligament, for all flexion angles tested. Only when both the ACL and the superficial and deep medial ligaments were sectioned simultaneously did anterior translation increase over that seen for isolated sectioning of the ACL. From this investigation it appeared that the posteromedial structures did not contribute significantly to the restraint of anterior translation of the tibia.[35]

Gollehon et al.[12] used an in vitro knee testing device to evaluate the contribution of the lateral structures to the restraint of translation and rotation of the tibia. Sectioning of the lateral collateral ligament, popliteus, and arcuate complex allowed a significant increase in posterior translation of the knee at 0° and 30° of knee flexion. This translation was not significantly changed by sectioning of the PCL at 0° and 30°. However, when evaluated at 60° and 90°, section of the posterior cruciate ligament allowed a significant increase in posterior translation over that seen after section of the lateral collateral ligament, the popliteus, and the arcuate complex alone. When both the popliteus and arcuate complex and the lateral collateral ligament were sectioned, the varus rotation resulting from a varus torque applied at 0° and 30° of knee flexion increased significantly over that seen with isolated

Fig. 6-8. Characteristic force/displacement response at 90° of knee flexion. Sectioning the medial side structures (*M.S.*) did not change the force/displacement response from that seen in the intact knee. However, when sectioning of the medial side structures followed sectioning of the anterior cruciate ligament *(ACL + M.S.)* the displacement increased over that previously noted after isolated sectioning of the anterior cruciate ligament *(ACL).* (Sullivan D, Levy IM, Sheskier S et al: Medial restraints to anterior–posterior motion of the knee. J Bone Joint Surg 66A:930–936, 1984.)

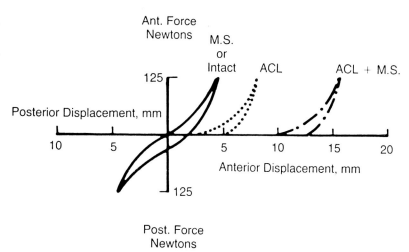

sectioning of the lateral collateral ligament. Forced external rotation of the tibia increased dramatically over the intact knee after sectioning of the lateral collateral ligament, the popliteus, and the arcuate complex at 0° and 30°

REFERENCES

1. Arnoczky SP, Warren RF: Microvasculature of the human meniscus. Am J Sports Med 10:90–95, 1982
2. Arnoczky SP: The blood supply of the meniscus and its role in healing and repair. pp. 94–110. In Finerman G (ed): A.A.O.S. Symposium on Sports Medicine: The Knee. CV Mosby, St. Louis, 1985
3. Brantigan OC, Voshell AF: The relationship of the ligament of Humphry to the ligament of Wrisberg. J Bone Joint Surg 28A:66–67, 1946
4. Bullough PG, Munuera L, Murphy J, Weinstein AM: The strength of the menisci of the knee as it relates to their fine structure. J Bone Joint Surg 52B:564–570, 1970
5. Cameron HU, McNab I: The structure of the meniscus of the human knee joint. Clin Orthop 89:215–219, 1972
6. Cox JS, Nye CE, Schaeffer WW, Woodstein IJ: The degenerative effects of partial and total resection of the medial meniscus in dog's knees. Clin Orthop 109:178–183, 1975
7. Cox JS, Cordell LD: The degenerative effects of medial meniscus tears in dog's knees. Clin Orthop 125:236–242, 1977
8. Fairbank TJ: Knee joint changes after meniscectomy. J Bone Joint Surg 30B:664–670, 1948
9. Freiberger RH, Kaye JJ: Arthrography. Appleton & Lange, New York, 1979, pp. 31–53
10. Fukubayashi T, Kurosawa H, Kimizuka A, Miyanaga Y: The contact area and pressure distribution pattern of the knee relating to the weight bearing function of the menisci. Acta Orthop Scand 51:871–879, 1980
11. Goldner RD, Kulund DN, McCue FC: The "blind side" of the medial meniscus. Am J Sports Med 8:337–341, 1980
12. Gollehon DL, Torzilli PA, Warren RF: The role of posterolateral and cruciate ligaments in human knee stability (a biomechanical study). Transactions of the 31st O.R.S., 10:270, 1985
13. Gould JD, Torzilli PA, Adams TC, et al: The effect of lateral meniscectomy on knee motion. Transactions of the 30th O.R.S., 9:25, 1984
14. Warwick R, Williams PL (eds): Gray's Anatomy of the Human Body, ed. 35. WB Saunders, Philadelphia 1973
15. Grood ES, Noyes FR, Butler DL, Suntay WJ: Ligamentous and capsular restraints preventing straight medial and lateral laxity in intact human cadaver knees. J Bone Joint Surg 63A:1257–1269, 1981
16. Hsieh HH, Walker PS: Stabilizing mechanisms of the loaded and unloaded knee joint. J Bone Joint Surg 58A:87–93, 1976
17. Huckell JR: Is meniscectomy a benign procedure? A long-term follow up study. Can J Surg 8:254–260, 1965
18. Hughston JE, Eilers AF: The role of the posterior oblique ligament in repairs of acute medial (collat-

eral) ligament tears of the knee. J Bone Joint Surg 55A:923–940, 1973

19. Inoue H, Isomaki AM, Oka M, Vainio K: Scanning electron microscopic studies: fibrocartilage degeneration in rheumatoid arthritis. Acta Rheum Scand 17:187–194, 1971

20. Insall JN: Surgery of the Knee. Churchill Livingstone, New York, 1984

21. Jelaso DV: The fascicles of the lateral meniscus: an anatomic-arthrographic correlation. Radiology 144: 335–339, 1979

22. Johnson RJ, Kettelkamp DB, Clark W, Leaverton P: Factors affecting late results after meniscectomy. J Bone Joint Surg 56A:719–729, 1974

23. Kaplan EB: Some aspects of functional anatomy of the human knee joint. Clin Orthop 23:18, 1962

24. Kaplan EB: Surgical approach to the lateral (peroneal) side of the knee joint. Surg Gynecol Obstet 104:346–356, 1957

25. Kennedy JC: The Injured Adolescent Knee. Williams & Wilkins, Baltimore, 1979

26. King D: The function of the semilunar cartilages. J Bone Joint Surg 18:1069–1076, 1936

27. Last RJ: The popliteus muscle and the lateral meniscus. J Bone Joint Surg 32B:93–99, 1950

28. Levy IM, Torzilli PA, Warren RF: The effect of medial meniscectomy on anterior-posterior motion of the knee. J Bone Joint Surg 64A:883–888, 1982

29. Levy IM, Levin PE, Torzilli PA: A method for classifying the passive pathomechanics of the knee: a new and precise classification system of knee instability using anatomical and mechanical terms. Presented at the American Orthopaedic Society for Sports Medicine. Nashville, Tenn., July 1985

30. Markolf KL, Bargar WL, Shoemaker SC, Amstutz HC: The role of joint load in knee stability. J Bone Joint Surg 63A:570–585, 1981

31. Maquet PG, Van De Berg AJ, Simonet JC: Femorotibial weight-bearing areas. J Bone Joint Surg 57A:766–771, 1975

32. Müller W: The Knee: Form, Function and Ligament Reconstruction. Springer-Verlag, New York, 1983

33. Seale KS, Haynes DW, Nelson CL, et al: The effect of meniscectomy on knee stability. Transactions of the 27th O.R.S. 6:236, 1981

34. Seebacher JR, Inglish AE, Marshall JL, Warren RF: The structures of the posterolateral aspect of the knee. J Bone Joint Surg 64A:536–541, 1982

35. Sullivan D, Levy IM, Sheskier S et al: Medial restraints to anterior-posterior knee motion. J Bone Joint Surg 66A:930–936, 1984

36. Walker PS, Hajek JV: The load-bearing area in the knee joint. J Biomech 5:581–589, 1972

37. Walker PS, Erkman MJ: The role of the menisci in force transmission across the knee. Clin Orthop 109:184–192, 1975

38. Wang CJ, Walker PS: Rotatory laxity of the human knee joint. J Bone Joint Surg 56A:161–170, 1974

39. Warren LR, Marshall JL, Girgis F: The prime static stabilizer of the medial side of the knee. J Bone Joint Surg 56A:665–674, 1974

40. Warren LF, Marshall JL: The supporting structures and layers on the medial side of the knee: an anatomical analysis. J Bone Joint Surg 61A:56–62, 1979

7
Kinematics of the Cruciate Ligaments

WERNER MÜLLER

The basic mechanism of movement between the femur and tibia is a combination of rolling and gliding. On closer analysis, it becomes difficult to discern the exact mix of rolling and gliding in the individual phases of movement. Automatic initial and terminal rotation as well as voluntary rotation are superimposed on the basic flexion and extension movements. However, if we reduce the problem to one involving a single plane, the sagittal, it becomes easy to demonstrate and understand how the femoral condyle rolls and glides simultaneously on the tibia.

In this chapter, I will delineate the basic kinematic principles of motion of the knee joint, which are represented by the crossed four-bar linkage and rolling–gliding motion. Also, I will discuss the Burmester curve. The cruciate ligaments, the foundation of knee joint kinematics, are subject to the crossed four-bar linkage principle. The Burmester curve is the ideal construct for the collateral ligaments. Sections of the chapter expand on the effects of reinsertion of the avulsed anterior cruciate ligament (ACL), the lateral pivot shift phenomenon, the collateral ligaments, and relationships of the structures within the knee. The kinematic principles provide an understanding of complex pathologic joint motion problems created by ligamentous lesions within the knee.

THE CROSSED FOUR-BAR LINKAGE AND ROLLING–GLIDING PRINCIPLE

Kapandji,[14] Huson,[13] and Menschik[16-19] were able to show that the basic kinematic principle of motion in the knee joint can be represented by the mechanism of the crossed four-bar linkage. Following their diagrams, we can demonstrate the crossed four-bar linkage by constructing a simple apparatus consisting of a sheet of drawing paper on which two rods are hinged at one end which intersect the longitudinal axis at a 40° angle through one of the points. One of the crossed rods is longer than the other; their length ratio is equal to that of the normal anterior and posterior cruciate ligaments. The free ends of the rods are linked by a movable rectangular plastic bar. This bar forms the coupler as it is moved through its various positions to generate tangents which delineate a curve. This "coupler envelope curve" (Fig. 7-1) approximates the contour of a sagittal section through the posterior half of the femoral condyle.

If, instead of a straight coupler, we use a concave or convex coupler corresponding closely to the actual contour of the upper tibial surface, we obtain a slightly different coupler envelope curve. This curve approximates the natural contour of the femoral condyle. However, this scheme holds theoretically only for motion in a single plane without allowance for rotation.

With the straight-coupler model, we can demonstrate the obligatory shift of the contact points during articulator motion. The obligatory sequence will remain unchanged if we move the envelope curve obtained with the coupler fixed horizontally or if we move the coupler itself (Fig. 7-1). But with the coupler as the stationary member, the system's intrinsic backward shift of the contact point on the coupler becomes more obvious. With the obligatory shift of contact points, the peculiar overhanging of the posterior tibial plateau, observed by Meyer[20] as early as 1853, can be understood. The knee can be flexed without the femoral shaft impacting on the posterior tibial plateau at the flexion-end-point.

The ratio of rolling to gliding does not remain constant through all degrees of flexion. This ratio is approximately 1:2 in early flexion and about 1:4 by the end of flexion. Only the posterior portion of the femoral condyle is subject to the rolling–gliding principle. The validity of the law ends where the femoropatellar joint surface begins.

When hyperextension occurs, it is not a sign of the continuation of rotational gliding but, instead, it is an angulation in the terminal sulcus of the femoral condyle between the femorotibial and femoropatellar articular surfaces. In ligamentous laxity of the knee joint with ACL insufficiency and corresponding hyperextensibility, an impression often forms on the femoral condyle. Strasser[26] recognized this feature in 1917. He called it "impressio terminalis." The impression may be the result of either an acute or chronic pressure. An analogous phenomenon occurs in knee joints with idiopathic laxity and hypermobility.[25]

THE CRUCIATE LIGAMENTS: FOUNDATION OF KNEE JOINT KINEMATICS

In 1974, Tillman[27] showed with histologic sections that the cruciate ligaments were present in the human embryo at 10 weeks. Also, the basic contour of the femoral condyle and the intercondylar roof angle of 40° were apparent. Distinct menisci were present, discoid in shape and fused with the upper tibial surface. When joint motion begins, the menisci separate from the tibia so that they can follow the excursion of the femur. Tillman's findings[27] suggest that the function of the cruciate ligaments and the shape of the condyles are closely interrelated. Apparently, the motion of the articular surfaces is predetermined to a large degree by the presence of the cruciate ligaments at this embryonic developmental stage.

The functional role of the cruciate ligaments begins early in the development of the human knee. Joint congruence can be maintained in later life only if the ligaments continue to perform their function to a sufficient degree. The ligaments convert a

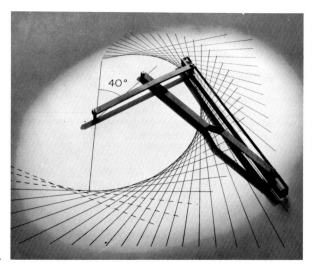

Fig. 7-1. (**A**) Model of crossed four-bar linkage. The cruciate ligaments are represented by rigid rods that are hinged on a line set at a 40° angle to a given perpendicular. The tibial plateau is represented by the "coupler," consisting of a rectangular plastic bar. *(Figure continues.)*

A

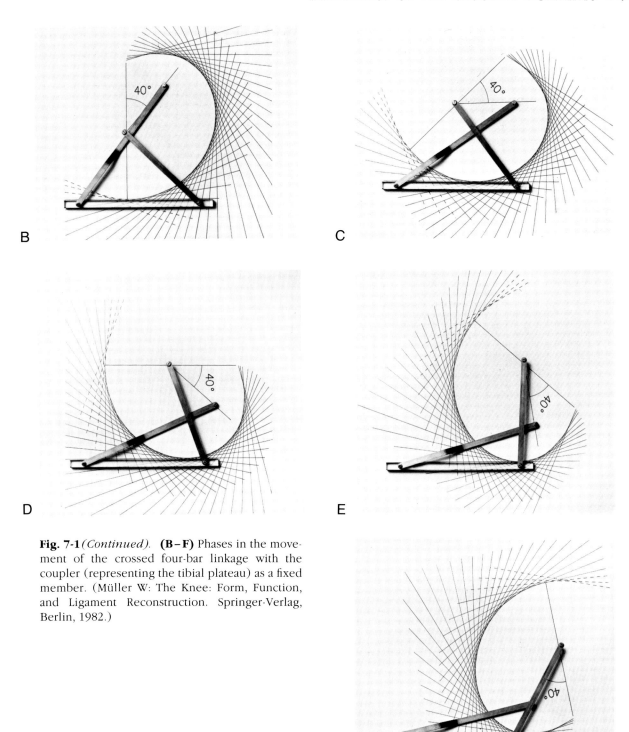

Fig. 7-1 *(Continued).* **(B–F)** Phases in the movement of the crossed four-bar linkage with the coupler (representing the tibial plateau) as a fixed member. (Müller W: The Knee: Form, Function, and Ligament Reconstruction. Springer-Verlag, Berlin, 1982.)

simple rotational movement into a more complex movement of the coupler. The cruciate ligaments perform the function of a true gear mechanism and form the nucleus of knee joint kinematics.[13,16-19] Rupture of a cruciate ligament abolishes the gear mechanism. The mechanism cannot be replaced satisfactorily by the peripheral ligaments and joint capsule.

PHYSIOLOGY AND PATHOPHYSIOLOGY OF THE LIGAMENTS DEPENDING ON THE KINEMATICS OF THE CRUCIATES

The laws of the four-bar linkage, which determine the obligatory motion of the joint surfaces with the posterior shift of the contact point, are solely responsible for the cruciates' functional sequence. Even if the collateral ligaments are lost and the extension and flexion movements between femur and tibia occur in one plane, the consequences of the laws affecting the sequence remain operative.

In the simple scheme of uniplanar motion, the cruciate ligaments can be used as radii (of constant length) to trace small circular arcs. With the tibia fixed, their end-points on the femur lie on a circle. Conversely, if the tibia is moved and the femur is fixed, the femoral end-point forms the center of the circle. This model is valid only if we view the cruciate ligaments as an ideal line. However, in reality, not all the fibers fit the ideal line.

To allow the normal mobility of 5° to 0° to 145°, the femoral origins of the cruciate ligaments must lie on a line which forms a 40° angle with the long axis of the femur. The roof of the intercondylar notch forms a 40° angle with the long axis.

The cruciate ligaments act to limit extension and prevent hyperextension. If the knee is forced into hyperextension, the posterior cruciate ligament (PCL) is not as vulnerable to injury as the ACL. However, if a patient has a chronic ACL insufficiency, pathologic hyperextensibility is always present.

REINSERTION OF AN AVULSED ACL

A ruptured cruciate ligament reinserted too far anteriorly in the vault of the intercondylar notch (Fig. 7-2) will be too short during flexion. Hence, the forces generated by the muscles and lever arms will cause the ligament either to rupture or to elongate during flexion. The forces affect not only the ligament but also the fixation wire.

Hyperextension and the ACL

The ACL can be injured at the anterior border of the intercondylar roof if the patient experiences passive trauma in hyperextension or active, violent hyperextension of the knee when it is internally rotated. According to Grant and Basmajian,[10] there is a notch into which the ACL fits when the knee is extended. When the knee is hyperextended, the ACL becomes kinked and torn at the edge of this "notch of Grant." The synergistic ligament structures (the semimembranosus corner on the medial side and the popliteus corner on the lateral side) only become stretched.

The ACL and the Menisci

ACL insufficiency results in disintegration of the rolling–gliding movement and causes the femoral condyle to roll excessively before it glides.[1] The menisci must move out of the way of the femoral condyles during knee motion so that they will not become "caught between the wheels" of the cruciate gear mechanism when the contact point moves anteriorly or posteriorly. When the ACL is torn, the femur rolls up onto the meniscus and its posterior horn when the knee is flexed. Then the femur skids back (Fig. 7-3). This sequence leads to disintegration of the rolling–gliding movement[1] and subsequently to the well-known pattern of clinical deterioration described by Chalandre in 1977.[3]

In 1972, Olsson et al.[22] described the formation of reactive degenerative osteophytes in dogs after ACL rupture. A vicious cycle developed with progression from ligamentous insufficiency to arthrosis.

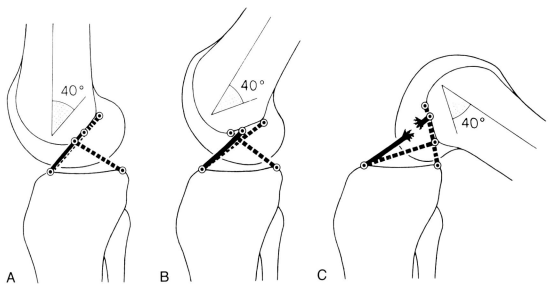

Fig. 7-2. Improperly inserted, the cruciate ligaments cannot trace out circular arcs during flexion. Thus, an ACL reinserted too far anteriorly **(A)** becomes lax at about 40° of flexion **(B)** and at 120° of flexion it is too short and must tear **(C)**. (Müller W: The Knee: Form, Function, and Ligament Reconstruction. Springer-Verlag, Berlin, 1982.)

Also in 1972, Gudde and Wagenknecht[12] reported poor results in 50 patients who underwent medial meniscectomy but had untreated ACL lesions. On follow-up evaluations, the patients had abnormal passive hyperextensibility, an anterior Drawer sign of 10 to 20 mm, and degenerative osteophytes.

The experience of other clinicians[1,5,12,22] support my observations in earlier cases as well as late-referred cases.

ACL INSUFFICIENCY AND THE LATERAL PIVOT SHIFT PHENOMENON

In 1968, Slocum and Larson[24] pointed out the abnormal freedom of rotation in complex instabilities of the knee. In 1972, Galway et al.[9] wrote their now-famous report putting forth the added dimension to the study of the effects of individual ligamentous ruptures reported 4 years earlier and calling the concept "lateral pivot shift." Galway[8] wrote also about the lateral pivot shift being a sign and symptom of ACL insufficiency. A whole syndrome of associated changes, such as flattening of the femoral condyle, cartilage erosion, and lateral meniscal ruptures has been attributed to ACL insufficiency. Ségal et al.[23] gave a topographic and chronologic description of the inevitable progress of these secondary changes. The investigators[9,23,24] strongly suspected that the insufficiency of the ACL was responsible for this subluxation phenomenon.

To test the hypothesis about the effects of ACL insufficiency, Chapchal[4] described how Jakob and Noesberger sectioned the ACL in a stable cadaveric knee. The lateral pivot shift was present. When they also sectioned the medial deep posterior ligament (semimembranosus corner) and lateral structure, the phenomenon was accentuated.

MacIntosh Test

The MacIntosh test helps to elucidate the lateral pivot shift phenomenon. In performing this test, the extended knee is slowly brought to 30° to 40° of

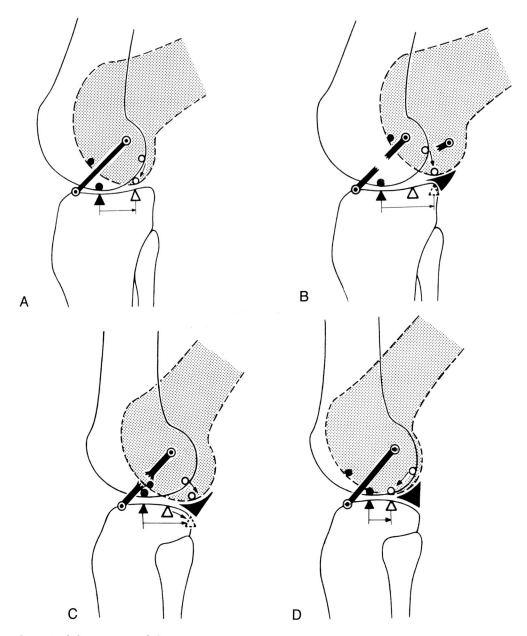

Fig. 7-3. (A) Function of the intact ACL. **(B)** Loss of the ACL leads to excessive femoral rolling, resulting in an abnormal posterior shift of the femoral contact point on both the medial and lateral sides. The posterior horns of the menisci are severely stressed as they act to brake this rolling movement, and are subject to chronic attrition. (△) Normal contact point in flexion; (⊿) abnormal contact points in anterior cruciate insufficiency. **(C–D)** If the ACL is insufficient, the femur can easily roll down beyond the posterior half of the tibial plateau. This phenomenon also underlies the "lateral pivot shift," a clinical sign of ACL insufficiency. (Müller W: The Knee: Form, Function, and Ligament Reconstruction. Springer-Verlag, Berlin, 1982.)

flexion under valgus stress and internal rotation. If the ACL is incompetent, a distinct "subluxation snap" occurs. Shortly before the snapping point, the anterior subluxation of the tibia increases. This subluxation reduces abruptly as soon as the snap occurs. After this reduction, the femur and tibia are again in normal relation to each other through the remainder of the range of motion. The phenomenon clearly demonstrates the disintegration of the rolling–gliding movement as a consequence of the ACL insufficiency.

The disintegration was demonstrated in a different context by Wirth and Artmann.[28] They proved the possibility that disintegration could occur in the presence of ACL insufficiency. They showed that in an ACL-deficient knee the femur rolled without any gliding to 30° of flexion and lay too far posteriorly on the tibial plateau. This effect is aided by the superior convexity of the lateral tibial plateau. The lateral pivot shift is driven by strong valgus pressure, favoring rolling over gliding when the iliotibial tract is stretched taut by internal rotation of the tibia. The tract, with its Y-shaped expansion directed posteriorly, pushes the lateral femoral condyle backward on the tibia as it rolls until it crosses the momentary flexion axis (at 30° to 40° flexion). Although at that moment the femur can appear to snap forward into its normal position relative to the tibia, actually it is the tibia that snaps back into place relative to the femur (Fig. 7-4).

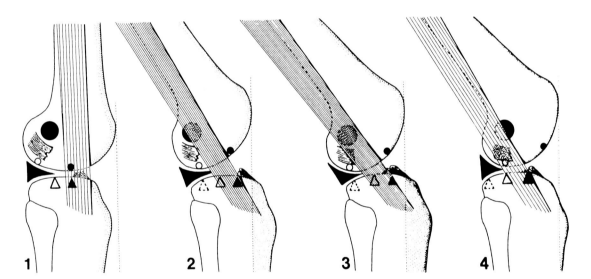

Fig. 7-4. Four-phase schematic representation of the lateral pivot shift phenomenon in ACL insufficiency. *Phase 1:* normal starting position in extension. *Phase 2:* increased posterior rolling of the femur due to ACL insufficiency. The iliotibial tract is still in front of the transverse flexion axis and lateral epicondyle. The tibia is in the anterior Drawer position. *Phase 3:* at this moment the iliotibial tract snaps across the flexion axis and epicondyle. The tract is under maximum tension, and anterior displacement of the tibia is also maximal. *Phase 4:* the tract is now behind the transverse flexion axis and epicondyle. The femur was able to snap back anteriorly, occupying a position on the tibia appropriate for the angle of flexion. The tibia has performed an opposite movement, snapping back from its anterior Drawer position into a normal relation with the femur; this movement is more obvious than that of the femur. The superior convexity of the lateral tibial plateau is recognized as another enabling factor in the pivot shift phenomenon, together with ACL insufficiency and the pathophysiology of the iliotibial tract. ●, Symbol for flexion axis. (Müller W: The Knee, Form, Function, and Ligament Reconstruction. Springer-Verlag, Berlin, 1982.)

Interrelationship of the Iliotibial Tract

The iliotibial tract has a complex task and performs several functions. It acts as an extensor when the knee is in 0° to 30° of flexion and becomes a flexor when the knee is flexed beyond 40°. The iliotibial tract has a neutral role between 30° and 40° (which is also explicit in Slocum's test for the anterior and posterior Drawer sign).

The iliotibial tract, a tendon of the tensor fasciae latae muscle, is an excellent example of a "dynamized" ligament. It incorporates extensions of the intermuscular septum (femorotibial ligamentous fibers which extend from the proximal part of the femoral condyle to the tubercle of Gerdy). In anterolateral instability of the knee, this ligamentous extension is no longer competent. The less competent the femorotibial component of the iliotibial tract and the greater the insufficiency of the ACL, the farther posteriorly the femur can roll. Thus the lateral pivot shift phenomenon (subluxation) will exhibit itself prominently.

COLLATERAL LIGAMENTS

The collateral ligaments can be represented by an ideal construct, the Burmester curve, just as the cruciate ligaments can be represented by an ideal construct, the crossed four-bar linkage. The collateral ligaments also follow an approximately circular path during the kinematic sequence. The path corresponds to a short circular arc when the femur is in motion and to a somewhat larger arc when the tibia

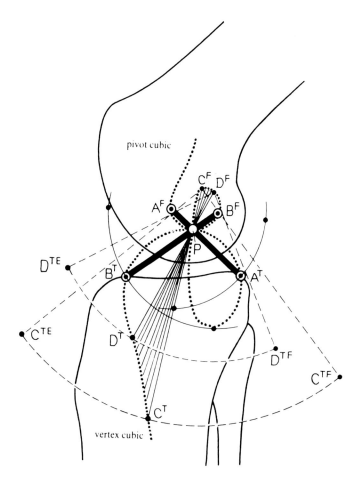

Fig. 7-5. The theoretical course of the MCL and its position in relation to the Burmester curve. In our simplified scheme after Menschik, the tibia is moved relative to the stationary femur. If a point C^F on the pivot cubic is connected with a point C^T on the vertex cube through the center P, the point C^T will follow an approximately circular path when the tibia is moved (hereafter we will assume this path is truly circular to simplify the drawings). Thus, the point C^T (tibia) belonging to C^F (femur) traces out a circular arc when passing from C^{TE} (extension) to C^{TF} flexion). An analogous path is followed by the boundary points D of the collateral ligament. The endpoints of the cruciate ligaments on the tibia, A^T and B^T, also follow circular paths in the present uniplanar scheme of motion (without rotation). (Müller W: The Knee: Form, Function, and Ligament Reconstruction. Springer-Verlag, Berlin, 1982.)

is in motion. The excursions of these arcs have not been determined; however, we have asked physicists to study them and provide us with a definitive answer.

Burmester Curve

Burmester, a mathematician from Munich, published a textbook on kinematics in 1888. In the 1970s, Menschik[16-19] brought Burmester's curve to the attention of knee surgeons. The Burmester curve is a curve comprised of two third-order curves, the *vertex cubic* and the *pivot cubic*. The Burmester curve is fundamental to the sites of insertion of the knee collateral ligaments. If we draw a straight line on the vertex cubic through the crossing point *P* of the four-bar linkage to a point on the pivot cubic, the two points will follow approximately circular paths when the linkage is moved. Their distance from each other on the straight line appears to remain practically constant. Whether the paths are precisely circular or not does not really concern us here, insofar as nature has confirmed the validity of the laws by the actual size of the ligament insertions.

Application of the Burmester Curve

In Figure 7-5, we see that if, in 43° of knee flexion,[16-19] we connect several points on the pivot cubic loop through center *P* with corresponding points on the descending limb of the vertex cubic, we obtain a construction that corresponds closely to the natural form and length of the medial collateral ligament (MCL). It even possesses the decussation characteristic of the ligament's fibers. This appears to be a type of crossed four-bar linkage system. The fibrous strands always intersect at the "pole"[16-19] which is located on the transverse flexion axis, and radiate out from the center like the spokes of a wheel (Fig. 7-6). Here we see the MCL and ACL grouped on one side and the lateral collateral liga-

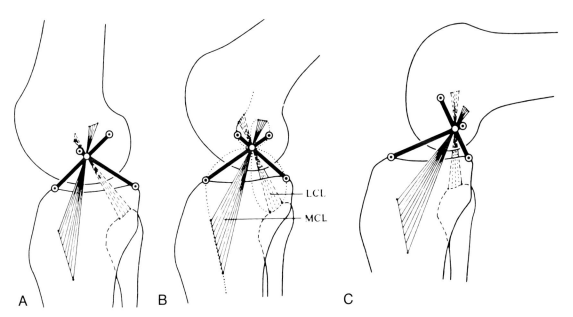

Fig. 7-6. This crossing point can be maintained in extension **(A)** and in flexion **(B)** and probably also represents the point where the flexion axis passes through the femur. In **(C)** the cruciate ligaments are represented by a crossed four-bar linkage, and the MCL and LCL by the principles of the Burmester curve. All elements intersect at the crossing point of the four-bar linkage. (Müller W: The Knee: Form, Function, and Ligament Reconstruction. Springer-Verlag, Berlin, 1982. After Menschik A: Mechanik des Kniegelenkes. Teil 3. Sailer, Vienna, 1974.)

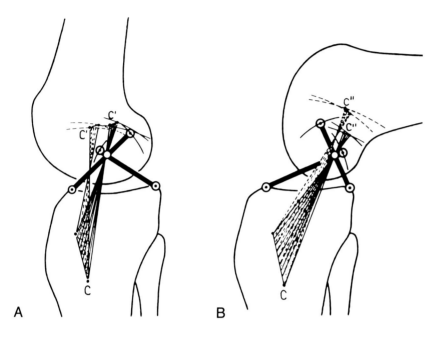

A

B

Fig. 7-7. If we mistakenly reinsert the MCL too far forward on the femur, as represented by the ligament (---) in the left half of **(A)**, it violates the law of the Burmester curve and becomes overstretched during flexion. (Müller W: The Knee: Form, Function, and Ligament Reconstruction. Springer-Verlag, Berlin, 1982.

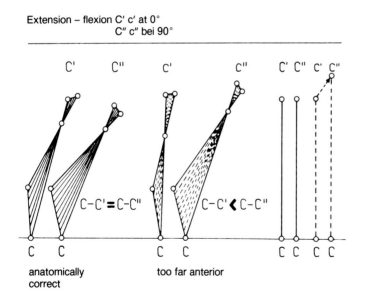

Extension – flexion C' c' at 0°
C" c" bei 90°

C-C' = C-C"

C-C' < C-C"

anatomically correct

too far anterior

ment (LCL) and the PCL grouped on the other side. The distribution of the spokes is somewhat uneven.

The spoked-wheel principle is well described in the theories of others[6,7,11,21] although the position of the flexion axis and instant center was calculated differently and represented by different models than the one described by Menschik.[16-19] Topo-graphically, all the axes are located close to the center of motion in the Menschik model. The essential difference between the Menschik model and the other models is that Menschik's model provides a unique solution for each individual knee; the other models do not offer such an alternative. Beauchamp et al.[2] have shown different length relations of the two cruciate ligaments. This condition results in individually different condylar profiles. Both profiles taken together yield a unique position on the Burmester curve. Likewise, the lengths of the collateral ligaments, which vary from person to person, will yield different positions on the curve. These individual differences, particularly if both the cruciate ligaments and the collateral ligaments are injured, have tremendous impact upon considerations by the surgeon during the ligamentous repair procedures.

LOSS OF ISOMETRY FROM FAULTY LIGAMENT INSERTION

With the aid of the Menschik model, we can approach the serious consequences of shifting the ligament insertion even just 1 cm anteriorly during the surgical repair. Such faulty ligament insertion affects ligament length changes during flexion and extension. Figure 7-7 shows that the ligament is stretched 16.7 percent. During the surgical procedure, the physician can test to see if the sutures have been properly placed. If they have not been placed on the correct line, during trial flexion and extension of the knee the falsely placed suture will promptly tear.

The knee joint is surrounded by a number of triangular structures, of which the fiber systems connecting the tibia–MCL–femur and femur–posterior oblique ligament–tibia are examples. Frequently, stresses that displace the tibia (Fig. 7-8) place great stress on the meniscotibial fibers of the posterior oblique ligament (POL) that form part of the coronary ligament. The importance of these fibers is particularly well demonstrated by the rare rupture of the meniscotibial ligament. In a situation where the semimembranosus corner remains essentially intact, but the surgeon knows the tibia is not restrained, he will need only two or three interrupted sutures to repair the meniscotibial connection to the semimembranosus corner and thus restore complete anteroposterior stability to the medial half of the joint. The stabilizing effect of these initial sutures is so great that, besides preventing the anterior Drawer sign, they also abolish any valgus laxity

in the extended knee long before the MCL and ACL have been repaired. In contrast, in the course of reconstructive operations for fresh injuries, we have repeatedly shown how accurate repair of the semimembranosus corner, with due regard for fiber isometry, is in itself sufficient to correct any anterior Drawer sign and anteromedial rotational Drawer sign long before the first cruciate suture is in place. In this context, I am presuming that the femorotibial band of the iliotibial tract is present as a lateral synergist to form the third element of the anterior stabilization[15] in combination with the meniscotibial ligament and the intact (or repaired) semimembranosus corner.

In most cases, the synergistic structures are con-

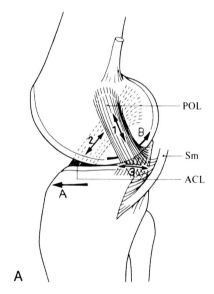

Fig. 7-8. (A) The POL is a synergist of the ACL *(2)*. When the tibia is displaced anteriorly *(arrow A)* relative to the femur, the ACL comes under tension. But at the same time, the femoral condyle must push the meniscus backward or ride up upon it *(arrow B)*. Because the meniscus is firmly attached to the tibia via the meniscotibial fibers of the POL *(3)*, its backward displacement is checked by these fibers. Thus it functions together with the femoromeniscal portion of the POL *(1)*, which also comes under strong tension, as a wedge brake against anterior tibial displacement. This structurally important system functions properly only if the POL, posterior meniscus horn, and semimembranous attachment form an intact unit. Even a small lesion leads to the first stage of anteromedial rotatory instability. *(Figure continues).*

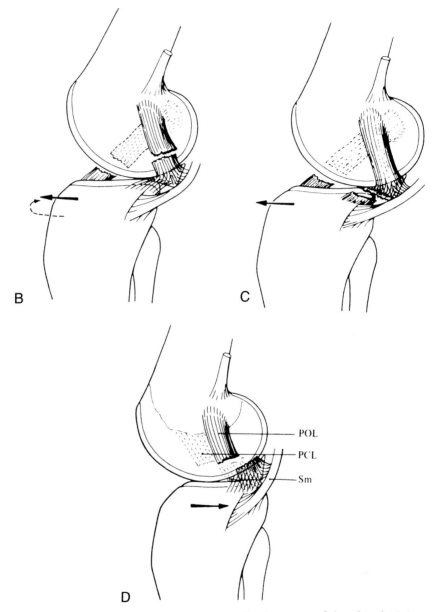

B

C

POL

PCL

Sm

D

Fig. 7-8 *(Continued).* **(B,C)** An anterior Drawer-type displacement of the tibia *(solid arrow)* combined with external rotation *(dashed arrow)* causes tearing of the ACL and POL **(B)**. The POL may be torn proximal or distal to the posterior meniscus horn **(C)**. Occasionally, both portions of the ligament, proximal and distal, may become detached from the meniscus horn. The clinical picture in such cases is that of a meniscal injury. However, the lesion is located not in the cartilaginous meniscus, but farther peripherally in the region of its capsuloligamentous attachment. Thus, the injury involves a ligamentous lesion that must be sutured, rather than a meniscus lesion; a meniscectomy in such cases is both unjustified and contraindicated. **(D)** Posterior displacement of the tibia *(arrow)*, if extensive, causes a rupture of the PCL and POL. This demonstrates the synergism of these two ligaments. The fact that the POL can be a synergist of both the ACL and PCL derives from the ability of the meniscus to transmit and redirect forces from both directions. (Müller W: The Knee: Form, Function, and Ligament Reconstruction. Springer-Verlag, Berlin, 1982.)

Fig. 7-9. If the femur is sawed in half along the sagittal plane exactly between the attachments of the cruciate ligaments and separated, these ligaments act as "medial collateral ligaments," each stabilizing its respective joint half. The lateral stability of the medial and lateral compartments thus created is surprisingly well maintained even during flexion and extension of the individual femur halves (V. Hochstetter). (Müller W: The Knee: Form, Function, and Ligament Reconstruction. Springer-Verlag, Berlin, 1982.)

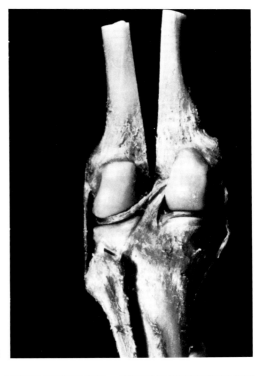

A

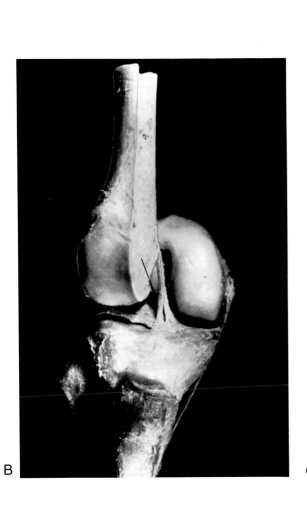

B

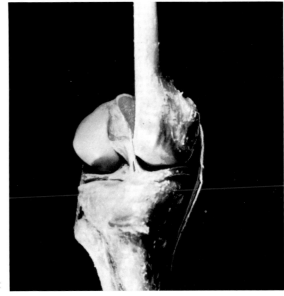

C

jointly injured. While an ACL injury is almost invariably associated with a lesion of the semimembranosus corner, the femorotibial band of the iliotibial tract has an intrinsic reserve of dynamic mobility that often enables it to escape concomitant injury. However, the surgeon must learn to appreciate the isometry of the knee structures and tune his repair of the structures so as to reestablish this isometry.

THE CRUCIATES: CENTRAL COLLATERAL LIGAMENTS FOR RESPECTIVE CONDYLES

A clinician can gain an excellent insight into knee function by splitting an anatomic specimen of the femur longitudinally in the sagittal plane down to the central pivot and studying the movement of the femur in relation to the tibia. One cruciate is retained on each half of the femur (Fig. 7-9A). He can flex and extend each half independently (Fig. 7-9B). The lesson learned is that each cruciate ligament acts as a collateral ligament for its respective condyle.

In extension, the two femoral halves can be spread apart only a small distance. Thus, if a lateral or medial ligament is incompetent because of a sprain or rupture, the cruciate ligaments can stabilize the knee against varus and valgus stresses from the center, both alone and in concert with the remaining ligaments. If there is a valgus or varus opening of the joint (more than 1+ or 2+, i.e., up to 10 mm) a lesion of the central pivot must be included in the diagnosis.

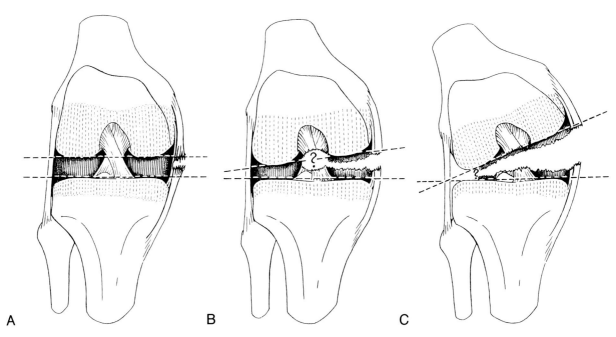

A   B   C

Fig. 7-10. The ligamentous lesion and associated passive instability. **(A)** If the tear is confined to the MCL and the posterior "corner" and posterior capsule (shaded) are intact, then a valgus stress applied to the extended knee will not cause medial opening of the joint. This is possible only when the knee is flexed about 30° to relax the posterior capsule, thereby eliminating its lateral stabilizing action. **(B)** If the knee shows medial opening in extension, involvement of the cruciate ligaments is a possibility, even if no significant Drawer sign can be elicited. **(C)** If the valgus instability extends across to the lateral side of both flexion and extension, there is no question that both cruciate ligaments are torn. The only question that remains is the degree of involvement of the posteromedial corner and femorotibial iliotibial tract fibers. (Müller W: The Knee: Form, Function, and Ligament Reconstruction. Springer-Verlag, Berlin, 1982.)

PATHOLOGIC JOINT MOTION

Five peripheral ligaments, together with the two cruciate ligaments, stabilize the knee passively. The five peripheral ligaments are the MCL, the POL–semimembranosus corner including the meniscus medialis; the arcuate–popliteus corner including

the meniscus lateralis; the LCL, and the anterolateral femorotibial ligament. If only one of these ligaments is cut or ruptured, then the measurable pathologic motion is not big (Fig. 7-10A and B). However, the functional instability may be great because the knee has lost an important restraint. The loss of one out of seven means an important break through the

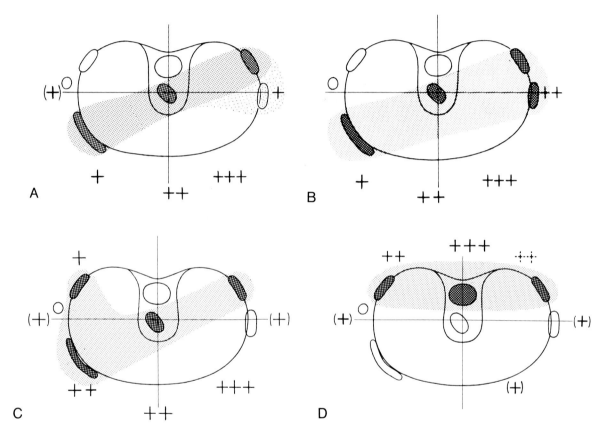

Fig. 7-11. (A) The "global anterior instability" is usually a result of chronic anterior instability and involves injuries of the POL, ACL, and ALFTL. It causes a 3+ anteromedial rotatory instability, 2+ anterior Drawer sign in neutral rotation (NR), 1+ anterolateral rotatory instability, valgus instability, varus instability, 1+ lateral pivot shift, and 1+ recurvatum. **(B)** The tetrad involves injury to the POL, ACL, anterolateral femorotibial ligament, and MCL; it causes a 3+ anteromedial rotatory instability, 2+ anterior Drawer sign in NR, 1+ anterolateral rotatory instability, 2+ valgus instability, 1+ lateral pivot shift, and a 1+ recurvatum. **(C)** A combined injury of the POL, ACL, anterolateral femorotibial ligament, and popliteus (popliteus corner) leads to a 3+ anteromedial rotatory instability, 2+ anterior Drawer sign in NR, 2+ anterolateral rotatory instability, 1+ valgus instability, (1+) varus instability, 1+ posterolateral rotatory instability, 1+ lateral pivot shift, and 1+ recurvatum. **(D)** The "global" posterior instability" involves a combined injury of the POL (semimembranosus corner), PCL and popliteus (popliteus corner). It creates a 2+ posteromedial instability, 3+ posterior Drawer sign in NR, 2+ posterolateral instability, 1+ valgus instability, 1+ varus instability, 1+ anteromedial rotatory instability, and a 1+ recurvatum. (Müller W: The Knee: Form, Function, and Ligament Reconstruction. Springer-Verlag, Berlin, 1982.)

first line of defense of the passive "roundabout stabilizing system" — the inner shell of passive stability. The pathologic motion, not more than 5 mm, may consist of (1) increased rotation (lesion of popliteus corner or the semimembranosus corner); (2) increased (i.e., 1+) opening for varus or valgus deformation (LCM, LCL lesions); or (3) increased translation mainly in the anteroposterior direction (LCL, LCP lesions).

As long as the "gear-like" mechanism of the cruciates is still intact and functioning so that they can take the physiological strain, the five peripheral ligaments may have a good chance to scar over and function well as healed tissues without surgical repair. However, if a cruciate is largely or completely ruptured, the chance for a functionally correct healing of the periphery is markedly less.

In the case of a combined lesion involving one ruptured ligament in the periphery and one in the central pivot, the patient has a break through the "second line of defense." Marked increase of combined pathologic motion follows, i.e., varus–valgus opening, translation, and rotation (Fig. 7-10B). Rotation can be described as an asymmetrical translation of the medial and lateral compartments (Fig. 7-11). As long as no muscle activity (tonus or controlled active innervation) is included (for example, in cadaveric studies), the pivot point may be located even outside the joint, which leads to more of a translation-type movement. Active muscle function pulls and pushes the pivot point back into the joint, and this leads again more to a rotational motion rather than a pure translation.

A combined lesion involving three or more ligaments, including one of the central pivot ligaments (Fig. 10C) is a break through the next line of defense, and creates the possibility of complex pathologic motion, often with mediolateral translation in a frontal plane. The axes of these motions can migrate in a much greater space after such a lesion than after a two-ligament lesion. They are now steered primarily by external forces and the reacting extrinsic muscle forces; as long as the axes were kept in the restricted area of the normal inner shell of stability, they were controlled primarily by all seven ligaments and secondarily by the active muscle forces and the additional external forces. The inner shell of stability allows the normal motion of extension-flexion-rotation, and, because of its "elastic re-

serve," permits some individual additional "play" in translational movements. Within every outer shell of stability they can move more freely because of the elongated ligaments, fasciae, tendons, and ruptured structures. With every added ligament rupture, a further "line of defense" is broken through, and the outer shell of stability gets a step wider.

The pathologic outer shell of stability, which corresponds to the "envelope of motion" (as described by Frank Noyes) with its increase of varus–valgus-opening, translation-and-rotation possibilities, is strictly related to the number and the localization of the ruptured anatomical structures which are involved (Fig. 7-11).

SUMMARY

The kinematics of the cruciate ligaments can be explained by Menschik's[16-19] crossed four-bar linkage model. The collateral ligaments have an ideal construct in the Burmester curve, which Menschik[16-19] brought to the attention of the orthopaedic surgeons in 1974. Given an understanding of these principles, the surgeon can appreciate the lateral pivot shift as a result of ACL insufficiency and can identify the site for correct reinsertion of avulsed cruciate ligaments. Faulty ligament insertion results in loss of isometry. The pathologic motion is strictly related to the number and location of the ruptured anatomical structures. As long as the gear-like mechanism of the cruciates is still intact, the joint may be functionally effective. With the loss of cruciate integrity, and the combined lesion of three or more ligaments, complex pathologic instability is inevitable without surgical intervention, and disability will probably ensue.

REFERENCES*

1. Artmann M, Wirth CJ: Untersuchung uber den funktionsgerechten Verlauf der vorderen Kreuzbandplastik. Z Orthop 112:160–161, 1974

---

* Addition reading and references are given in Müller W: The Knee. Form, Function, and Ligament Reconstruction. Springer-Verlag, Berlin, 1982; New York, 1983.

2. Beauchamp P, Laurin CA, Bailon JP: Etudes des propriétés mécaniques des ligaments croisés en vue de
   leur remplacement prothétique. Rev Chir Orthop
   65:197–207, 1979

3. Chalandre P: Le remplacement du ligament croisé
   antérieur du genou par le procédé de Lindemann.
   Mémoire du C.E.S. de Biologie et de Médecine du
   Sport, Université de Grenoble, 1977

4. Chapchal G (ed): Injuries of the Ligaments and Their
   Repair. Thieme, Stuttgart, 1977

5. Del Pizzo W, Norwood LA, Kerlan RK, et al: Analysis
   of 100 patients with anterolateral rotatory instability
   of the knee. Clin Orthop 122:178–180, 1977

6. Frankel VH: Biomechanics of the knee. Orthop Clin
   North Am 2:175–190, 1971

7. Frankel VH, Burstein AH, Brooks DB: Orthopaedic
   Biomechanics. Lea & Febiger, Philadelphia, 1971

8. Galway R: Pivot shift syndrome. J Bone Joint Surg
   54B:558, 1972 [Abstract]

9. Galway R, Beaupré A, McIntosh DL: Pivot shift: A clinical sign of symptomatic anterior cruciate insufficiency. J Bone Joint Surg 54B:763, 1972 [Abstract]

10. Grant JCB, Basmajian JV: Grant's method of Anatomy.
    Williams & Wilkins, Baltimore, 1965

11. Groh W: Kinematische Untersuchungen des mensch-
    lichen Kniegelenkes und einige Prothesen-Kniekon-
    struktionen, die als ''physiologische'' Kniegelenke
    bezeichnet werden. Arch Orthop Unfallchir 47:637–
    645, 1955

12. Gudde P, Wagenknecht R: Untersuchungsergebnisse
    bei 50 Patienten 10–12 Jahres nach der Innenmeni-
    scusoperation bei gleichzeitig vorliegender Ruptur
    des vorderen Kreuzbandes. Z Orthop 3:369–372,
    1973

13. Huson A: Biomechanische Probleme des Kniege-
    lenkes. Orthopaede 3:119–126, 1974

14. Kapandji IA: The Physiology of the Joints. Vol II.
    Churchill Livingstone, New York, 1970

15. Kaplan EB: Iliotibial band. Morphology, function.
    Anat Rec 121:319, 1955

16. Menschik A: Mechanik des Kniegelenkes. Teil 1. Z
    Orthop 112:481–495, 1974

17. Menschik A: Mechanik des Kniegelenkes. Teil 3,
    Sailer, Wien, 1974

18. Menschik A: The basic kinematic principle of the col-
    lateral ligaments, demonstrated on the knee joint. pp.
    9–16. In Chapchal G (ed): Injuries of the Ligaments
    and Their Repair. Thieme, Stuttgart, 1977

19. Menschik A: Mechanik des Kniegelenkes. Teil 2. Z
    Orthop 133:380–400, 1975

20. Meyer H: Die Mechanik des Kniegelenkes. Arch Anat
    Phys Wiss Med 1853, pp. 497–547

21. Nietert M: Untersuchungen zur Kinematik des
    menschlichen Kniegelenkes im Hinblick auf ihre Ap-
    proximation in der Prothetik. Dissertation, Tech-
    nische Universität, Berlin, 1975

22. Olsson SE, Marshall JL, Story E: Osteophytosis of the
    knee joint in the dog. A sign of instability. Acta Radiol
    (Stockh) (Suppl) 319:165–167, 1972

23. Ségal P, Lallement JJ, Raquet M, Jacob M, Gérard Y:
    Les lésions ostéo-cartilagineuses de la laxité antéro-
    interne du genou. Rev Chir Orthop 66:357–365, 1980

24. Slocum DB, Larson RL: Rotatory instability of the
    knee. J Bone Joint Surg 50A:211–225, 1968

25. Smillie IS: Injuries of the Knee Joint. 4th ed. Williams
    & Wilkins, Baltimore, 1970

26. Strasser H: Lehre der Muskel-und Gelenkmechanik.
    Springer, Berlin, 1917

27. Tillman B: Zur funktionellen Morphologie der Ge-
    lenkentwicklung. Orthop Prax 1210:691–697, 1974

28. Wirth CJ, Artmann M: Verhalten der Roll-Gleit-Bewe-
    gung des belasteten Kniegelenkes bei Verlust und
    Ersatz des vorderen Kreuzbandes. Arch Orthop Un-
    fallchir 78:356–361, 1974

8

A Biomechanical Function of the ACL: Prevention of Medial Translation of the Tibia

J. TIMOTHY BRYANT
T. DEREK V. COOKE

Over the past decade, a great deal of biomechanical information has been published on the role of the anterior cruciate ligament (ACL) in knee stability. It is generally accepted that this ligament, composed of two interactive parts, limits anterior translation of the tibia with respect to the femur.

The main body of the ligament has an oblique orientation, arising from the anteromedial portion of the tibial eminence and extending posterolaterally to its insertion on the posteromedial aspect of the lateral femoral condyle. This orientation prevents hyperextension of the joint, while the interactive anteromedial and posterolateral segments provide for tension of at least some part of the complex during all phases of motion. As the knee extends, internal rotation of the tibia is especially restricted in keeping with the alignment of its parts and with the progressive forward rolling of the tibia beneath the femoral condyles.[3,22]

In cadaver studies, Girgis et al.[9] demonstrated that absence of the anterior cruciate ligament permitted hyperextension by an average of 25°. Anterior Drawer increased by 5.7 mm. Internal rotation with the knee in extension increased by 8°. These authors also demonstrated that in 120° of flexion the loss of the ACL had a much smaller effect on rotation of the tibia. These rotation changes correlated with the observation that only the anteromedial band of the ACL was taut in deep flexion. How-

ever, anterior Drawer changes in this position were similar to those observed in the extended range. These observations are supported by more recent studies of knee kinematics using standardized mechanical tests in a cadaver, and instrumented tests in patients with known ACL disruption.[1,2,4–8,10–18,20,21,23–29]

Disruption of the ACL may occur as one of several lesions sustained in an injury, for example, as in the triad in which the two ligaments (anterior cruciate and medial collateral) and the medial meniscus disrupt simultaneously. Arthroscopic studies have shown that the isolated injury of the ACL also may occur. While a great deal more is known now about the role of the ACL in knee stability, several important questions about the lesion in isolation remain unanswered. Through our mechanical knee testing analyses, we have gained some additional insight into the biomechanics of the ACL-deficient knee.

BACKGROUND

The advent of mechanical knee testing has further documented biomechanical changes in the joint of patients with ACL-deficient knees.[6,14,17,21,26,28] These tests have quantified measurements of anterior Drawer and internal–external rotation. Mechanical testing is not only of use in diagnosis but also is

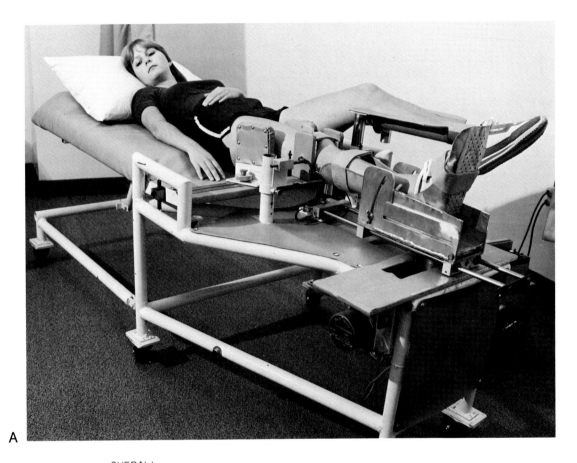

A

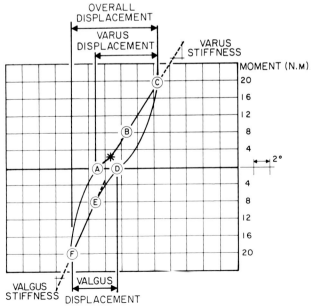

B

Fig. 8-1. (A) The knee analyzer. Patient is supine with the femur clamped at the thigh and the epicondyles. The tibia is placed in an aluminum cradle which is rotated about a pivot located below the knee. In the testing procedures, the tibia is cycled sideways between preset moment limits. Simultaneous measurements of tibial displacement and resisting moment at the knee allow quantification of the standard orthopaedic varus–valgus laxity test. **(B)** Typical moment-displacement curve for the knee. Starting at point *A*, the knee moves inward while the curve passes through points *B* and *C*. At *C*, reversal takes place and outward displacement of the tibia produces valgus displacement. The five indicated parameters are used to describe the curve.

important in the documentation of progressive laxity. While most studies of rotation have examined the characteristics of the knee in some range of flexion, few have been applied in the extended range. Only recently have these studies assessed stability of the ACL-deficient knee in varus–valgus rotation in an extended position.

Our observations on the ACL-deficient knee were serendipitous. Our first intention, using mechanical testing device, was to assess the stability of the collateral ligament structures in vivo. To our surprise, our studies documented biomechanical changes in varus–valgus rotation of knees with isolated ACL lesions. Specifically, changes were observed in the varus–valgus displacement and stiffness of the joint at 0° of flexion. The results correlated with postulated biomechanical roles of this ligament. However, these roles were not defined until the advent of suitable mechanical knee testing apparatus.

BIOMECHANICAL DOCUMENTATION OF VARUS–VALGUS DISPLACEMENT IN ACL-DEFICIENT KNEES

Test Sequence

The knee analyzer (Fig. 8-1A) was developed by Lowe and Saunders.[19] The device is based on a standard clinical test for varus–valgus stability and is constrained to quantify this assessment. The patient is supine with the femur clamped at the thigh and epicondyles. The tibia is placed in an aluminum splint that moves in the coronal plane. The splint is free to move axially. It rotates about a pivot located below the knee. A linear drive moves the ankle sideways, thereby displacing the tibia with respect to the femur. The drive system is instrumented to measure resisting moment about the knee. Sideways displacement of the tibia is measured with a potentiometer. Plotting moment (in newton-meters) against varus–valgus angle (in degrees) gives the typical moment–displacement curve shown in Fig. 8-1B.

Patient Population

Two groups, totalling 25 patients, were selected from those referred to the Orthopaedic Clinic of Kingston General Hospital. The first group of 12 included patients diagnosed with isolated ACL disruption. The second group contained 13 patients with ACL disruption with an associated pathologic conditions. Each patient had one knee without demonstrable pathologic change or history of injury to serve as an asymptomatic control. Clinical diagnosis of cruciate disruption was based on a positive pivot shift, a positive anterior Drawer, and the Lachman maneuver. Diagnosis of other injuries was based on standard tests for meniscus, collateral ligament, and capsular involvement.

Moment–displacement curves for one man in the isolated ACL disruption group are shown in Fig. 8-2. The asymptomatic (curved mirror image) and pathologic curves are superimposed to show the differences between the two curves. Varus displacement was obviously greater in the pathologic knee than in the asymptomatic knee. A smaller increase in valgus displacement was also observed.

Data for all the patients were analyzed by comparing curve parameters obtained from pathologic and

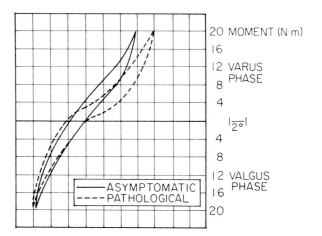

Fig. 8-2. Moment-displacement curve for participant in study (a man). Curves from the asymptomatic and pathologic knees are superimposed to illustrate differences. Large changes in the varus phase of the response are observed compared to the smaller changes observed in the valgus phase.

Table 8-1. Varus–Valgus Displacement and Stiffness (n = 25)

		Mean	SEM	Units
Pathologic knee				
Varus	Displacement	9.20	0.49	deg
	Stiffness	2.83	0.15	Nm/deg
Valgus	Displacement	6.63	0.37	deg
	Stiffness	3.68	0.20	Nm/deg
	Overall displacement	13.79	0.67	deg
Asymptomatic knee				
Varus	Displacement	7.99	0.36	deg
	Stiffness	2.98	0.17	Nm/deg
Valgus	Displacement	5.92	0.30	deg
	Stiffness	3.82	0.20	Nm/deg
	Overall displacement	12.16	0.54	deg
Difference (pathologic − asymptomatic)				
Varus	Displacement	1.21[a] (+18%)[b]	0.45 (6%)	deg
	Stiffness	−0.15 (−2%)	0.10 (4%)	Nm/deg
Valgus	Displacement	0.71[a] (+14%)[b]	0.28 (5%)	deg
	Stiffness	−0.14 (−2%)	0.11 (3%)	Nm/deg
	Overall displacement	1.63 (+15%)[c]	0.52 (4%)	deg

[a] Significantly greater than zero; $P < 0.01$
[b] Significantly greater than zero; $P < 0.005$
[c] Significantly greater than zero; $P < 0.001$
Values in parentheses are expressed as percent differences computed individually for each subject, not as a percentage of the mean value for the group.

asymptomatic joints (Table 8-1). There were no significant differences between mean parameter values from the two groups. Thus, it was appropriate to combine the data for all 25 patients. In order to account for differences in raw values for curve parameter, differences between the two groups are expressed as percentages. Three differences between symptomatic and asymptomatic joints were significant at $P < 0.01$. Varus displacement was 18 percent greater in the pathologic knee compared to the asymptomatic knee ($P < 0.005$); valgus displacement was 14 percent greater ($P < 0.005$); and overall displacement was 15 percent greater ($P < 0.001$).

JOINT BIOMECHANICAL IMPLICATIONS

The in vivo results from our studies correspond well with those predicted by our previous in vitro experiments. Furthermore, the observations support the theory of Piziali et al.[24] that, the anatomic alignment of the ACL will prevent medial translation of the tibia with respect to the femur. A mechanical model is presented in Figure 8-3 to illustrate this theory.

When the knee analyzer displaces the tibia medially, both a varus moment and a medially directed shear force are transmitted to the knee. The hypothesis is that initial resistance to medial shear is provided by the ACL. Thus sideways motion of the joint is restrained during the *initial* phase of medial loading (Fig. 8-3A). During this phase, contact occurs on the lateral side of the tibial eminence and on the medial tibial condyle. When contact forces are sufficient, pivoting begins, thereby stretching the lateral collateral structures (Fig. 8-3B). This resistance provides the clinically observed firm end point in the varus–valgus stress test. It also corresponds to the linear region (Fig. 8-1B) of the knee analyzer moment–displacement curves.

In the absence of the ACL, the initial medial force displaces the tibia medially with respect to the femur (Fig. 8-3C). In this situation, contact only

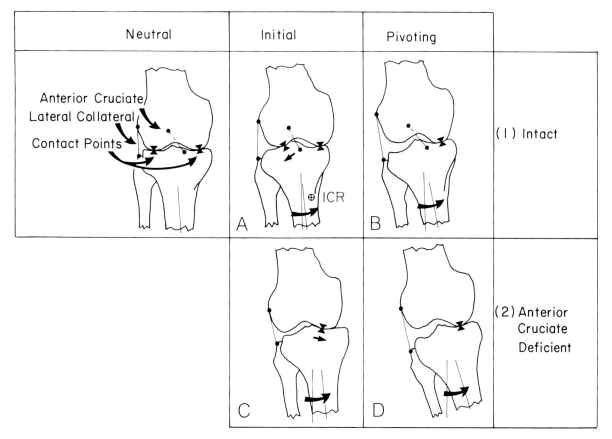

Fig. 8-3. Representation of events during the varus phase of testing on the knee analyzer. **(A)** Intact joint. During initial movement, resistance of the ACL produces contact between lateral tibial eminence and lateral femoral condyle. This is in addition to contact in the medial compartment. **(B)** Pivoting occurs when contact forces in the medial compartment are sufficient to require extension of the lateral collateral ligament. This is clinically observed as an "end-point." **(C)** ACL-deficient knee. In the absence of the ACL, translation of the tibia with respect to the femur is permitted. This allows varus displacement without contact between the tibial eminence and the lateral femoral condyle. **(D)** As the lateral collateral ligament becomes tight, contact forces in the medial compartment increase. This results in pivoting with a pattern of increased resistive moment and end-point similar to the intact joint.

occurs on the medial tibial condyle. When contact forces are again sufficient, pivoting occurs (Fig. 8-3D). Since the pivoting action involves the same structures as in the intact case, the firm end point (and stiffness of the curve) do not change in the absence of the ACL. However, before pivoting, the tibia slides medially a significant amount. In the moment–rotation curve, this is seen as an increase in varus displacement in the absence of the ACL.

The observation of a small but significant increase in valgus displacement of the tibia in the ACL-deficient knee may be due to a changed "neutral" position of the joint. Since at 0° flexion the ACL is normally under tension, its absence would permit the tibia to seek a more medial, "neutral" position.

The excessive varus–valgus displacement of the tibia portrayed by these mechanical tests has a clinical correlation. Thus the clinical observation of mild

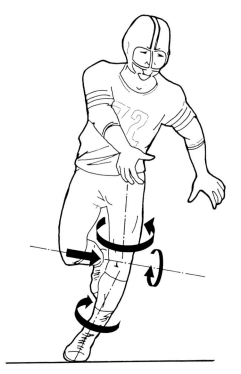

Fig. 8-4. Postulated pathomechanics of isolated ACL injury. The knee is near full extension and is loaded with two key components: internal rotation of the tibia and varus angulation of the tibia. If, in addition, posterior motion of the femur with respect to the tibia also takes place, the effect of tightening the ACL is exaggerated.

but definite increase in side-to-side laxity of the knee with firm end points tested in slight flexion reflects the abnormal side-to-side (varus more than valgus) translation of the tibia.

Based on anatomic studies, clinical observations, and tests defining the mechanical characteristics of the joint, one may speculate on the role of the ACL when the knee is near the extended position. The mechanisms for control of internal rotation of the tibia with respect to the femur, hyperextension of the joint, and anterior Drawer are known. However, our biomechanical studies suggest a further role of the ACL in preventing medial translation of the tibia with respect to the femur in the extended knee. This newly defined restraint has implications for the pathomechanics of the isolated ACL injury, its diagnosis and assessment, and on patterns of dysfunction that occur over time and which may lead to

secondary osteoarthritis or protect the joint from osteoarthritis.

A possible explanation of the pathomechanics of an isolated ACL injury is illustrated in Figure 8-4. This composite drawing includes the three main roles of the anterior cruciate in stabilizing the joint. A dynamic situation is posed during which an outward cutting maneuver is undertaken. Here, the foot is solidly planted as the player cuts outward and thrusts the tibia into extension. In the attempt to move the body, the femur rotates externally, and so the tibia becomes internally rotated with respect to the femur. At the same time the knee assumes a varus angulation. Together these actions provide a medial shear, anterior shear, and internal rotation movement to the tibia and thus maximally load the ACL to failure. In this situation one might further envision contact with the lower limb, which accentuates posterolateral displacement of the femur (or anteromedial displacement of the tibia). We consider that any situation that gives rise to these three critical factors simultaneously places the ACL in jeopardy.

CLINICAL IMPLICATIONS

The clinical assessment of an isolated ACL lesion may be aided by the assessment of medial translation of the tibia when the knee is extended (Fig. 8-5). During the standard varus–valgus stress test undertaken in a few degrees of flexion, a definite difference in medial translation of the tibia may be noted between the pathologic and asymptomatic joint. The medial shift is most readily detected when the patient's leg is suspended by the ankle held on the examiner's pelvis by the elbow. With both the examiner's hands free, the knee is brought to a few degrees of flexion and is in a "neutral" varus–valgus position. Thrust on the medial aspect of the femur in an outward direction will easily define an apparent "opening" of the knee laterally, and then a firm end point. However, the opening represents medial sliding of the tibia that lacks the restraint of the ACL. The firm end point indicates the increasing resistance to stretch imposed by the lateral collateral ligament. Careful attention to detail also may reveal an apparent medial opening of the joint tested under the same conditions when a force

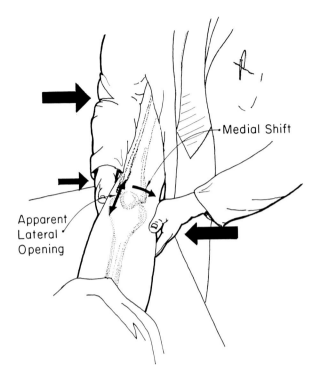

Fig. 8-5. The medial shift test. In the absence of the ACL, it is possible to detect a medial shift in the knee. With the knee in a few degrees of flexion, an outward-directed thrust on the medial aspect of the femur is applied. The optimal method for demonstrating the medial shift involves suspending the ankle on the examiner's pelvis by the elbow. A less preferred method is to support the knee in one hand and the ankle in the other. While marked opening is detected, it is easily misread as collateral laxity.

is applied to the knee on the lateral side. This "opening" probably represents the slight lateral sliding of the tibia from its new "neutral" position afforded by the loss of the ACL.

The medial shift may also be tested by supporting the knee in one hand and the tibia (ankle) in the other hand. The position of the knee is not as easily controlled (as it is in the position described above) and the varus–valgus shifts are easily misread as "collateral laxity."

The loss of the ACL (and thus the loss of control of medial sliding of the tibia with respect to the femur) may be important in the pathomechanics of gait. This may be especially so during stance phase when the knee approaches and leaves near-zero flexion,

because high joint contact forces are transmitted between 0° and 20° of flexion. In limbs with a varus alignment of the knee, the loss of a stabilizing ACL in an extended position may contribute to excessive abnormal mediolateral sliding between the joint surfaces. Normally the knee is constrained to roll, with consequent reduction in shear motion. Abnormal anterior and medial displacement may result in high shear forces, leading ultimately to cartilage degeneration. Such forces would be accentuated by progressive alteration of secondary ligamentous and meniscal restraints. In addition, limb varus–valgus alignment may positively or negatively influence subsequent outcome of the ACL-deficient knee.

These ideas, although speculative at this stage, have important clinical and biomechanical correlates in the ACL-deficient knee. The information may be of considerable use in diagnostic assessment and treatment as well as in preventive measures aimed at lessening the incidence of instability-induced osteoarthritis.

CONCLUSIONS

The ACL is a short, strong ligament directed in a proximal posterior and outward direction within the knee. It is composed of anteromedial and posterolateral bundles. In flexion, the entire ligament transmits force in the normal knee, whereas in full extension only the anteromedial band is tight. In an extended range, the ACL resists internal rotation of the tibia with respect to the femur and anterior displacement of the tibia. The ACL also resists medial translation of the tibia with respect to the femur, which we have demonstrated by our biomechanical studies. All three roles are demonstrable in instrumented test apparati and are readily defined in patients with an isolated ACL disruption. By the medial shift test, the passive medial translation of the tibia in slight flexion can be felt and measured. Our observations suggest that these three biomechanical functions of the ligament are involved in the pathomechanics of an isolated lesion of the anterior cruciate ligament. Furthermore, the absence of the ACL is likely to induce excessive joint contact forces and ligamentous forces during the highly loaded phases of gait nearing extension in stance phase.

These data also suggest that the ACL-deficient knee will be highly vulnerable to aberrations of limb alignment.

REFERENCES

1. Butler DL, Noyes FR, Grood ES: Ligamentous restraints to anterior-posterior drawer in the human knee. A biomechanical study. J Bone Joint Surg 62A:259–270, 1980
2. Brantigan OC, Voshell AF: The mechanics of the ligaments and menisci of the knee joint. J Bone Joint Surg 23A:44–66, 1941
3. Cabaud EH: Biomechanics of the anterior cruciate ligament. Clin Orthop 172:26–31, 1983
4. Crowninshield R, Pope MH, Johnson RJ: An analytical model of the knee. J Biomech 2:397–405, 1976
5. Detenbeck LC: Function of the cruciate ligaments in knee stability. J Sports Med 22:217–221, 1974
6. Edixhoven P, Huiskes R, van Rens TJG, Slooff TJ: Accuracy and reproducibility of an instrumented knee-drawer tester. Proc Orthop Res Soc, 31st Annual Meeting, Las Vegas, January 1985
7. Fukubayashi T, Torzilli PA, Sherman MF, Warren RF: An in vitro biomechanical evaluation of anterior-posterior motion of the knee. Tibial displacement, rotation, and torque. J Bone Joint Surg 64A:258–264, 1982
8. Furman W, Marshall JL, Girgis FG: The anterior cruciate ligament. J Bone Joint Surg 64A:258–264, 1976
9. Girgis FG, Marshall JL, Al Monajem ARS: The cruciate ligaments of the knee joint. Clin Orthop 106:216–231, 1975
10. Grood ES, Noyes FR, Butler DL, Suntay WJ: Ligamentous and capsular restraints preventing straight medial and lateral laxity in intact human cadaver knees. J Bone Joint Surg 63A:1257–1269, 1981
11. Hallen LG, Lindahl O: Rotation in the knee-joint in experimental injury to the ligaments. Acta Orthop Scand 36:400–407, 1965
12. Hughston JC, Andrews JR, Cross MJ, Moschi A: Classification of knee ligament instabilities. Part I. The medial compartment and cruciate ligaments. J Bone Joint Surg 58A:159–172, 1976
13. Hughston JC, Andrews JR, Cross MJ, Moschi A: Classification of knee ligament instabilities. Part II. The lateral compartment. J Bone Joint Surg 58A:173–179, 1976
14. Jacobsen K: Gonylaxometry. Stress radiographic measurement of passive stability in the knee joints of normal subjects and patients with ligament injuries. Acta Orthop Scand 52 (Suppl 194):1981
15. Kennedy JC, Fowler PJ: Medial and anterior instability of knee. J Bone Joint Surg 53A:1257–1270; 1971
16. Kennedy JC, Weinberg HW, Wilston AS: The anatomy and function of the anterior cruciate ligament. J Bone Joint Surg 56A:223–235, 1974
17. Levy MI, Torzilli PA, Warren RF: The effect of medial meniscectomy on anterior-posterior motion of the knee. J Bone Joint Surg 64A:883–888, 1982
18. Lipke JM, Janecki CJ, Nelson CL et al: The role of incompetence of the anterior cruciate and lateral ligaments in anterolateral and anteromedial instability. A biomechanical study of cadaver knees. J Bone Joint Surg 63A:954–960, 1981
19. Lowe PJ, Saunders GAB: Knee analyser. An objective method of evaluating mediolateral stability in the knee. Med Biol Eng Comput 15:548–552, 1977
20. Markolf KL, Graff-Radford A, Amstutz HC: In vivo knee stability. A quantitative assessment using an instrumented clinical testing apparatus. J Bone Joint Surg 60A:664–674, 1978
21. Markolf KL, Kochan A, Amstutz HC: Measurement of knee stiffness and laxity in patients with documented absence of the anterior cruciate ligament. J Bone Joint Surg 66A:242–252, 1984
22. Müller W: The Knee. Form, Function, and Ligament Reconstruction. Springer-Verlag, New York, 1983
23. Piziali RL, Rastegar JC, Nagel DA, Shurman DJ: Effects of fixed axes of rotation on the varus-valgus and torsional load displacement characteristics of the in vitro human knee. J Biomech Eng 101:134–140, 1979
24. Piziali RL, Seering WP, Nagel DA, Schurman DJ: The function of the primary ligaments of the knee in anterior-posterior and medial-lateral motions. J Biomech 13:777–784, 1980
25. Seering WP, Piziali RL, Nagel DA, Shurman DJ: The function of the primary ligaments of the knee in varus-valgus and axial rotation. J Biomech 13:785–794, 1980
26. Sherman O, Markolf KL, Weibel W, Ferkel R: Instrumented testing of normal and ACL deficient knees. A comparison of two devices. Proc Orthop Res Soc, 31st Annual Meeting, Las Vegas, January 1985
27. Slocum DB, Larson RL: Rotary instability of the knee. J Bone Joint Surg 50A:211–225, 1968
28. Torzilli PA, Greenberg RL, Insall J: An in vivo biomechanical evaluation of anterior-posterior motion of the knee. J Bone Joint Surg 63A:960–968, 1981
29. Wang C, Walker PS, Wolf B: The effects of flexion and rotation on the length patterns of the ligaments of the knee. J Biomech 6:587–596, 1977

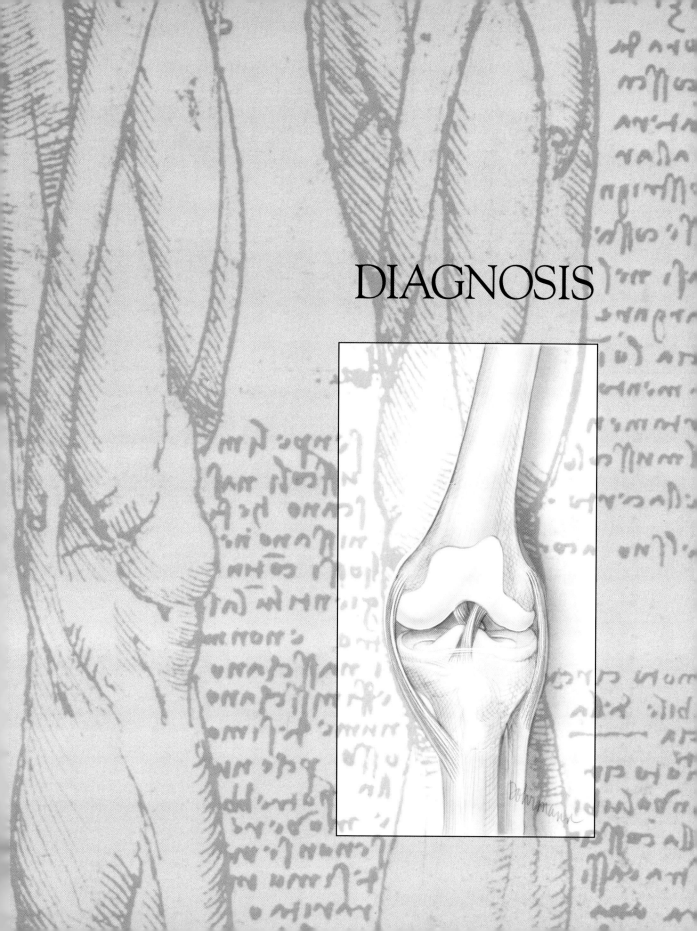

DIAGNOSIS

9

Diagnosis of Knee Ligament Injuries: Biomechanical Precepts

EDWARD S. GROOD
FRANK R. NOYES

Ligaments of the knee serve the mechanical function of limiting motion between the tibia and femur. The loss of this function, partial or complete, causes the position of the tibia at the limits of motion to change. The altered tibial positions (subluxations) at each of the limits indicate the specific structures injured. Diagnosis of ligament injury should be based on the altered limits observed during the physical examination.

To date, because of the complex and interdependent way the ligaments work together in limiting motion, a consensus does not exist on the significance of all abnormal joint motions. One result is the practice of listing groups of ligaments that may be injured if a particular abnormal knee motion is present. However the goal of diagnosis is to determine which specific structures are injured and how severe the injury is to each one.

In this chapter we present the biomechanical principles upon which we base our approach to differential diagnosis of knee ligament injuries. First, we review the three properties of ligaments that determine their function in limiting motion; second, we describe joint motion; third, we apply these precepts to develop a logical basis for differential diagnosis; fourth, we present a "bumper model" of the knee that we have found useful in interpreting laboratory data required for accurate diagnosis. At the time of writing, some important biomechanical

data are not yet available — not due to any limitation in experimental techniques but because of time factors. We expect the missing data to be available within the next 10 years.

BIOMECHANICAL PRECEPTS

Properties of Ligaments

Ligaments have two distinct mechanical functions. First, they help limit the amount of motion between bones. Second, they help determine the motions that occur between opposing cartilage surfaces. These are interdependent functions and both are important.

We address the limits to joint motion that the ligaments provide. We focus on the limits of motion because loss of this function (resulting in abnormal laxity) and consequent subluxation are the underlying deficits in ligament-injured knees. Furthermore, the change in limits of motion is the primary basis of diagnosis.

The ability of ligaments to limit motion between bones is important because it sets up the geometric conditions within which the neuromuscular system is able to control the position of the knee during activity so that the lower limbs can support the body. Sometimes a person can compensate for an increase in joint laxity by improving neuromuscular coordination. Similarly, the disability resulting from ligament injury can be made worse through muscle atrophy and loss of coordination due to inactivity or pain.

Although we are focusing on the mechanical function of the ligaments and capsular structures, the reader should be cognizant of the potentially important role of ligaments in providing sensory feedback to the neuromuscular system.[6,11]

Ligaments have three properties that affect their ability to limit joint motion: the location of their attachment on the bones, their just-taut length, and their stiffness.

Attachment Location

Tibial motion is limited by the action of the ligaments limiting the motion of their tibial attachments. The limitation is along the line that connects the ligament's tibial and femoral attachments in the direction that stretches the ligament. Ligaments are not able to limit motions perpendicular to their orientation or motions that cause them to become slack. At least two ligaments are required to limit translation—one for each sense (direction). For example, the anterior cruciate ligament (ACL) resists anterior translation but not posterior translation.[1,2,8] The opposite is true for the posterior cruciate ligament (PCL).

The fact that ligaments only limit translation of their attachments by applying a resisting force back along the ligament axis has an impact upon how they limit joint rotations. First, a single ligament acting alone is unable to resist rotation since the bone can always rotate freely about the attachments. As shown in Figure 9-1, the medial collateral ligament (MCL) is able to limit abduction–adduction only because of the compressive joint contact force that occurs in the opposite compartment. The ligamentous force (resisting distraction) and the joint contact force (resisting compression) act in opposite directions. Together these forces produce an internal moment that counteracts the external applied moments tending to rotate the knee.

As illustrated in Figure 9-2A and B, at least two soft tissue structures are required to limit each direction of tibial rotation. An increased rotation does not directly indicate which of the two ligaments is injured. To diagnose the injury, it is necessary to determine which of the two attachments has an in-

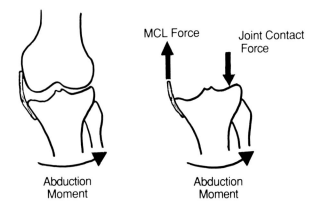

Fig. 9-1. Forces limiting knee abduction. An abduction moment will induce a valgus rotation of the tibia. This rotation is limited by two forces, the MCL force, a proximally oriented force at the medial aspect of the joint, and a joint contact force acting distally on the lateral plateau.

creased excursion. This can be determined from the subluxations that occur in the medial and lateral compartments. Detecting abnormal compartment subluxation and combining this with biomechanical data on which specific ligaments resist these motions form the basis for diagnosing injury of ligamentous restraints that limit tibial rotations.

Length

Just-taut length, the second property, is a determinant of joint laxity because it controls the amount of motion before the ligament can begin to provide a resisting force. Since the two cruciate ligaments are required to limit anterior–posterior (AP) translation, total AP translation is determined by the just-taut length of both ligaments. Injury to either will produce an increase in total AP translation. The direction (sense) of the increase will depend on which of the ligaments is injured. For tibial rotation, at least two structures are involved for each limit: two that limit internal rotation and two that limit external rotation. An increase in tibial rotation will occur if any of the structures are injured. The sense of the increase does not indicate the specific injury because at least two ligaments limit each direction.

Stiffness

Ligamentous stiffness, the third property, controls how much additional joint movement is required (after the ligament has become taut) to create a

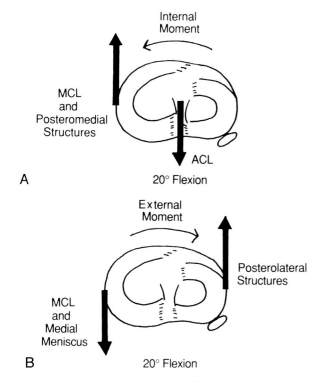

Fig. 9-2. Forces limiting internal/external rotation. **(A)** When the knee is at 20° flexion, internal rotation is resisted by forces in the ACL directed posteriorly and by anterior-directed forces provided by the MCL and posteromedial structures. **(B)** External rotation is resisted by structures on both the lateral and medial sides of the knee. The lateral structures include the lateral collateral ligament, popliteal tendon, and arcuate complex. The medial structures include the medial meniscus and MCL.

force large enough for the ligament to resist the applied load. For example, ligament stiffness is the factor that determines the difference in AP laxity between a 10 and 25-pound Lachman test. Decreased ligament stiffness produces an increase in laxity because a greater motion is required before the ligament can develop a sufficient restraining force.

Description of Joint Motion

Since diagnosis is based on the changes in the limits of motion of the knee, it is important to have a clear understanding of all the possible types of motions as well as of the properties of the ligaments that affect

their function. This knowledge will aid the examiner in performing the manual stress tests, in determining the specific abnormality in motion in the knee joint, and in interpreting the significance of the abnormal motion.

Degrees of Freedom

In three dimensions, six possible motions can occur. Each of these six motions — three rotation, three translation — is a distinct and separate motion, independent of the other five motions. Each independent motion is called a "degree of freedom." To describe these six motions requires three axes, one fixed in each bone and one that moves relative to both.[5] Each axis helps describe two degrees of freedom. One is a rotation (in which all particles of the bone move in circular paths about the axis) and the other is a translation (in which all particles in the bone move along identical paths parallel to the axis).

The three rotations are illustrated in Figure 9-3 and the translations are illustrated in Figure 9-4. The three rotational degrees of freedom correspond to the clinical motions of flexion–extension, abduction–adduction, and internal–external rotation. The three translational degrees of freedom are medial–lateral translation of the tibia in the direction of the flexion–extension axis; compression–distraction translation in the direction of the tibial rotation axis; and anterior–posterior translation in the direction of the abduction–adduction rotation axis.

The first of the three axes, the flexion–extension axis, is located in the femur and oriented in a pure medial–lateral direction so that it is perpendicular to the femoral sagittal plane. Rotation of the tibia about this axis is flexion–extension without any associated internal–external rotation or abduction–adduction motions.[5] Since all of these motions occur during flexion of a normal knee, the flexion–extension axis of Figure 9-3 does not correspond to the functional flexion axis. While the flexion axis has a pure medial–lateral orientation, the functional flexion axis is skewed in the knee and even changes its orientation as the knee is flexed.[15] The skewed orientation of the functional axis accounts for the combined motions of flexion, abduction, and tibial rotation that occur together.

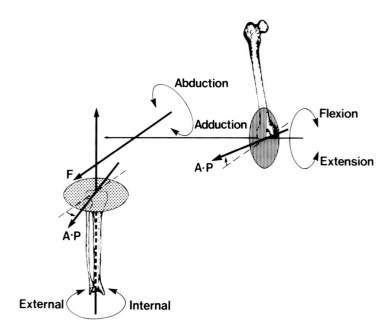

Fig. 9-3. Joint rotations. The three independent rotations of the knee occur about the three axes shown. Flexion–extension occurs on a medial–lateral oriented axis located in the femur. Internal–external tibial rotation occurs about an axis parallel to the shaft of the tibia. Abduction occurs about a third axis, which is parallel to both the femoral sagittal plane and the tibial transverse plane. (Modified from ref. 5, with permission.)

The second axis, shown in Figure 9-3, is located in the tibia. It is parallel to the tibial shaft and perpendicular to the tibial transverse plane. Rotations about this axis are pure internal and external rotation motions without any associated abduction–adduction or flexion–extension.[5]

The third axis is for abduction–adduction rotations. It is slightly more difficult to visualize because it is not part of either bone and its orientation can change relative to both. The abduction–adduction axis is always perpendicular to the flexion axis and, consequently it is always parallel to the femoral sagittal plane.[5] When the knee is flexed the orientation of the abduction axis changes relative to the femur as it rotates in the sagittal plane. The motion of this axis can be thought of as similar to the motion of the second hand on a clock. The face of the clock is the sagittal plane and the abduction axis is the second hand. The motion of the axis, however, is controlled by changes in the flexion angle, not changes in time. Similarly, the abduction axis is perpendicular to the tibial rotation axis and parallel to the tibial transverse plane. When the tibia is internally or externally rotated, the orientation of the axis changes relative to the tibia as the axis rotates in the transverse plane in an identical manner to that described for the motion in the sagittal plane. Rotations about this third axis are pure abduction–

adduction motions without concurrent changes in either knee flexion or tibial rotation.

Combined Rotations and Translations

Although there are six degrees of freedom, the manual stress examinations are designed to test the limits to just one or two at a time. We consider here the special situation when only one rotation — tibial rotation — is combined with anterior–posterior translation. Combinations of these motions are particularly important to the diagnosis of knee ligament injury because they occur during many of the manual stress examinations.

To understand combined rotations and translations we first recognize that translations of a rigid body such as one of the bones comprising the knee is described by the motion of an arbitrarily selected point on the body. Typically, AP translation is described by the motion of a point located midway between the medial and lateral margins of the tibia. If only translation motions occur, the amount of motion does not depend upon which point is chosen, that is, whether the point is at the center of the knee or at the medial or lateral joint margin. This is because all points will move along parallel paths. However, when rotation and translation motions are

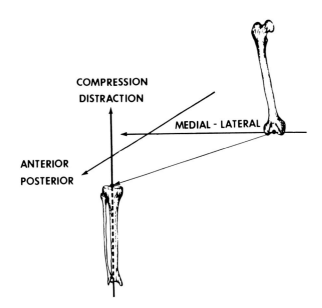

Fig. 9-4. Knee translations. The three translations of the knee are motions of a point on the tibia parallel to each of the three axes. The point on the tibia we use is located midway between the spines of the intercondylar eminence. Its location is indicated by the arrow originating at a point on the femur and ending at a point on the tibia. Medial–lateral translation is motion of the tibial point parallel to the flexion–extension axis. Anterior–posterior translation is motion of the tibial point parallel to the abduction–adduction axis, and compression–distraction translation is motion of the point along the internal–external rotation axis. (Modified from ref. 5, with permission.)

combined, the amount of translation does depend upon which point is used. This can be seen by considering the four cases illustrated in Figure 9-5A–D.

Figure 9-5B shows an anterior translation of 10 mm without associated tibial rotation. All points move anteriorly by the same amount.

Figure 9-5C shows an internal rotation of 15° about an axis located midway between the spines of the intercondylar eminence. The point on the rotation axis is stationary while the lateral joint margin (edge) moves anteriorly and the medial margin posteriorly.* This illustrates that when translation is

---

* The amount of anterior and posterior motion of the points at the joint margin depends upon the amount of rotation and how far they are away from the rotation axis (center of rotation).

measured in the presence of a concurrent rotation it is important to know at what point the translation was measured.

Figure 9-5D shows the motions of B and C combined. The medial joint margin is nearly stationary while the joint center moves 10 mm anteriorly and the lateral margin moves 20 mm anteriorly. This combined motion is equivalent to a pure 15° rotation about an axis located at the medial joint line.

While the dependence of translations upon rotations may at first seem confusing, a common clinical application in knee diagnosis illustrates this graphically: the abduction stress test. During this test, the clinician causes a rotation of the tibia to produce a joint opening or distraction translation between the medial tibial plateau and corresponding femoral condyle. This distraction stresses the medial ligaments, and thus tests their integrity. During the abduction stress test, the rotation axis is located in the lateral femoral condyle[3] such that medial distraction is accompanied by relative compression at the lateral joint line, which causes the lateral structures to become slightly lax. The benefit of this result is that it allows the clinician to stress the medial ligaments that limit joint distraction independently from the lateral ligaments that also limit joint distraction.

In an exactly analogous manner, we apply this concept to internal and external tibial rotations performed in combination with anterior and posterior Drawer forces. This combination of tibial rotation plus translation applied together is designed to allow anterior and posterior Drawer tests to be performed separately on the medial and lateral tibiofemoral compartments in order to isolate and test separately the medial and lateral ligamentous and capsular structures that resist anterior and posterior translation of each plateau.

As an example, we refer to Figure 9-5D where an anterior translation and internal rotation are combined. This combined motion allows us to stress the lateral ligaments without stressing the medial ligaments. This approach is similar to the Slocum-Larson drawer tests at 90° where the tibia is prerotated either internally or externally before applying the Drawer motion. It is also different from the Slocum-Larson tests (1968)[12] in that (1) we recommend that the foot not be fixed so that tibial rotation is not restricted; (2) the maximum amount of Drawer at

A. Reduced Position

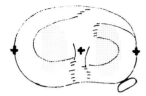

B. 10mm Anterior Translation

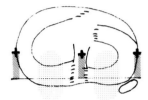

C. 15° Rotation About Joint Center

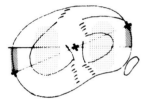

D. Combined Translation and Rotation

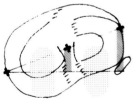

Fig. 9-5. Combined anterior translation and tibial rotation. **(A)** The tibial plateau is shown along with the contact area on the femur indicated by the shaded regions. The tibia is in a reduced position. **(B)** Anterior tibial translation of 10 mm produces a posterior displacement of the tibial–femoral contact. The amount of translation, shown by the vertical bars, is the same at the medial and lateral joint margins as it is at the center of the joint. **(C)** 15° internal rotation about the joint center. Contact is posterior on the lateral plateau and anterior on the medial plateau. The bars show the amount and direction of its translation at the medial lateral joint lines and the center of the joints. Note that the lateral margin translates anteriorly while the medial margin translates posteriorly. The amount of translation is approximately 10 mm in an average knee 80 mm wide. There is no translation at the center of the joint where the rotation axis is located. **(D)** Combined tibial translation and rotation. A 10 mm anterior translation is combined with a 15° internal rotation about the joint center. The medial joint line does not translate, due to equal but opposite effects of the two motions. The center of the tibia translates anteriorly 10 mm, while the lateral joint margin translates 20 mm anteriorly.

the margins be obtained by forcibly rotating the tibia to its limit of rotation motion, as in the abduction test, at the same time anterior or posterior forces are applied; (3) the tests should be done for all four corners where Slocum-Larson[12] described them for only the anterior direction; and (4) we stress the importance of performing these tests at both 30° and 90° of flexion. The tests are performed at both flexion angles so as to isolate individual ligamentous structures to test their integrity more reliably.

APPLICATION OF PRECEPTS TO DIAGNOSIS OF KNEE INJURY

Differential Diagnosis

Since there are six knee motions (degrees of freedom), there are six possible joint laxities or conditions of increased motion. Together, the ligaments and joint geometry provide two limits (opposite directions) for each degree of freedom. All together there are 12 possible limits of motion of the knee, which are listed in Table 9-1 along with the struc-

Table 9-1. Twelve Limits of Joint Motion

Motion Limit	Structures Limiting the Motion
Flexion	Ligaments, leg and thigh shape
Extension	Ligaments and joint compression
Abduction	Ligaments and lateral joint compression
Adduction	Ligaments and medial joint compression
Internal rotation	Ligaments and menisci
External rotation	Ligaments and menisci
Medial translation	Bone (spines interlocking with femoral condyles) and ligaments (to prevent distraction)
Lateral translation	Bone (spines interlocking with femoral condyles) and ligaments (to prevent distraction)
Anterior translation	Ligaments
Posterior translation	Ligaments
Joint distraction	Ligaments
Joint compression	Bone, menisci, and cartilage

tures that limit each motion. Injury to these tissues alters the limits of each motion, increasing joint laxity. It is not really the amount of laxity but the position of the joint at the final limits of motions (reflecting the position of ligament attachment sites) that provides the information needed for diagnosis. From a diagnostic standpoint, it would be ideal if each of the 12 limits of motion were controlled by a single ligamentous structure. Differential diagnosis could then be performed by evaluating each of the 12 limits separately. Clearly, this ideal situation does not exist. The ligaments, capsular structures, and joint geometry all work together and each contributes to limiting more than one motion. Thus

The problem of diagnosing knee injuries reduces to determining how to apply individual or combination motions to lengthen primarily a single ligament or capsular structure so that structure can be evaluated independently.

The ability to isolate each structure is the key to differential diagnosis of individual ligament injuries. The isolation of a structure is accomplished by placing the knee at the proper joint position, specifically, knee flexion angle and tibial rotation position, before the clinical stress test is performed. Joint position is recognized as important to diagnosis of

an injury to the medial extraarticular structures. The abduction stress test is performed both in full extension and at 20° to 30° of flexion. In the flexed position the posterior capsule becomes slack, thus allowing the examiner to isolate the MCL better. Diagnosis of injury to specific ligaments is best done at a joint position where the other structures are most lax and least able to block the abnormal subluxations that occur when the ligament being tested is injured. This is a direct application of the precepts discussed under ligament function. The approach is to shorten the distance between attachments of the secondary restraints. This makes them become slack so a larger joint motion can be applied before they become taut and begin to resist further joint motion. Thus

Isolating a ligament so its integrity may be individually tested requires placing the knee in a position in which other supporting structures are slack.

An example of isolating a ligament is the evaluation of the ACL at 20° of knee flexion[14] as opposed to the 90° position commonly used 10 years ago.[9] Now it is recognized that the 20° position more often results in increased anterior subluxation following ACL injury because secondary restraining structures are more slack and less able to block this motion.

Another example of the importance of joint position can be seen in the evaluation of the PCL. Figure 9-6 shows the amount of increased posterior tibial translation that occurs when the PCL is removed.[2,4] The increase in posterior translation is two to three times greater at 90° of flexion than at 20° of flexion. This phenomenon is easily understood when it is realized that the amount of joint motion after a ligament is injured depends on the role and function of the remaining ligaments that must ultimately limit the joint motion. Thus

The increase in joint laxity that occurs when a ligament is injured reflects the amount of additional joint motion required before the remaining intact ligaments become stretched and are able to limit further motion.

A corollary to this is

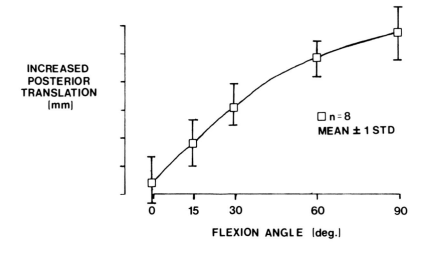

Fig. 9-6. Increased posterior translation with isolated PCL injury. Average increase in posterior translation under a 100 N posterior force when the PCL was removed along with any associated ligaments of Wrisberg and Humphry. Note that the increased translation at 90° is much greater than at 15° and 30° flexion.

INCREASED POSTERIOR TRANSLATION (mm)

□ n = 8
MEAN ± 1 STD

FLEXION ANGLE (deg.)

The increased laxity that occurs following ligament rupture depends upon how slack the remaining intact ligaments (secondary restraints) are.

Following rupture of the PCL, only a small posterior translation near full extension is required before the remaining ligaments limit further motion. As the knee is flexed, larger amounts of joint motion are required. Thus the increase in posterior translation with flexion reflects a slackening of the secondary restraints and an increased joint motion before they become taut. This pattern is consistent with the slackening of the posterior capsule that occurs with knee flexion. By inference we conclude that the posterior capsule is an important secondary restraint to posterior Drawer near full extension. The validity of this inference has, in fact, been demonstrated by the further increases in posterior translation when the posterolateral capsule is also sectioned.[4]

Subluxation versus Laxity

When performing diagnosis of knee ligament injuries from information obtained during the manual stress examinations, it is important to distinguish between the final position of the bones at the limit of motion (subluxation) and the amount of motion (normal and abnormal). Ligament injury changes the limits of motion, thus resulting in an abnormal subluxation. While the amount of motion (laxity) will also increase, this alone is not sufficient for diagnosis because it does not indicate which limit (for example, anterior or posterior) is abnormal. To determine the limits, the physician must also know the position of the tibia (relative to the femur) at the start of the examination.

The starting position is also referred to as the neutral position of the knee. Each motion has its own neutral position. The difficulty in defining this position is widely acknowledged in both the clinical and biomechanical literature. The classic clinical example is the false-positive anterior Drawer test that occurs in the presence of a PCL injury.[1,10] In this case, correct diagnosis can only be made if it is recognized that the starting position is really abnormally posterior and the anterior Drawer sign is really a posterior Drawer test in reverse. The point is that

Diagnosis must ultimately be made not on the amount of laxity present but on the final subluxation position and whether or not that final position is abnormal compared to the contralateral knee.

The final subluxation position indicates which ligament attachments are able to be placed in abnormal position indicating injury to the corresponding ligament.

The final subluxation position of a joint can be determined in ways other than measuring the amount of joint motion and the corresponding neutral position. One way is to palpate the stepoff between the femoral condyles and the anterior edge of the tibia. The amount of the stepoff, in fact, gives a direct measure of the amount of tibial subluxation and is used by many skilled examiners as a method of determining whether an increased AP translation is occurring in the anterior or posterior direction.

The difference between the final subluxation position of the knee and the amount of laxity is also important to consider when using any of the current devices for quantitating AP translation. With each of these devices the significance of the amount of AP translation measured always depends upon knowledge of the starting position. One advantage of these devices is that they provide information besides laxity—specifically, joint stiffness—which is a secondary indication of the direction in which the increased motion occurs. Thus it is often possible to determine whether an increased AP translation is anterior or posterior by looking at the terminal stiffness (i.e., whether there is a hard or soft end point). A soft end point, indicating a reduced stiffness, is often noted during the manual examination. A soft

end point usually, although not always, occurs in the direction of the increased motion.

"BUMPER MODEL" OF THE KNEE

We developed a model of the knee that we find useful in understanding how the ligamentous and capsular structures limit AP translation and internal–external rotation. It also helps us to determine the types of subluxations that occur when ligaments are injured. We call this the "bumper model" of the knee because we have replaced the ligamentous and capsular restraints with rubber bumpers that limit tibial motion.

The model is illustrated in Figure 9-7. The tibia is represented by the line (or plank) whose AP and internal–external rotational motion is limited by six bumpers. Two of the bumpers are located centrally to account for the restraints of the cruciate ligaments. The remaining bumpers are located at the four corners of the knee and account for the re-

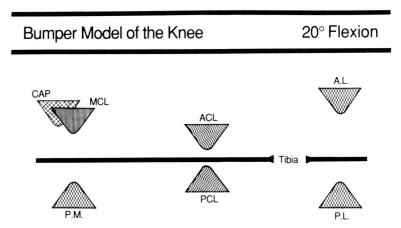

Fig. 9-7. Bumper model of the knee. The bumper model is used to show how the various structures about the knee limit internal and external rotation and anterior–posterior translation, both at the joint center and at the medial and lateral joint margins. The tibia is represented by the horizontal line whose motion is limited by the bumpers. Six bumpers are shown, which replace the limiting action of the ligaments, capsular structures, and menisci. The two central bumpers account for the limiting action of the ACL (above) and the PCL (below). The bumpers in the four quadrants are the A.M. (anteromedial restraints, in this diagram represented by the capsule (CAP) and medial collateral ligament (MCL)), A.L. (anterolateral restraints), P.M. (posteromedial restraints), and P.L. (posterolateral restraints). These bumpers include the combined effects of several ligamentous and capsular structures and are not meant to designate single anatomic entities. (From ref. 9a, with permission.)

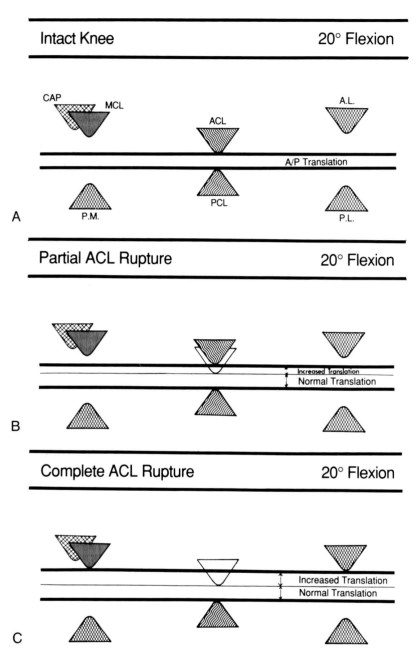

Fig. 9-8. Anterior–posterior translation. **(A)** The total AP translation of the knee is limited by the ACL and PCL in the absence of any tibial rotations. **(B)** Partial ACL injury. A partial injury to the ACL resulting in a stretching causes the bumper to be displaced anteriorly. This results in an increase in anterior translation over that in the normal intact knee. **(C)** Depending on the extent of injury to the ACL, it is possible that translation of the medial and lateral plateaus could be limited by extraarticular restraints and the menisci. (For abbreviations, see Fig. 9-7 legend.)

straints provided by the extraarticular structures and menisci. As shown for the anteromedial corner, the bumpers in each corner are really composed of bumpers representing several structures. A more complete model would include the bumpers for each structure.

Figure 9-8A shows that total AP laxity during a straight Drawer test is just the distance between the two central cruciate bumpers. The position of the bumpers is determined by the slack length of the ligaments. This is one of the ligament properties we described earlier that determines knee laxity. If the

ACL is stretched due to partial injury, its slack length will increase and its corresponding bumper will be moved anteriorly, as shown in Figure 9-8B. This anterior movement of the bumper produces increased anterior tibial translation. Relationships of the bumpers after complete ACL rupture is illustrated in Figure 9-8C.

In our bumper model, we have replaced the tethering effect of the ligaments and the restraining force they apply when stretched by a bumper that provides an identical restraining force when compressed. The bumper is located so that it stops the motion of the tibia at the same position as the ligament would when it reached its just-taut length.

The amount of slack in each ligament changes with knee flexion due to changes in the distance between the tibial and femoral attachments. This change in ligament slackness with flexion causes joint laxity to vary with flexion. In the bumper model this is described by a change in the position of the bumper with a change in knee flexion. For example, the largest amount of AP translation in many knees occurs around 30° of flexion and then reduces as the knee is flexed toward 90°. Figure 9-9 shows this behavior in one of the knees we tested. The change in AP translation reflects the total amount of slack that exists in both cruciate ligaments. Thus a bumper model drawn for the knee in

the 30° flexion position will have a greater distance between the anterior and posterior cruciate bumpers than the model drawn for the same knee at the 90° flexion position.

A second example of the effect of flexion angle involves the changes knee flexion produces in the amount of slack in the posteromedial and posterolateral capsule. Near full extension, these structures are tight and the corresponding bumpers are located close to the position of the PCL (Fig. 9-10). As the knee is flexed, however, these structures become progressively slack and a substantial amount of posterior subluxation is required before they are able to resist further posterior motion. Thus, at 90° the bumpers are located more posteriorly than they are at 30° of knee flexion.

The increasing slack of the posterior capsule can be seen in Figure 9-6, which shows the increase in posterior translation when the posterior cruciate is cut. The greater increase at 90° than at 30° results from the posterior capsule becoming slack with flexion as the distance between its tibial and femoral attachments becomes shorter. In the flexed position a greater posterior displacement is thus required before the capsule becomes taut and resists further posterior motion. This effect is shown in Figure 9-10 by the two sets of posterior capsular bumpers, one at 30° and the other (more posterior)

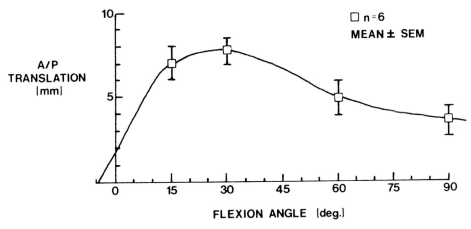

Fig. 9-9. Total AP translation. This figure shows the total AP translation in six intact knees under forces of 67 N applied posteriorly and anteriorly. In these six knees, the total AP translation was greatest at 30° and less at 90°. The curve represents the results from a seventh knee, which fortunately was near the average of the other six.

Effect of Knee Flexion on Posterior Bumpers

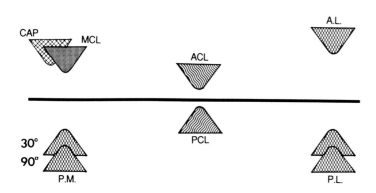

Fig. 9-10. Effect of knee flexion on posterior bumpers. As the knee is flexed, the posterior capsular structures become slack and require increased tibial displacement before they limit posterior translation. This is shown in the model by the more posterior position of the PM and PL bumpers at 90° as compared to 30° of knee flexion. (For abbreviations, see Fig. 9-7 legend.)

at 90°. The distance between the 30° and 90° bumpers reflects the additional posterior translation required at 90° before the capsule becomes taut and resists further translation.

While the bumper model can be used to explain the limits to anterior and posterior translation, it is most useful when one is trying to understand the limits to tibial rotations and the combined motions of rotation and translation. We studied the changes that occur in the amount of tibial internal and external rotations when ligaments are cut. The results we are presenting were obtained in two studies[4,13] in which we used the entire lower limb of cadavers and a three-dimensional (six degrees of freedom) electrogoniometer to measure total knee motion. In the first study,[13] the ACL and anterolateral extraarticular structures were sectioned alone and in combination. The anterolateral structures were the iliotibial band and the midlateral capsule. In the second study[4] the PCL and posterolateral structures were sectioned alone and in combination. The posterolateral structures included the lateral collateral ligament, the popliteus tendon at its femoral attachment, and the arcuate complex.

Figure 9-11 illustrates our results for internal rotation. At 30° flexion (Fig. 9-11A), the limits to internal rotation were provided by the posteromedial structures, the anterolateral structures, and the ACL all working together. Sectioning either the ACL or the anterolateral structures produced a small increase in internal rotation. When both were cut to-

gether a larger increase in internal rotation occurred, but not more than 7° in any of the six knees we tested. The further limits to internal rotation were not determined but are likely to be the lateral collateral ligament (LCL), based upon its anatomy and studies by Lipke et al.[7] This is illustrated by the bumper marked LCL. Note that this bumper does not come into play until the ACL and the iliotibial band are both injured.

At flexion angles less than 30° the ACL dominated, whereas at flexion angles greater than 30° the anterolateral structures dominated. This can be explained by considering the changes that occur in ligament slackness with flexion and extension. As the knee is extended past 20°, the amount of AP translation rapidly decreases due to reduction in the combined slackness of both cruciate ligaments. This brings these bumpers closer together. The posteromedial capsule also tightens, moving its bumper anteriorly. This combination (Fig. 9-11B) results in a decreased role of the anterolateral structures since the tibia can no longer rotate to the point where they become taut.

With flexion beyond 30°, the anterolateral structures become progressively tighter while the posteromedial structures become progressively slack. This combination causes internal rotation to be limited first by the extraarticular restraints. This is consistent with our results that sectioning the ACL alone did not increase internal rotation when the knee was flexed between 40° and 80°.

Fig. 9-11. Limits to internal rotation. **(A)** At 30° of flexion, internal rotation is limited by the ACL centrally and the anterolateral restraints. These structures limit anterior translation. In addition, the posterior translation of the medial plateau is limited by the posteromedial restraints. **(B)** At 10° of flexion, the posterior bumpers move in closer towards the PCL due to a reduction in the slack present in the posterior capsule. In addition, the ACL bumper moves posteriorly as a result of tightening the ACL/PCL complex. Because of this, internal rotation of the tibia is now limited by the ACL centrally and the posteromedial restraints alone. The tibia can no longer rotate far enough to engage the anterolateral restraints. **(C)** At 80° flexion, the posterior bumpers move further posterior, reflecting the increased slack in the posterior capsule. In addition, the distance between the ACL and PCL bumpers has increased slightly to reflect the increased laxity of these structures. The anteromedial/anterolateral structures are now moved posteriorly due to tightening of the extraarticular restraints with knee flexion. Internal rotation is now limited by the anterolateral and posteromedial restraints without direct involvement with the ACL. (For abbreviations, see Fig. 9-7 legend.)

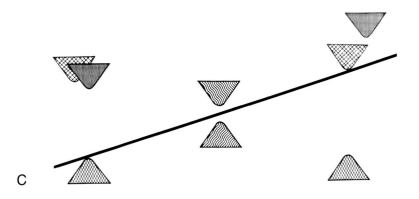

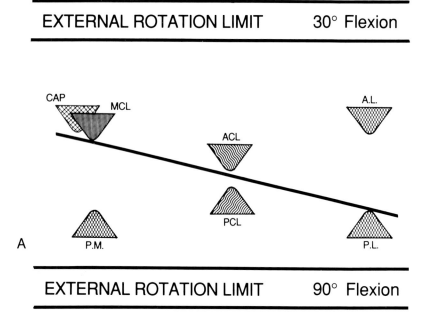

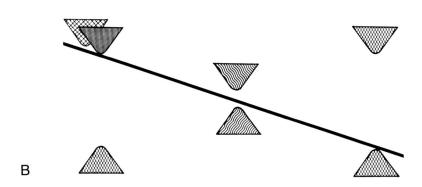

Fig. 9-12. Limits to external rotation. **(A)** At 30° flexion the external rotation of the tibia is limited by the bumpers, which stop anterior translation of the medial plateau and posterior translation of the lateral plateau. Due to the position of the structures, there is no direct involvement of either the ACL or PCL in limiting external rotation. **(B)** At 90° flexion, the posterior bumpers are moved posterior, reflecting the increased slack in the posterior capsule. Because of this, the PCL is nearly taut at the limit of external rotation. After removing the posterolateral restraints there, only a small increase in external rotation occurs at this flexion angle. (For abbreviations, see Fig. 9-7 legend.)

Our results for external rotation are illustrated in Figure 9-12. At 30° flexion, external rotation is limited only by the extraarticular restraints. On the lateral side we found that this included all the structures in the posterior corner, which acted at a unit. Large increases in rotation were not found until all structures were cut. While we have not yet investigated the medial restraints to external rotation, we believe that the medial meniscus and MCL are important to resisting anterior translation of the medial tibial plateau. Figure 9-12A illustrates our finding

that sectioning the ACL or PCL has no effect on external tibial rotation at 30° flexion. This is because the external rotation is limited by the meniscus and extraarticular restraints before the cruciates can become taut.

The limits to external rotation at 90° are illustrated in Figure 9-12B. At this knee position the posterior capsule has become so slack that the PCL can now block significant increases in external rotation when the posterolateral structure is totally sectioned. This is consistent with our finding that external rotation increased an average of only 5.3 ± 2.6° when the entire posterolateral corner was sectioned and the PCL was intact. Sectioning the PCL as well did produce a large additional increase in external rotation ranging from 15° to 20° with the combined cuts. The medial structures limiting external rotation and anterior translation of the medial tibial plateau were not determined but are most likely the medial meniscus, the MCL, and the posterior oblique ligament.

While the bumper model above does not account for all ligament restraints and clinical laxities, we have found it extremely helpful in understanding how the ligamentous and capsular structures work together to limit both AP translation and internal–external rotation, alone and in combination. The model needs further refinement, and more biomechanical data must be analyzed to allow us to understand completely the interaction of the ligament(s) during clinical examination. We do not think of the bumpers as representing the physical anatomical structures but rather as simulating the effect each structure has on limiting motions of the tibia. We hope this model will be useful to others as they undertake the complex task of diagnosing ligament injury.

SUMMARY

We have presented the physical factors that govern the way ligaments limit knee motion. These factors are important because they directly affect the way an examiner must approach the differential diagnosis of individual ligamentous and capsular structures. Although the knee is a complex mechanism and the ligaments work interdependently, we believe that differential diagnosis can be accomplished by a relatively small number of clinical tests that allow evaluation of the integrity of the individual structures. The tests performed must take into account the changing amount of slack in the ligament with knee flexion in a way that allows, as much as possible, the isolation of individual structures. The specific tests performed need to be chosen so that they displace the attachment of the ligament being tested in a direction that causes the ligament to become

longer. Finally, the amount of motion of the ligament's attachment must be inferred from the final subluxated position of the joint and not from the amount of motion (translations and rotations) elicited during the manual stress test.

We have not tried to provide the reader with a cookbook method for diagnosing ligament injury. Rather our goal is to provide biomechanical precepts, since they are the keys to understanding the meaning of the clinical findings obtained during laxity examinations and permit accurate inferences as to the injuries present. The ability to diagnose injury accurately also depends upon biomechanical data that document the motions limited by each ligament and the knee position where the ligaments act alone. Not all the data required for complete diagnosis are currently available, but we are confident that they will be, due to the efforts of many investigators currently conducting research on knee ligament function.

REFERENCES

1. Butler DL, Noyes FR, Grood ES: Ligamentous restraints to anterior-posterior drawer in the human knee, A biomechanical study. J Bone Joint Surg 62A:259–270, 1980
2. Fukubayashi Y, Torzilli PA, Sherman MF, Warren RF: An in vitro biomechanical evaluation of anterior-posterior motion in the knee. J Bone Joint Surg 64A:258–264, 1982
3. Grood ES, Noyes FR, Butler DL, Suntay WJ: Ligamentous and capsular restraints preventing straight medial and lateral laxity in intact human knees. J Bone Joint Surg 63A:125'–1269, 1981
4. Grood ES, Stowers SF, Noyes FR: Laxity limits in the human knee. Effect of sectioning the posterior cruciate and posterolateral structures. J Bone Joint Surg (in press, 1987)
5. Grood ES, Suntay WJ: A joint coordinate system for the clinical description of three-dimensional motion. Application to the knee. J Biomech Eng 105:136–144, 1983
6. Kennedy JC, Alexander IA, Hayes KC: Nerve supply of the human knee and its functional significance. Am J Sports Med 10:329–335, 1982
7. Lipke JM, Janecki CJ, Nelson CL et al: The role of incompetence of the anterior cruciate and lateral liga-

ments in anterolateral and anteromedial instability. J Bone Joint Surg 63A:954–960, 1981

8. Markolf KL, Mensch JS, Amstutz HC: Stiffness and laxity of the knee. The contributions of the supporting structures. J Bone Joint Surg 58A:583–594, 1976

9. Marshall JL, Wang JB, Furman W et al: The anterior Drawer sign. What is it? Am J Sports Med 3:152–158, 1975

9a. Noyes FR, Grood ES: Classification of ligament injuries: Why an anterolateral laxity or anteromedial laxity is not a diagnostic entity. pp. 185–200. In Griffin PP (ed): Instructional Course Lectures. American Academy of Orthopaedic Surgeons, Park Ridge, IL, 1987

10. Noyes FR, Grood ES, Butler DL, Paulos L: Clinical biomechanics of the knee. Ligament restraints and functional stability. In Funk FJ (ed): Symposium on the Athlete's Knee. Surgical Repair and Reconstruction. CV Mosby, St Louis, 1980

11. Schultz RA, Miller DC, Kerr CS, Micheli L: Mechanoreceptors in human cruciate ligaments. A histological study. J Bone Joint Surg 66A:1072–1076, 1984

12. Slocum DB, Larson RL: Rotatory instability of the knee. J Bone Joint Surg 50A:211–225, 1968

13. Suntay WJ: Three Dimensional Kinematics in the Human Knee. Application to the Clinical Laxity Exam and the Leg Extension Exercise. Doctoral Dissertation, University of Cincinnati, Department of Mechanical Engineering, 1982

14. Torg JS, Conrad W, Kalen V: Clinical diagnosis of anterior cruciate ligament instability in the athlete. Am J Sports Med 4:84–93, 1976

15. Van Dijk R: The Behaviour of the Cruciate Ligaments in the Human Knee. Rodopi, Amsterdam, 1983

10

Diagnosis of Knee Ligament Injuries: Clinical Concepts

FRANK R. NOYES
EDWARD S. GROOD

Our goal is to present a logical scheme for the diagnosis and classification of knee ligament injuries. In this chapter the scientific (biomechanical) precepts contained in Chapter 9 will be applied to different types of anterior knee subluxations that result after injury to the anterior cruciate ligament (ACL) and extraarticular ligament restraints. A significant controversy exists in this area and is readily apparent from the several different classification schemes that have been proposed.[3,5-7,11-13,16-24,28-31] Most of the current schemes are not based on kinematic or biomechanical principles and, in our opinion, are scientifically flawed. New concepts about knee motions and ligament function have evolved over the past 5 years.[8-10,31] The concepts we advance here are based on prior work by us and others and also contain new information based on biomechanical data gathered in our laboratory and clinic.

This chapter will review four concepts which we believe the clinician must understand in order to diagnose knee ligament injuries. After listing these concepts, we will expand on each in the text.

> Concept I: The diagnosis of a ligament injury must be expressed as a specific anatomic defect.
>
> Concept II: The clinical ligament examination must be performed and interpreted using knowledge of the three-dimensional motions of the knee.

> Concept III: The so-called "rotatory instabilities" can be characterized by the separate subluxations that occur to the medial and lateral tibial plateaus.
>
> Concept IV: The diagnosis of ligament and capsular defects requires the use of selected laxity tests for which the primary and secondary ligamentous restraints have been experimentally determined.

CONCEPT I: The diagnosis of a ligament injury must be expressed as a specific anatomic defect.

To communicate the diagnosis of a ligament injury correctly and clearly, the examiner must describe the anatomic defect in unambiguous terms (Table 10-1). When specifying a diagnosis, the ambiguous use of the terms *instability, laxity,* and *subluxation* cause confusion and uncertainty.

In the literature, *instability* is used in two ways: to describe an event (symptom) and to describe a condition (sign). In the former context, *instability* or *functional instability* can refer to one of three distinct events. It may indicate total knee collapse or giving way, partial giving way without complete collapse of the joint, or merely the subjective sensation of instability perceived by the patient. One does not know under what specific conditions (running, jumping, twisting, or turning) the instability

261

Table 10-1. Definition of Terms

Term	Common Use	Preferred Use
Instability	Symptom: Giving way, collapse of knee joint	Describe specific symptom, i.e., "complete giving way with jumping activities"
	Symptom: Functional instability	Describe specified event
	Sign: Increased joint mobility on clinical testing	General term requires specific degree of freedom to be further described
		Correct use of general classification systems for knee instability
Laxity	Slack, loose, decreased tension	Specify normal or abnormal laxity of the ligament structure
	Normal motion or greater than normal motion	Specify motion (degree of freedom), i.e., anterior translation rather than anterior laxity

occurs, nor what the instability event represents (full or partial giving way). Unless the instability is further defined in the context of the report, the reader cannot know which event the author is describing. The author must clarify precisely the meaning of the general terms to avoid ambiguity.

More commonly, the term *instability,* as it is used in the literature, indicates a condition (physical sign) characterized by increased mobility, excessive motion, or increased play in the knee joint. In this context, the use of the term is similar to that in the literature on spinal injuries, in which excessive mobility of the cervical vertebra is referred to as "cervical instability." Several problems arise when the term is used to indicate a condition. First, although common, it is incorrect to specify an anatomical structure, as in "ligamentous instability," "ACL instability" or "posterolateral ligament instability." Rather, the author should indicate which specific ligament defect (abnormal ligament laxity) contributes to the excessive motion (instability) of the joint. Note that when one refers to an "ACL instability" one presumes and/or implies that the ligament alone causes the instability. In fact, it is com-

monly acknowledged that the conditions of stability and instability result from the dynamic interaction of many factors (ligamentous restraints, weight-bearing compressive forces, meniscus structures, and neuromuscular control mechanisms).

Most classification systems are based upon the term *instability;* the abnormal motion or abnormal position of the knee joint is referred to as an instability. But *stability* and *instability* are general terms and do not convey sufficient information to define the type of instability. Thus, if the instability refers to a particular type of abnormal motion, the author must clarify, with great precision, the degree of freedom that is abnormal and any abnormalities in the other degrees of freedom. Confusion arises when the authors of classification systems fail to establish specific inclusionary criteria for specific types of instability. Systems based on general criteria cannot be used in a uniform manner and thus are often used inconsistently. In contrast, systems that provide specific criteria for specific instabilities allow examiners to understand the unique conditions of various instabilities, and, consequently, to apply these systems consistently.

The term *instability,* when used to describe an event, should be further clarified as to the event itself (total knee collapse, partial giving way, or the joint instability perceived by the patient), thereby avoiding ambiguity. We strongly recommend that the term *instability* be used only in a general sense to indicate excessive motion or mobility of the knee joint.

The term *laxity,* in the orthopaedic literature, has two general meanings: looseness or slackness (a characteristic of a ligament) and motion (as of a joint). Problems have arisen from each of these usages.

When applied to a ligament, *laxity* indicates looseness or slackness. But since all ligaments exhibit a certain amount of looseness, and the degree of slackness varies among individuals, laxity may be normal or abnormal. An abnormal (or pathologic) laxity may result after a partial ligament injury or it may be congenital. Too often, authors have used *laxity* to indicate abnormal looseness when the correct term would have been *abnormal laxity.*

The orthopaedic literature contains many instances in which the term *laxity* is applied to a joint; commonly, the term indicates some degree of motion, generally unrestricted and free motion (play). The *International Dictionary of Medicine and Biology* (Wiley, New York, 1986) defines *laxity,* in part, as either normal free motion or greater than normal motion, as of a joint. But the use of *laxity* in this context is often problematic, since the factor that allows the joint to move freely—the looseness of the ligaments—is not identified. Moreover, the specific type of motion is rarely stated or, if stated, is nonetheless ambiguous. For example, does "anterior laxity" of the knee joint refer to a general anterior displacement of the tibia or to the specific amount of anterior tibial translation? If used to indicate displacement, the overall displacement should be further specified, since the anterior Drawer motion is composed of both anterior translation and internal tibial rotation. If, on the other hand, "anterior laxity" describes only the translation component of the Drawer motion, it would be better to say "anterior translation." This term avoids ambiguity; the amount of anterior translation under the specific loads applied may be specified in millimeters.

It is interesting to note that the engineering literature refers to the *play,* rather than the *laxity,* of a machine or a part. In this context, *play* means free or unimpeded motion, as of a part of machinery, and implies that the part can move or function freely within prescribed limits. One example is the normal play of a piston rod within a cylinder in an engine. It is entirely acceptable to refer to the *play* of the knee joint, and to refer to *increased play* as denoting the greater than normal play that may occur after a ligament injury.

We recommend that *laxity* be used only in a general sense to indicate slackness or looseness of a ligament. When referring to the laxity of a specific ligament, it should be specified whether the laxity is normal or abnormal. When *laxity* is used to describe joint motion it is preferable that the motion itself be specified. The use of *laxity* as a synonym for *joint motion* is unnecessary and vague.

Classification systems should be based on the term *instability* (which refers to the condition of increased mobility of the knee joint rather than *laxity*) because it is more precise to say that the joint

demonstrates a *state of increased mobility* rather than a *state of increased slackness* or *decreased tension* (as the term *laxity* indicates).

In the literature, *subluxation* has been defined as an instability, an abnormal motion, or an abnormal laxity. Since *instability* means excessive mobility or motion of the joint, it is more precise to say that an instability results in an altered position or subluxation of the joint. Similarly, it is incorrect to equate abnormal knee motion and subluxation, since increased knee motion does not always produce a joint subluxation. Less frequently, *subluxation* has been defined as abnormal laxity. Because *laxity* is a general term meaning slackness, it cannot denote a specific abnormal position.

Generally, *subluxation* is defined as an incomplete or partial dislocation. Difficulty arises in quantitating or demonstrating when a subluxation has occurred. Note that the term does not have units; therefore, the author must establish and define criteria for the occurrence of a subluxation. For example, one criterion might define an anterior subluxation of the tibia, indicating an abnormal relationship between the medial and lateral tibial femoral compartment, as the result of a specific number of millimeters of anterior tibial translation. Moreover, there are different types of anterior subluxations, depending on the position of the medial and lateral tibial plateaus. Hence, when using the term *anterior subluxation,* the author must also specify the degree to which the medial or lateral plateau is involved.

Although a clinical sign may be diagnostic of a specific ligament defect, it does not itself represent the diagnosis. This is true of physical diagnosis in general. For example, a cardiologist may detect the clinical sign of a grade III systolic ejection murmur with the stethoscope. This clinical sign would be recorded as a finding observed during examination. However, the diagnosis of aortic valvular stenosis would be recorded separately. Note that the diagnosis indicates the anatomic part affected. In a similar way, the sign of an abnormal joint motion must not stand as the final diagnosis. It would be incorrect for the clinician to record as a diagnosis "anterior subluxation of the knee." Instead, the specific anatomic defect of the ACL and any other associated ligamentous or capsular structures should be recorded as the diagnosis. In the past, abnormal motions (clinical signs) have been rendered as diagnoses and have led to confusion as to what is representative of the exact ligamentous and capsular defect.

The diagnosis of ligament defects is accomplished through a clinical laxity examination, which consists of four parts: (1) the examiner applies a set of forces, (2) the knee joint undergoes motions described by individual degrees of freedom, (3) the examiner determines position of the joint (normal or subluxed), and (4) the examiner then diagnoses the ligament defect.

CONCEPT II: The clinical ligament examination must be performed and interpreted using knowledge of the three-dimensional motions of the knee.

We believe that major problems exist with current classification systems. In our opinion, most classification systems are not diagnostic for a specific ligament defect. For example, among the "rotatory instabilities," the terms *anterolateral instability* and *anteromedial instability* are highly imprecise and do not represent a specific motion or set of motions that is definable. In some classification systems only one degree of freedom, internal–external tibial rotation, is used to describe the "rotatory instabilities." In other classification systems the term implies combinations of two motions: anterior tibial translation and internal–external tibial rotation.

The American Orthopaedic Society for Sports Medicine (AOSSM) classification[19] defines *anteromedial instability* as comprising three motions: tibial abduction, external tibial rotation, and anterior tibial translation. An infinite number of different combinations of joint motions could theoretically occur in anteromedial instabilities, depending upon the abnormalities in any one, two, or three of the degrees of freedom. The same is true for *anterolateral instability* or *posterolateral instability.* These terms are imprecise and do not define the specific change in each degree of freedom of motion involved. Obviously this results in a significant problem in communicating the results of treatment when the pathologic condition under treatment is ambiguously defined.

The correct way to analyze and communicate abnormal increase in joint motions is in terms of the six independent degrees of freedom. These consist of three rotations (flexion–extension, abduction–adduction, internal–external rotation) and three translations (anterior–posterior, medial–lateral, and compression–distraction). We want to emphasize three points related to these six degrees of freedom. First, the specific increase in motion (amount and sense) of each degree of freedom that is clinically relevant should be determined. Second, both the amount of increased motion and resulting subluxation of the tibial plateaus depend strongly on the position of the knee joint, which is also defined in terms of the six degrees of freedom. Third, there commonly exists, after ligament injury, an abnormal position in the axis of tibial internal–external rotation that may be clinically detected and is helpful for diagnosis of the ligament defect.

The axes and motions that comprise the six degrees of freedom are described and illustrated in Chapter 9. In many instances, the knee joint functions with coupled motions, such as the combination of anterior translation with internal tibial rotation that occurs during the Lachman-type anterior translation test. For proper diagnosis it is necessary to understand the effect the ligament injury has upon both anteroposterior (AP) translation and tibial rotation since one or both may be increased. This will be disussed below.

In order to interpret the results of the clinical laxity test, a clear distinction must be made between abnormalities in joint motion and abnormalities in joint position (subluxation) at the limit of the test (Table 10-1). As a result of an abnormality in one or more motion limits, the knee joint may be displaced into an abnormal position (subluxation). The precise position will depend on the direction and magnitude of the loads applied. Clinical laxity tests are used to detect both abnormal (increased) motions and the final abnormal joint position.

The term *subluxation* means an incomplete or partial dislocation. The laxity examination usually produces subluxations rather than a complete non-contact position of both tibiofemoral compartments (a *dislocation*).

These motion concepts will now be applied to understanding what often occurs after an ACL tear.

Fig. 10-1. Anterior translation vs. tibial rotation is shown during the anterior Drawer test at 15° and 90° of flexion. (Straight pull, force applied in an anterior direction alone; straight pull + int. rot., anterior force plus internal rotation torque.) (Top graph from ref. 19a, with permission.)

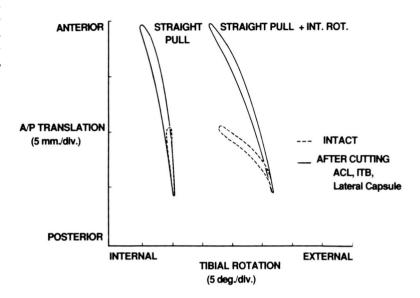

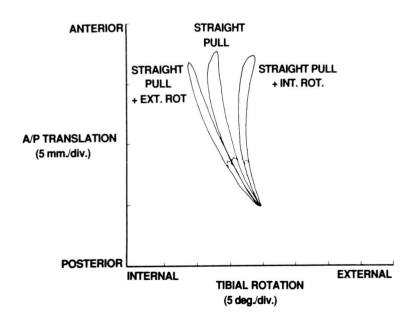

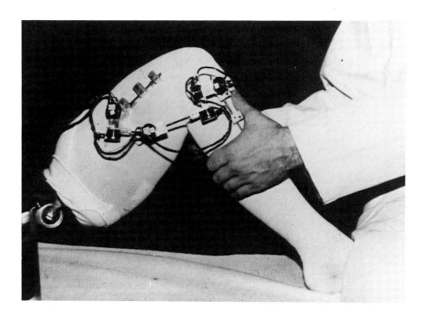

Fig. 10-2. The six-degree-of-freedom electrogoniometer provides the clinician immediate feedback of the motions induced during the laxity test. (From ref. 8, with permission.)

We found in cadaver knees that, after the ACL was cut, an abnormal increase in both anterior tibial translation and internal tibial rotation occurred. However, the increase in anterior tibial translation was the primary abnormality. Anterior tibial translation increased approximately 100 percent, whereas internal rotation increased only 15 percent with the knee at 20° flexion.

In Figure 10-1, the data are shown for a Lachman-type anterior Drawer test conducted at 15° of knee flexion. The amount of anterior tibial translation that occurred during the test is plotted against the position of tibial rotation. Tibial translation was measured at a point midway between the spines of the intercondylar eminence. As shown in Figure 10-2, we used a six-degrees-of-freedom electrogoniometer to measure knee motion in whole cadaver legs. The actual knee motions during the laxity test were displayed on a monitor.[9,10,31] First note, in Figure 10-3, that with an anterior load a few degrees of internal tibial rotation occurred. This is an example of coupled motions due to the manner in which the physician performs the examination. After the ACL and lateral extraarticular structures were cut, the coupled motions still occurred; however, the in-

crease in anterior tibial translation was the predominant abnormality. Such coupled motions can be caused by factors intrinsic to the knee or by the methods used to perform the clinical test. The amount of internal tibial rotation that occurred depended on the internal rotation torque applied by the clinician. That is one reason why obtaining reproducible results is so difficult. Thus, the Lachman test, like other clinical laxity tests, is highly variable in terms of the ways it may be performed and the results interpreted.

Figure 10-3 shows another phenomenon the clinician must understand about the amount of tibial translation that occurs with ACL injuries. The amount of anterior translation depends on the position of internal or external tibial rotation at the start of the test. This occurs because the tibial rotation position determines the tautness of the extraarticular restraints. In the example in Figure 10-3, only the ACL was cut. The greatest amount of anterior translation occurred when the test was conducted in a neutral rotation position. Note that the amount of tibial translation markedly decreased when the tibia was rotated internally before starting the test. Small amounts of additional internal rotation during the

Fig. 10-3. The amount of anteroposterior translation depends on the rotation position of the tibia at the beginning of the anterior Drawer test. (From ref. 19a, with permission.)

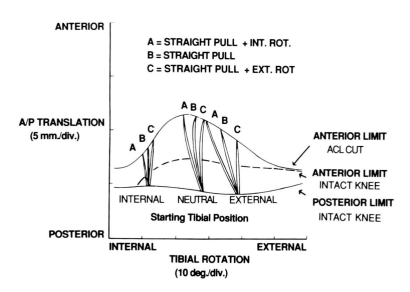

ANTERIOR DRAWER 90° FLEXION

A = STRAIGHT PULL + INT. ROT.
B = STRAIGHT PULL
C = STRAIGHT PULL + EXT. ROT

test reduced the amount of tibial translation. A similiar but opposite effect occurs when a position of external tibial rotation is selcted before the test.

These results show that the examiner controls the amount of translation by varying the initial rotational position of the tibia and the rotation moment imposed during the test. It is for this reason that the clinician must be as consistent as possible in the way the laxity tests are performed. Clinicians must minimize the technique-related differences seen from test to test or between right and left limbs.

We routinely use all of the various laxity tests, and believe no one single test is sufficient for every knee. The Lachman anterior Drawer test, performed at 20° to 30° of knee flexion, is the most reliable test for us in detecting the increased anterior tibial translation due to ACL injury.

Newer diagnostic knee-measuring devices have already been found useful in making this measurement more objective and could become the standard for diagnosis and reporting treatment results. The finding of even a few millimeters of increased anterior translation indicates complete ACL disruption, with the secondary ligamentous restraints blocking further translation.

When performing anterior translation-type tests we routinely palpate the medial and lateral tibofemoral compartments to estimate the amount of translation of the individual compartments.

We first perform the Lachman test, attempting to block any associated internal tibial rotation. When the ACL is intact (Fig. 10-4A), the amount of translation is limited by this ligament alone. Any subtle increase is due to damage to this ligament. With an ACL tear, the next structures to resist anterior translation are those that limit motion of the medial tibiofemoral compartment. Note in Figure 10-4B that the lateral bumpers are not restraining tibial translation as long as the examiner prevents internal rotation. We then repeat the test with an anterior force plus internal tibial rotation moment to allow further anterior translation of the lateral tibial plateau and to test for the lateral extraarticular restraints, as shown in Figure 10-4C. With this added rotation, the full anterior subluxation position of the lateral compartment is reached. This is one advantage of the flexion–rotation Drawer test when the knee is not constrained during the test and the full anterior subluxation of both the medial and lateral tibial plateaus is usually reached.

The end point "hardness" or terminal stiffness provides added information in the Lachman test, but

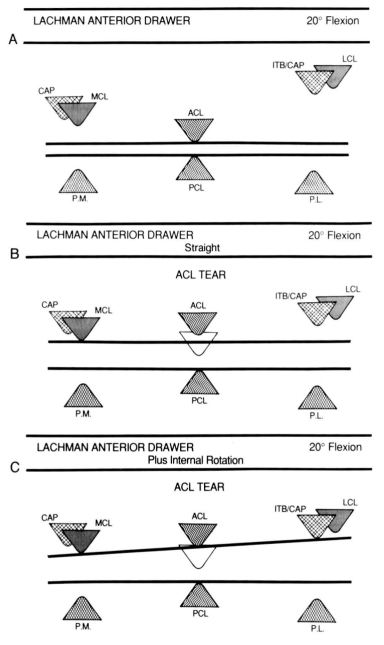

Fig. 10-4. The different types of anterior Drawer tests. **(A)** A straight anterior Drawer alone tests the ACL. **(B)** After ACL rupture, a straight anterior Drawer tests the medial ligamentous structures that control the amount of subluxation. **(C)** After ACL rupture an anterior Drawer plus internal rotation is required to reach the maximum anterior subluxation to the lateral tibial plateau. (*ACL,* anterior cruciate ligament; *CAP,* capsule; *ITB,* iliotibial band; *LCL,* lateral collateral ligament; *MCL,* medial collateral ligament; *PCL,* posterior cruciate ligament; *P.L.,* posterolateral restraints; *P.M.,* posteromedial restraints.)

a word of caution is warranted. A hard end point may be produced by a nonfunctional and elongated ACL. Also, intact secondary ligamentous restraints may occasionally give the sensation of a hard end point.

For the traditional anterior Drawer test conducted at 90° of knee flexion, our laboratory studies show that an increase in external or internal tibial rotation before the test will reduce the amount of tibial translation obtained. We believe that rotating the tibia internally (blocking test) tightens the iliotibial band and blocks anterior translation, producing a false-negative test even in knees without an ACL.

The type of 90° Drawer test that we routinely perform is similar to the test conducted at 20° flexion. The tibia is placed in a neutral starting position before the test. The first maneuver is to apply an anterior load without any associated internal or external rotational torque. The second maneuver is to apply an anterior load and then internally or externally rotate the tibia, palpating the increase in anterior displacement of each tibiofemoral compartment. These maneuvers should be performed so as to obtain maximum subluxation of the medial and lateral tibial plateaus. We prefer not to sit on the foot during the test so as not to constrain tibial rotations. Any increase in anterior translation of the tibia indicates injury to the laxity of the ACL, with further increases in the respective compartments being due to involvement of the secondary medial and lateral restraints.[2]

The pivot shift and flexion–rotation Drawer tests[6,7,25] involve a rather complex set of tibial rotations and translations that have not previously been measured using a six-degrees-of-freedom (three-dimensional) system. Figure 10-5 shows the technique for performing the flexion–rotation Drawer test. Figure 10-6 shows the sequence of motions that occur during the test. The results presented here are based on prior studies[28] using whole lower limbs and a three-dimensional electrogoniometer to measure total knee motion. At the start of the tests (position A), the lower extremity is simply supported against gravity. After ligament sectioning, an increase in anterior tibial translation and internal rotation is noted as the femur drops back and rotates externally, into a subluxated position. This position is accentuated as the tibia is lifted anteriorly (position B). At approximately 30° of knee flexion the tibia is pushed posteriorly, reducing the tibia into a normal relationship with the femur (position C). This is the limit of posterior translation, which is resisted primarily by the posterior cruciate ligament (PCL). From position C to position A, the knee is extended to again produce the subluxated position.

The examiner may purposely accentuate the rotational component of the test by inducing a rolling motion of the femur. It is not necessary to produce

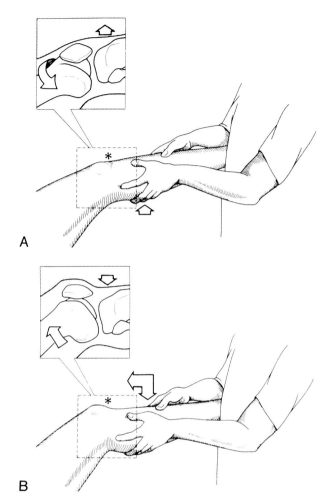

Fig. 10-5. (A) Flexion–rotation Drawer test in subluxated position. With the leg held in neutral rotation, the weight of the thigh causes the femur to drop back posteriorly and, more importantly, to rotate externally, producing anterior subluxation of the lateral tibial plateau. **(B)** Flexion–rotation Drawer test in reduced position. Gentle flexion and a downward push on the leg (as in a posterior Drawer test) reduce the subluxation. This test assesses the function of the ACL in the control of both translation and rotation. (Noyes FR, Basset RW, Grood ES, et al : Arthroscopy in acute traumatic hemarthrosis of the knee. J Bone Joint Surg 62A:687–695, 1980.)

joint compression or add an abduction movement as in the pivot shift test. This avoids the pain sometimes associated with the latter test. A finger is placed along the anterior aspect of the lateral and

FLEXION ROTATION DRAWER

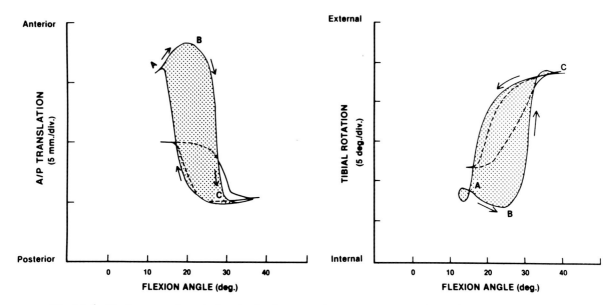

Fig. 10-6. The knee motions during the flexion–rotation Drawer test are shown for tibial translation vs. knee flexion and for tibial rotation vs. knee flexion. The laxity test is shown for the normal knee (open curve) and after ligament sectioning (shaded curve). The ligaments sectioned were the ACL, iliotibial band, and lateral capsule. Position A equals the starting position of the test, B is maximum subluxated position, and C indicates the reduced position. (From ref. 19a, with permission.)

medial tibial plateaus to estimate the millimeters of anterior subluxation from the tibiofemoral step-off. However, the main aspect of the test is to detect visually the translation and rotation movement rather than to determine the magnitude of the motions. Tibial translation is detected in a manner similar to the Lachman test by observing the forward motion of the tibial plateaus. Rotation is observed by watching the patella rotate externally with the femur in the subluxated position and internally in the reduced position.

Figure 10-7 shows the sequence of knee motions during the pivot shift test. The test starts at position A. The maximum subluxated postion is reached at position B. The sudden reduction phenomenon occurs between position B and position C. This motion produces the characteristic "thud" sensation. With knee extension after reduction, there is an increase in anterior tibial translation at about 10° of knee flexion. Tibial rotation returns to normal, but this may be altered during the test depending on

whether or not an external tibial rotation is applied as the knee goes to extension. A truly normal reduced position is only obtained in the pivot shift test at position C, and not at position A, since as the knee approaches extension there is still an abnormal anterior tibial translation.

The amount of tibial rotation was greater during the pivot shift test than in the other laxity tests studied. This was due to the manner in which the tibia is used to apply rotational torques during the test. The jerk test represents the reverse of the pivot shift test; it goes from the flexion-reduced position (position C) to the subluxated position (position B) with knee extension.

The bumper model shown in Figure 10-8A is helpful in understanding the overall effect of the combined rotation and translation that occur during the pivot shift test. In this illustration the ACL bumper has been removed as a restraint and the medial and lateral bumpers are shown for an average normal knee. In Figure 10-8A the pivot shift and

PIVOT SHIFT

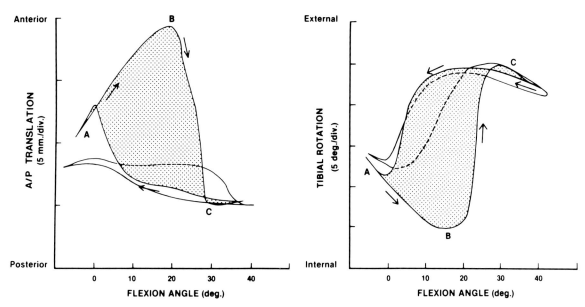

Fig. 10-7. The knee motions during the pivot shift test are shown for the parameters of tibial translation and tibial rotation vs. knee flexion before ligament sectioning (open curve) and after ligament section-ing (shaded curve). For positions A, B, and C see Figure 10-6 legend.

flexion – rotation Drawer tests have produced an anterior subluxation of both the medial and lateral tibiofemoral compartments. To reach the maximum position, it is necessary to apply an anterior force on the tibia while the tibia is simultaneously forced to rotate to its internal limit of rotation. These forces and moments are applied by the examiner's hand on the leg during the test. In Figure 10-8B the internal rotation torque alone is applied without the anterior force. This technique is sometimes used; however, there is a problem in that the internal rotation torque reduces the medial compartment into a normal tibiofemoral relationship. Therefore, the added anterior subluxation of the medial tibial plateau would not be detected.

The pivot shift and flexion – rotation Drawer tests are graded only qualitatively, since it is difficult to estimate with any degree of accuracy the true amounts of internal tibial rotation or anterior translation present.

The subjective difference in the pivot shift phenomenon used to grade qualitatively the different

types of anterior subluxations is shown in Table 10-2. A fully positive pivot shift test (grade IV) indicates a gross subluxation of the lateral and medial tibial plateaus. This amount of anterior subluxation indicates not only ACL laxity but also that secondary extraarticular ligament restraints are not providing resistance. Since the lateral tibial plateau has the greater subluxation in a positive pivot shift test, the lateral extraarticular secondary restraints (iliotibial band, lateral capsule) are not functionally tight, or they would block the pivot shift test. This does not mean that associated injury to the lateral extraarticular ligaments has occurred, since this slackness normally appears at the knee flexion position used in the pivot shift test. This allows most knees with an ACL tear alone to have a positive pivot shift phenomenon (grade III).

Occasionally the classic subjective phenomenon of the "thud" or "clunk" of the pivot shift test will be absent with ACL tears. The experienced examiner will still detect an increased slipping sensation (grade II). This is due to tight extraarticular second-

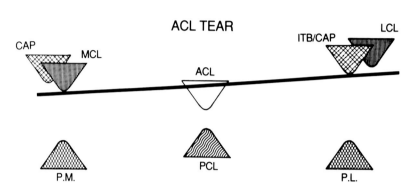

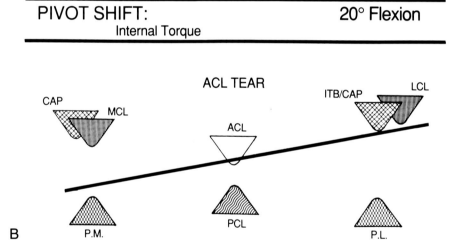

Fig. 10-8. The bumper model is shown for the pivot shift and flexion–rotation Drawer-type tests. **(A)** An anterior force is combined with internal tibial rotation to reach a maximum anterior subluxation of the medial and lateral tibiofemoral compartments. **(B)** Only an internal rotation motion is used, as is sometimes done in the pivot shift test. This reduces the medial tibiofemoral compartment and is therefore less useful for diagnosis. (For abbreviations see Fig. 10-4 legend.)

ary restraints that limit the amount of anterior tibial subluxation even though the ACL is torn. We have found the Lachman test and flexion–rotation Drawer test to be the most sensitive in picking up these subtle types of anterior subluxation.

The type IV subluxation is characterized by a loss of the medial and lateral secondary ligamentous restraints. If the amount of anterior subluxation of the tibia is large enough, the posterior margin of the lateral tibial plateau actually impinges on the femo-

Table 10-2. Classification of Pivot-Shift-Type Tests

Laxity Grade	Structures Involved			Positive Test	Comments
	ACL	Iliotibial Band, Lateral Capsule	Medial Ligaments, Capsule		
Normal (grade I)	−	−	−	−	Physiologic laxity (motion) normally present
Moderate (grade II)	+	−	−	Lachman test Flexion–rotation drawer Losee test, ALRI Pivot shift "slip" but not "jerk"	Subtle subluxation–reduction phenomena Secondary ligamentous restraints limit the amount of joint subluxation but may stretch out later with repeated injury Pivot shift and jerk tests do not show obvious jump, thud, or jerk, although the subluxation may be detected as a "slip" with experience
Severe (grade III)	+	+	−	All tests positive	Hallmark is an obvious jump, thud, or jerk with gross subluxation–reduction during the test. This indicates laxity of other ligamentous restraints, either a normal physiologic laxity (lateral capsule, iliotibial band), or injured secondary restraints
Gross (grade IV)	+	++	++	All tests positive	Hallmark is a gross subluxation with impingement of the posterior aspect of the lateral tibial plateau against the femoral condyle. The examiner must effect reduction to allow further knee flexion

+, Ligamentous structure is loose; −, ligamentous structure is not loose.
(Modified from ref. 19a, with permission.)

ral condyle, blocking knee flexion during the pivot shift test. It is important to impose both an anterior force and forcible internal tibial rotation to reach the maximum subluxation position. It is easy to hypothesize that such a knee has the worst prognosis. We previously discussed treatment implications for a type IV subluxation in considering acute augmented repairs in acute knees and the possibility of a combined intraarticular and extraarticular surgical approach in chronic knees.[26] Since this grading is not exact, the amount of anterior tibial translation (medial, lateral, or central translation) measured by clinical testing devices has greater accuracy and should be used for reporting clinical results.

CONCEPT III: The so-called "rotatory instabilities" can be characterized by the separate subluxations that occur to the medial and lateral tibial plateaus.

Up to this point, we have described abnormalities in anterior tibial translation and internal tibial rotation that occur in knees with ACL disruption. We noted that the clinician must be aware of both mo-

tions when performing laxity tests in order to interpret properly which motions are increased. A simple unifying concept will now be presented that combines the abnormal motions that occur after ACL disruption. The concept states that the amount of anterior and posterior translation of each tibiofemoral compartment may be used to classify the rotatory subluxations. The scientific basis for this assertion has been presented in Chapter 9. Now we wish to apply these precepts to the clinical examination. Figure 10-9 shows an analogy to a Lachman test performed on a knee in which the combined motions of tibial translation and internal tibial rotation occur about a rotation axis located medially. In this ideal test (where only planar motion occurs), rupture of the ACL doubles anterior translation and slightly increases the internal tibial rotation, as previously noted. This results in a medial shift of the rotation axis. The ratio of tibial translation to degrees of internal tibial rotation determines how far medially the axis of rotation is located.

The abnormalities in tibial rotation and translation are easily expressed in terms of the separate

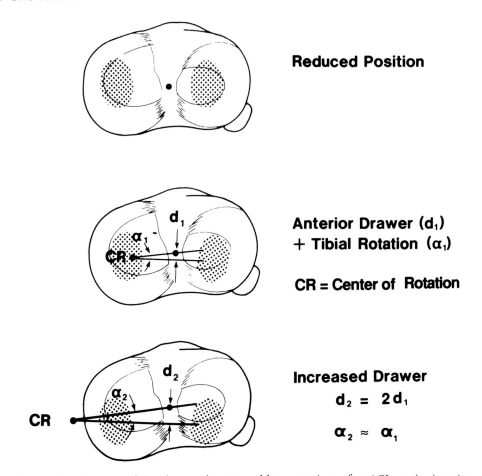

Reduced Position

Anterior Drawer (d₁)
+ Tibial Rotation (α₁)

CR = Center of Rotation

Increased Drawer
$$d_2 = 2d_1$$
$$\alpha_2 \approx \alpha_1$$

Fig. 10-9. A simplification of the abnormal increased knee motions after ACL sectioning. An understanding of rotatory subluxations requires specifying changes in position of the vertical axis of rotation and the displacement of the medial and lateral tibiofemoral compartments separately. The normal or subluxated position of the joint is determined by the degrees of rotation and the amount of translation. In this analogy, an anterior pull is applied to the knee with an intact ACL. There is a normal anterior translation (d_1) and internal tibial rotation (α_1) about the center of rotation (CR). After ACL sectioning there is a 100 percent increase in tibial translation (d_2) along with only a slight (15 percent) increase in internal tibial rotation (α_2). This shifts the axis of rotation medially and produces the subluxation of the lateral compartment and medial compartment as demonstrated (shaded area represents tibiofemoral contact area). Loss of the medial extraarticular restraints would result in a further medial shift in the axis of rotation. This would increase the anterior subluxation of the medial tibial plateau and the lateral tibial plateau. (From ref. 19a, with permission.)

amount of anterior translation that occurs to the medial and lateral compartments. This anterior translation of each tibial plateau can be palpated and observed visually during the clinical laxity tests. We believe that characterizing the medial and lateral plateau AP translations is much simpler than having to define specifically the individual components of translation, rotation, and rotation axis location that led to the anterior subluxation. This agrees with the precepts advanced in Chapter 9, where it was shown that the rotations and translations combine to amplify and reduce the motions of the medial and lateral tibial plateaus. This phenomenon determines the separate translations of the medial and lateral tibiofemoral compartments.

To appreciate the difference in anterior transla-

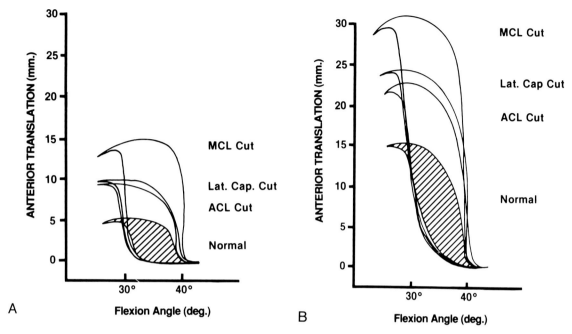

Fig. 10-10. The amount of anterior tibial translation is shown separately for the **(A)** medial and **(B)** lateral tibial plateau (reference point at joint margin) during the flexion–rotation Drawer test.

tion between the medial and lateral compartments, the results of one cadaveric knee specimen are shown in Figure 10-10. This figure shows the amount of tibial translation measured separately for the medial and lateral joint margins. The ligaments sectioned include the ACL, lateral capsule, and tibial collateral ligament. The flexion–rotation Drawer test was performed after sectioning each ligament. The increase in translation for the lateral compartment during the test is greater than the translation of the medial compartment. A further increase in translation, principally to the lateral compartment, occurs after the lateral capsule and iliotibial tract are sectioned. The final increase in translation of both compartments is shown after the tibial collateral ligament is sectioned. The important clinical point is that it is necessary to palpate separately the lateral and medial tibial plateaus to characterize the type of anterior subluxation that occurs.

Table 10-3 shows the secondary restraints that resist anterior tibial subluxation after the ACL is sectioned. The amount of anterior subluxation of the lateral compartment depends on the integrity of the lateral meniscus and lateral extraarticular restraints. Similarly, the amount of anterior subluxation of the medial compartment depends upon the intactness of the medial meniscus and medial extraarticular restraints.

We previously determined that the type of rota-

Table 10-3. Comparison of Secondary Structures at Increased Anterior Displacement (%)[a]

	Iliotibial Tract and Band	Midmedial Capsule	Midlateral Capsule	Medial Collateral Ligament	Lateral Collateral Ligament
Mean ± S.E.M.	24.8 ± 4.7	22.3 ± 6.9	20.8 ± 5.4	16.3 ± 2.9	12.4 ± 3.3
Minimum	9.8	3.4	1.6	8.1	7.0
Maximum	44.4	43.6	36.9	29.4	25.2

[a] n = 6; anterior Drawer of 12.2 to 16.3 mm at 90° of knee flexion. By Duncan's multiple range test, no statistical difference was found among the percentages for any of the structures shown (P > 0.05). (Butler DL, Noyes FR, Grood ES: Ligamentous restraints to anterior–posterior Drawer in the human knee: a biomechanical study. J Bone Joint Surg 62A: 264, 1980.)

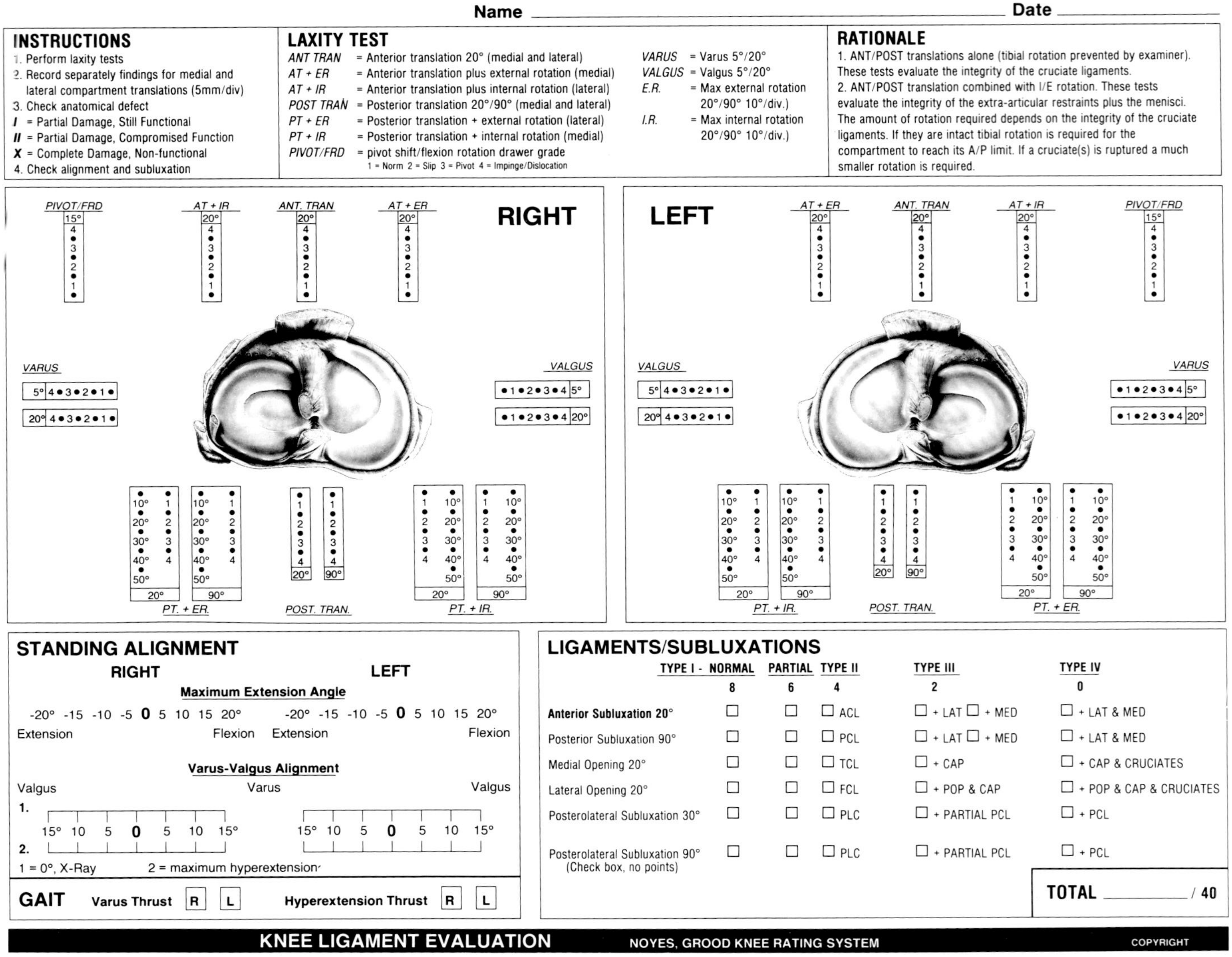

INSTRUCTIONS

1. Perform laxity tests
2. Record separately findings for medial and lateral compartment translations (5mm/div)
3. Check anatomical defect
   - I = Partial Damage, Still Functional
   - II = Partial Damage, Compromised Function
   - X = Complete Damage, Non-functional
4. Check alignment and subluxation

LAXITY TEST

ANT TRAN	= Anterior translation 20° (medial and lateral)
AT + ER	= Anterior translation plus external rotation (medial)
AT + IR	= Anterior translation plus internal rotation (lateral)
POST TRAN	= Posterior translation 20°/90° (medial and lateral)
PT + ER	= Posterior translation + external rotation (lateral)
PT + IR	= Posterior translation + internal rotation (medial)
PIVOT/FRD	= pivot shift/flexion rotation drawer grade
	1 = Norm 2 = Slip 3 = Pivot 4 = Impinge/Dislocation

VARUS	= Varus 5°/20°
VALGUS	= Valgus 5°/20°
E.R.	= Max external rotation 20°/90° 10°/div.)
I.R.	= Max internal rotation 20°/90° 10°/div.)

RATIONALE

1. ANT/POST translations alone (tibial rotation prevented by examiner). These tests evaluate the integrity of the cruciate ligaments.
2. ANT/POST translation combined with I/E rotation. These tests evaluate the integrity of the extra-articular restraints plus the menisci. The amount of rotation required depends on the integrity of the cruciate ligaments. If they are intact tibial rotation is required for the compartment to reach its A/P limit. If a cruciate(s) is ruptured a much smaller rotation is required.

RIGHT

LEFT

STANDING ALIGNMENT

RIGHT

Maximum Extension Angle

-20° -15 -10 -5 0 5 10 15 20°

Flexion   Extension

Varus-Valgus Alignment

Varus

15° 10 5 0 5 10 15°

Valgus

1.

2.

1 = 0°, X-Ray   2 = maximum hyperextension·

LEFT

Maximum Extension Angle

-20° -15 -10 -5 0 5 10 15 20°

Extension   Flexion

Varus-Valgus Alignment

Varus

15° 10 5 0 5 10 15°

Valgus

GAIT   Varus Thrust R L   Hyperextension Thrust R L

LIGAMENTS/SUBLUXATIONS

	TYPE I - NORMAL	PARTIAL	TYPE II		TYPE III		TYPE IV
	8	6	4		2		0
Anterior Subluxation 20°	☐	☐	☐ ACL	☐ + LAT ☐ + MED	☐ + LAT & MED	☐ + LAT & MED
Posterior Subluxation 90°	☐	☐	☐ PCL	☐ + LAT ☐ + MED	☐ + CAP & CRUCIATES
Medial Opening 20°	☐	☐	☐ TCL	☐ + CAP	☐ + POP & CAP & CRUCIATES
Lateral Opening 20°	☐	☐	☐ FCL	☐ + POP & CAP	
Posterolateral Subluxation 30°	☐	☐	☐ PLC	☐ + PARTIAL PCL	☐ + PCL
Posterolateral Subluxation 90° (Check box, no points)	☐	☐	☐ PLC	☐ + PARTIAL PCL	☐ + PCL

TOTAL _____ / 40

KNEE LIGAMENT EVALUATION   NOYES, GROOD KNEE RATING SYSTEM   COPYRIGHT

Fig. 10-11. Knee ligament evaluation form used in the Noyes/Grood rating system. (From ref. 19a, with permission.)

Table 10-4. Primary and Secondary Ligamentous Restraints to Laxity Tests

Laxity Test	Primary Restraint				Secondary Restraint		
	Medial	Central	Lateral		Medial	Central	Leteral
A. Anterior Drawer	—	ACL	—	20°/90°	TCL + MM	—	ALS
B. Anterior Drawer + internal rotation	—	ACL	ALS	20°/90°	—	—	FCL + PLS
C. Anterior Drawer + exterior rotation	TCL + MM	ACL	—	20°/90°	PMS	—	—
D. FRD, pivot shift	—	ACL	—	15°	MM + TCL + PMS	—	ALS + FCL
E. Posterior Drawer	—	PCL	—	20°/90°	PMS + TCL	—	FCL + PLS
F. Posterior Drawer + external rotation	—	—	FCL + PLS	30°	—	PCL	—
	—	PCL	FCL + PLS	90°	—	—	—
G. Posterior Drawer + internal rotation	TCL + PMS	—	—	20°	--	ACL + PCL	—
	TCL + POL	PCL	—	90°	—	ACL	—
H. Valgus	TCL + PMS	—	Bone	5°	—	PCL + ACL	—
	TCL	—	Bone	20°	PMS	PCL	—
I. Varus	Bone	—	FCL + PLS	5°	—	ACL + PCL	—
	Bone	—	FCL	20°	—	ACL	PLS
J. External rotation	PMS + TCL	—	FCL + PLS	30°	MM	PCL	—
	MM + TCL	PCL	FCL + PLS	90°	PMS	—	—
K. Internal rotation	TCL + PMS	ACL	ALS	20°	—	PCL	FCL
	TCL + POL	ACL + PCL	ALS	90°	—	—	FCL

ALS, iliotibial band plus anterior plus midlateral capsule
PLS, popliteus, posterolateral capsule
PMS, posterior oblique ligament plus posteromedial capsule
MM, medial meniscus
POL, posterior oblique ligament
TCL, tibial collateral ligament
FCL, fibular collateral ligament
(From ref. 19a, with permission.)

tory subluxation that can occur depends not only on the injury but also on the knee flexion position. One of the problems of some classification systems is that the rotational subluxations are recorded at only one knee position (90°), and in other systems the knee flexion position is simply not stated. We wish to advance the concept that the subluxation of the medial and lateral tibiofemoral compartments must be recorded at both 20° to 30° and 90° flexion.

CONCEPT IV: The diagnosis of ligament and capsular defects requires the use of selected laxity tests for which the primary and secondary ligamentous restraints have been experimentally determined.

We have discussed the abnormal motion limits and resulting joint subluxations that occur after ACL

tears and injury to the extraarticular ligamentous and capsular structures. The anterior Drawer, pivot shift, and flexion–rotation Drawer-type tests provide the basic signs necessary to determine which ligamentous and capsular structures are injured. This is based on the experimental determination of the ligaments that resist these selected laxity tests. Our approach is to perform compartmental anterior–posterior and rotation tests, choosing select knee positions in which the secondary restraints are "out of the way." This allows for the maximum excursion of the joint to test individual ligaments. It is not possible to guess which ligaments are acting as functional restraints. Major discrepancies exist in ligament-cutting studies due to differences in methodology we have described elsewhere.[2,8,21,32]

The scheme we use for recording the findings of the ligament laxity tests and the diagnosis is shown in Figure 10-11. Brief instructions for use of the form are given in the upper left-hand column. First, a laxity test is selected for which the primary and secondary resisting ligament restraints have been experimentally determined. The major tests we use are shown in Figure 10-11, and the primary and secondary ligamentous restraints to each test are shown in Table 10-4. The basic set of laxity tests is the anteroposterior translation test, the pivot shift type of tests, abduction–adduction tests, and the external rotation tests. They provide the information necessary to detect most knee ligament defects. However, more complex knee instabilties require the additional laxity tests, and therefore appropriate scoring of these tests are provided in the form (Fig. 10-11). The clinical findings are marked on the anatomic drawing for each knee (Fig. 10-11). A scale is provided for this; each major division equals 5 mm translation and each minor division is half of this amount. The maximal amount of translation is recorded for each tibial plateau. In essence the medial and lateral compartments can go forward, backward, or open up sideways. Also shown is a scale to give the maximum amount of internal and external tibial rotation. However, increases in tibial rotation may be due to medial or lateral ligament injuries, so the translation of each tibiofemoral compartment must always be determined.

In most acute knee cases, an increase in one grade of translation to the anterior–posterior or varus–valgus tests represents a third-degree or complete ligament injury to the primary restraint.[1,21] Each subsequent grade represents damage to the secondary restraints.

The extent of damage to each structure is recorded by placing an appropriate slash mark

Table 10-5. Functional Capacity of Injured Ligament

Extent of Failure	Sprain	Damage[a]	Joint Motion, Subluxation	Residual Strength	Residual Functional Length	Residual Functional Capacity
Minimal	First degree	Less than 1/3 of fibers failed; includes most sprains with few to some fibers failed; microtears also exist	None	Retained or slightly decreased	Normal	Retained
Partial	Second degree	1/3 to 2/3 ligament damage; significant damage but parts of the ligament are still functional Microtears may exist	In general no or minimal increased motion. Remaining fibers in ligament resist opening	Marked decrease At risk for complete failure	Increased, still within functional range but may later act as a check rein rather than subtle control of joint motions	Marked compromise, requires healing to regain function
Complete	Third degree	Over 2/3 to complete failure; continuity remains in part	Depends on secondary restraints	Little to none	Lost	Severely compromised or lost
		Continuity lost and gross separation between fibers	Depends on secondary restraints	None	Lost	Lost

[a] Estimate of damage is often difficult, however, the different types listed can usually be differentiated. Anterior and posterior cruciate tears commonly exist with little to no abnormal laxity. The examination for medial and lateral ligamentous injury is usually more accurate.

(Modified from *Athletic Training and Sports Medicine,* American Academy of Orthopaedic Surgeons, Chicago, IL, 1984, p. 232.)

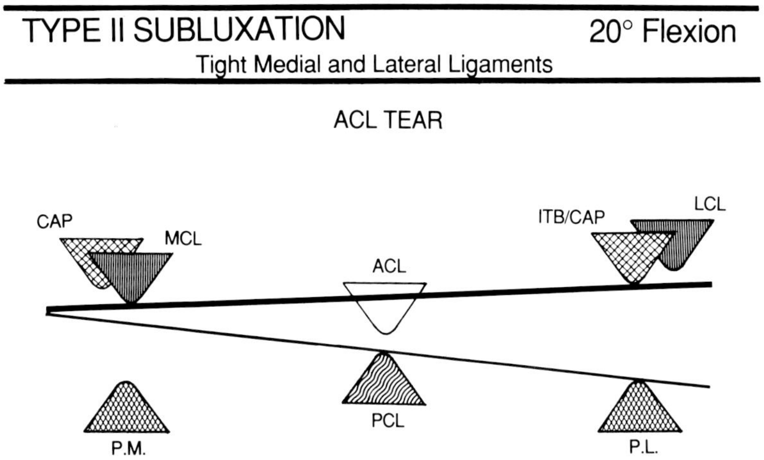

Fig. 10-12. In type II subluxation there is an abnormal tightness (restraining function) of one or both compartments. This can be detected by palpating the amount of anterior excursion of the medial and lateral tibial plateau during the Lachman and flexion–rotation Drawer tests. The lesion involves the ACL alone, which is indicated. The lower line represents the posterior limit of tibial excursion with a posterior Drawer plus external rotation and is used as a reference line throughout (Figs. 10-12 to 10-14). The upper line represents the anterior limit of tibial excursion resisted by the appropriate ligament bumpers. (For abbreviations see Fig. 10-4 legend.) (From ref. 19a, with permission.)

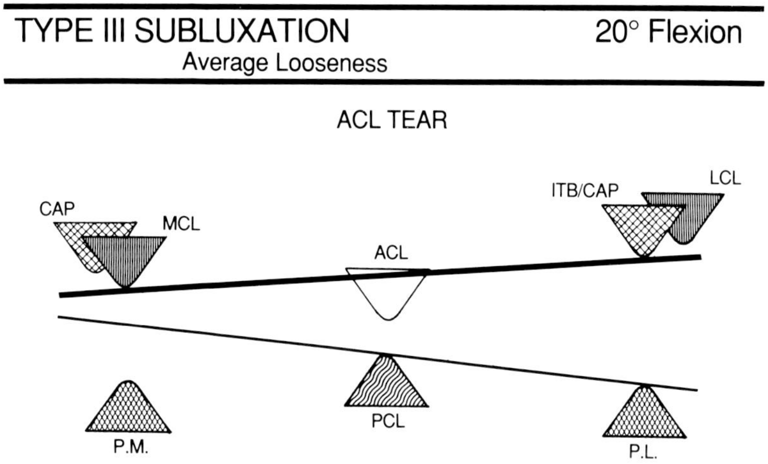

Fig. 10-13. Type III anterior subluxation is shown. This is the usual finding after ACL disruption. The lateral extraarticular structures are physiologically lax between 0° and 45° knee flexion, allowing for increased anterior translation of the lateral tibial plateau. The lesion involves laxity of both the ACL and secondary restraints. The bumper model shows that the relative increase in medial compartment translation is actually greater than that of the lateral compartment. This is because the normal position for the medial tibial plateau is actually posteriorly positioned, resting on the posteromedial bumper. (For abbreviations see Fig. 10-4 legend.) (From ref. 19a, with permission.)

Fig. 10-14. Type IV anterior subluxation is shown. There is associated laxity of both the medial and lateral extraarticular restraints. This allows for a gross subluxation of both the medial and lateral tibial plateaus that is easily palpable during the Lachman and flexion–rotation Drawer tests. (For abbreviations see Fig. 10–4 legend.) (From ref. 19a, with permission.)

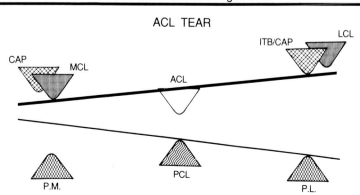

TYPE II SUBLUXATION · 20° Flexion
Tight Medial and Lateral Ligaments
ACL TEAR

TYPE III SUBLUXATION · 20° Flexion
Average Looseness
ACL TEAR

TYPE IV SUBLUXATION · 20° Flexion
Loose Medial and Lateral Ligaments
ACL TEAR

Table 10-6. Anterior Knee Subluxations Following ACL Rupture

Type	ACL	Medial Ligaments and Capsule	Anterior Translation[a]	Lateral Ligaments and Capsule	Anterior Translation[a]	Rotation Axis[b]	Characteristics	Laxity Test	Treatment Considerations
Type I (normal pattern)	Intact	—	Medial tibial plateau	—	Lateral tibial plateau	Central	Normal pattern ACL maintains central restraint	Normal AP Translation	—
Type II	No	Tight[c]	—	Intact	↑	Medial compartment	One or both extraarticular restraints limit compartment translation (less than 10% of knees with ACL disruption)	Positive Lachman and flexion-rotation Drawer grade amount of translation separately for medial and lateral compartments; Grade II pivot shift (slipping sensation)	Secondary restraints provide stability if protected from repeat injury; Generally best prognosis; consider nonoperative approach in less athletically active individuals; Still warrants acute augmented repair in fully competitive athlete since primary restraint is disrupted
	No	Intact	↑	Tight[c]	—	Lateral compartment			
	No	Tight[c]	—	Tight[c]	—	Central			
Type III	No	Intact	↑↑	Intact	↑↑↑	Outside knee medially	Typical pattern after ACL disruption	Positive Lachman and flexion-rotation Drawer; Grade III pivot shift (thud, clunk, jerk phenomena)	Avoid repeat giving-way injuries to protect secondary restraints; Acute augmented repair in active athletic individual

| Type IV | No | Lax[a] | ↑↑↑ | Lax[a] | ↑↑↑↑ | Outside knee medially | Gross anterior subluxation due to involvement of one or both extraarticular restraints (approximately 20–30% of ACL-deficient knees)

Commonly has associated increased varus or valgus opening or posterolateral subluxation | Obvious anterior subluxation of both compartments

Grade IV pivot shift (impingement) | Extra-articular procedure may convert to Type II subluxation but does not restore stability

Severe functional disability for any kind of athletics

Often produces giving-way with activities of daily living

Extra-articular procedure alone not warranted: would only effect lateral tibiofemoral compartment translation

In acute and chronic cases consider need to restore lateral extraarticular restraints |

[a] Refers to anterior translation of the medial or lateral tibial plateau during laxity test.
[b] During Lachman-type anterior Drawer test or flexion-rotation Drawer test.
[c] Refers to physiologic tightness of structure or result of operative treatment.
[d] Refers to abnormal laxity caused by injury or to physiological laxity.
(Data from works of Noyes and associates.[2,5,23–27])

through the structure on the drawing. The biomechanical information on the functional capacity of ligaments and their mechanisms of failure does allow for the approximate classification of injury, as we have previously described[1,20,21] (Table 10-5). The residual ability of a ligament to resist joint subluxation is estimated from the fraction of the ligament torn (one third, two thirds, complete), increases in functional length of the ligament (just-taut length), and joint stiffness. The estimate is also based on knowledge of the failure properties of the individual ligaments and capsular structures.[20-22] The assessment of the functional capacity of the damaged ligamentous and capsular structures is only an approximation. As we discussed in Chapter 9, to be more precise, a quantitative measurement of joint stiffness or compliance would provide added information.[4,14,15] It will ultimately be necessary to measure the stiffness of each one of the ligamentous systems (or functional "bumpers"). The goal here is for the physician to arrive at an approximation of the extent to which the individual structures have been damaged.

For completeness, the type of subluxation is checked in the lower right-hand corner. This will be demonstrated next using the bumper models. Also included in the form is the evaluation for the standing alignment of the knee joint as to degrees of varus–valgus angulation and degrees of hyperextension.

The form allows one to record both the clinical signs and diagnosis on one page. The reporting of surgical treatment results must be in quantifiable, measurable parameters. All of the concepts presented here can be applied in either a qualitative or quantitative manner.

There are at least three types of anterior knee subluxations that can occur following rupture of the ACL and which we believe can be clinically identified. These types are illustrated in Figures 10-12 to 10-14 and listed in Table 10-6. The data are based on experiments conducted on cadaveric lower limbs, in which the three-dimensional motions and resultant joint subluxations were measured before and after ligament sectioning.

Figure 10-12 shows the results after only the ACL was removed. This is for a knee with very tight medial and lateral extraarticular restraints that limit the amount of anterior translation of both tibiofemoral compartments (type II subluxation). The tight medial extraarticular restraints function to hold the center of rotation close to the medial aspect of the knee joint. There is only a slight increase in the amount of central and lateral tibial translation. The "bumper model" indicates the function of these anterior restraints during the flexion–rotation Drawer test, in which the maximal anterior excursion of the medial and lateral tibial plateaus is allowed. In the diagnostic map (Fig. 10-11) the amount of subluxation to the medial and lateral compartments would be estimated during different anterior translation tests, performed first with translation alone and then with internal or external rotation as previously described. The qualitative estimate for the pivot shift phenomenon would be listed as a grade II (Table 10-2).

Figure 10-13 shows the type of anterior subluxation (type III) most common after an ACL injury. The center of rotation shifts far medially outside of the knee joint and an increase in translation of both the medial and lateral tibial plateaus occurs. The diagnostic map indicates the anterior subluxation of both compartments (greatest in the lateral compartment). The qualitative estimate of the pivot shift test is a grade III (Table 10-2). The anatomic lesion involves the ACL and the lateral extraarticular restraints. These structures are functionally lax since they do not provide resistance in limiting the anterior subluxation of the lateral compartment. However, as previously discussed, the lateral extraarticular structures are physiologically loose at this knee flexion position.

The gross type of anterior subluxation (type IV) is shown in Figure 10-14. In this case there is increased translation and resultant subluxation to both the medial and lateral tibial plateaus, with a subsequent shift in the rotation axis even further medially outside the knee joint. The qualitative estimate of the pivot shift test is a grade IV, which indicates gross subluxation with impingement of the posterior aspect of the tibia against the lateral femoral condyle. In the diagnostic map (Fig. 10-11) the associated functional involvement of the medial extraarticular restraints to allow for the amount of anterior subluxation of the medial compartment would be indicated as a second-degree partial damage. This means that the medial ligamentous structures are still providing some resistance. If there was a significant increase in medial tibiofemoral joint opening under valgus stress, testing a third-degree lesion of the medial structures would be indicated.

The clinical significance of identifying these three types of anterior subluxations rests in the different natural histories and treatment programs we believe exist[2,5,23-27] (Table 10-6). The type II subluxation in which there is associated tight extraarticular structures has a better prognosis, and the abnormal motions may not increase if there are no further episodes of giving way to damage the secondary restraints. The type III subluxation, which is the most common, has an anterior subluxation of the medial and lateral tibial compartments, with the subluxation to the lateral compartment being greater due to associated increases in internal rotation. In those patients with a functional impairment we recommend ACL reconstruction alone and not a lateral extraarticular reconstruction alone or in combination with an intraarticular procedure. In essence a lateral extraarticular procedure may limit anterior subluxation of the lateral compartment but would not have a significant effect on the medial compartment.

In our clinical experience, a patient with a type IV anterior subluxation may frequently have giving way episodes with normal activities of daily living. The natural history in these knees is rather poor since the patient has a limited ability to compensate for this magnitude of potential subluxation. Patients are advised that the knee joint is significantly at risk for future giving-way episodes. A recommendation in acute knee injuries to perform acute augmented repair of the ACL is made. Attention is also directed to restoring any associated damaged ligamentous structures, particularly the lateral extraarticular tissues. In the chronically unstable knee with similar anatomic defects, we commonly advise both an intraarticular and lateral extraarticular procedure in view of the gross anterior subluxation that exists. Whether or not this is the correct treatment for these types of subluxations will require careful long-term analysis. The reporting of surgical results should define the types of anterior subluxation that exist. Newer knee motion testing systems allow for the actual measurement of the anterior subluxation of the medial and lateral compartment to quantify separately these different types of anterior subluxation and provide for the additional data that are still needed in this area.

CONCLUSIONS

When we first began the task several years ago of applying the data from clinical laxity tests to the diagnosis of ligament defects we found many problems and scientific inconsistencies. To resolve these problems it has been necessary to conduct a variety of biomechanical and kinematic studies and to establish a more precise definition of terms and nomenclature. We believe that this provides the basis for defining abnormalities in knee joint motions (increased limits), joint positions (subluxations), and diagnostic categories of specific ligament defects, on the basis of which treatment

Table 10-7. Diagnosis of Ligament Injury

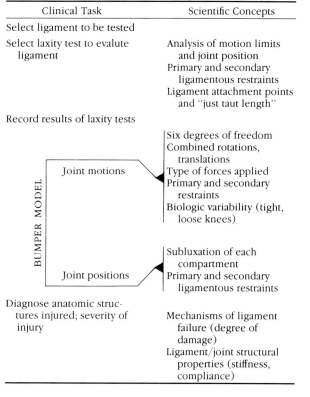

Clinical Task	Scientific Concepts
Select ligament to be tested	
Select laxity test to evaluate ligament	Analysis of motion limits and joint position Primary and secondary ligamentous restraints Ligament attachment points and "just taut length"
Record results of laxity tests	
Joint motions	Six degrees of freedom Combined rotations, translations Type of forces applied Primary and secondary restraints Biologic variability (tight, loose knees)
Joint positions	Subluxation of each compartment Primary and secondary ligamentous restraints
Diagnose anatomic structures injured; severity of injury	Mechanisms of ligament failure (degree of damage) Ligament/joint structural properties (stiffness, compliance)

programs and surgical results may be analyzed, recorded, and communicated.

To accomplish these diagnostic tasks it is necessary to apply certain scientific concepts, which have been presented in this chapter. The scheme that shows the ordering or progression of the diagnostic process is summarized in Table 10-7. Note that the entry level is to define which specific ligamentous or capsular structure is to be evaluated in terms of its functional integrity. The end of the process is the definition of the anatomic defects present. A series of clinical tests is used to determine abnormalities in motion limits and resultant joint subluxations that can occur. These clinical signs are used to determine the injuries present. The subluxations are not diagnostic entities themselves since so many different types exist that depend on the forces and moments applied, the position of the joint (flexion and tibial rotation), and the injury present. The bumper model provides a useful tool that embodies these concepts and allows the function of the primary and secondary ligamentous restraints to be understood.

Other scientific principles that the clinician must understand deal with how ligaments and capsular structures fail (mechanisms of failure). For example, the collateral ligaments demonstrate an abrupt failure process at relatively minor joint displacements due to their parallel collagen fiber arrangement. The cruciate ligaments have a more sequential failure of the fiber bundles due to a less parallel fiber microgeometry. These and many other factors influence ligament function[22] and are important in assessing the degree of damage and residual functional capacity. The diagnosis of ligament damage and the resulting joint subluxations is a difficult clinical task; however, the scientific basis for accomplishing this task is now becoming apparent.

ACKNOWLEDGMENTS

This work is supported in part by grant AM 21172, from the National Institute of Arthritis, Diabetes, Digestive and Kidney Diseases and the Cincinnati Sportsmedicine and Orthopaedic Research and Education Foundation.

REFERENCES

1. Athletic Training and Sports Medicine. The American Academy of Orthopaedic Surgeons, Chicago, Illinois, 1984
2. Butler DL, Noyes FR, Grood ES: Ligamentous restraints to anterior–posterior drawer in the human knee. A biomechanical study. J Bone Joint Surg 62A:259–270, 1980
3. Cabaud HE, Slocum DB: The diagnosis of chronic anterolateral rotary instability of the knee. Am J Sports Med 5:99–105, 1977
4. Daniel DM, Malcom LL, Losse G et al: Instrumented measurement of anterior laxity of the knee. J Bone Joint Surg 67A:720–726, 1985
5. Fetto JF, Marshall JL: Injury to the anterior cruciate ligament producing the pivot-shift sign. An experimental study on cadaver specimens. J Bone Joint Surg 61A:710–714, 1979
6. Galway HR, Beaupré A, MacIntosh DL: Pivot shift: a clinical sign of anterior cruciate ligament insufficiency. Proc Can Orthop Assoc, J Bone Joint Surg 54B:763, 1972 (abstr)
7. Galway HR, MacIntosh DL: The lateral pivot shift: a symptom and sign of anterior cruciate ligament insufficiency. Clin Orthop 147:45–50, 1980
8. Grood ES, Noyes FR, Butler DL, Suntay WJ: Ligamentous and capsular restraints preventing straight medial and lateral laxity in intact human cadaver knees. J Bone Joint Surg 63A:1257–1269, 1981
9. Grood ES, Suntay WJ, Noyes FR et al: Total Motion Measurement During Knee Laxity Tests. Transaction of the 25th Annual Orthopaedic Research Society, p. 80, 1979
10. Grood ES, Suntay WJ: A joint coordinate system for the clinical description of three dimensional motions: application of the knee. ASME Trans, J Biomech Eng 105:136–144, 1983
11. Hughston JC, Andrews JR, Cross MJ, Moschi A: Classification of knee ligament instabilities. Part I. The medial compartment and cruciate ligaments. J Bone Joint Surg 58A:159–172, 1976
12. Hughston JC, Andrews JR, Cross MJ, Moschi A: Classification of knee ligament instabilities. Part II. The medial compartment and cruciate ligaments. J Bone Joint Surg 58A:173–179, 1976
13. Kennedy JC, Fowler RJ: Medial and anterior instability of the knee. J Bone Joint Surg 53A:1257–1270, 1971
14. Markolf KL, Mensch JS, Amstutz HC: Stiffness and laxity of the knee — the contributions of the supporting structures. J Bone Joint Surg 58A:583–594, 1976

15. Markolf KL, Graff-Radfor A, Amstutz HC: In vivo knee stability. A quantative assessment using an instrumented clinical testing apparatus. J Bone Joint Surg 60A:664–674, 1978
16. Marshall JL, Rubin RM, Wang JB, et al: The anterior cruciate ligament, the diagnosis and treatment of its injuries and their serious prognostic implications. Orthop Rev 7:35–46, 1978
17. Müller W: The Knee: Form, Function, and Ligament Reconstruction. Springer-Verlag, Berlin, Heidelberg, 1982
18. Nicholas JA: Lateral instability of the knee. Orthop Rev 6:33–44, 1977
19. Nicholas JA: Report of the Committee on Research and Education. Am J Sports Med 6:295–304, 1978
19a. Noyes FR, Grood ES: Classification of ligament injuries: Why an anterolateral laxity or anteromedial laxity is not a diagnostic entity. pp. 185–200. In Griffin PP (ed): Instructional Course Lectures. American Academy of Orthopaedic Surgeons, Park Ridge, IL, 1987
20. Noyes FR, Grood ES, Butler DL, Malek M: Clinical laxity tests and functional stability of the knee: biomechanical concepts. Clin Orthop 146:84–89, 1980
21. Noyes FR, Grood ES, Butler DL, Paulos LE: Clinical biomechanics of the knee–ligament restraints and functional stability. In Funk FJ (ed): AAOS: Symposium on the Athlete's Knee: Surgical Repair and Reconstruction. CV Mosby, St. Louis, 1980
22. Noyes FR, Keller CS, Grood ES, Butler DL: Advances in the understanding of knee ligament injury, repair, and rehabilitation. Med Sci Sports Exer. 16:427–443, 1984
23. Noyes FR, McGinniss GH: Controversy about treatment of the knee with anterior cruciate laxity. Clin Orthop 198:61–76, 1985
24. Noyes FR, McGinniss GH, Mooar LA: Functional disability in the anterior cruciate insufficient knee syndrome, review of knee rating systems and projected risk factors in determining treatment. Sports Med 1:278–302, 1984
25. Noyes FR, Butler DL, Paulos LE, Grood ES: Intra-articular cruciate reconstruction. Part I: Perspectives on graft strength, vascularization and immediate motion after replacement. Clin Orthop 172:71–77, 1983
26. Noyes FR, Mooar PA, Matthews DS, Butler DL: The symptomatic anterior cruciate deficient knee. Part I: The long-term functional disability in athletically active individuals. J Bone Joint Surg 65A:154–162, 1983
27. Noyes FR, Matthews DS, Mooar PA, Grood ES: Symptomatic anterior cruciate deficient knee. Part II: The success of rehabilitation activity modification and counseling in functional disability. J Bone Joint Surg 65A:163–174, 1983
28. Noyes FR, Grood ES, Suntay WJ, Butler DL: The three dimensional laxity of the anterior cruciate deficient knee as determined by clinical laxity tests. Iowa Orthop J 3:32–44, 1983
29. Slocum DB, Larson RL: Rotatory instability of the knee. J Bone Joint Surg 50A:211–255, 1968
30. Slocum DB, James SL, Larson RL, Singer KM: Clinical test for anterolateral rotary instability of the knee. Clin Orthop 118:63–69, 1976
31. Suntay WJ, Grood ES, Hefzy MS et al: Error analysis of a system for measuring three-dimensional motion. ASME Trans J Biomech Eng 105:127–135, 1983
32. Torzilli PA, Greenberg RL, Insall J: An in-vivo biomechanical evaluation of anterior–posterior motion of the knee, roentgenographic measurement technique, stress machine, and stable population. J Bone Joint Surg 63A:960–968, 1981

11

Diagnosis of Knee Ligament Injury: Tests and Measurements of Joint Laxity

DALE M. DANIEL
MARY LOU STONE

Ligaments have been defined as tough fibrous tissue structures that tie or bind the bones together. Ligament and ligature have the same Latin root "liga," meaning to bind or tie. Definitions of ligament use words such as bind, tie, connect, support, and strengthen, but ligaments also allow motion. These words conjure up the image of a tether or a leash which suggests that ligaments (1) allow a certain range of motion without being loaded and (2) are under load only to limit undesired motion.

Recent studies support the concept that ligaments do more than allow and limit motion; they guide motion.[1,2,5,26] The position of a joint depends on the joint surface contours, muscle forces, ligament/capsule restraints, and external forces. Joint surfaces are coated with hyaline cartilage, which has a low coefficient of friction and therefore produces negligible resistance against shear forces. The joint surfaces essentially only resist compressive forces. Ligaments, capsular structures, and tendons, like rope, are loaded under tension. The ligaments function as guys. They might be compared to the guys of a tent. The position of a tent is dependent on the central pole, which, like the joint surface, is principally loaded in compression and the guy ropes on either side, which, like the tendons and ligaments, are loaded under tension. External forces will alter the position of the tent and the loads on the various supporting structures. Injury to one of the guy ropes

will alter the position of the tent and the position change resulting from external forces. Likewise, knee position depends on the integrity of the ligaments, tendons, and the applied external forces. Ligament integrity may therefore be evaluated by assessing joint motion, either qualitatively or quantitively. Because the changes in motion resulting from ligament injury may be small, it is important that the conditions of testing be precisely defined and that the examiner be aware of the sensitivity and limitations of the testing system, be it a manual or instrumented examination.

In this chapter we will discuss knee motion, primary qualitative tests of knee ligament disruption, and quantitative measurements of knee laxity.

KNEE MOTION

The motion of the knee or any other system can be described in terms of rotations about or translations along some set of axes. Rotation is simply turning about an axis and translation is sliding along an axis. Translation is more precisely defined as a motion whereby all lines in the body remain parallel to their original position. The ability to rotate or translate along or about a particular axis is called a "degree of freedom." Free motion about or along the three mutually perpendicular axes used to define a space

Axis	Rotation	Translation

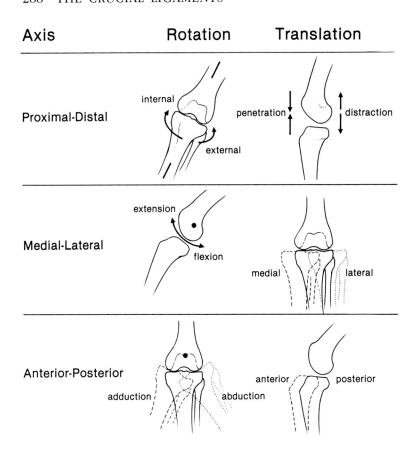

Fig. 11-1. The three knee axes. Around each axis there is rotation and along each axis there is a translation to give a total of six degrees of freedom (6 DOF).

represents "six degrees of freedom." In this condition a body is completely free to move. Motion of the knee has usually been described as motion of the tibia in relation to a fixed femur. Figure 11-1 shows the three knee axes and their associated motions.

Natural knee motions and the motions resulting from clinical laxity tests are not limited to one degree of freedom. For example "knee flexion" during normal gait requires the knee to rotate about the medial/lateral axis, translate along and rotate about the anterior/posterior axis, and rotate about the proximal/distal axis. When an anterior displacement force is applied in performing the 30° anterior displacement tests, the tibia translates anteriorly and rotates internally. When a posterior displacement force is applied, the tibia externally rotates and posteriorly translates. These linked or joined motions are referred to as "coupled motion" (Fig. 11-2). Constraining one motion of the couple will limit the other.

Whether testing joints in the laboratory or the clinic, one must take care not to apply inappropriate constraints. Joint laxity tests frequently focus on one motion. The tester, however, must be aware that the constraint of the testing system on associated motions (coupled motions) may have a major effect on the movement being measured. For example, if joint rotation is constrained by the testing system when performing the 30° anterior displacement tests, the tibia's anterior translation will be significantly diminished.

LIGAMENT INJURY TESTS

Over the past half century numerous authors have reported their correlations between the clinical knee examination and pathologic findings noted at surgery. A system for classifying knee joint instability (pathologic laxity) has evolved based on joint motion detected by the clinical examination.[12,17]

Fig. 11-2. Linked or joined motions are referred to as *coupled motions.* This figure shows coupled motion in the anterior displacement and internal rotation of the tibia that results from an anterior tibial displacement force. A posterior displacement force also results in coupled motion, posterior displacement, and external rotation of the tibia.

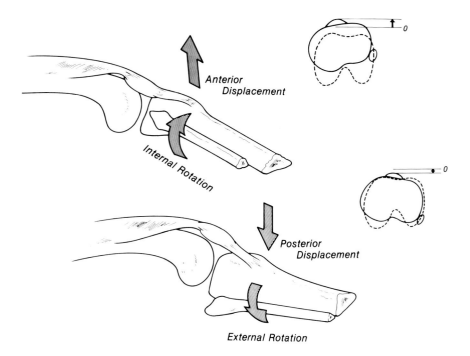

The strength of the classification system is that it emphasizes the complexity of pathologic knee motion resulting from knee ligament injuries. The weakness of the system is that there has been no objective testing system to validate, contradict, or refine the clinical observations. In recent years, laboratory studies on joint motion have been published and frequently have been at odds with reported clinical concepts of pathologic knee motion. The following are three examples.

Based on the clinical examination and surgical observation, Hughston et al.[12] stated that anteromedial rotatory instability, defined as "the medial plateau of the tibia rotates anteriorly with the joint opening on the medial side,"[17] results from a "tear of the medial compartment ligaments, including the posterior oblique ligament." Laboratory studies by Sullivan et al.[32] did not demonstrate anterior subluxation of tibia when ligament sectioning was confined to the medial compartment ligaments. Only when the anterior cruciate ligament (ACL) was disrupted did they measure an increase in anterior tibial motion, which was enhanced with sectioning of the medial compartment ligaments.

A second example is the clinical diagnosis of anterolateral rotatory instability (anterior subluxa-tion of the lateral tibial plateau) resulting from "a tear of the middle third of the lateral capsular ligament."[12] This clinical observation was not confirmed in laboratory studies by Lipke et al.[19] Significant increase in tibial internal rotation occurred only when the anterior cruciate ligament was sectioned. The increased rotation resulting from sectioning of the ACL was enhanced by sectioning the lateral ligament structures.

The third example involves the posterior cruciate ligament (PCL). Based on clinical examination and surgical observations, Hughston and Norwood[13] reported that tibial external rotation with a posterior displacement force occurs with disruption of the posterior lateral structures but not when in association with a disrupted PCL:

> It is possible to have an injury to the arcuate ligament complex and to the posterior cruciate ligament in the same knee. However, the tibial rotation of the posterolateral rotatory instability will not be present, because the posterior cruciate ligament pivot for rotation is absent.

In vitro studies[11,31] support the observation that disruption of the popliteal/arcuate ligament complex results in an increase in tibial external rotation with posterior subluxation of the lateral tibial plateau. The studies[11,31] do not support a negating of this motion when the PCL is then sectioned; on the contrary, there is an enhancement of the tibial external rotation.

The question of the precise alteration of knee motion after ligament injury is unresolved. On the one hand, the clinician does not have the joint measurement tools to document precisely joint motion and delineate pathologic motion. On the other hand, laboratory scientists have the testing tools. However, the in vitro ligament sectioning study may not simulate the in vivo injury condition. Although the technology is not available in the clinic or the operating room to measure pathologic knee motion along and around three axes, the experienced clinician has been able to use certain clinical laxity tests to predict specific ligament injuries with a high degree of accuracy. The pathologic motion resulting from certain tests is associated with specific ligaments or ligament complexes. The following tests we use as primary tests of ligament disruption. The test will render pathologic motion only if the specific ligament in question is injured. The injury of other ligaments may increase the pathologic motion being tested, provided the primary ligament is disrupted. For each of the five major ligament/ligament complexes, the laxity tests we have found most predictive of an injury to that structure are presented in the following paragraphs.

Anterior Cruciate Ligament

The *Lachman test* is a clinical test to assess anterior knee laxity and stiffness of the knee in about 20° of flexion. The examiner applies a manual anterior displacement force to the proximal calf and perceives tibial displacement both manually and visually and "end point stiffness" manually. The examiner then grades the laxity of the knee in relation to the patient's normal knee. Our review of instrumented joint displacement measurements with a manually applied displacement force similar to the Lachman test compared to Lachman test grade in the same patients revealed that the Lachman test grade has only fair correlation with measured displacement. However, the Lachman test has proven a reliable test in the hands of experienced clinicians to detect ab-

normal joint motion.[16,33] Of the two changes resulting from an anterior cruciate ligament injury, an increase in anterior joint laxity and a decrease in anterior end point stiffness (increase in compliance), the clinician's manual test is probably more sensitive to changes in end point stiffness.

Pivot shift tests have been described by a number of authors as pivot shift test,[9,10] Losee test,[20] sidelying test,[30] and flexion-rotation Drawer test.[24] The tests produce anterior subluxation and reduction of the tibia with knee flexion and extension from 10° to 40° as a sequela of an ACL disruption. The tests are performed by lifting the tibia and allowing the femur to sublux posteriorly[10,24] or pushing the tibia forward.[20,30] As the knee is flexed and the iliotibial tract moves from a position anterior to the axis of knee flexion to a position posterior to the axis of knee flexion, the anteriorly subluxed tibia reduces. Due to greater laxity in the normal posterior lateral capsular structure and greater mobility of the lateral meniscus compared to the posterior medial structures, there is more lateral tibial plateau motion than medial plateau motion. This results in internal rotation of the tibia with anterior joint subluxation and external rotation of the tibia with joint reduction.[25] The pivot shift test is consistently positive in the relaxed patient with a chronic ACL disruption and in the acutely injured anesthetized patient with an ACL disruption. In patients with a medial collateral ligament disruption resulting in valgus laxity of the knee and in patients with prior iliotibial tract surgery, the tension and/or orientation of the tract may be altered. The reduction of the tibia with knee flexion may then occur gradually and the test's findings will be less dramatic. Surgery of the iliotibial tract may also serve to constrain lateral tibial plateau anterior displacement.

Posterior Cruciate Ligament

The 90° quadriceps active test is performed with the patient in the supine position with the hip flexed 45°, the foot on the table, and the knee flexed 90°. In this position the tibia is supported from sagging posteriorly by the PCL. If the PCL is intact, the patella ligament in this position is oriented posteriorly as it passes up from the tibia to the patella. Therefore, contraction of the quadriceps moves the tibia slightly posterior (0 to 2 mm). If the PCL is disrupted, the tibia sags posteriorly. The patellar ligament orientation is then anterior as it passes from the tibial tubercle to the patella. Contraction of the quadriceps results in anterior tibial translation. The test is performed as shown in Figure 11-3. The patient is supine with the knee flexed 90°. The examiner sits beside the table with eyes at the level of the knee. The examiner rests an elbow on the table and supports the patient's thigh. With the supporting hand the examiner can palpate the hamstrings and the quadriceps to monitor muscle tone. The examiner's other hand supports the foot. While watching tibial motion, the examiner asks the patient to gently try to slide his foot down the table. The examiner resists this motion with a hand on the patient's foot. It is important that the patient execute a quadriceps contraction only. A simultaneous hamstring contraction would check the forward tibial motion. Anterior tibial motion with the quadriceps

contraction is a positive test and is indicative of posterior tibial subluxation seen consistently with a PCL disruption. Alterations of the normal patellar ligament/tibia anatomy (e.g., patellectomy, tibial tubercle elevation, or proximal tibia fracture) will alter the test. For validation of the test, it should be done on both of the patient's knees. The normal knee will demonstrate no motion or backward tibial excursion with contraction of the quadriceps and the PCL-injured knee will move anteriorly.

The *posterior Drawer test* is less diagnostic of PCL disruption than the 90° quadriceps active test, which documents posterior tibia subluxation. The posterior Drawer is less diagnostic because not all chronic PCL injured knees displace posteriorly significantly from their subluxed resting position. However, in acutely injured patients with partial PCL tears or patients who are unable to flex the knee past 45° to 60°, the evaluation of posterior tibial displacement and end point stiffness with a posterior tibial displacement force may be a helpful indicator of PCL injury.

Medial Collateral Complex

The *abduction stress test* evaluates the knee for medial collateral ligament (MCL) injury. The clinical test is most effectively performed with the patient supine, the thigh resting on the examining table, and the knee gently flexed 30° over the side of the table with the foot and leg supported by the examiner. The normal knee is examined first and the laxity on valgus stress of the injured knee is compared to the normal knee. An MCL injury is demonstrated by an increase in medial joint line opening, an increase in limb valgus, and a decrease in end point stiffness. With the knee in 30° of flexion to relax the posterior capsule, the MCL is the primary stabilizer against valgus stress. Other medial stabilizers are the medial capsule and posterior oblique ligament.

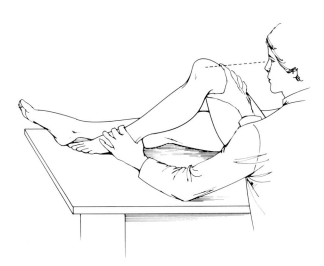

Fig. 11-3. The 90° quadriceps active test. The patient is supine. The examiner sits beside the table with the patient's knee flexed 90° and at eye level. When testing the left leg, the right elbow rests on the table and the right hand supports the thigh and palpates the quadriceps and biceps to monitor muscle tone. The left hand stabilizes the foot. The patient is asked "try gently to slide your foot down the table." The hand on the ankle prevents the foot from moving. The examiner watches for anterior translation of the tibia, which occurs when the tibia is posteriorly subluxed secondary to a PCL disruption.

Lateral Ligament Complex

The *adduction stress test* evaluates the knee for lateral collateral ligament injury. With the knee in 30° of flexion, the lateral collateral ligament and associated lateral structures (lateral capsule, iliotibial band, and lateral capsular ligament) are stressed. The examination is performed similarly to the valgus stress test except that a varus stress is applied. A lateral ligament complex injury is demonstrated by an increase in lateral joint space opening, increase in limb varus, and a decrease in end point stiffness.

Posterior Lateral Ligament Complex

The *reverse pivot shift test* is the primary test for injury to the posterior lateral ligament complex.[15] The associated pathologic laxity, which has been termed posterior lateral rotatory instability, is the least understood of the ligament laxities. The primary restraining structures are the popliteus tendon/arcuate ligament complex, lateral collateral ligament, and PCL.[11,15,31]

We begin the test by supporting the limb with a hand under the heel, placing the knee in full extension and neutral rotation. With the examiner's second hand on the lateral aspect of the calf, a mild valgus stress is applied and the knee is flexed. In a positive test, at about 20° to 30° of flexion the tibia will externally rotate and the lateral tibial plateau will sublux posteriorly and remain in this position during further flexion. When the knee is then extended, the tibia reduces. In the standard pivot shift the tibia is anteriorly subluxed in early flexion and then reduces between 20° and 40° of flexion. In the reverse pivot shift the tibia is initially reduced and then the lateral tibial plateau posteriorly subluxes at 20° to 30° of flexion. In a patient with a combined ACL and posterior lateral injury, one may observe the tibia go from an anterior subluxed position to a reduced position and then on to a posterior subluxed position. We have found the reverse pivot shift test to be helpful in the clinic if a patient has a chronic injury, but if the knee is acutely injured the patient is unable to relax and allow the test to be performed. Therefore in the acutely injured patient with pathologic laxity on varus testing or a posterior tibial sag or Drawer, especially with associated lateral tenderness, the possibility of injury to the posterior lateral ligament complex must be considered.

To establish the diagnosis more accurately, the patient should be examined under anesthesia.

Other tests helpful in identifying posterolateral ligament complex injuries are tibial external rotation in 30° of flexion,[11,31] and the external rotation–recurvatum test.[12]

The above five ligament/ligament complex injuries may occur in isolation. For each there is a laxity test specific for that complex (Table 11-1). When more than one ligament/ligament complex is injured, the laxity increases in both tests. For example, if the ACL and the MCL complex are both injured, the laxity on the Lachman test will increase, the laxity to a valgus stress will increase, and there will be increased external rotation of the tibia. Surgical restoration of the joint involves the repair or reconstruction of all injured structures identified at the time of surgery and would include the posterior oblique ligament, MCL (deep and superficial portions), and the ACL.

A system that documents pathologic joint motion along and around all three axes of motion will certainly greatly advance our knowledge of knee pathomechanics. We have that technology in the laboratory at this time but not in the clinic or operating room. The presentation of concepts and hypotheses of joint pathomechanics that result from clinical observations from ligament injury provide food for thought and direction for investigation. However, it is important to acknowledge the limitation of our present understanding of knee pathomechanics and press on in the clinic, the operating room, and the laboratory to place motion/laxity measurements on a more objective foundation.

The system of primary laxity tests is simple; its simplicity may lead the clinician to think that the alteration in joint motion resulting from a ligament injury is limited to one translation or one rotation. This is an error. Pathologic motion resulting from ligament injuries is complex. The primary laxity tests are each keyed to one of the pathologic motions that result from an injury to the structure being tested. The primary laxity test system can be confirmed by the clinician. The results of the laxity test are either positive, equivocal, or negative. When an operation is performed, the ligament in question is either normal, injured but in continuity, or completely disrupted.

Table 11-1. Primary Laxity Tests for the Five Ligament/Ligament Complex Injuries that May Occur in Isolation

Test	Ligament/Ligament Complex Isolated Injury[a]				
	ACL	PCL	MCC	LCC	PLC
Lachman	■				
Pivot shift	■				
Tibia posterior subluxation		■			
Posterior Drawer		■			
Abduction (30°)			■		
Adduction (30°)				■	
Reverse pivot shift					■

[a] The height of the box indicates the relative accuracy of the test.
MCC, medial collateral complex; LCC, lateral collateral complex, PLC, posterolateral complex.

MEASUREMENT OF JOINT LAXITY

When you can measure what you are speaking about, and express it in numbers, you know something about it; when you cannot measure it — when you cannot express it in numbers — your knowledge is a meager and unsatisfactory kind: it may be the beginning of knowledge, but you have scarcely, in your thoughts, advanced to the stage of science.

William Thomson Lord Kelvin,
popular lectures and addresses,
1891–1894,
as quoted by Bartlett.[3]

Over the past two decades, in the pursuit of placing measurements of knee laxity on a more objective foundation, numerous investigators[4,6,18,19,21–23,25–29,32,34] have described various instrumented systems. In all systems, knee joint motion resulting from a known displacement force is measured. The resulting motion is dependent on the joint starting position, applied force (point of application, direction, load), and constraints to motion applied by limb supports, force applicators, and motion sensors. Also, the resulting motion is dependent on bone contours, soft tissue restraints (ligament, capsule, menisci), and muscle activity.

We offer three examples of the effect of joint starting position on anterior–posterior measurements.

Example 1. A 20 lb anterior tibial displacement force applied to the proximal tibia with the knee in 30° of flexion will reveal an increase in anterior laxity consistently in the ACL injured knee.[7] However, we have found when the knee is flexed to 70° to 90° of flexion only 20 percent of the patients with an ACL disruption demonstrated pathologic laxity.

Example 2. When the PCL is disrupted the tibia subluxes posteriorly. If an anterior–posterior test is performed from the patient's resting position (a posteriorly subluxed position), an increased anterior knee laxity will be measured instead of increased posterior laxity.

Example 3. With the knee in 30° of flexion the patella ligament is oriented anteriorly as it passes from tibial tubercle to patella. A slight contraction of the quadriceps (such as when the patient is not relaxed) will translate the tibia anteriorly. An anterior laxity measurement performed from an anterior starting position will diminish the measured anterior laxity, and pathologic anterior laxity in an ACL injured knee may not be revealed.

When comparing displacement results with similar loads applied to two knees or with two testing systems, the point of application of the load must be compared. An anterior force applied to the tibia at the level of the ankle will result in knee extension, whereas a force applied at the level of the knee joint line will result in anterior tibial translation. The extension moment and translation effect of an anterior-applied force will depend on the point of application on the tibia. The effect of an applied force on translation or rotation will depend on the direction of the force as well as the point of application. The restraining soft tissues are compliant: the greater the load, the greater the displacement.

Knee motion may occur along and around three axes; therefore, there are six degrees of freedom (DOF)—three translations and three rotations (Fig. 11-1). Many of the motions are linked or coupled. If one motion is constrained it will diminish the displacement in the linked motion(s). For example, laboratory studies of anterior displacement of the tibia after sectioning of the ACL show a small increase in anterior laxity when the specimen is tested in a device with one DOF[4] compared to tests of specimens in a device with four DOFs. Tests of the same specimens with four DOFs revealed different results than tests with five DOFs.[32] A comparison of the UCLA Instrumented Clinical Testing Apparatus (which uses a limb support system that stabilizes "the femur quite rigidly" and a footrest that holds "the ankle rigidly" [22]) with the KT-1000 arthrometer testing system (which applies less limb constraints[28]) revealed that the UCLA apparatus

measured less anterior laxity in the same patients than the KT-1000 arthrometer. The lesson is important: when evaluating test results, be aware of the constraints on joint motion imparted by the testing system.

Muscle activity may have two effects on laxity measurements. First, it may alter the joint starting position as previously discussed. Second, it may have a significant effect on total joint displacement. Markolf et al.[22] documented that in anterior–posterior testing, muscle activity decreases joint laxity up to 50 percent of the normal value. All muscle groups crossing the joint can alter joint laxity measurements. Therefore, a testing system should be comfortable to the patient. The examiner must assess muscle relaxation and assist the patient in muscle relaxation. We have found that the lack of muscle relaxation is the major cause of spurious measurements of ligamentous systems.

INSTRUMENTED TESTING SYSTEMS

Overview of the Systems

Instrumented testing systems consist of a limb support system, a force application device, and a motion sensor. Kennedy and Fowler[18] were the first to report using a clinical testing machine for in vivo measurements of tibial–femoral displacement. Their device was used for both anterior laxity measurements and varus–valgus laxity measurements. The patient sat in the machine, which looked like a golf cart. Anterior displacement loads were applied with the patient's knee in 90° of flexion and varus–valgus loads were applied with the knee in slight flexion. The motion sensor technique was radiographic. Radiographs were taken in the unstressed and stressed state. The radiographs were compared and the joint displacement was measured. Others[8, 14,34] have radiographically documented joint change with applied stress. Torzilli et al.[34] reported a technique to differentiate translation from rotation when measuring anterior–posterior laxity. Tria and associates (in exhibit, American Academy of Orthopaedic Surgeons, Las Vegas, 1985) demonstrated a radiographic index for medial knee injuries.

Markolf et al.,[22] Malcom et al.,[21] Daniel et al.,[6]

Fig. 11-4. Arthrometer model KT-1000. *A*, force handle; *B*, patellar sensor pad; *C*, tibial tubercle sensor pad; *D*, Velcro strap; *E*, arthrometer case; *F*, displacement dial indicator; *G*, thigh support; *H*, foot support. *1*, A constant pressure of 4 to 6 lb applied to the patella sensor pad keeps it in contact with the patella; *2*, posterior force is applied; *3*, anterior force is applied.

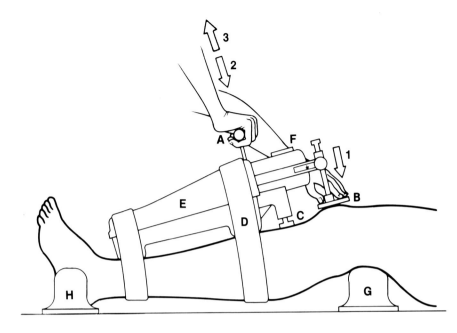

Shino et al.,[29] and Dilworth Cannon (personal communication, 1984) have developed anterior–posterior laxity testing instruments with mechanical sensing systems. Oliver and Raab[27] reported a computerized measurement device designed to measure joint flexion–extension, varus–valgus, anterior–posterior translation, and internal–external rotation. To date, the devices that have been most widely used or reported are the UCLA Instrumented Clinical Testing Apparatus[22,23,28] and the MEDmetric Arthrometer models KT-1000[7,21] and KT-2000.[7] For the past 4 years we have used the MEDmetric arthrometers.[5-8,21] We will summarize our experience with that testing system (Fig. 11-4).

Documented Testing with the MEDmetric Arthrometer KT-1000

Anterior–Posterior Laxity Testing of Normal Knees

The arthrometer (KT-1000) is placed on the anterior aspect of the leg and held in place by two circumferential Velcro straps. There are two sensor pads: one in contact with the patella and the other in contact with the tibial tubercle. These move freely in the anterior–posterior plane in relation to the arthrometer case. The instrument detects the rela-

tive motion in millimeters between the two sensor pads and, therefore, motion of the arthrometer case (as the calf compresses under the Velcro straps) does not affect the instrument's output. Displacement loads are applied through a force sensing handle which is located 10 cm distal to the joint line.

The first test performed on the normal knee is the *90-degree quadriceps test.* The examination is performed with the patient supine. The examiner sits lightly on the patient's foot to stabilize the limb. The knee is flexed 90° (the same as when performing the 90° Drawer test). The arthrometer is placed on the leg. With the hand stabilizing the arthrometer patella sensor pad, the examiner also supports the patient's knee so that the patient may relax the leg musculature (Fig. 11-5). In larger patients, frequently we have an assistant sit by the side of the table and support the limb, as seen in Fig. 11-3. It is critical that the muscle units crossing the knee be completely relaxed. The testing reference position is established: the resting position after a 20 lb posterior force is applied and then released. The patient then performs an isolated quadriceps contraction. We have found that the most helpful command to the patient is "Try to slide your foot gently down the examining table." The examiner palpates the hamstring tendons to confirm that there is no ham-

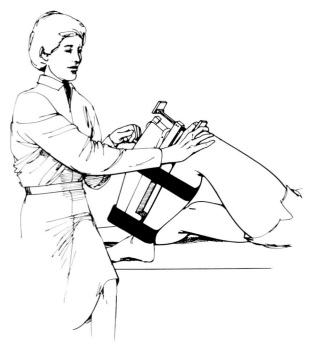

Fig. 11-5. Arthrometer position for testing at the quadriceps neutral angle (mean = 70°).

string contraction. The test is repeated until the patient performs an isolated quadricep's contraction without concomitant knee extension. The arthrometer documents the anterior or posterior tibial displacement. Anterior tibial motion greater than 1 mm is abnormal and probably indicates a PCL injury. If the anterior tibial motion is greater than 1 mm, then, the quadriceps *neutral angle test* should be performed (see below). If there is no anterior tibial motion, posterior laxity is normal and the examination should proceed to the 30° laxity tests.

The quadriceps neutral angle (QNA) of the normal knee is located by placing the normal knee at an angle at which the quadriceps contraction does not result in either an anterior or posterior tibial shift (mean QNA = 70°). The quadriceps active test is then performed in the involved knee at the same degree of flexion. The resulting anterior tibial shift with quadriceps contraction is equal to the posterior tibial subluxation. The position of the tibia at the QNA with an isolated quadriceps contraction is termed the quadriceps active position. From the quadriceps active position, the examiner can then perform 20 lb anterior and posterior displacement tests and compare them to displacement tests at the resting position in the normal knee.

For the 30° flexion test, the examiner places an 11 cm support under the thigh and adjusts the footrest so that both limbs are in an equal position of flexion and rotation (30 ± 5° flexion; 0° to 20° of external rotation). If insufficient flexion is obtained by the 11 cm thigh support to stabilize the patella in the femoral trochlea, the examiner can place a board under the thigh support to obtain further knee flexion. The positioning supports do not constrain tibial internal rotation. The lateral aspect of the foot rests against the foot support, which partially constrains tibial external rotation. When performing displacement measurements, it is important that the patient be comfortable and relaxed. Gentle manual anterior–posterior Drawer oscillation may assist in obtaining muscle relaxation. The arthrometer is applied to the leg oriented in a position so that pressure on the patellar sensor pad is maintained throughout the testing. The patellar pad pressure must remain constant during the test; variation in the patella pad pressure will alter the position of the patellar sensor pad secondary to soft tissue and cartilage compression and will result in spurious displacement measurements. The measurement reference position is then obtained by applying a 20 lb posterior load and releasing it several times until a reproducible unloaded knee position is obtained. The instrument dial is set at 0. A 20 lb anterior force (89 N) followed by a 20 lb posterior force is then applied and the displacements are read directly off the dial. When the posterior force is released, the dial should return to 0 ± 0.5 mm at the end of each cycle. The mean of three consecutive tests rounded to 0.5 is recorded as the measurement.

Five measurements are recorded for each limb at 30°: (1) posterior excursion from the measurement reference position with a 20 lb push (the 20 lb posterior displacement test); (2) anterior excursion from the measurement reference position with a 15 lb pull (the 15 lb anterior displacement test); (3) anterior excursion from the measurement reference position with a 20 lb pull (the 20 lb anterior displacement test); (4) anterior displacement with a high anterior force applied directly to the proximal calf just distal to the knee joint line (manual maximum anterior displacement test); and (5) anterior displacement as heel leaves table (30-degree quadriceps active test).

The difference between the anterior excursion with a 15 lb displacement force and a 20 lb displacement force in the same cycle is an indication of the compliance of the structures resisting displacement. This is the *compliance index*. Then, to perform the manual maximum test, the limbs are positioned with the support system, the arthrometer is applied, and the testing reference position is obtained in the standard way. While the patellar sensor pad is stabilized with one hand, the other hand applies a strong anterior force directly to the proximal calf (as opposed to using the force handle), as shown in Figure 11-6. Care is taken that the knee is not extended. The tibial displacement is then read off the dial. In our clinic, manual loads applied are between 30 and 40 lb. Before performing the quadriceps active test, the examiner confirms that the thigh muscles are relaxed by noting minimal resistance to the anterior–posterior oscillation of the tibia and by palpating the thigh muscles. The *testing reference position* is established and the instrument dial is set at 0. The patient is then asked to lift his or her heel gently off the table. The anterior displacement as the heel leaves the table is recorded.

Anterior–Posterior Laxity Measurements after Cruciate Ligament Disruptions

These have been documented in our laboratory. We conducted in vitro studies[6] that consistently demonstrated an increase in anterior knee laxity after sectioning the ACL. The 30° – 20 lb anterior laxity measurements in patient with a unilateral ACL disruption showed that anterior displacement in the injured limb was 2 mm or more greater than in the patient's normal limb in 96 percent of patients (mean 5.6 mm).[6] In patients with an acute ACL disruption, measurements in the clinic were indicative or diagnostic of an ACL disruption in 90 percent of patients and, when the patients were measured under anesthesia, displacement measurements were diagnostic in all patients.[7] The manual maximum test, with a high manually applied load of 30 to 40 lb, proved to be the most diagnostic test for an ACL injury.

In a group of 50 patients in a multicenter study of ACL reconstruction with Marshall-MacIntosh/LAD procedure, the mean anterior displacement side-to-side difference was 6 mm with a 20 lb displacement load and 9 mm with the manual maximum test. Measured in the operating room at the end of the reconstruction procedure, the mean injured minus normal knee difference was −1.5 mm with the 20-lb test and −0.5 on the manual maximum test. The 1 year follow-up measurements revealed a mean in-

Fig. 11-6. Manual maximum anterior displacement test. A high anterior displacement force is applied directly to the proximal calf and the displacement is measured with the arthrometer.

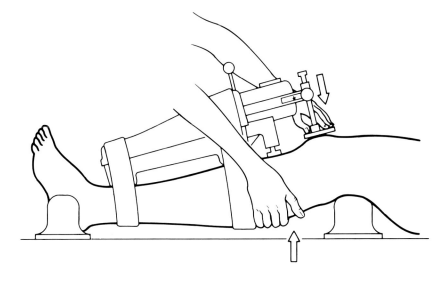

jured minus normal difference of 1.5 with the 20 lb test and 2.5 with the manual maximum test. The anterior laxity measurements allow the surgeon to document pathologic anterior laxity before surgery and to determine whether the procedure has returned the anterior laxity to a normal level, and sub-

sequent measurements permit monitoring of the anterior laxity.

Laboratory studies[2] of sectioning of the PCL with the knee supported in a position similar to the 90° Drawer test consistently reveal posterior subluxation of the tibia. When tension is placed on the

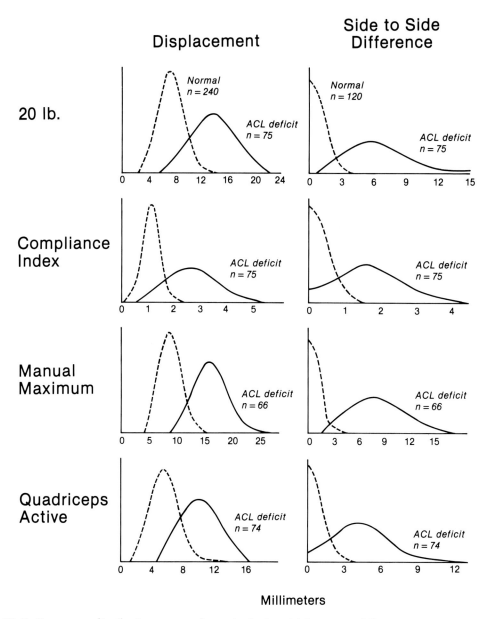

Fig. 11-7. Frequency distribution curves of anterior laxity with knee in 30° flexion in normal subjects and in patients with a unilateral chronic ACL disruption.

quadriceps tendon, the tibia is translated anteriorly. We have found anterior translation of the tibia with a quadriceps contraction a consistent finding in patients with a PCL disruption. Measured at the quadriceps neutral angle, the anterior translation with quadriceps contraction is usually 4 to 10 mm in the patient with a chronic PCL disruption and 2 to 6 mm in a patient with an acute PCL disruption with normal varus – valgus laxity. The posterior displacement from the resting subluxed position is frequently only 2 or 3 mm. Unless the examiner uses the quadriceps test or some other means such as lateral view x-ray studies to establish the anatomic neutral position, PCL ligament injuries will frequently not be diagnosed or be misdiagnosed as knees with pathologic anterior laxity.

The essential step in evaluating patients with pathologic anterior – posterior laxity is the establishment of the neutral position: the active quadriceps position at the quadriceps neutral angle. The anterior and posterior laxity measurements are then calculated from this position. The other test that is useful in deciding if a patient with an increase in total anterior – posterior knee laxity has injured both cruciates or only one cruciate is the comparison of the anterior and posterior compliance index to the values measured in the patient's normal knee.

Figure 11-7 presents anterior – posterior laxity measurements of patients with cruciate ligament disruption.

SUMMARY

Ligament integrity may be evaluated by assessing joint motion both qualitatively or quantitatively. Changes in knee motion following ligament injury may be small; therefore, testing must be precise and the examiner must be aware of the limitations of the testing system. Knee motion is described in terms of rotations about axes or translations along some set of axes. The constraint of the testing system on coupled motions, whether the system is manual or instrumented, may have a major effect on the movement being measured. Clinical tests are specific for detecting ligamentous injury. Thus, this chapter includes descriptions of the applicable tests for each ligament. Measurement of joint laxity depends on joint starting position, applied force, motion constraints, bone contours, soft tissue restraints, and muscle activity. Instrumented testing systems, such as the KT-1000 arthrometer, reflect modern technology that can be used as an adjunct to the physician's manual examination. The KT-1000 arthrometer provides precise testing, accurate (reproducible) measurements, and reveals to the physician any existing pathologic laxity.

REFERENCES

1. Arms SW, Pope MH, Johnson RJ et al: The biomechanics of anterior cruciate ligament rehabilitation and reconstruction. Am J Sports Med 12:8–18, 1984
2. Barnett P, Daniel D, Biden E et al: Posterior cruciate ligament/quadriceps interaction. Orthop Trans 8:258, 1984
3. Bartlett J: Familiar Quotations, 15th edition. Little Brown, Boston, 1980
4. Butler DL, Noyes FR, Grood ES: Ligamentous restraints to anterior – posterior drawer in the human knee. J Bone Joint Surg 62A:260–270, 1980
5. Daniel D, Lawler J, Malcom L et al: The quadriceps anterior cruciate interaction. Orthop Trans 6:199–200, 1982
6. Daniel DM, Malcom LL, Losse G et al: Instrumented measurement of anterior laxity of the knee. J Bone Joint Surg 67A:720–726, 1985
7. Daniel DM, Sachs R, Stone ML et al: Instrumented measurement of anterior laxity in patients with acute ACL disruption. Am J Sports Med 13:401–407, 1985
8. Daniel DM, Stuart C, Stone ML et al: Controlled mobilization after acute knee ligament repair. Orthop Trans 7:73, 1983
9. Fetto JF, Marshal JL: Injury to the anterior cruciate ligament producing the pivot-shift sign. J Bone Joint Surg 61A:710–714, 1979
10. Galway HR, MacIntosh DL: The lateral pivot shift: a symptom and sign of anterior cruciate ligament insufficiency. Clin Orthop 147:45–50, 1980
11. Gollehon DL, Torzilli PA, Warren RF: The function of posterolateral and cruciate ligaments in human knee stability (a biomechanical study). Orthop Trans 9:328, 1985
12. Hughston JC, Andrews JR, Cross JC, Moschi A: Classification of knee ligament instabilities. Part I. The medial compartment and cruciate ligaments. J Bone Joint Surg 58A:159–172, 1976
13. Hughston JC, Norwood LA: The posterolateral drawer

test and external rotational recurvatum test for posterolateral rotatory instability of the knee. Clin Orthop 147:82–87, 1980

14. Jacobsen K: Stress radiographical measurement of the anteroposterior, medial and lateral stability of the knee joint. Acta Orthop Scand 47:335–344, 1976

15. Jakobs RP: Observations on rotatory instability of the lateral compartment of the knee. Acta Orthop Scand 52 (Suppl 191): 1981

16. Jonsson T, Althoff B, Peterson L, Renstrom P: Clinical diagnosis of ruptures of the anterior cruciate ligament: a comparative study of the Lachman test and the anterior drawer sign. Am J Sports Med 10:100–102, 1982

17. Kennedy JC: The Injured Adolescent Knee. Williams & Wilkins, Baltimore, 1979

18. Kennedy JC, Fowler PJ: Medial and anterior instability of the knee. An anatomical and clinical study using stress machines. 53A:1257–1270, 1971

19. Lipke JM, Janecki CJ, Nelson CL et al: The role of incompetence of the anterior cruciate and lateral ligaments in anterolateral and anteromedial instability. J Bone Joint Surg 63A:954–960, 1981

20. Losee RE, Johnson TR, Southwick WO: Anterior subluxation of the lateral tibial plateau. A diagnostic test and operative repair. J Bone Joint Surg 60A:1015–1030, 1978

21. Malcom LL, Daniel DM, Sachs R, Stone ML: The measurement of anterior knee laxity after ACL reconstructive surgery. Clin Orthop 196:35–41, 1985

22. Markolf KL, Graff-Radford A, Amstutz HC: In vivo knee stability. A quantitative assessment using an instrumented clinical testing apparatus. J Bone Joint Surg 60A:664–674, 1978

23. Markolf KL, Kochan A, Amstutz HC: Measurement of knee stiffness and laxity in patients with documented absence of the anterior cruciate ligament. J Bone Joint Surg 66A:242–252, 1984

24. Noyes FR, Bassett RW, Grood ES, Butler DL: Arthroscopy in acute traumatic hemarthroses of the knee. J Bone Joint Surg 62A:687–695, 1980

25. Noyes FR, Keller CS, Grood ES, Butler BL: Advances in the understanding of knee ligament injury repair and rehabilitation. Med Sci Sports Exerc 16:427–443, 1984

26. O'Connor JJ, Goodfellow JW, Young SK et al: Mechanical interaction between the muscles and the cruciate ligaments in the knee. Orthop Trans 9:271, 1985

27. Oliver JH, Raab S: A new device for in vivo knee stability measurement: the Genucom knee analysis system. Presented at the interim meeting of the American Orthopaedic Society for Sports Medicine, Las Vegas, 1985

28. Sherman O, Markolf K, Weibel W, Ferkel R: Instrumented testing of normal and ACL deficient knees: a comparison of two devices. Orthop Trans 9:330, 1985

29. Shino K, Ohta N, Horibe S, Ono K: In vivo measurement of A-P instability in the ACL-disrupted knees. Trans Orthop Res Soc 9:394, 1984

30. Slocum DB, James SL, Larson RL, Singer KM: Clinical test for anterolateral rotatory instability of the knee. Clin Orthop 118:63–69, 1976

31. Stowers SF, Grood ES, Noyes FR: Differential diagnosis of knee ligament injuries producing posterolateral subluxation. Transactions of the 31st Annual Meeting. Orthop Res Soc 10:271, 1985

32. Sullivan D, Levy IM, Sheskier S et al: Medial restraints to anterior–posterior knee motion. J Bone Joint Surg 66A:930–936, 1984

33. Torg JS, Conrad W, Kalen V: Clinical diagnosis of anterior cruciate ligament instability in the athlete. Am J Sports Med 4:84–93, 1976

34. Torzilli PA, Greenberg RL, Insall J: An in vivo biomechanical evaluation of anterior–posterior motion of the knee. Roentgenographic measurement technique, stress machine, and stable population. J Bone Joint Surg 63A:960–968, 1981

12
The Pivot Shift

RONALD E. LOSEE

The pivot shift is not merely a diagnostic sign of the anterior cruciate ligament (ACL) deficient knee; it is a common, troublesome, and incapacitating dysfunction resulting from anterior cruciate and secondary restraining ligament deficiencies. This chapter will emphasize the description and analysis of the mechanisms of the pivot shift. Methods of testing[16] will then be described, and finally clinical applications of the pivot shift.

HISTORICAL ANECDOTE

Before June 16, 1969, I repeatedly heard from patients the complaint "My knee goes out." This was exceedingly disturbing because of my appalling ignorance of some yet unknown (to me) dysfunction. On this day a 29-year-old man enlightened me somewhat, as the following case history will show. He had injured his knee 2 years previously when he jumped off a fence, landed on a rock, and internally twisted the flexed knee. His case history reads:

> He has to operate this joint manually. . . . he has to think with every step. The main thing is the fear of an episode. He states he would give a year of his life to have a good stable knee again. He notices he has a rotational instability. He does not feel that the entire joint dislocates. It seems to be the same mechanism every time. He knows it always goes out if he jumps a ditch. It has never gone out and stuck. Many minor episodes of going out. . . . once in a while a major one when the joint will be sore and swollen for 2 weeks.

The examination indicated no sign of patellar or meniscus dysfunction and no lateral instability.

There was a definite anterior Drawer sign and a suspicion of hyperextension of the joint. As usual, I was perplexed. At the time, I can't say why, I was making an anterior Drawer test with the knee in a slightly flexed position. I simultaneously and accidentally forced it into a valgus position. It dramatically subluxed, which was an entirely new and disturbing sensation to me. The patient suddenly sat up erect on the table; grabbed his knee and exclaimed, "That's it!" The record continues:

> The major finding here, and it is very interesting, is that when the knee is partially flexed, internally rotated, and abducted, the entire femoral (–tibial) joint subluxates. I was unable at this time to figure whether the pivot was holding laterally and the tibia was rotating posteriorly on the medial aspect of the joint; or was pivoting and holding and that the lateral aspect of the joint capsule was relaxed allowing the tibia to rotate. In spite of the fact that I was able to do this two or three times . . . I haven't quite figured it out.

Two weeks later, upon reexamination, the record continues:

> I could again and again repeat the subluxation of his knee. It is done by flexion, abduction, and internal rotation of the tibia . . . could not demonstrate to my satisfaction whether the medial aspect of the tibia comes out anteriorly, but seems to be an impossible thing as I am internally rotating the tibia. On one of the pictures [roentgenogram] I had my thumb directly on the head of the fibula [Fig. 12-1]. It is my impression that this man has old capsular damage and relaxation and complete cruciate rupture. I am sure the anterior cruciate is gone. Whether the posterior cruciate is gone, I am not quite sure.

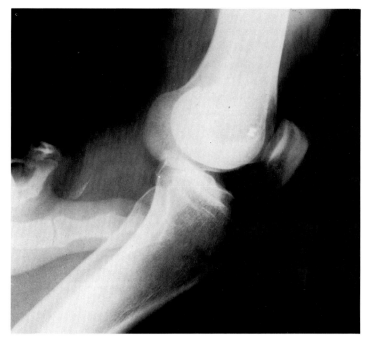

Fig. 12-1. Roentgenogram of subluxed left knee of a 29-year-old man taken 2 years after an injury. The lead skin markers indicate "medial" and "lateral" and the author's thumb is over the fibular head.

It took another 2½ years to devise a surgical remedy for the problem. Through correspondence with Kennedy (1971–1981), I included in the remedy both his ideas [12] and those of Galway, Beaupre, and MacIntosh.[5,6] Let us not forget that Lemaire[14] had already reported a similar operation for this syndrome in 1967.

LAXITY AND INSTABILITY

The terms *laxity* and *instability* must be defined to provide improved understanding of the pivot shift. Noyes et al.[24] have defined them for us. We shall lean on their words of wisdom:

> The word *laxity* is used in this paper to denote a slackness or displacement of the joint that is quantifiable and specific as to the type of displacement. A laxity may be either normal or abnormal depending on the degree, the type of laxity, and the variation between knees. The word *instability* is used in a general sense, implying unsturdiness, and may be due to a variety of causes including a specific joint

laxity. An instability is always pathological. The term laxity is more specific for ligament problems and is usually preferred unless one is talking of a general condition affecting the joint of a general clinical syndrome.

Pivot shift with its definite laxities falls more accurately into the category of an instability. Occasionally it will be necessary to use either *anterolateral rotatory instability* or *laxity* synonymously with *pivot shift* because, historically, different authorities appear to use the terms interchangeably. I prefer the term *pivot shift*. It signifies a dysfunction of the knee with varying degrees of laxity caused by deficient ACL and secondary ligamentous restraints.

Anterolateral rotatory laxity is the major directionally defined laxity of the pivot shift.

Anteromedial rotatory laxity and anterolateral rotatory laxity are frequently detected in the same knee with a pivot shift. We operated on 50 patients to overcome the dysfunction of the pivot shift that we termed *anterior subluxation of the lateral tibial plateau.*[17] We documented that 33 of the 50 patients had not only anterolateral rotatory laxity with the pivot shift but also anteromedial rotatory laxity.

Posterolateral rotatory laxity can cause a false-positive pivot shift sign. It is the major directional laxity in the clinical instability syndrome now termed by Jakob et al.[10] the *reversed pivot shift*. It is a troublesome instability that requires therapeutic and surgical methods different from those used to treat the pivot shift; its further discussion is not in the scope of this chapter.[9,17]

PATHOLOGY

Galway and MacIntosh[7] state unequivocally that the sine qua non of the lateral pivot shift phenomenon is a torn ACL.

Fetto and Marshall[4] sectioned only the ACLs in 37 fresh cadaver knee specimens and produced a positive pivot shift in 33 of them. They found that

. . . There was a 13 percent incidence of positive pivot shift tests in 37 knees, in the presence of an intact anterior cruciate ligament. These positive tests were all in lax knees.

Continuing the 1978 series[17] in 1983, I reported that 95 of 181 patients who had operations to correct pivot shift dysfunction also had arthrotomies of their knees.[15] All 95 patients had ACL lesions.

Noyes et al.[22] state that most knees with ACL tears alone will have a pivot shift.

Snydor and Andrews[25] recently reported that of 69 knees (68 patients) treated surgically for acute anterolateral rotatory instability, all had ACL disruption with 35 medial and 21 lateral capsular lesions, 12 of these being combined medial and lateral injuries.

Hughston et al.,[8] in 1976, reported that the middle third of the lateral capsule was torn in five of six knees with acute anterolateral rotatory instability. All 20 knees with the severe type of chronic instability had laxity of the middle one-third of the lateral capsular ligament. In 1980 Norwood and Hughston[20] stated that only 2 of the 47 consecutive knees with acute anterolateral rotatory instability had a normal midthird lateral capsular ligament and ilio-

Table 12-1. Classification of Anterolateral Rotatory Laxity

	Structures Involved			
Laxity Grade	Anterior Cruciate	Iliotibial Band, Lateral Capsule	Positive Tests	Comments
Mild (grade I)	−	−	Lachman test Flexion-rotation Drawer test	Physiologic laxity normally present and usually correlates with up to 5 mm of straight anterior Drawer.
Moderate (grade II)	+	−	Lachman test Flexion-rotation Drawer test Losee test ALRI Pivot shift "slip" but not "jerk"	Subtle subluxation-reduction phenomena may require testing in two planes, Drawer and rotation, such as in the flexion-rotation Drawer or Losee tests. This grade usually correlates with 5–10 mm of anterior Drawer. Secondary ligament restraints provide a false sense of stability and may stretch out later.
				Pivot shift and jerk tests do not show obvious jump, thud, or jerk, although the laxity may be detected as a "slip" with experience.
Severe (grade III)	+	+	All tests positive	Hallmark is an obvious jump, thud, or jerk with the gross subluxation-reduction during the test. This indicates laxity of other ligament restraints, either a normal physiologic laxity, as is the usual case, or injured secondary restraints. This grade usually correlates with over 10 mm of straight anterior Drawer.
Gross (grade IV)	+	++	All tests positive	Hallmark is a gross impingement of the lateral tibial-femoral articulation during the subluxation which requires the examiner to back off during the pivot shift test to effect reduction. The grade usually correlates with over 15 mm of straight anterior Drawer.

+, ligamentous structure is lax; −, ligamentous structure is not lax.
(Noyes FR, Grood ES, Suntay WJ, Butler DL: The three dimensional laxity of the anterior cruciate deficient knee as determined by clinical laxity tests. Iowa Orthop 3:32–44, 1983.)

tibial tract with a torn ACL, and 6 of the 47 knees had torn lateral capsular ligaments and grossly normal ACLs.

Noyes et al.[22] wrote in 1983:

> A positive pivot shift test indicates a gross subluxation of the lateral tibial–femoral articulation and, importantly, that there is also an increased forward displacement of the medial tibial condyle due to the associated increase in anterior translation as already discussed. This gross amount of anterolateral subluxation indicates not only anterior cruciate laxity, but also that secondary extra-articular ligament restraints are not providing resistance [Table 12-1]. Since it is the lateral tibial plateau which has the greater subluxation in a positive pivot shift test, the lateral extra-articular secondary restraints (iliotibial band,[*] lateral capsule) are not functionally tight. A fully positive pivot shift test does not, however, necessarily imply associated injury to the lateral extra-articular ligament restraints since they normally have a certain amount of physiological laxity.

DESCRIPTION AND ANALYSIS OF THE PIVOT SHIFT

The pivot shift is either a subluxation, a reduction, or both in rapid sequence of an axially loaded knee joint. A twist subluxes or reduces the partially flexed knee. The femur is externally and the tibia is internally twisted during subluxation (Fig. 12-2). Complete extension stabilizes it. Flexion beyond 40°, with the iliotibial tract functioning, prohibits its subluxation.[1,15]

During the pivot shift, the whole joint subluxes with more shifting in the lateral than the medial compartment of the knee. Compression during the reduction–subluxation–reduction pathologic motion causes impingement of the misfitting lateral femoral–tibial articular parts. This compression is needed to make the pivot shift a symptomatic dysfunction. The medial ligamentous structures can

---

* In this chapter, *iliotibial tract* is used synonymously with *iliotibial band.* The author would include the lateral and posterolateral capsule to be extraarticular secondary restraints,[15] but qualifies the effect of the iliotibial tract later in this chapter.

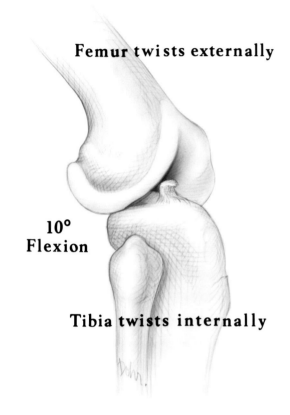

Fig. 12-2. The right knee is subluxed during a pivot shift dysfunction.

also stretch during the pivot shift and cause medial capsular pain.

The Twist

One example of several ways to twist the knee about a vertical axis into or out of subluxation is to twist the body while standing with the same foot planted. The unstable knee subluxes when the femur twists externally; it reduces again when the femur twists internally (Fig. 12-3).

Conversely, when clinicians examine the patient in a supine position, they feel the free tibia twisting on the femur as they sublux the knee. It is from this point of view that we have historically artificially titled the rotatory laxities of the knee to be *anteromedial, anterolateral,* and *posterolateral* rotatory laxities (or "instabilities," at times used synony-

Fig. 12-3. The subluxed right knee reduces during a pivot shift dysfunction. Note the direction of the twist, the slight knee flexion, and the axial loading of the lateral compartment of the joint.

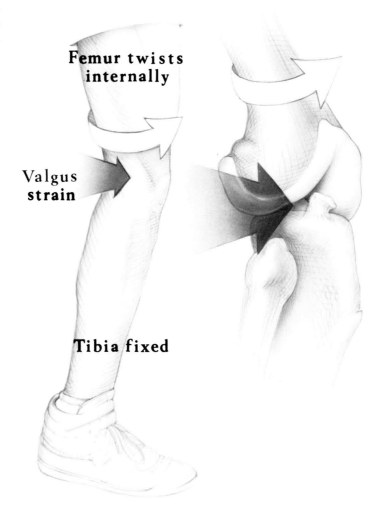

Femur twists internally

Valgus strain

Tibia fixed

mously). These terms are now even replaced with the acronyms AMRI, ALRI, and PLRI.

Complete extension tightens the posterior capsule, which causes the subluxed knee to twist back into reduction. The contracting quadriceps makes a patellofemoral joint reaction force that pushes the lateral femoral condyle posteriorly during the pivot shift. This twists the femur externally and subluxes the knee when the tibia is fixed. For this force to be effective the posterior capsule must be relaxed by flexing the knee 15° to 20°. This is the "slingshot effect" of the quadriceps (Fig. 12-4).[15] Feagin and Lambert[3] noted the basics of this effect when they

started that the quadriceps is antagonistic to the ACL during the athlete's deceleration and change of direction. Independently, in 1977, Feagin[2] had noted that deceleration was a mechanism of rupture of the ACL.

A functioning iliotibial tract, through its attachment at Gerdy's tubercle, twists the tibia externally if it is free to rotate while the patient is being examined in the supine position. When the subluxed knee is flexed during a pivot shift test it causes the iliotibial tract to tighten. Flexion beyond 40° tightens the iliotibial tract to the extent that it pulls the lateral tibial tubercle of Gerdy and twists the

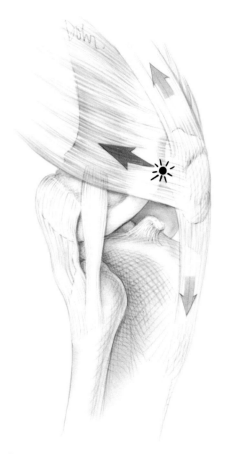

Fig. 12-4. "Slingshot effect" of the contracting quadriceps that subluxes the knee during the pivot shift dysfunction. The ACL is deficient. The slightly flexed knee slackens the posterior capsule. The foot and tibia are fixed. The posteriorly directed patellofemoral joint reaction force *(dot)* twists the femur externally to sublux the lateral femoral condyle.

tibia externally, causing a sudden reduction of the subluxed knee.

Extension

The completely extended knee tightens the posterior capsule and provides stability.[1,15] The patient can then comfortably twist the body to and fro on the vertical axis while standing one-legged on the dysfunctioning limb. The pivot shift occurs when the knee is flexed 10° to 20°; therefore, body twisting in this range of flexion causes apprehension.

Flexion

Rotational stability of the knee is regained when it is flexed beyond 40°. An intact iliotibial tract helps to reduce the subluxed knee at this angle. The greater curvature of the femoral condyles now articulates with the tibial surfaces when the knee is in this flexed position. The femoral–tibial articular surfaces are not as parallel as when the joint is approaching full extension. The patellofemoral joint reaction force is at a directional disadvantage and cannot effectively push the lateral femoral condyle posteriorly at 40° of knee flexion.

Articular Dysfunction

Further flexion, which is made possible by the gliding of the articular surfaces, is interrupted if the knee subluxes at 10° flexion. This dysfunction is exaggerated when the lateral articular surfaces are squeezed together. Instead of continuing the flexion in a proper smooth glide, the posteriorly displaced lateral femoral condyle (in the standing patient) jams itself into the posterolateral articular margin of the tibia, which resembles a wedge. This wedging forms a fulcrum that is impacted between the greater and lesser curvature of the lateral femoral condyle in the area of the anatomic notch. Further flexion causes the femoral and tibial articular surfaces to gape open anteriorly like a book. This levering pulls the insertion of the iliotibial tract at Gerdy's tubercle distally and palpably tightens it (Fig. 12-5).

In one series, I observed the surgically exposed iliotibial tract of 59 patients who underwent an extraarticular reconstruction of the ACL.[15] The exposed lateral area was watched while the knee was allowed to sublux when the joint was flexed 10°. Force was applied to the lateral side of the joint and it was flexed further. This made the iliotibial tract tighten and protrude. In some patients the tract appeared and felt as if a smooth willow branch had been tucked under it in the direction of its fibers. At 40° of flexion (range, 30 to 50°) 57 of the 59 knees suddenly reduced and the iliotibial tract relaxed. The tract was then surgically lifted off the side of the joint and left attached to Gerdy's tubercle in preparation for the operation. The same test was performed. This time there was no reduction in 58

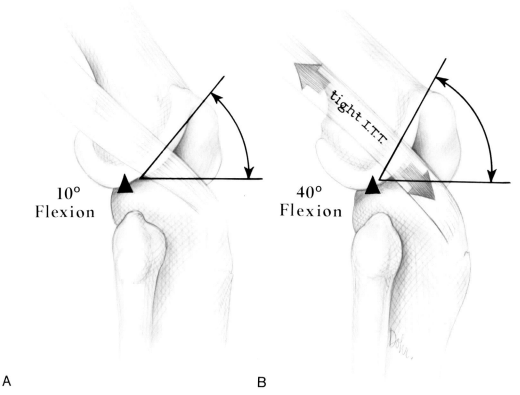

Fig. 12-5. Articular dysfunction of the flexing subluxed knee during the pivot shift. **(A)** When there is axial loading of the lateral joint compartment, the posteriorly displaced lateral femoral condyle jams itself into the posterolateral articular margin of the tibia, forming a fulcrum. **(B)** Instead of the lateral condyle gliding, further flexion causes the femoral and tibial articular surfaces to gape open anteriorly like a book. The gaping displaces Gerdy's tubercle distally, which palpably tightens the iliotibial tract.

knees. They remained subluxed even though they were flexed to 110°. This observation suggests that the iliotibial tract is influential in the reduction of a subluxed knee during flexion.[15]

Compressing the Lateral Joint Compartment

When a stress is applied to the patient's knee in a way that causes a valgus strain, the lateral femoral–tibial articular surfaces are compressed. If the anterior cruciate and secondary restraining ligaments are deficient, a twisting force about the vertical axis of the knee will cause excessive rotatory slippage between the femoral and tibial articular surfaces.

(The knee must be less than completely extended, for example, 10 to 20 degrees, or the tightened posterior capsule prevents the slippage). There is more rotatory slip between the lateral than the medial joint surfaces. When the lateral joint is compressed during the excessive rotatory slippage the deforming forces are compounded. The unsturdiness is pathologic; it is the pivot shift. The lateral compression of the axially loaded joint causes the tibial–femoral impaction with its plowing and impingement during the twisting, flexing and extending, subluxing, and reducing movements. This impingement is a critical clinical factor since it causes pain and sometimes damage to the meniscus and/or articular surfaces of the patient's knee.[7,17,24]

VARYING DEGREES OF PIVOT SHIFT

The pivot shift dysfunction can be determined to be either present or absent in a given knee. The dysfunction is the instability. When it is present, varying severity of the dysfunction among different patients is appreciated by the clinician. Upon examination, the variation discovered depends upon multiple factors: the force applied by the examiner during the examination; the resistance to the examination exercised by the patient; the amount of compression applied to the lateral compartment of the knee by the examiner when testing; the laxity of the joint; and the presence or absence of impingement during the subluxation and reduction that occurs in the pivot shift. Attempting to grade the degree of pivot shift as trace, 1, 2, 3, and 4 is confusing, meaningless, and nonquantitative. I do recognize a lesser and greater degree of the pivot shift that may be clinically meaningful when indicating severity. In both severities the sense of instability and "giving way" is reproduced during the test and is recognized by both the patient and the examiner. The difference is determined by the presence or absence of an impingement between the joint surfaces of the lateral compartment that occurs during the test. The greater degree of pivot shift had this impingement, has more laxity, and is more symptomatic than the lesser.

An example of the lesser variant would be the knee of the patient who has a positive anterior drawer or Lachman test, whose activity is limited, and who has had no further episodes of giving way since the original incident. This patient has a positive pivot shift sign that reproduces the original giving way, but there is neither jamming of the joint nor painful impingement when testing. The patient is not interested in an operation, even though aware of knee imperfection and instability.

The greater and more symptomatic variant of the pivot shift is to be found in the knee of the active person who cannot engage in sports without fear of the knee giving way and who wants to have an operation to eliminate the problem. This knee will have painful impingement and jamming upon examination as the joint is manipulated into and out of subluxation. Both the examiner and the patient will recognize the magnitude and severity of the pivot shift, which recapitulates the dysfunction with more subjective distress than the lesser variant.

The difference in laxity between these two qualitative variants of the pivot shift is potentially measurable: increased laxity is a factor that potentiates increased severity of the pivot shift. Noyes et al.[22] have provided a classification of anterolateral rotatory laxity and relate this to the pivot shift instability. Their classification is also qualitative at this time and their system encourages the examiner to estimate the laxity in 5 mm intervals. They expect more objective measurements to be available in time. Their classification is reproduced in Table 12-1.

TESTING FOR THE PIVOT SHIFT

Zarins and Nemeth[27] advised us to "remember that the phenomenon that occurs during the pivot shift is the same no matter which testing method is used." However, let us remember that either a subluxation or a reduction of the knee may be emphasized in the different tests.[1,15] When testing, think of basics. The knee both reduces in complete extension and, if the iliotibial tract is intact, reduces in flexion beyond 40°; the unstable joint subluxes readily in the 10° to 20° range of flexion. Test while compressing the lateral compartment; think of quadriceps and iliotibial tract action while testing; and estimate the amplitude of the positive test. False-positive testing is uncommon. Test the patient in the supine position.

Testing by Extending the Knee from a Reduced to a Subluxed Position

Stand and face the side of the knee to be tested. Grasp and control the patient's right foot with your right hand to examine the right knee (Fig. 12-6). With the left hand assisting on the lateral side of the knee, flex it to 45°. Compress the lateral compartment of the knee by pulling the foot laterally and pushing the knee medially. Firmly maintain this force that makes a valgus strain and let the knee extend. Feel the pathologic slip of the joint that occurs as the knee extends between 20° and 10°.

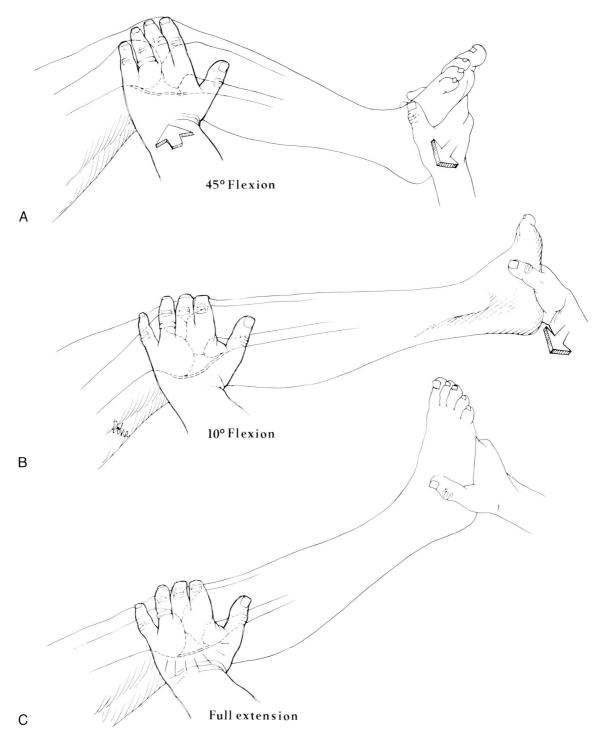

Fig. 12-6. Losee's test for the pivot shift by extending the knee from a reduced to a subluxed position. **(A)** The 45° flexed knee is reduced with the foot and tibia twisted externally. Push the knee and pull the foot to compress the lateral joint compartment. **(B)** Let the knee extend while maintaining strong lateral compartment compression. Let the tibia twist internally as the joint subluxes with a thud between 20 and 10°. **(C)** Complete extension quietly reduces the knee as the posterior capsule tightens.

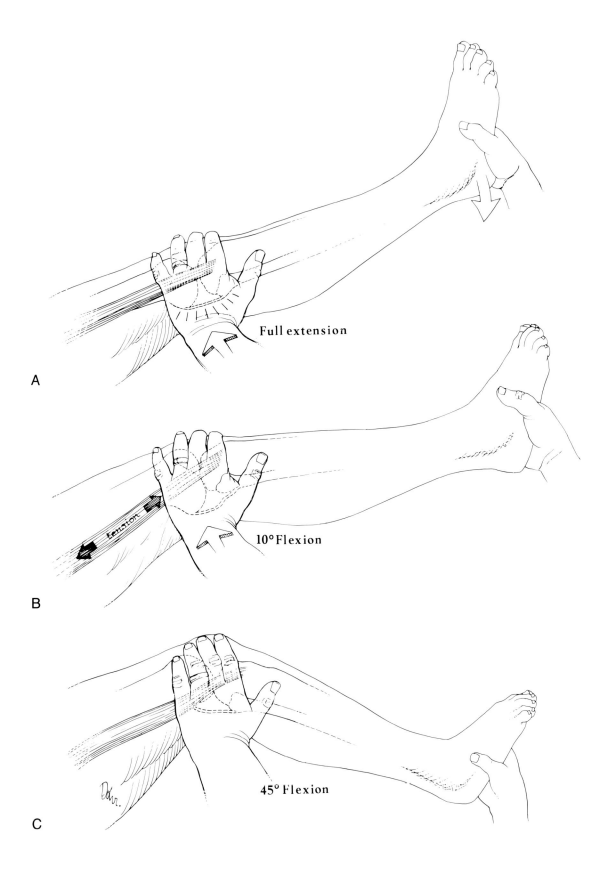

A

Full extension

B

tension

10° Flexion

C

45° Flexion

You are reproducing the dysfunction that the patient will recognize if he or she has the pivot shift. At full extension the knee is reduced again, but without any sensation of slip or jarring: the joint quietly twists together again. To test the left knee, control the patient's left foot with your left hand.

Testing by Flexing the Knee from a Subluxed to a Reduced Position

Lift the foot off the examining table with the knee extended until the hip is flexed to 40° (Fig. 12-7). Strongly compress the lateral side of the joint by pulling the foot laterally and pushing the knee medially. Maintain this force and flex the knee 10°. Feel the lateral femoral condyle subluxing posteriorly if there is a pivot shift. (Gravity causes this.) Continue flexion in this manner. (At 30° the patient may complain of pain.) By 45° of knee flexion there will be a reduction if there is a pivot shift. (The knee joint will not reduce if the iliotibial tract has been effectively lengthened by trauma or surgery.) Palpate the iliotibial tract to see if it protrudes when the knee is flexed 30° to 40°. Note impingement or jamming during reduction. Do not force the knee if there is a painful jamming! Think of false-negative testing (see below); if this is suspected, test for pivot shift by twisting the tibia externally to reduce the subluxed knee.

Testing by Twisting the Tibia Externally to Reduce the Subluxed Knee

Lift the foot with the knee extended to flex the hip. Flex the knee ten degrees. Let gravity drop the lateral femoral condyle posteriorly if the knee is unstable (Fig. 12-8). Forcefully compress the lateral compartment as described above by pulling the foot and pushing the knee. Twist the tibia externally. (This reproduces an impinging reduction of the knee that the patient recognizes. It happens after the knee has subluxed and then the patient twists the body toward the opposite side from the dysfunctioning knee with the same foot fixed and in a way that compresses the lateral joint compartment) (Fig. 12-3).

Testing the Slingshot Effect of the Quadriceps

Repeat the test that extends the knee from a reduced to a subluxed position (Fig. 12-6). Instead of letting the knee passively extend, have the patient kick the knee into extension while you compress the joint laterally. If there is a pivot shift, the patient will apprehensively refrain from making the kick or will kick and recognize the subluxation that occurs. The patient may indicate that the pain of subluxation was much more distressing during a jumping episode when the knee was axially loaded than during the examination.

False-Negative Pivot Shift Sign

A pivot shift sign is false-negative if it cannot be performed until the patient is under anesthesia. The frequency of false-negative testing is not accurately known because of variations in evaluations among different authors.[4,18,19] Noyes et al.[21] indicate a high frequency of false-negative pivot shift testing when they correlate their "flexion-rotation drawer" modification of the MacIntosh[7] test for the pivot shift with arthroscopic findings. Although 32 of 36 knees with acute complete disruption of the ACL had positive signs when the patient was tested under anesthesia,

Fig. 12-7. MacIntosh's test for the pivot shift by flexing the knee from a subluxed to a reduced position. **(A)** Start with the extended and reduced knee (with tight posterior capsule). Strongly compress the lateral joint compartment by pushing the knee and pulling the foot. **(B)** Continue the compression and flex the knee. Gravity lets the lateral femoral condyle sublux posteriorly. Further flexion jams the joint and tightens an intact iliotibial tract, as also illustrated in Fig. 12-5. **(C)** Continue the compression and flexion. By 45° the subluxed knee will suddenly reduce unless the iliotibial tract is deficient. This illustration shows the knee reduced and the previously tightened iliotibial tract now relaxed.

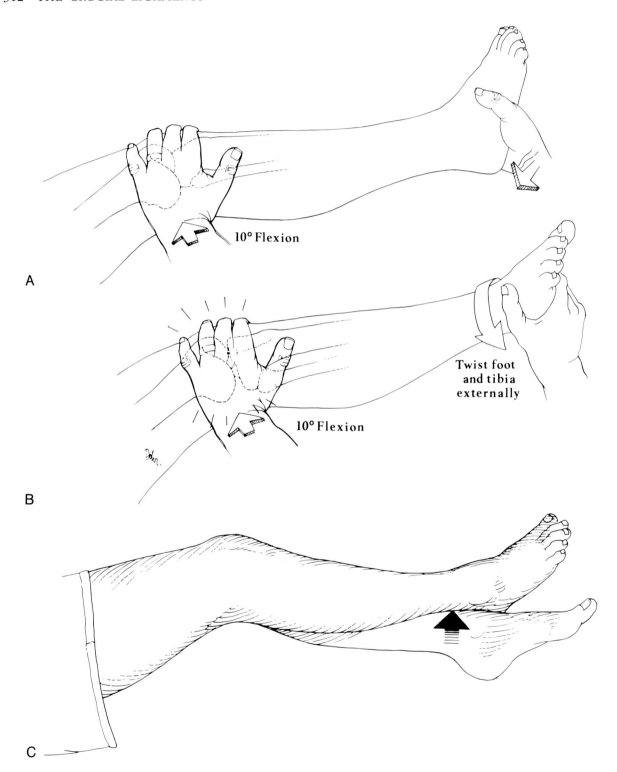

10° Flexion

10° Flexion

Twist foot
and tibia
externally

A

B

C

only 14 of the 37 knees tested in this group had positive signs before the operation. Continuing our series[17] to include consecutively 300 patients operated on to eliminate the pivot shift, I discovered that only 13 had a false-negative pivot shift test that was later shown to be positive during examination under anesthesia. Both the extending and flexing testing methods (described above) were used to evaluate these patients.

Causes of false-negative tests are obstruction of the joint from displacement of torn meniscus (e.g., 10 of the 13 patients in our series had displacement of torn meniscus that obstructed their knee joint and prevented discovery of the pivot shift before they were operated on); tense hemarthrosis; apprehension and the patient's ability to control the knee instability; and failure to recognize a false-negative pivot shift sign when testing the knee by flexing it from a subluxed to a reduced position in the presence of a stretched iliotibial tract.

A pivot shift instability sign can sometimes be discovered before examining the patient under anesthesia by testing the knee again while extending it from a reduced to a subluxed position (but using more force to maintain the valgus strain than previously), or testing by twisting the tibia externally to reduce the subluxed knee.

USE OF THE PIVOT SHIFT

Application of the results of the pivot shift helps the surgeon choose between operative and nonoperative management of the instability.[11,18] Patients with grade III and grade IV anterolateral rotatory laxity,[22] can be said to have a troublesome pivot shift instability. When the symptoms cannot be tolerated, when the patient is unwilling to modify his or her activities, when repeated major instability episodes threaten joint deterioration, or when a damaged me-

niscus obstructs knee motion or causes unpleasant symptoms, an operation is indicated.[23]

Pivot shift testing is essential during anterior cruciate ligament repair or reconstruction operations to assure that the pathologic instability caused by the deficient ligament and secondary restraints has been properly corrected.

An operation designed to eliminate the instability of the pivot shift fails if it does not correct the dysfunction. Patients who have been operated on for the dysfunction and continue to have subjective symptoms of giving way and show the positive pivot shift sign with impingement and grade III and IV anterolateral rotatory laxity (Table 12-1)[22] have had a failed procedure. *The pivot shift sign should be used to judge the success of an ACL repair or reconstruction operation.*

Teaching Patients the Principles of the Pivot Shift

Some patients who repeatedly experience the pivot shift dysfunction decline surgery. Others, for medical reasons, should be advised not to have an operation for this. These people can be helped if they are taught the principles of the pivot shift. It is true that knee "blowouts" are so painful that it does not take long for the victims to master preventive techniques. They can be helped if they are shown the mechanisms and actually practice the unstable stances and maneuvers. Then they will know what to avoid and how to modify certain actions.

Teach the principle that lateral compartment compression hurts during a twist.

Have the patient stand and abduct the opposite hip so that he or she is standing one-legged on the symptomatic side. Flex the unstable knee 10°. Twist the body about a vertical axis from side to side. (This causes apprehension.) Now "decompress" the lateral compartment of the unstable knee by adducting

Fig. 12-8. Test for the pivot shift by externally twisting the tibia to reduce the subluxed knee. **(A)** Flex the knee 10°. Allow gravity to drop the lateral femoral condyle posteriorly. **(B)** Assist this by internally twisting the foot. Forcefully compress the lateral joint compartment by pushing the knee and pulling the foot. **(C)** Externally twist the foot with the tibia to cause an impinging reduction of the knee that the patient will recognize and relate to the dysfunction illustrated in Fig. 12-3.

the same hip. Have the patient drop the hip and pelvis on the opposite side and again twist the body to and fro axially. (The knee will sublux, but it will not impinge painfully.)

Teach the patient to avoid the twist.

Teach "walking around" instead of pivoting. Talk about reducing "shoe/floor friction": (use of cleats on shoes and rubber soles, and "swivel shoes" in sports functions).[26]

Teach stable positions of the knee in the sagittal plane.

Have the patient do the above twisting maneuvers with the symptomatic knee stiffly extended and then repeat with the knee flexed as much as is practical. (Twisting is possible in these positions.)

Teach the "slingshot" effect of the quadriceps mechanism (Fig. 12-4)

Use Larson's[13] "leaning hop test" to do this. Ask the patient to abduct the opposite hip while he or she jumps up and down on the symptomatic limb. This will cause apprehension; it is a maneuver to avoid. Teach decelerating in a crouching position. Have horseback riders shorten the stirrups. When pushing a heavy object (e.g., a car stuck in the snow), have the patient push with the ipsilateral shoulder and contralateral lower limb. Teach the jumper with the pivot shift to land either on the stable limb or in a crouch-kneed position.

Bracing

It is impractical for the athlete to use a brace that limits extension of the knee. Insufficient leverage is available to make derotation systems practical in bracing. Therefore, if the knee is going to twist into and out of subluxation in spite of bracing, let it do so without the pain and damage that results from lateral joint compartment compression. Let the brace prevent valgus angulation strain of the knee (in the frontal plane) as efficiently as possible. Stout inside and outside hinges are needed. The brace must be rigid and strong, yet as light and comfortable as possible. The brace must be attached to a wide paddle that pushes against the side of the thigh to prevent it from sinking into the soft tissues: This lessens lateral joint compression. Its length should approach the crotch and ankle as close as engineering and practicality permit. Bulk on the medial side must be minimized for obvious reasons.

CONCLUSION

The epithet *pivot shift* first appeared in an article by Galway[5] in 1971. It vividly expresses the characteristic dysfunction of the knee that occurs with the combination of anterior cruciate ligament and secondary restraining ligament deficiencies. Pivot shift is a sudden twist of the 10 to 20° flexed knee that shifts (mainly the lateral portion of the joint), into and/or out of subluxation.

Axial loading and compression of the lateral articular surfaces of the knee joint during the twist magnify the symptoms and threaten further joint damage. By being aware of the pivot shift the clinician can now test to discover the knee dysfunction, test to ensure its elimination at operation, and test to judge the success of the operation. With knowledge about the pivot shift, the clinician can rationally and helpfully advise the patient with this troublesome knee dysfunction.

ACKNOWLEDGMENTS

Generous support was provided by The Dallas Foundation for Health, Education and Research, The King Foundation, Mr. and Mrs. Robert A. Wilson, and my colleague, Thomas R. Johnson, M.D.

REFERENCES

1. Ellison AE: The pathogenesis and treatment of anterolateral rotary instability. Clin Orthop 147:51–55, 1980
2. Feagin JA Jr: The syndrome of the torn anterior cruciate ligament. Orthop Clin North Am 10:81–90, 1979
3. Feagin JA Jr, Lambert KL: Mechanism of injury and pathology of anterior cruciate ligament injuries. Orthop Clin North Am 16:41–45, 1985
4. Fetto JF, Marshall JL: Injury to the anterior cruciate ligament producing the pivot-shift sign, an experimental study on cadaver specimens. J Bone Joint Surg 61A:710–714, 1979
5. Galway R: Lateral pivot shift injury of the knee. J Bone Joint Surg 53B:772, 1971
6. Galway RD, Beaupre A, MacIntosh DL: Pivot shift: A clinical sign of symptomatic anterior cruciate insufficiency. J Bone Joint Surg 54B:763, 1972

7. Galway HR, MacIntosh DL: The lateral pivot shift: a symptom and sign of anterior cruciate ligament insufficiency. Clin Orthop 147:45–50, 1980

8. Hughston JC, Andrews JR, Cross MJ, Moshi A: Classification of knee ligament instabilities. Part II: The lateral compartment. J Bone Joint Surg 58:173–179, 1976

9. Hughston JC, Jacobson KE: Chronic posterolateral rotatory instability of the knee. J Bone Joint Surg 67A:351–359, 1985

10. Jakob RP, Hassler H, Staeubli H-U: Observations on rotatory instability of the lateral compartment of the knee. Acta Orthop Scand 52(Suppl 191):1–32, 1981

11. Jokl P, Kaplan N, Stovell P, Keggi K: Non-operative treatment of severe injuries to the medial and anterior cruciate ligaments of the knee. J Bone Joint Surg 66A:741–744, 1984

12. Kennedy JC, Swan WJ: Lateral instability of the knee following lateral compartment injury. J Bone Joint Surg 54B:763, 1972

13. Larson RL: Physical examination in the diagnosis of rotatory instability. Clin Orthop 172:38–44, 1983

14. Lemaire M: Ruptures anciennes du ligament croise anterieur du genou. J Chir (Paris) 93:311–320, 1967

15. Losee RE: Concepts of the pivot shift. Clin Orthop 172:45–51, 1983

16. Losee RE: Diagnosis of chronic injury to the anterior cruciate ligament. Orthop Clin North Am 16:83–97, 1985

17. Losee RE, Johnson TR, Southwick WO: Anterior subluxation of the lateral tibial plateau, a diagnostic test and operative repair. J Bone Joint Surg 60A:1015–1030, 1978

18. McDaniel WJ, Dameron TB: Untreated ruptures of the anterior cruciate ligament: a follow-up study. J Bone Joint Surg 62A:696–705, 1980

19. Norwood LA, Andrews JR, Meisterling RC, Glancy GL: Acute anterolateral rotatory instability of the knee. J Bone Joint Surg 61A:704–709, 1979

20. Norwood LA, Hughston JC: Combined anterolateral-anteromedial rotary instability of the knee. Clin Orthop 147:62–67, 1980

21. Noyes FR, Bassett RW, Grood ES, Butler DIO: Arthroscopy in acute traumatic hemarthrosis of the knee. J Bone Joint Surg 62A:687–695, 1980

22. Noyes FR, Grood ES, Suntay WJ, Butler DL: The three dimensional laxity of the anterior cruciate deficient knee as determined by clinical laxity tests. Iowa Orthop 3:32–44, 1983

23. Noyes FR, Matthews DS, Mooar PA, Grood ES: The symptomatic anterior cruciate-deficient knee. Part II: The results of rehabilitation, activity modification, and counseling on functional disability. J Bone Joint Surg 65A:163–174, 1983

24. Noyes FR, Mooar PA, Matthews DS, Butler DL: The symptomatic anterior cruciate-deficient knee. Part I: The long term functional disability in athletically active individuals. J Bone Joint Surg 65A:154–162, 1983

25. Snydor RW, Andrews JR: Combined arthroscopy and minireconstruction techniques in the acutely torn anterior cruciate ligament. Orthop Clin North Am 16:171–179, 1985

26. Yamamoto SK, Hartman CW, Feagin JA Jr, Kimball G: Functional rehabilitation of the knee. A preliminary study. Am J Sports Med, 3:288–291, 1975

27. Zarins B, Nemeth VA: Acute injuries in athletes. Orthop Clin North Am 16:285–302, 1985

13

Imaging

Radiographic Indicators of Anterior Cruciate Ligament Injury

BERNARD R. BACH, JR.
RUSSELL F. WARREN

A careful history and physical examination are the most crucial elements in the diagnosis of acute or chronic anterior cruciate ligament (ACL) injuries. Radiographs are mostly used to exclude fractures involving the femoral condyle and tibial plateau regions, as well as to exclude tibial eminence avulsion fractures. An anteroposterior (AP) view, lateral view, patellar-trochlear view (skyline, Merchant, and others), and notch views make up a complete knee series. Oblique views aid in the diagnosis of a tibial plateau fracture. AP and lateral tomograms or a 10° caudal-directed AP view may aid further in the diagnosis of tibial plateau fractures. The patellar-trochlear view excludes patellar facet avulsion and osteochondral fractures of the patellofemoral joint.

There are, however, radiographic findings consistent with, or suggestive of, acute or chronic ACL deficiency. These findings will be the topic of this discussion, which will address the Segond fracture (lateral capsular avulsion fracture), lateral notch fracture, arthrographic findings suggestive of ACL injury, and specific radiographic findings seen in chronic ACL deficiency.

RADIOGRAPHIC FINDINGS SUGGESTIVE OF ACL INJURY

The Segond Fracture (AP View)

The Segond fracture (Fig. 13-1A,B) is an avulsion fracture of the lateral tibial plateau located at or near the midlateral joint line posterior to the insertion of the iliotibial band on Gerdy's tubercle. This marginal fracture is variable in size, usually several millimeters in diameter, minimally displaced, and is generally oriented vertically. This fracture is best seen on an AP radiograph. Segond,[8] in 1879, described this fracture and experimentally produced it in 18 of 34 cadaver knees with flexion and varying amounts of rotation to the knee joint.[8] This fracture, also known as the "lateral capsular avulsion fracture," was also discussed by Milch[6] in 1934 in a series of case reports of "Segond's fractures." He did not specifically correlate this finding with ACL injury, but did note that the ACL was disrupted in one of the four patients he reported. In 1979, Johnson[2] reported on the "lateral capsular ligament complex" and its anatomic and surgical considera-

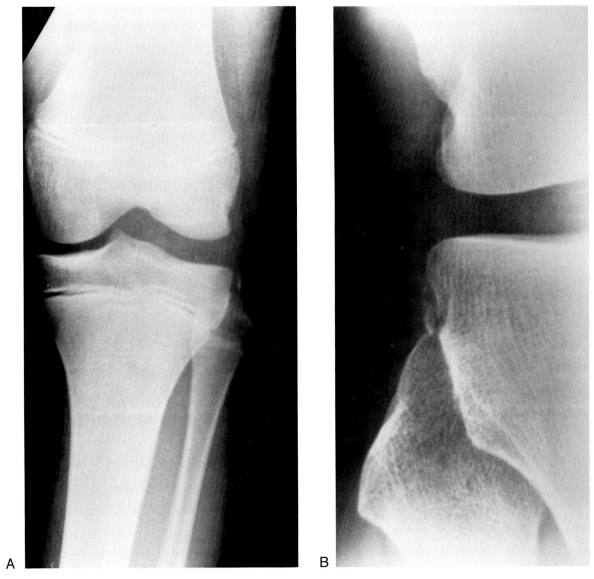

Fig. 13-1. (A) A lateral capsular sign or Segond fracture is noted in this patient with open epiphyses. **(B)** Lateral capsular sign is readily apparent in this anteroposterior (AP) radiograph.

tions. In cadaver specimens he surgically created these lesions and noted the resulting instability. Based on his observations, he advocated distal and inferior reattachment of the avulsion fracture. He subsequently noted the lesion in seven patients over a 29-month period. Woods et al.[11] in 1979 discussed the "lateral capsular sign" and its clinical significance. They presented two illustrative case reports of patients with a Segond fracture who intra-

operatively had extensive knee injury involving the ACL, lateral capsular complex, and medial collateral ligament. They mentioned four additional patients all of whom had complete ACL injuries. They maintained that the lateral capsular sign represents but is not limited to a repairable disruption of the middle third of the lateral capsule and an ACL tear. Losee et al.,[3] in a review of 84 patients treated with the "sling and reef" technique, noted Segond fractures in three of these patients. They noted that this lesion was much less common than the "lateral notch" fracture involving the lateral intraarticular aspect of the lateral femoral condyle. The avulsion fracture must be differentiated from a loose body or avulsion fracture of the fibular head. Pathoanatomically it represents disruption of the meniscotibial portion of the middle third of the lateral capsule. Although it is an uncommon radiographic finding, we believe it is direct evidence of lateral capsular injury and indirect evidence of ACL injury.

The Lateral Notch Fracture (Lateral or Oblique Views)

The "lateral notch" sign (Fig. 13-2A – E) is an area of fracture or degeneration that occurs at the site of normal lateral femoral condyle indentation. It may represent either an acute or a chronic ACL deficiency. This sign is best seen radiographically on a lateral or oblique view. Losee et al.[3] noted this abnormality in 15 of 84 patients, and believed it resulted from anterior subluxation of the lateral tibial plateau and represented impingement of the lateral or posterolateral tibial margin. They compared it to the Hill-Sachs lesion seen on the posterolateral aspect of the proximal humerus in recurrent anterior shoulder dislocation. MacIntosh and Darby[4] noted the notch in 32 of 50 knees. It was 1 to 2 mm in depth on either lateral or oblique radiograph. They maintained that the notch was "pathologic" when the articular cartilage in the notch was fissured, fragmented or eroded, or when the lateral or posterolateral tibial margin could be placed within the notch at arthrotomy. They believed that this area represented an area of impingement.

Warren et al.[10] investigated the lateral notch sign in populations of normal, acute, and chronic ACL-deficient patients. They determined the depth of the notch by drawing a tangent across the lesion,

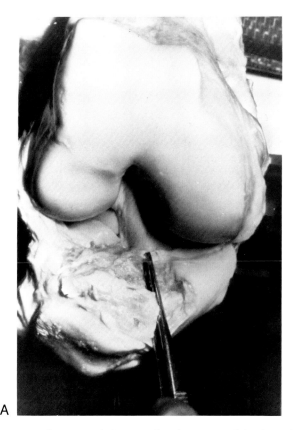

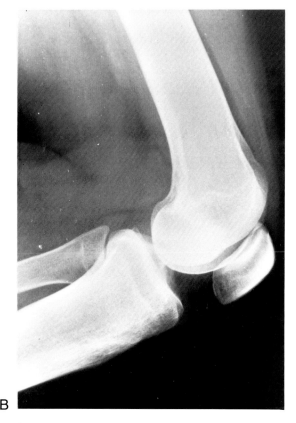

Fig. 13-2. (A) Normal indentation of the lateral femoral condyle is noted. **(B)** Lateral radiograph of normal indentation within lateral femoral condyle. *(Figure continues.)*

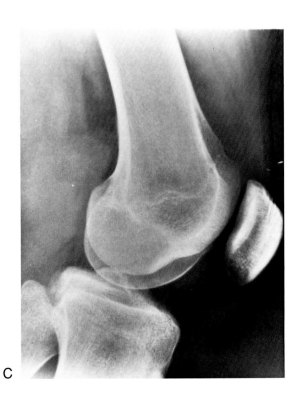

C

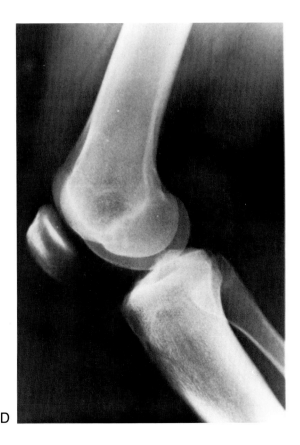

D

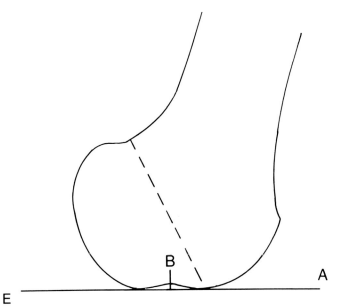

E

Fig. 13-2 *(Continued)*. **(C)** Abnormal lateral notch sign in a patient with an acute ACL injury. **(D)** Abnormal lateral notch sign in a patient with a chronic ACL insufficiency. **(E)** Method for determining depth of lateral notch. A tangent *A* is drawn across the indentation and a perpendicular *B* is dropped to its depth. The lateral notch is posterior to Blumensatt's line.

Fig. 13-3. (A) Double-contrast arthrogram reveals "ruler straight" or normal ACL. **(B)** Double-contrast arthrogram reveals a concave bow anteriorly, consistent with a "lax but intact" ACL. *(Figure continues.)*

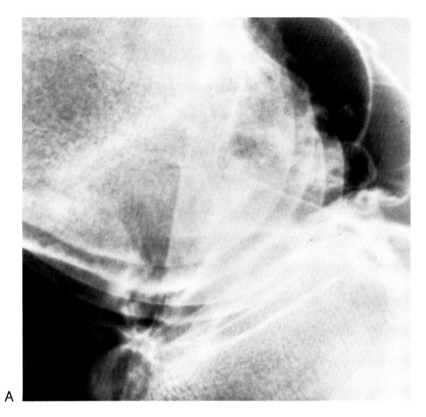

A

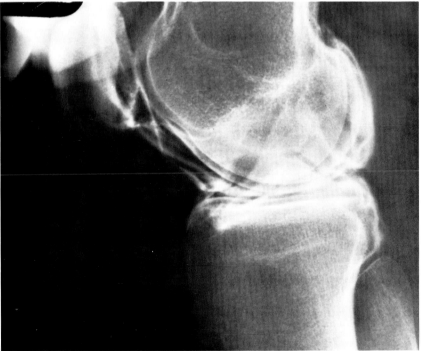

B

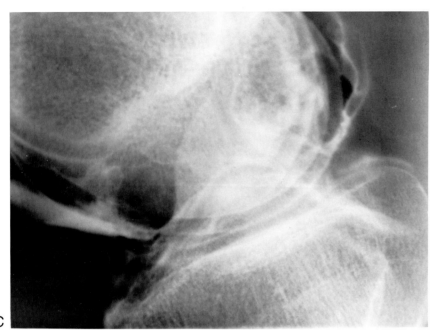

C

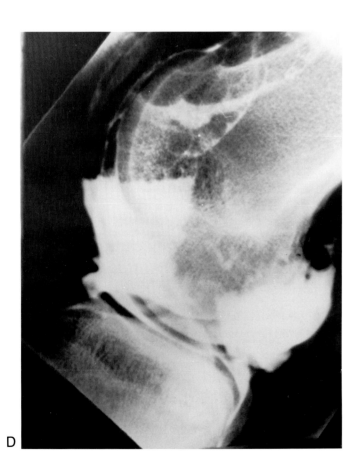

D

Fig. 13-3 *(Continued).* **(C)** Double-contrast arthrogram reveals a "wavy and lumpy" anterior synovial surface consistent with a torn ACL with intact synovial sleeve. **(D)** Double-contrast arthrogram reveals pooling of the contrast medium and is interpreted as torn or absent ACL.

dropping a perpendicular line at its deepest point, and measuring the depth of the defect (Fig. 13-2E). In a group of 47 normal patients with an intact ACL determined by normal Lachman, pivot shift, and anterior Drawer test, only one patient had a notch greater than 1 mm in depth. Two patients with acute ACL injuries had notches $\geq$ 1.5 mm. Thirteen of 101 patients with chronic ACL injuries had notches $\geq$ 1.5 mm, of which 8 patients had defect $\geq$ 2 mm. The depth of the notch appeared to be time related: the eight patients with notches $\geq$ 2 mm had average injury intervals of 71 months.

It is unknown whether this lateral notch adversely affects ACL reconstruction or primary repair end results, or whether the patient with an ACL injury and abnormal notch should have an early repair to prevent progressive deepening of the defect. *The lateral notch sign is an exaggeration of the normal lateral femoral condyle indentation, is an abnormal finding when greater than 2.0 mm on the lateral radiograph, and may be seen in acute or chronic ACL-deficient knees.* It is an inconstant finding that is more readily and commonly seen in chronic ACL-deficient knees. It must be differentiated from an osteochondral fracture as well as osteochondritis dissecans.

Arthrographic Findings

Double-contrast arthrographic evaluation of the menisci is recognized as an accurate method of interpreting meniscal pathology. When strictly interpreted and accompanied by specific radiographs, it can be an equally effective method for diagnosis of ACL injuries. Pavlov et al.[7] retrospectively reviewed 163 patients using a double-contrast technique. Two stress lateral projections, a horizontal cross table, and fluoroscopic spot radiograph were employed. They employed the fluoroscopic method described by numerous authors. After aspiration of all intraarticular fluid, they injected 5 ml of Reno-M-60, 0.3 ml of epinephrine, and 50 ml of room air. They found that the normal ACL appears ruler straight (Fig. 13-3A). If the line is bowed but concave anteriorly, it is "lax but intact" (Fig. 13-3B). If the anterior synovial surface is "wavy and lumpy" it is interpreted as a torn ACL with intact synovial tissue (Fig. 13-3C). The ACL is presumed torn or absent if the anterior synovial surface is acutely an-

gled, not demonstrated, or if there is pooling of the contrast medium (Fig. 13-3D). In their study the arthrographic diagnoses matched the surgical diagnosis in 95 percent of the patients. *Double-contrast arthrography is an accurate technique for assessing ACL injury when it is performed by a skilled radiologist with an interest in ligamentous injuries of the knee.*

We consider that the arthrogram provides useful information on the ACL but, more importantly, it provides information concerning the status of the medial and lateral menisci. The arthrogram may document medial or lateral meniscal tears associated with ACL injury and thus direct the orthopaedist towards arthroscopy in the conservatively treated ACL patient, or it may document a tear that might later extend, or it may confirm a peripheral meniscal tear that may be amenable to meniscal repair.

ANALYSIS OF RADIOGRAPHIC FINDINGS

Controversies concerning the ACL have involved many arenas. In the last decade dramatic improvements in our understanding of anatomy, biomechanics, vascular supply, and pathoanatomy of rotational instabilities have evolved. A multitude of surgical techniques have been and are still used for the treatment of acute and chronic ACL deficiency. A technically well executed ACL reconstruction with excellent and appropriate rehabilitation may eliminate functional instability. We do not know of any study that shows whether ACL reconstruction prevents degenerative arthritic changes.

Feagin et al.[1] addressed the radiographic signs of unsuccessful ACL repair with rotatory instability of the knee. They noted five radiographic changes that occurred within 6 to 12 months of injury: (1) intercondylar tubercle peaking, (2) intercondylar eminence spurring and hypertrophy, (3) inferior facet patellar osteophyte formation, (4) intercondylar notch narrowing, and (5) joint space narrowing with buttressing osteophytosis ("rim sign") (Fig. 13-4).

Marshall's experimental canine study,[5] in which he performed selective ACL cutting, demonstrated periarticular proliferative changes and minimal articular degenerative changes within 3 months. He

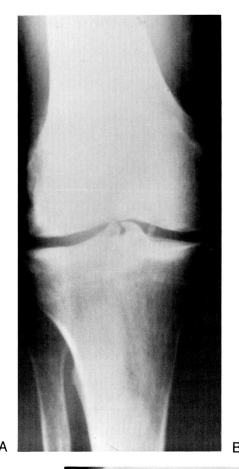

A

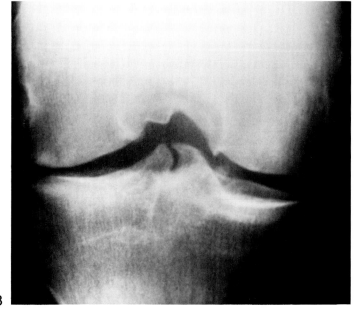

B

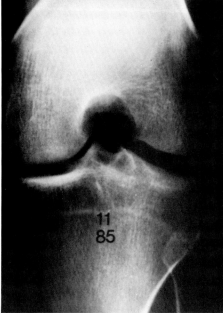

11
85

C

Fig. 13-4. (A) AP radiograph shows inter-condylar tubercle spurring. **(B)** Tunnel view demonstrates intercondylar tubercle and in-tercondylar notch osteophytes. **(C)** Early in-tercondylar notch osteophytes in a patient with isolated ACL insufficiency confirmed ar-throscopically. *(Figure continues.)*

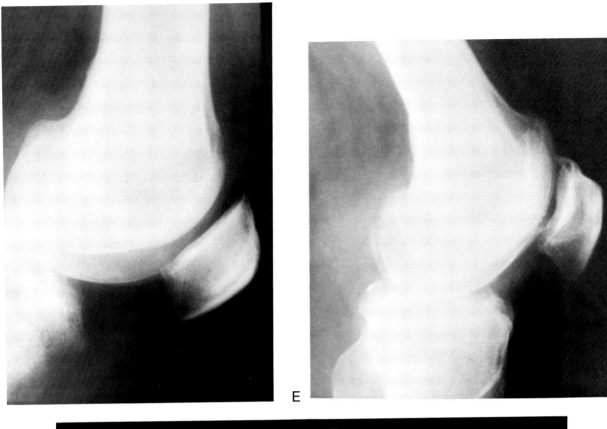

D

E

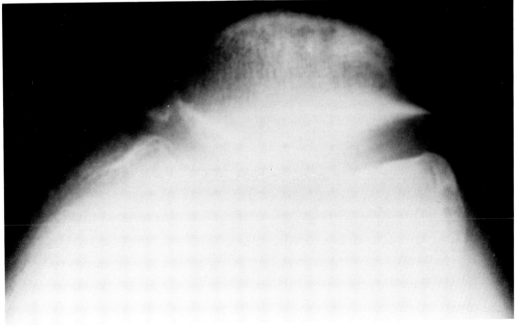

F

Fig. 13-4 *(Continued).* **(D)** Lateral view showing normal lateral notch and superior and inferior patellar spurring in a patient with arthroscopically documented ACL insufficiency and patellar pain syndrome. **(E)** Lateral view demonstrating severe patellar spurring superiorly and inferiorly in a patient with arthroscopically documented ACL insufficiency. **(F)** Merchant patellofemoral view shows peripatellar osteophytes in a patient with ACL insufficiency.

suggested that these periarticular changes are a reaction to instability and not to true degeneration.

In a series of symptomatic ACL-deficient knees, Sherman et al.[9] demonstrated a natural progression towards degenerative osteoarthritis. Periarticular osteophytes predominate early, along the condylar ridges, tibial plateau, and femoral intercondylar region. Periarticular changes predominate early, but as the time interval from injury increases true degeneration becomes apparent.

Sherman, Warren and colleagues[9] reviewed 127 ACL-deficient knees including the following subgroups: (1) ACL-deficient knees (25 percent); (2) ACL deficiency and absent medial and/or lateral meniscus (12.1 percent); (3) ACL deficiency with documented meniscal tear that had not undergone meniscectomy (10 percent); (4) ACL deficiencies associated with collateral ligament insufficiency without meniscal damage or meniscectomy (26 percent); (5) ACL deficiency with associated collateral insufficiencies and absent menisci (19 percent); and (6) ACL deficiency with documented meniscal tear and collateral ligament insufficiency (8 percent).

They established a radiographic score (T score) based on a sum of the periarticular score (P score) and the degenerative radiographic score (D score). The P score ranged from 0 to 10 points (normal) and was based on the amount of patellar and intercondylar spurring, and the size of medial or lateral osteophytes. The D score was determined by the degree of medial and/or lateral sclerosis, joint space narrowing, subchondral sclerosis, loose bodies, and varus or valgus angulation. This score ranged from 0 to 18 points with 18 points considered normal. A normal knee, therefore, received a score of 28 points. In this series,[9] 74 percent of the patients were male; right knees and left knees were affected equally, and the mean age was 28. The time between the initial ACL injury and the evaluation was 6 months to 43 years, with a mean interval of 79 months. Forty-seven patients had intervals greater than 5 years, 28 greater than 10 years, and 12 greater than 20 years.

Table 13-1 summarizes the radiographic changes seen for the entire population.[9] Several important observations were noted in this study.[9] First, the time from initial injury correlated most strongly with deteriorating roentgenographic changes. The

Table 13-1. Summary of Radiographic Changes[9]

Findings	Percent of Population
Medial tibial osteophyte	72
Tibial spine spurring	69
Patella spurring	56
Lateral tibial osteophyte	31
Tibial sclerosis (19% medial, 9% lateral)	28
Joint space narrowing (21% medial, 5% lateral)	26
Loose bodies	6
Tibial cysts	3
Significant angulation (all varus)	4

postmeniscectomy ACL-deficient knee had significantly lower radiographic scores ($P < 0.01$). Second, all radiographic scores of the six subgroups deteriorated with time, although by 10 years after injury the groups had similar radiographic scores. Third, there was a correlation between the radiographic score and the Hospital for Special Surgery knee diagnostic score (KDS) based on subjective complaints, functional ability, and objective clinical findings. Knees with a poor KDS had the lowest radiographic scores, and also had the longest time interval from injury. Fourth, there was no relationship beween the patient's age and the radiographic score.

Radiographic degeneration was seen in 65 percent of the patients followed up for 10 years, and in 83 percent of patients followed up for longer than 20 years. However, these statistics do not separate the patients who had meniscectomies from those who did not have meniscectomies.

In their series, Sherman et al.[9] noted that by 18 months periarticular changes were consistently present and worsened with time. Although other series suggest that degenerative changes were more likely related to meniscal injuries than ACL instability, at 10 years all subgroups in this series[9] had similar radiographic changes.

SUMMARY

ACL injury may be diagnosed radiographically. The Segond lateral capsular sign implies severe knee injury involving at least lateral complex and ACL injury. The "lateral notch" sign is an exaggeration of the normal indentation within the lateral femoral condyle and is seen infrequently in acute ACL injuries and more commonly in chronic ACL injuries. A double-contrast arthrography has been helpful in documenting ACL laxity and disruption in conjunction with meniscal injuries. Characteristic degenerative radiographic findings are seen in chronic ACL-deficient knees. We have had no experience using magnetic resonance imaging.

REFERENCES

1. Feagin JA, Cabaud HE, Curl WW: The anterior cruciate ligament: radiographic and clinical signs of successful and unsuccessful repairs. Clin Orthop 164:54–58, 1982
2. Johnson LL: Lateral capsular ligament complex: anatomical and surgical considerations. Am J Sports Med 7:156–160, 1979
3. Losee RE, Johnson TR, Southwick WO: Anterior subluxation of the lateral tibial plateau. J Bone Joint Surg 60A:1015–1030, 1978
4. MacIntosh DL, Darby T: Paper read at the Annual Meeting of Canadian Orthopaedic Association, Toronto, Canada, 1977.
5. Marshall JL: Periarticular osteophytes. Initiation and formation of the knee of the dog. Clin Orthop 62:37–47, 1969
6. Milch H: Cortical avulsion fracture of the lateral tibial condyle. J Bone Joint Surg 18:159–164, 1936
7. Pavlov H, Warren RF, Sherman MF, Cayea PD: The accuracy of double contrast arthrographic evaluation of the anterior cruciate ligament. J Bone Joint Surg 65A:175–183, 1983
8. Segond P: Récherches cliniques et expérimentales sur les épanchements sanguins du genou par entorse. Prog Med (Paris) 7:297, 1879
9. Sherman MF, Marshall JL, Warren RF, Savatsky GJ: A clinical and radiographic analysis of 127 anterior cruciate insufficient knees. Submitted for publication.
10. Warren RF, Kaplan N, Bach BR: The lateral notch sign of anterior cruciate ligament insufficiency. Submitted for publication.
11. Woods GW, Stanley RF, Tullos HS: Lateral capsular sign: x-ray clue of a significant knee instability. Am J Sports Med 7:27–33, 1979

Magnetic Resonance Imaging of the Cruciate Ligaments

DAVID W. POLLY, JR.
JOHN J. CALLAGHAN

Magnetic resonance imaging (MRI) is a new clinical imaging modality that results from manipulating atoms containing unpaired protons, especially hydrogen atoms. The patient is placed inside a strong magnetic field which causes the unpaired protons to align their spin with the magnetic field. A specific radiofrequency wave is then pulsed through the body, causing the unpaired protons to shift out of phase with the magnetic field. After the pulse is complete, the protons realign with the magnetic field, emitting energy in the form of a radiowave. This new radiowave signal is recovered by an antenna and converted by computer to a pictorial image similar to a computed tomography scan. Various radiofrequency pulse sequences can be used to yield different information about the imaged tissue. Terms used to describe these pulse sequences include

TE—time to echo (in a spin echo sequence, the time between the 90° pulse and spin echo production)

TR—time to repetition for the radiopulse

T1—imaging sequence with a short TR

T2—imaging sequence with a long TR

Magnetic resonance imaging is appealing for use in the knee because it is totally noninvasive and poses no ionizing radiation hazard. MRI is capable of imaging bone, tendons, and ligaments.[6] It can be a physiologic study, with the ability to detect hemorrhage and edema, and to detect avascular bone earlier than any other imaging modality.[5]

To image the cruciate ligaments the patient is placed supine inside the scanner and either a planar surface coil or a saddle coil is used.[1,4] Surface coils are used to image superficial anatomy. Saddle coils, which are still being developed, wrap around the body part to be imaged and have the theoretical advantage of greater resolution. Various sequences can be used; the T1 technique provides the greatest amount of information concerning the integrity of the cruciate ligaments and the menisci (Table 13-2), whereas T2 imaging may yield additional information about hemorrhage, effusion, and edema. The greater the number of imaging planes, the higher the sensitivity, specificity, and accuracy, but also the cost. The most useful imaging plane to delineate cruciate ligament anatomy is the modified sagittal plane. In a true sagittal plane the posterior cruciate ligament (PCL) is imaged well but the anterior cruciate ligament (ACL), because of its oblique

Table 13-2. Structures in the Knee Giving Low and High Signals on T1 MRI

Low Signal	High Signal
Ligaments	Fat
Menisci	Cancellous bone
Cortical bone	Joint fluid
Articular cartilage	
Tendons	

course, is not regularly imaged. By placing the foot in 20° of external rotation the ACL is usually (75 to 80 percent of the time) brought into alignment with the sagittal imaging plane (Fig. 13-5). Additional imaging in the coronal plane is useful in evaluating the collateral ligaments, osteochondritis dissecans, and the patterns of meniscal tears, but is not as useful in identifying cruciate ligament pathology.

The intact ACL appears on MRI as a dark, low-signal structure that is continuous from its origin to its insertion without disruption or an intervening high signal (Fig. 13-6). MRI can identify an attenuated or one-bundle ACL compared to the normal state (Fig. 13-7). Identifying a completely torn ACL is more difficult (Fig. 13-8). The region must be imaged in the precise plane of the ACL, and if no continuous, low-signal, obliquely-oriented structure is visualized, a complete disruption is diagnosed. If the intact or disrupted ACL cannot be visualized, the rotation of the foot must be altered or a different imaging plane used (i.e., coronal).

The intact PCL is quite regularly and reliably visualized in the modified sagittal plane (with the foot in 20° of external rotation (Fig. 13-9). The PCL is visible as a wide, continuous, low-signal structure in

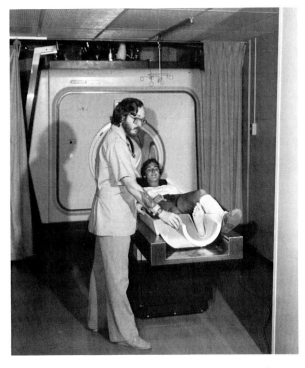

Fig. 13-5. The patient's foot is positioned in 20° of external rotation in order to bring the ACL into a more truly sagittal alignment.

Fig. 13-6. The intact ACL is well visualized as a homogenous low-signal (i.e., dark) structure extending from the medial aspect of the lateral femoral condyle to the anterior tibial plateau.

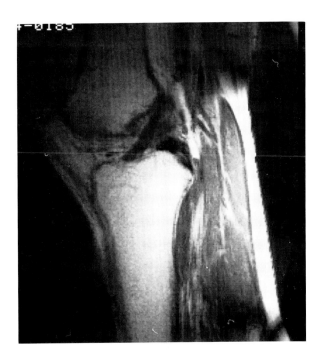

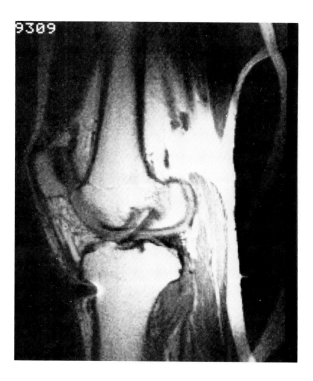

Fig. 13-7. A one-bundle ACL, which is obviously attenuated compared to the normal one shown in Fig. 13-6. There is a continuous structure extending from the medial aspect of the lateral femoral condyle to the anterior tibial plateau, so the ACL cannot be completely disrupted.

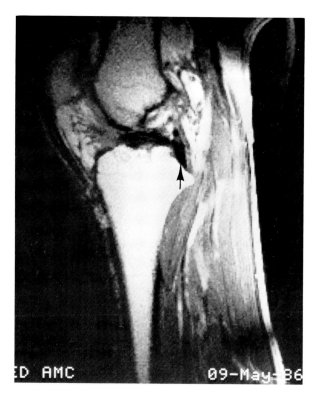

Fig. 13-8. This ACL is completely disrupted. This image is located in the lateral aspect of the intercondylar notch and the origin of the PCL is just beginning to appear *(arrow)*. There is no continuous low-signal structure where the ACL should be located.

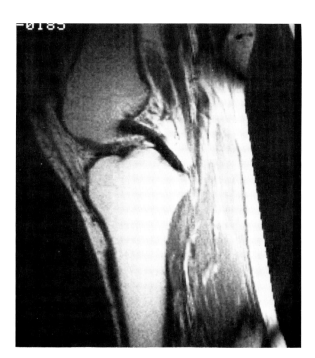

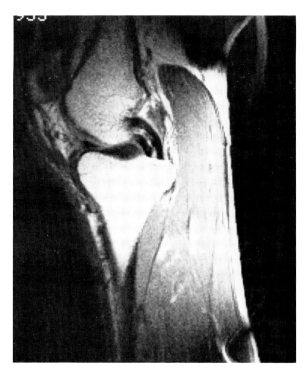

Fig. 13-9. The intact PCL is a continuous low-signal structure extending from the lateral aspect of the medial femoral condyle to the posteroinferior aspect of the tibial plateau. It is very reliably imaged by this technique.

Fig. 13-10. This image clearly demonstrates a large ligament of Humphry located just anterior to the PCL. It has the same MRI signal characteristics as the PCL and also has an adjoining origin and insertion.

the posterior aspect of the intercondylar notch, originating from the lateral aspect of the medial femoral condyle and inserting on the tibia. The ligament of Humphry is frequently imaged anterior to the PCL and may approach the PCL in size (Fig. 13-10). When the PCL is seen not to be continuous along its entire course, it is disrupted (Fig. 13-11). When attenuated or partially torn, the PCL appears thinner (occasionally interspersed with areas of high signal) or more redundant in its course. MRI is the imaging modality of choice for visualizing the PCL.

While MRI has several attractive features such as no ionizing radiation exposure, pain-free examination, and noninvasiveness, it can be expensive, especially when multiple imaging planes are used. A selective sequence has been developed that can be performed in 15 minutes of scanner time. It costs about the same as or less than arthrography. This selective sequence uses a surface coil and requires only a single modified sagittal scan (foot placed in

20° of external rotation) with images interleaved at 4 mm. This sequence will visualize the PCL 100 percent of the time and the ACL 76 to 80 percent of the time. When adequately visualized, PCL accuracy was 100 percent and ACL accuracy 97.3 percent.[4]

MRI provides a useful noninvasive method for diagnosis of cruciate and/or meniscal pathology. It has the potential to allow the surgeon more informed preoperative counseling of the patient and it allows better preoperative planning.[2,3] An example might be a patient with a probable ACL tear (i.e., a hemarthrosis and a positive Lachman test). If the MRI reveals preoperatively a meniscal tear in addition to the ACL tear, the surgeon can better discuss with the patient the rehabilitative implications of meniscal repair in addition to ACL augmentation versus partial menisectomy and rehabilitation.

The contraindications to MRI are few. The absolute contraindications are cardiac pacemakers and certain intracranial metallic aneurysmal clips. Pace-

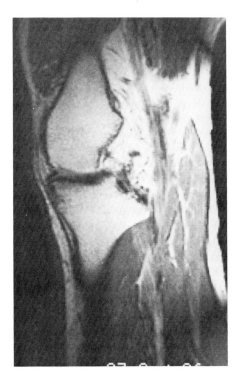

Fig. 13-11. This image demonstrates a completely disrupted PCL. The plane of the image is through the medial aspect of the intercondylar notch, and there is no continuous low-signal structure present.

maker settings are altered by the strong magnetic field of the scanner. Intracranial aneurysmal clips could conceivably be caused to align with the magnetic field and possibly be torn off the vessel. Claus-

trophobia is a relative contraindication. Because of the shape of the scanner some patients (apparently less than 1 percent) become claustrophobic. Metallic devices in the area of interest are also a relative contraindication. The more ferromagnetic the device, the more it will distort the image. Often, however, it is still possible to obtain the desired information.

REFERENCES

1. Burke DL, Kanal E, Brunberg JA et al: 1.5-T surface coil MRI of the knee. Am J Roentgenol 147:293–300, 1986
2. Kean DM, Preston BJ, McKim-Thomas H, Hawkes RC: Nuclear magnetic resonance imaging of the knee: Examples of normal anatomy and pathology. Br J Radiol 56:355–364, 1983
3. Mandelbaum BR, Finerman GAM, Reicher MA et al: Magnetic resonance imaging as a tool for evaluation of traumatic knee injuries. Anatomical and pathoanatomical correlations. Am J Sports Med 14:361–370, 1986
4. Polly DW, Callaghan JJ, Sikes RA et al: The accuracy of selective magnetic resonance imaging as compared with arthroscopy of the knee. J Bone Joint Surg (in press, 1987)
5. Reicher MA, Bassett LW, Gold RH: High-resolution magnetic resonance imaging of the knee joint: Pathologic correlations. Am J Roentgenol 145:903–909, 1985
6. Reicher MA, Rauschning W, Gold RH, et al: High-resolution magnetic resonance imaging of the knee joint: Normal anatomy. Am J Roentgenol 145:895–902, 1985

14

Arthroscopy in the Cruciate-Injured Knee

KENNETH E. DEHAVEN

Arthroscopy has been used routinely in several sports medicine centers for the past 15 years and has earned a rightful place in the diagnosis and treatment of cruciate ligament injuries. Arthroscopic procedures can be satisfactorily performed for either acute or chronic injuries. The types and relative frequencies of associated pathological conditions which can be encountered have been documented by several studies.[2,5,6,8] The important issues of whether arthroscopy should be performed in acute and chronic cruciate injury and when it should be used, as well as some technical aspects, will be discussed in this chapter.

ACUTE INJURIES OF THE CRUCIATE LIGAMENTS

Clinical Evaluation

The diagnosis of acute anterior (ACL) or posterior (PCL) cruciate ligament rupture is made or suspected on the basis of careful clinical evaluation including history, physical examination, and routine radiographs. The arthroscopic examination always follows careful examination under anesthesia, which should be definitive for diagnosis of ACL injuries but is not always definitive for PCL injuries.

Acute injuries to the ACL and PCL are associated with significant acute trauma to the knee in athletic, occupational, or vehicular injuries; they result in immediate disability due to pain and, frequently, instability, and in swelling (hemarthrosis) in the knee wtihin 1 to 4 hours after injury. A careful physical examination should be carried out as permitted by pain and muscular guarding. Although examination can be difficult and limited under these circumstances, a great deal of important information can be obtained.

Of the clinical tests for ACL integrity (Lachman, anterior Drawer, anteromedial rotatory instability, lateral pivotshift), by far the most informative in acute cases without anesthesia is the Lachman test (which has been positive in 85 percent of our cases in waking patients). Under anesthesia the Lachman test is virtually 100 percent reliable, although it is also positive in cases wtih partial tears of the ligaments. The lateral pivot shift test is also highly reliable in patients under anesthesia (85 to 95 percent) but requires relaxation and usually cannot be demonstrated without anesthesia. The classic anterior Drawer and anteromedial rotatory instability tests are positive in only 10 to 25 percent of cases without anesthesia and are only 50 percent positive at best under anesthesia.

The most common mechanisms of injury for acute "isolated" PCL injuries are a direct blow to the anterior aspect of the tibia with the knee flexed ("dashboard injury"), hyperextension, and a fall on the flexed knee with the foot and ankle in plantar flexion. Hemarthrosis may not be as marked as it is in ACL injuries since a posterior capsular injury may also occur which permits extravasation of the hemarthrosis. In contrast to ACL injuries, in which the classic anterior Drawer sign is not very reliable, the classic posterior Drawer sign is usually positive in acute PCL rupture, but can be misinterpreted as a positive Drawer sign. The test is normally performed with the knee flexed 70° to 90° and the foot supported on the examining table. In this position the tibia sags posteriorly; when pulled back to the neutral position by the examiner, it is mistaken for an anterior Drawer. Two helpful maneuvers to avoid this misinterpretation are the "sag sign" (placing the legs in relaxed position with knees and hips flexed 90 degrees and the heels supported while observing the prominence of the tibial tubercles) or the "thumb sign" advocated by Clancy (WG Clancy, M.D., University of Wisconsin, personal communication, 1984). The reverse Lachman sign is also usually positive.

It has been documented, however, that cases of complete PCL disruption do occur with negative posterior Drawer sign. The posterior laxity may be demonstrated with examination under anesthesia; however, in a few instances, the posterior Drawer sign remains negative under anesthesia with complete PCL disruption.

For patients with PCL tears, it is extremely important to assess the posterolateral structures, since combined posterior cruciate-posterolateral injuries have a much poorer prognosis (especially with nonoperative treatment) than "isolated" PCL tears. The clinical tests include varus stress at 30 of flexion, posterolateral Drawer, reverse pivotshift, and the external rotation test at 30° and 90° of flexion. Anesthesia may be required to demonstrate these signs in the acutely injured patient, but the external rotation test can often be adequately performed without anesthesia.

Contributions of Arthroscopy: ACL Injuries

Following careful examination under anesthesia, it should be apparent in virtually every case that there has been damage to the ACL. The clinical examination alone cannot differentiate partial from complete tears, but this can be determined by arthroscopic examination including probing. It is important to assess the degree of disruption in partial tears, as 40 percent or less disruption can be confidently treated nonoperatively, while 50 percent or greater partial disruption should be considered functionally to be completely torn. In addition to defining the type and extent of ACL injury, arthroscopic examination can define associated meniscal pathology. Several studies[2,5,6,8] have documented a 50 to 70 percent incidence of meniscus tears associated with acute ACL tears. While some of these lesions are minor tears that can be left alone, many of them are significant peripheral and near-peripheral tears that can be successfully repaired,[1,3,4,7] or in some instances will heal spontaneously. Finally, arthroscopic examination may be the best way to visualize the associated articular cartilage injury, which was documented by Noyes et al.[8] in 20 percent of acute ACL cases. The presence or absence of significant articular damage at the time of injury is an important prognostic factor.

Contributions of Arthroscopy: PCL Injuries

Arthroscopic examination may be required to establish the diagnosis of PCL tears since the usual diagnostic tests for pathologic posterior laxity can be negative, as previously discussed. Gillquist et al.[6] have repeatedly emphasized that posterior visualization is usually necessary to evaluate adequately the status of the PCL arthroscopically. This can be accomplished by passing a 70 telescope through the intercondylar notch or by using posterior compartment portals. Evaluation of the PCL from an anterior approach can be misleading since the synovial sleeve and subsynovial fat covering the anterior (proximal) portion of the PCL may not be disrupted. In addition, Humphry's ligament running from the posterior horn of the lateral meniscus to the medial femoral condyle directly anterior to the PCL may not be disrupted, and if the palpating probe encounters an intact Humphry's ligament with excellent tension the erroneous impression may be given that the PCL is intact. Associated meniscal tears occur very infrequently with acute PCL tears, in marked contrast to acute ACL tears. Damage to the articular surfaces also seems unusual in acute PCL disruption, but the exact incidence has not been documented as for ACL injuries.

INDICATIONS AND TIMING FOR ARTHROSCOPY

Established Cruciate Ligament Tears

For those cases in which acute surgical treatment of the cruciate injury has been elected, evaluation under anesthesia and arthroscopy with possible arthroscopic surgery would be performed as a prelude to the acute ligament surgery, whether performed as an open or arthroscopic procedure. The question "Why bother with arthroscopy if extensive open surgery is to be carried out at the same time?" might seem appropriate. Arthroscopy should be performed before open surgery because it can allow visualization of the posterior portions of the joint, particularly the compartment opposite to the arthrotomy incision. Arthroscopic techniques are the most consistent way to perform partial meniscectomy as conservatively as possible under direct visual control. Also, depending upon the location of the meniscus tear and the type of open surgical procedure to be performed, arthroscopy may significantly decrease the extent of skin and capsular incisions.

For patients selected for nonsurgical treatment of the acute cruciate injury, there are two alternatives regarding arthroscopy. The first is to proceed with examination under anesthesia, arthroscopic examination, and possible arthoscopic surgery for any associated mensicus lesion, followed by nonoperative treatment of the cruciate injury itself. The other option is to proceed with nonoperative treatment of the cruciate injury, recognizing that arthroscopy and arthroscopic surgery and/or stabilization might be necessary later. The decision of which of these two options to pursue depends upon many factors, and should be made on an individual basis for each patient.

Suspected but not Definitive Cruciate Ligament Tears

If the patient profile (age, sex, level of demand, degree of laxity, associated lesions, patient factors) places the person in the "high-risk" category (meaning that acute surgical treatment would be carried out if the diagnosis is established), one should proceed to evaluation under anesthesia, arthroscopy, and possible surgical treatment as promptly as possible. If the patient profile places that individual in the lower-risk category for which nonoperative treatment is recommended for the cruciate injury (if present), there are again two options. The first is to proceed with examination under anesthesia and arthroscopy to establish clearly the diagnosis and extent of injury, and then to proceed with nonoperative treatment regardless of the findings. There are occasional patients in whom the findings (such as severe degree of laxity or multiple associated lesions) could convert that patient from "lower risk" to "high risk." The other alternative is to proceed with nonoperative treatment recognizing the possible necessity of delayed arthroscopy and/or surgical treatment. Again, the decision should be made on an individual basis for each patient.

CONTRAINDICATIONS FOR ARTHROSCOPY

Arthroscopy is not recommended in cases where there is major collateral ligament disruption combined with cruciate ligament injury. With these injuries, there is no longer a closed capsular system. Arthroscopic irrigation fluid will extravasate into the area of collateral ligament rupture, which complicates the subsequent repair of the collateral ligament and frequently makes arthroscopic visualization difficult. Additionally, there is the potential for massive extravasation of fluid into the adjacent soft tissues with neurovascular compression. Visualization of the internal structures of the knee should be adequate with the surgical exposure required for repair.

ARTHROSCOPIC TECHNIQUE FOR HEMARTHROSIS

General or spinal anesthesia should be used to provide optimal conditions for examination of the ligaments. Every attempt should be made to avoid inflation of the tourniquet so that tourniquet time can be saved for any subsequent open surgical procedure. A diagnostic-size telescope (4 to 5 mm) should be utilized. After insertion of the arthroscope sleeve, the knee should be irrigated through the sleeve until the hemarthrosis has cleared. A constant flow irrigation system is usually required, with inflow through the arthroscope sleeve and outflow through a multiply perforated cannula in the suprapatellar pouch attached to suction generally providing the best visualization. If constant flow is not necessary for clear viewing, shutting off the outflow will provide maximum distension of the joint, which improves visualization. The more rapid the flow, the less distension is possible unless an arthroscopic pump is utilized. Routine use of a probe is essential to evaluate menisci for posterior horn and peripheral tears, and to palpate the cruciate ligaments. Posterior visualization should be carried out whenever necessary, using either separate posterior punctures or by viewing with the telescope passed through the intercondylar notch with 30° or 70° angled lenses. Whenever open surgery follows arthroscopy, it is recommended that the leg be reprepped and redraped, the surgical team change gowns and gloves, and another set of sterile instruments be used.

The anterior cruciate ligament is best visualized from an anterior approach combined with palpation with a probe. The intercondylar notch is frequently congested with hemorrhagic and edematous synovium in addition to the ligamentum mucosum and perhaps a prominent fat pad, making direct visualization of the torn ligament fibers difficult. It is helpful to flex the knee to nearly 90° and employ maximum distension as well as patience and persistence to obtain optimal assessment of the ligament. In subacute and chronic cases the torn ACL may reattach itself to the posterior cruciate synovium, and at first glance may appear normal. Careful attention should be paid to the lateral wall of the intercondylar notch posteriorly where the ACL should attach to the femur. Finding this area empty and devoid of any ligament fibers is pathognomonic for ACL disruption.

The PCL is much more difficult to evaluate from an anterior approach because of the large amount of synovium and subsynovial fat that obscures the ligament itself. Additionally, an intact Humphry's ligament can give the false impression of an intact PCL. The best way to assess the PCL is with posterior viewing. Through the intercondylar notch, the tele-scope can be passed into the posterior medial compartment, and with use of a 70° or greater optical angle, the telescope can be rotated to visualize the medial aspect of the PCL over a considerable portion of its length including the tibial attachment. The arthroscope can then be placed into the posterolateral compartment through the intercondylar notch, and the lens rotated to visualize the lateral border of the PCL. Posterior visualization can also be accomplished utilizing standard posteromedial and/or posterolateral portals and standard 10° or 30° diagnostic telescopes.

CHRONIC INJURIES OF THE CRUCIATE LIGAMENTS

Making the clinical diagnosis of chronic ACL or PCL insufficiency is usually not difficult. For the ACL, the typical history includes episodes of injury and reinjury with functional instability. The clinical tests for ACL integrity (Lachman, anterior Drawer, anteromedial rotatory instability, lateral pivotshift) are usually all positive but to varying degrees in individual cases. Patients with chronic PCL insufficiency may not complain of functional instability but only of disability from pain without recognizable instability. The clinical tests for PCL integrity are invariably positive (reverse Lachman, posterior Drawer sign, external rotation test), and it is essential to determine whether there is concomitant posterolateral rotatory instability.

Nonsurgical Management

Initial nonsurgical management is indicated when the degree of laxity and the level of demand are mild to moderate and there is no clinical evidence of meniscus pathology. The basic principles of nonsurgical management include comprehensive muscular rehabilitation of the quadriceps, hamstrings, and hip abductors, along with protective bracing for athletic activities or other strenuous activities. If the nonsurgical program is successful in managing the chronic cruciate ligament injury, arthroscopy is not necessary.

Minimal Surgical Intervention

Indications for minimal surgical intervention include mild to moderate laxity with mild to moderate demands on the knee, and clinical indications of an associated meniscus tear. Minimal surgical intervention includes evaluation under anesthesia to assess more completely the types and degree of laxity, followed by arthroscopic examination to define precisely the type of meniscus tear and to document the extent of damage of the articular cartilage. Any significant meniscus lesion is then treated as conservatively as possible by repair or partial meniscectomy. Traditional total meniscectomy is performed only when there is no other option. In chronic ACL insufficiency, meniscus repair without ligamentous stabilization has been associated with a high incidence of meniscus retears (40 percent)[3] and is recommended only in highly selected cases with mild laxity and relatively low levels of demand. Following surgical treatment of the meniscus lesion, the chronic cruciate insufficiency is managed nonsurgically according to the guidelines listed previously.

Ligamentous Reconstruction

If nonoperative or minimal surgical intervention is inappropriate or unsuccessful, ligamentous reconstruction is indicated. Preliminary arthroscopy is recommended to assess the menisci and articular surfaces. Any necessary menisus surgery can be performed before proceeding to the ligamentous procedure. Reprepping and draping, changing gowns and gloves, and using fresh instruments are strongly recommended, as are prophylactic antibiotics. Techniques are currently being developed and evaluated for arthroscopic placement of ACL and PCL reconstructions, which may prove to be the way of the future.

SUMMARY

Evaluation and management of cruciate ligament injuries pose several problems. For acute injuries, the essential factors are diagnosis of the cruciate injury and any associated injuries, and the choice of surgical or nonsurgical management. In chronic cases, diagnosis of the cruciate lesion is usually not difficult, and management depends upon the presence of functional instability or disability and associated meniscal pathology. Arthroscopy can play a significant role in the overall diagnosis and management of acute and chronic cruciate deficiencies, but is not an isolated procedure and cannot replace careful clinical evaluation, nor can it decrease the need for sound clinical judgement. Arthroscopic findings and techniques must be integrated into sound principles of evaluation and management but do provide means of refining and extending clinical evaluation and tradional treatment methods.

REFERENCES

1. Cassidy RE, Shaffer AJ: Repair of peripheral meniscus tears. A preliminary report. Am J Sports Med 9:209–214, 1981
2. DeHaven KE: Diagnosis of acute knee injuries with hemarthosis. Am J Sports Med 8:9–14, 1980
3. DeHaven KE: Peripheral meniscus repair. Three to seven years results. Presented at the Third Congress of the International Society of the Knee, Gleneagles, Scotland, 1983
4. Dolan WA: Peripheral meniscus repair. A clinical and histopathologic study. Presented at the 50th Annual Meeting, American Academy of Orthopaedic Surgeons, Anaheim, California, 1983
5. Eriksson E: Sports injuries of the knee ligaments. Their diagnosis, treatment, rehabilitation and prevention. Med Sci Sports 8:133–144, 1976
6. Gillquist J, Hagberg G, Oretorp N: Arthoroscopy in acute injuries of the knee joint. Acta Orthop Scand 48:190–196, 1977
7. Hamberg P, Gillquist J, Lysholm J: Suture of new and old peripheral meniscus tears. J Bone Joint Surg 65A:193–197, 1983
8. Noyes FR, Bassett RW, Grood ES, Butler DL: Arthroscopy in acute traumatic hemarthrosis of the knee. Incidence of anterior cruciate tears and other injuries. J Bone Joint Surg 62A:687–695, 1980

NATURAL
HISTORY
PREVENTION
COUNSELING

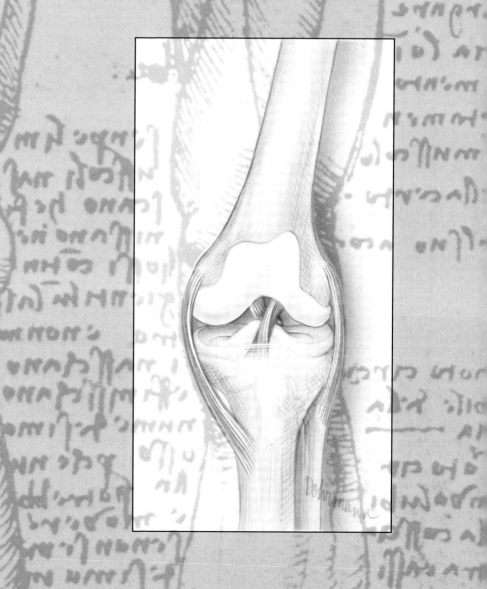

15

The Torn ACL: Natural History of Untreated Lesions and Rationale for Selective Treatment

ROBERT W. JACKSON

The catastrophic knee injury, with rupture of one or both of the collateral ligaments, disruption of the menisci, and tearing of the anterior cruciate ligament (ACL), whether due to sporting activities or motor vehicle accidents, is an easily recognizable clinical problem, with surgical repair being the generally accepted solution.

How often in the past, however, have orthopaedic surgeons heard the following story or a minor variation of it, recounted months or years after the event? The patient is usually a young athletic person who, while running, stopping suddenly, changing direction, or coming down from a jump, felt something "pop" in the knee and experienced severe pain. This was followed by rapid swelling and a feeling of instability. Almost invariably, the individual was unable to continue his or her activity and went to a hospital emergency ward where roentgenograms were taken and he or she was told there was no fracture. An elasticized wrap or splint was applied, crutches were supplied, and the patient returned home. After 2 to 3 weeks of relative rest and steadily increasing ambulation, he or she felt good enough to resume athletic activities. From then on, however, the knee tended to give way on certain movements. Some of these people learn to live with their trick knee because it only "goes out" with unguarded movements and only infrequently. Most of

them, however, modify their activity level and give up the sport that caused them the problem in the first place.

As orthopaedic surgeons, most of us immediately recognize this syndrome as a torn ACL, which may or may not be associated with damage to one or both of the menisci. We also recognize that if the problem goes untreated, there appears to be a natural sequela of arthritis and disability 20 or 30 years later.[17] For this reason, increasing emphasis has been placed on the early diagnosis and appropriate treatment of the ruptured ACL. We are all anxious to prevent the long-term adverse ill effects of such an injury. However, our treatment methods today must be compared against some standards based on past experience; otherwise, we do not know if we are actually helping the patient or merely providing yet another form of relatively ineffective treatment. We must, therefore, seek to establish the true natural history of the untreated ACL. Most of the studies published to date can be criticized because patients included, who are identified as having an ACL rupture, have come to some form of further treatment because they have trouble with their knees.[2,6,7,21]

In this chapter, I will describe the natural history of a group of patients who had ACL rupture and, for one reason or another, were left untreated. I will try to differentiate those knee injuries that must be treated by surgical repair and augmentation from those that can be treated without operative procedures. We and others[2,6,7,21] have not been able to identify patients who do *not*. have trouble after an ACL tear if, indeed, such patients exist. We advocate a selective approach to the treatment of the ACL based on two factors: the severity of the injury and the activity level of the patient. The *selection of treatment*, which forms the major portion of this chapter, leads to the conclusions that more than half of the patients we see can be treated adequately by nonoperative means with results equal to those obtained by surgical measures. Isolated and partial lesions of the cruciates are amenable to conservative treatment, but total rupture of the ACL and multistructural injury within the knee joint should be treated surgically.

NATURAL HISTORY OF UNTREATED ACL LESIONS

This is a report of a fairly unique experience in which patients with ACL ruptures, documented by arthroscopy or arthrotomy, were left untreated, and have since been evaluated in an effort to find out what really happened.[16] In view of our present knowledge, one might wonder why no attempt was made to treat the ACL in these cases. After an early, unpromising experience in attempting to repair anterior cruciates, we accepted the philosophy taught by the late J.C. Kennedy that surgical time should not be wasted on repairing the acutely torn cruciate, but spent instead on adequately repairing other torn structures around the knee joint. Consequently, over a period of 15 years, in all acute cases the collateral ligaments were repaired, the capsule was sutured, and the menisci were either removed or sutured back into position at the time of diagnosis. The ACL was either left untouched or, in some instances, actually excised. In instances where the ACL was seen to be torn at arthroscopy, and there was no other significant capsular, collateral ligament, or meniscal damage, the cruciate lesion was recorded as an "isolated" injury and was left untreated. A smaller group of patients included those whose injury had occurred months or years previously, and were seen and arthroscoped because of

the symptom of instability. In these cases also, any associated pathology was treated but the torn ACL was left untreated.

Our first review of these documented but untreated ACL lesions, revealed 63 cases with a follow-up from 2 to 23 years.[16] We classified the cases into two groups: those in whom the ACL lesion was combined with, or accompanied by damage to other structures in the knee; and those in which the ACL lesion appeared to be the *only significant* injury within the knee joint, (i.e., an isolated injury).

The largest group consisted of 42 knees in which there was documented associated damage to one or more of the other supporting structures. This group contained 37 knees with meniscal disorders, 15 with collateral ligament ruptures, and 3 with osteochondral fractures. The ACL pathology was recorded as a complete rupture in 65 percent and partially torn in 35 percent. Twenty-five percent of this group had undergone further knee surgery at some time following the original injury. Functionally, most were markedly disabled, with only 10 percent of the patients still involved in competitive sports. Forty-five percent had given up all sporting activity because of the injured knee, and stated that the knee was still deteriorating.

The second group consisted of 21 knees considered isolated ACL lesions. Ten of the knees showed complete rupture of the anterior cruciate and 11 showed partial rupture. This group, with a mean follow-up period of 10 years, appeared to be quite different from the group with combined injuries. Only one case (5 percent) had undergone any further surgical procedures, and 80 percent (16 cases) were still actively involved in sports. Several were functioning at a high level of competitive amateur or professional athletics.

Our impression from this review was that most knees in which the ACL is the only major structure damaged (isolated lesions) can function quite well without surgical treatment. If any of the secondary restraints to forward subluxation of the tibia are damaged at the same time as the ACL (combined lesions), the resultant instability can be severe enough to cause rapid deterioration of the joint. The difference between the two groups was striking. We believe, therefore, that this study,[16] although the numbers are small, represents the first documented long-term follow-up of isolated untreated ACL lesions. We also believe that throughout the country, unknown numbers of isolated ACL tears have been undiagnosed and, therefore, untreated in the past, with little adverse effect on the function of these knees. However, only a well-documented prospective study would reveal the true incidence of such cases. We consider this to be important, since with better diagnostic abilities (clinical acumen and arthroscopy) there might be a tendency to treat all torn ACLs in the same way, with aggressive surgery, thus subjecting some patients to unnecessary surgery.

Several series[4,10,12,22] have now demonstrated that an injury to a knee joint that is severe enough to cause a hemarthrosis will reveal an ACL tear in approximately 70 percent of cases. With the advent of arthroscopy as a diagnostic tool, an increasing number of acutely injured knees are being examined arthroscopically shortly after the injury. We believe this is an excellent principle to follow; the amount of damage to the knee should be determined early, the appropriate treatment instituted rapidly, and rehabilitation commenced as soon as possible to obtain the best possible result.[24] The old philosophy of splinting a knee and merely treating it symptomatically, while waiting to see whether or not any significant instability was the result, should not be condoned. However, an aggressive approach to diagnosis and the common use of arthroscopy in cases of hemarthrosis will lead to an increasing number of torn ACLs being diagnosed, of which 81 percent will be combined with damage to the menisci, capsule, or collateral ligaments and 19 percent will be isolated lesions.[20]

I believe that it is important to document not only the extent of damage to the knee joint but also the type of damage the ACL has sustained. Our studies[20] have shown that almost one third of the cruciate lesions (32 percent) are only partial tears, with some of the functional bands of that ligament being left intact. In other words, it is not always a complete rupture (the all-or-none phenomenon), but in a significant number the stress applied is dissipated in the rupturing of only a portion of the ligament, leaving some fibers intact. It is therefore quite possible that not all traumatic ruptures of the ACL require a major surgical reconstruction. Certainly, it would appear from both our experience and that of others, that a complete tear of the cruciate, associated with disruption of the secondary restraints of the joint, is best treated aggressively with surgical repair and augmentation, or a rapid downhill course may ensue, leading ultimately to the destruction of the joint. In a recent study, we found that 60 percent of freshly torn cruciate ligaments were associated with a torn meniscus (or menisci). This figure rose to 90 percent of knees that were primarily diagnosed 10 years or more after the initial injury.[20] Similarly, the incidence of articular cartilage lesions rose from 30 percent in fresh ACL cases to 69 percent in those diagnosed 10 years after injury.

It is our contention, however, that lesser degrees of damage to the anterior cruciate *do* occur and that in some instances conservative management or nonoperative management is not only possible but probably the wisest method of treatment. We therefore advocate a selective approach to the treatment of ACL injuries based on two major factors: the extent of pathology and the activity level of the patient. We tend to be surgically aggressive with younger patients and those with a higher functional demand, and much less aggressive with the elderly, and those who have little demand in terms of athletic performance.

ANATOMY AND FUNCTION OF THE ACL

Van Dijk, in his recent thesis[25] noted that an anatomic distinction between anterior and posterior bundles in the ACL was first proposed by the Weber brothers in 1836. Fick, in 1911, further developed the two band concept, describing an anteromedial-superior part and a posterolateral-inferior part. He also introduced the concept that part of the ACL was tense in all positions of the knee. Palmer (1938),[24] Brantigan and Voshell (1941),[3] Abbott et al. (1944),[1] Kennedy et al. (1974),[18] Girgis et al. (1975),[11] and Van Dijk (1983)[25] all added to our knowledge of the reciprocal function of these component bands. It is now apparent that the anteromedial band is tight throughout flexion and extension, and becomes even tighter as the knee is flexed. The posterolateral band is tight in extension and becomes quite relaxed as the knee is flexed. Therefore, the anteromedial band is the most isometric of the two bands. The posterolateral band adds additional stability when the knee is almost straight, when the supportive muscular action of the hamstrings is minimized by the loss of mechanical advantage in the extended position.

CLINICAL CORRELATION WITH ANTERIOR CRUCIATE PATHOLOGY

A study[14] correlating the clinical examination with the pathologic arthroscopic findings has supported the concept of functional banding of the ACL. When the knee is in extension, the posterolateral component of the cruciate is taut. As the knee flexes, the posterolateral band becomes relaxed with the anteromedial band becomes increasingly taut. This concept is reflected in the clinical findings one sees in relation to an ACL. If both the Lachman and Drawer tests are positive, one normally finds a complete rupture of the ACL. If the Lachman test alone is positive and the Drawer test is negative, one usually finds a rupture of the posterolateral band and an intact anteromedial band. Conversely, in a small number of instances, if the Drawer test is positive and the Lachman test is negative, one finds an isolated anteromedial band tear. The pivot shift test is positive when the poterolateral band is torn, either as a partial tear of the ligament or as part of a total tear.

A double-blind study[23] simulating an examination under anesthesia was conducted on 40 fresh cadaveric knees. Randomized sectioning of the functional bands, and independent examination by two observers, produced data on the three clinical tests (Drawer, Lachman, and pivot shift) and the cut bands. The data were controlled for confounding variables. *The anterior Drawer was found to be a specific test for the anteromedial band. The Lachman test was a good test for both bands, and the pivot shift test was preferential for the posterolateral band,* although it was positive in some anteromedial band tears. This study[23] supported the concept that the anteromedial band is taut in all ranges of flexion and extension and that the posterolateral band is relaxed in flexion and taut in extension only.

SELECTION OF TREATMENT

A selective approach to the treatment of the ACL problem, based on both the spectrum of pathology that one encounters and on the spectrum of patients that sustain these injuries, is advocated.[13] At the extreme end of the severity scale would be a total rupture of the ACL combined with other pathology in the knee. If such an injury is sustained by a young, aggressive, elite athlete, experience suggests that aggressive surgical treatment, with repair of all structures and augmentation of the repaired ACL, is the treatment of choice. At the other end of the severity scale would be an isolated partial rupture of the ACL with no other significant pathology in the knee joint. If such an injury is sustained by a middle-aged executive, or an athlete who only occasionally engages in sport, and who has no desire to be incapacitated by treatment for a prolonged period of time, the treatment could be nonoperative. Between these two extreme examples lie various combinations of pathology and athletic demand, which should lead the surgeon to choose either surgical treatment or nonoperative treatment, using bracing as a component of both types.

Therefore, the acute knee should be evaluated under anesthesia and by arthroscopy; treatment should be applied selectively (Table 15-1). Decisions regarding treatment are based on the severity of injury and the activity level of the patient. Isolated lesions tend to be treated nonoperatively whereas combined lesions are treated aggressively, with surgical repair of all torn structures and extraarticular augmentation.

The chronic knee is treated only slightly differently from the acutely injured knee. If a small meniscal fragment might be responsible for the feeling of instability, this should be resected under arthroscopic control. The knee is then treated conservatively with bracing, muscle rehabilitation, and reeducation of the patient regarding all physical activities. If the instability remains a problem, the patient is a candidate for surgery. Surgery in our hands is usually extraarticular, because this carries a predictable level of improvement with few complications. If there is a large meniscal fragment and a torn cruciate, we repair the meniscus at the same time that we perform an extraarticular surgical repair for the cruciate.

Table 15-1. Types of ACL Tear Treatment

| | Total Rupture | Partial Rupture | | | |
		Anteromedial Band	Posterolateral Band	Attenuated	
Nonoperative	81	12	23	16	132 (55%)
Early surgery (acute cases)	46	1	8	9	64 (26%)
Late surgery (chronic cases)	26	0	3	4	33 (14%)

Excluded are nine cases (5 percent) repaired elsewhere.

Nonoperative Treatment

Nonoperative treatment does not mean no treatment. After careful selection based on an examination under anesthesia and an arthroscopic evaluation of the extent of pathology, several specific steps in treatment are taken. Instability is experienced by the patient with an absent cruciate when the quadriceps contracts as the knee is at or near full extension. This occurs when landing from a jump or when trying to decelerate suddenly from running, either to stop or to change direction. However, if an athletic activity is performed with the knee in the flexed position, the hamstring muscles are quite capable of stabilizing the knee and preventing a forward shift of the tibia. Sports performed with the knee mainly flexed, such as skiing, skating, and bicycle riding, are quite consistent with prolonged and safe athletic activity in the absence of other pathology in the knee. However, sports such as basketball, volleyball, tennis, or squash place the knee at considerable risk because it comes into full extension frequently during these sports. Nonoperative treatment, therefore, includes not only the education of the patient in the types of sport that are relatively safe but also rehabilitation of the hamstring musculature, in an effort to produce a strong, quickly reactive, and resistant muscle, to overcome any tendency to anterior subluxation of the tibia. Bracing may be useful; the greatest value of a brace lies in the prevention of full extension through a block to extension at 15° to 20°. With such an extension stop, the athlete experiences a feedback mechanism that enables the hamstring muscles to come into play before a subluxation can occur.

Thus nonoperative treatment consists not only of careful selection of the case to be treated but also reeducation, hamstring rehabilitation, and bracing. Should, however, these nonoperative measures fail, and the patient have repeated episodes of the knee giving way, we then consider moving to an operative procedure.

Surgical Treatment—Acute ACL Injury

If the person's knee is selected for surgical treatment, the surgeon should attempt to repair or restore all of the damaged structures within the joint. In addition, he or she should augment the repair of the torn ACL with whatever technique he or she prefers. As studies have shown repeatedly, mere suturing of the ACL is insufficient to obtain sound healing and a stable knee. Various types of augmentation have been advocated, including intraarticular and extraarticular procedures, with autogenous, heterogenous, and synthetic materials. It is not the purpose of this paper to discuss the merits of these various surgical procedures since there are few long-term follow-up studies with sufficient cases to allow us to draw firm conclusions or make sound recommendations. However, the importance of stabilizing the joint by some means cannot be overemphasized. This involves the repair of both the primary and the secondary restraints. Because these structures often stretch in the healing phase with resultant chronic laxity, the additional stabilization afforded by some method of augmentation is strongly recommended.[13,19]

Surgical Treatment—Chronic ACL Insufficiency

Often the patient's first contact with an orthopaedic surgeon happens many months or years after injury to the knee.[2,5,9] The patient presents with a story of repeated episodes of the knee giving way. Physical examination should reveal the absence of cruciate stability. The possibility remains, however, that the giving way might be due to associated instability from a torn meniscus. Consequently, it is our practice to conduct an examination under anesthesia and an arthroscopic evaluation. If a torn meniscus is present, the surgeon is then faced with the problem of either removing the mobile fragment of meniscus or repairing it. The secondary restraints are best retained to provide additional stability of the knee. However, if the torn fragment of meniscus is mobile and unstable, it may be the main reason for the patient's instability. Accordingly, we resect a small fragment of meniscus that has less than a perfect chance of union if repaired. If the meniscal tear is extensive, vertical in type, and in the peripheral vascular area of the meniscus, a repair is carried out at the same time that the cruciate ligament is repaired. With this approach, we have been successful in eliminating the problem of instability in a significant number of cases. In a retrospective review of 100 consecutive instances in which partial meniscectomy was selectively performed at the time of arthroscopic evaluation and a torn cruciate ligament was present as an associated pathologic finding, 65 percent of the patients had undergone no further surgery at the time of follow-up and only 35 percent had required further stabilization.[15] Analysis of those who underwent further stabilizing surgery revealed most to be young women with large meniscal lesions. The increased instability due to removal of a large segment of meniscus and the inability to rehabilitate completely the surrounding musculature were considered the main reasons for further stabilizing surgery. With proper selection, (i.e., small meniscal fragments in motivated and compliant patients), arthroscopic partial meniscectomy can be an effective way to eliminate the symptom of instability.

Most of the patients with chronic ACL instability are candidates for surgical stabilization. Many of these patients present because of persisting and perhaps increasing problems due to the cruciate instability, which leads to further destruction of the menisci or articular cartilages within the knee. Accordingly, one should seriously consider this group of patients as candidates for surgery.

The type of surgical repair would again depend upon the individual surgeon's preference and the techniques with which he or she is most familiar. My personal preference is an extraarticular repair because it carries a predictable level of improvement and is associated with minimal complications.

Pivot Shift Repair

Our standard method of surgical stabilization over the past 20 years has been an extraarticular procedure using a strip of iliotibial band in a modification of MacIntosh's original procedure. A recent study of 37 patients with isolated ACL lesions, all treated by the same surgeon with the same procedure, and having a 2 year minimum follow-up, was conducted by an independent observer.[8] Any case with meniscal, chondral, or ligamentous pathologic conditions was excluded. Each patient was his or her own control: the preoperative signs and symptoms were compared with those postoperatively. An excellent result was a virtually normal knee, while a good result was a knee that was markedly improved but still had either minor subjective symptoms of instability or minimal objective signs of instability. A poor result was a knee that was neither better nor worse than preoperatively. There were more male (22) than female patients (17), with the average duration of symptoms preoperatively being 3.0 years. None of the patients had undergone further surgery. We could detect no correlation with the end result of either the time from injury to surgery or the type of pathology (i.e., partial or total ACL tear). Subjectively, 95 percent of patients were improved, with 76 percent stating they were definitely better, and 19 percent claiming slight improvement. The symptom of giving way was totally abolished in 32 percent and was present but not a problem in 41 percent. Occasional major episodes of giving way were reported by 22 percent. Only 5 percent stated they were worse than preoperatively. Objectively, 89 percent were either normal or had a grade I (minimal) pivot shift, and 11 percent had a pivot shift grade II (moderate) in severity. There were no grade III (marked) instabilities on objective testing. Combining both the subjective and objective findings, we considered that 35 percent could be considered excellent, 43 percent were good, 13 percent were fair, and 9 percent were poor results. There were no major complications such as infection, joint stiffness, or further meniscal tearing.

Because extraarticular repairs have been said to stretch out with time, we tried to gain some insight into this problem by looking into the main follow-up time of the good and excellent groups, and comparing it to the fair and poor groups. The good/excellent group had a mean followup of 4.4 years, and the fair/poor group, 6.7 years. This suggests that stretching and further instability might occur with time, or that we were not performing the surgical procedure as well in the earlier years.

We concluded that an extraarticular procedure can *improve* the knee in most cases (78 percent), but many of the resulting knees are not truly normal. The improvement is maintained for at least several years, and is obtained with virtually no complications. We believe that similar results are probably obtained as a result of most of the extraarticular procedures performed around the world, and that the beneficial effect of all of them is obtained through their tenodesis effect.

Rehabilitation

Our goal in rehabilitation is to achieve a functional range of motion with as much dynamic stability as possible contributed by the thigh muscles. We must remember, however, to protect the repaired cruciate until it matures. In addition to this local rehabilitation of the limb, we must also consider psychological rehabilitation and ultimately physiologic rehabilitation. Early mobilization appears to be of great value in preventing disuse atrophy of muscles and resultant stiffness of the joint. Consequently, either no immobilization or early mobilization in a protective fashion, using hinged casts, would appear to be the treatment of choice. Hinged casts should permit a range of motion from 30° to 90°, and active quadriceps exercises should be performed in this limited range until the repair has matured. Such protective mobilization is encouraged for at least 6 weeks, sometimes longer. One

can, perhaps, be more aggressive in rehabilitation if the secondary restraints are intact. Throughout the rehabilitation phase, hamstring reeducation is considered most important.

RESULTS OF TREATMENT

How effective is this selective approach to treatment? To determine this, we analyzed many factors, such as stability, swelling, and daily function at a minimum of 2 years after treatment. One parameter of function that was closely analyzed was the return to sporting activity of those so inclined.[20] Of 238 patients treated for ACL deficiency, 129 indicated a desire to participate in sports. Of this group, only 11 percent stated that instability prevented them from participating. Thirty percent were involved in nonstrenuous sports, and 59 precent were engaged in strenuous sports such as football, basketball, and squash. Those treated nonoperatively (after appropriate selection) amounted to 55 percent of the cases.

In analyzing those would-be athletes who were treated nonoperatively, 62 percent were engaged in strenuous sporting activities. Of those treated with early surgery (acute cases), 55 percent were engaged in strenuous sport activity; also 55 percent of those treated with late surgery (chronic cases) were involved in strenuous sport. (Table 15-2). All of the patients with isolated tears, whether partial or total and whether treated surgically or nonoperatively, had returned to some form of sport. It may be significant that 30 percent of those stabilized months or years after their injury (i.e., late surgery) were no longer participating in sport. This suggests that the development of degenerative changes will keep some people from further participation. It also emphasizes the need for early diagnosis and treatment before such degenerative changes have occurred.

Table 15-2. Participation in Sport after Treatment

Treatment	Percent Nonparticipation	Percent Nonstrenuous Sport	Percent Strenuous Sport
Nonoperative (72/132)	6	32	62
Early surgery (33/64)	9	36	55
Late surgery (20/33)	30	15	55

We believe that these results justify our continued use of nonoperative treatment in carefully selected cases.

SUMMARY AND CONCLUSIONS

Treatment of a torn ACL injury should be based on careful and complete evaluation of the extent of pathology, with consideration of the activity level of the patient. In our experience, slightly more than half the patients can be treated adequately by nonoperative means, with results that equal those obtained by surgical measures. Isolated and partial lesions of the cruciate are amenable to conservative treatment, whereas total ruptures, combined with damage to the menisci, capsule, or collateral ligaments, are prime candidates for surgical repair and augmentation. We therefore enter a plea for selective treatment based on the individual case.

REFERENCES

1. Abbott LC, Saunders JB, Bost FC, Anderson CE: Injuries to the ligament of the knee joint. J Bone Joint Surg 26A:503–521, 1944
2. Arnold JA, Coker TP, Heaton LM et al: Natural history of anterior cruciate tears. Am J Sports Med 7:305–313, 1979
3. Brantigan OC, Voshell AF: The mechanics of the ligaments and the menisci of the knee joint. J Bone Joint Surg 23A:44–66, 1941
4. DeHaven K: Diagnosis of acute knee injuries with hemarthrosis. Am J Sports Med 8:9–14, 1980
5. Feagin JA: The syndrome of the torn anterior cruciate ligament. Orthop Clin North Am 10:81–90, 1979
6. Feagin JA Jr, Curl WW: Isolated tear of the anterior cruciate ligament: 5-year follow-up study. Am J Sports Med 4:95–100, 1976
7. Fetto JD, Marshall JL: The natural history and diagnosis of anterior cruciate ligament insufficiency. Clin Orthop 147:29–38, 1980
8. Frank CB, Jackson RW: Late results of lateral pivot shift repair. Presented at Canad. Orthop. Assoc. Meeting, 1985
9. Galway RD, MacIntosh DL: The lateral pivot shift: A symptomatic sign of anterior cruciate insufficiency. Clin Orthop 147:45–50, 1980
10. Gillquist J, Hagberg G, Oretorp N: Arthroscopy in acute injuries of the knee joint. Acta Orthop Scand 48:190–196, 1977
11. Girgis FG, Marshall JL, Almonajem ARS: The cruciate ligaments of the knee joint: Anatomical functional and experimental analysis. Clin Orthop 106:216–231, 1975
12. Jackson RW: Lesions of the Ligaments. In Arthroscopy and Arthrography of the Knee. American Academy of Orthopaedic Surgeons. St Louis, CV Mosby, 1978
13. Jackson RW: Anterior cruciate ligament injuries. pp. 52–73. In Casscells SW (ed): Arthroscopy: Diagnostic and Surgical Practice. Lea & Febiger, Philadelphia, 1984
14. Jackson RW, Campbell AJ: Diagnosis of partial ruptures of the anterior cruciate ligament (abstract). Orthop Trans 5:441, 1981
15. Jackson RW, Johnson RG: Results following arthroscopic meniscectomy in anterior cruciate deficient knees. Presented at the Annual Meeting of the Arthroscopy Association of North America, 1982
16. Jackson RW, Peters RI, Marczyk RL: Late results of untreated anterior cruciate ligament rupture (abstract). J Bone Joint Surg 62B:127, 1980
17. Jacobsen K: Osteoarthrosis following insufficiency of the cruciate ligaments in man. Acta Orthop Scand 48:520–526, 1977
18. Kennedy JC, Weinberg HW, Wilson AS: The anatomy and function of the anterior cruciate ligament. As determined by clinical and morphological studies. J Bone Joint Surg 56A:223–235, 1974
19. Losee RE, Johnson TR, Southwick WO: Anterior subluxation of the lateral tibial plateau: a diagnostic test and operative repair. J Bone Joint Surg 60A:1015–1030, 1978
20. Maruyama K, Jackson RW: A perspective of anterior cruciate ligament injuries. Presented at International Knee Society Meeting, Gleneagles, Scotland, 1983
21. McDaniel WJ, Dameron TB: Untreated ruptures of the anterior cruciate ligament; a follow-up study. J Bone Joint Surg 62A:696–705, 1980
22. Noyes FR, Bassett RW, Grood ES, Butler DL: Arthroscopy in acute traumatic hemarthrosis of the knee. Incidence of anterior cruciate tears and other injuries. J Bone Joint Surg 62A:687–695, 1980
23. Paley D, Holtby R, Fornasier VL, Jackson RW: The relationship between the two bands of the anterior cruciate ligament and the pivot shift, Lachman and anterior Drawer tests (submitted for publication)
24. Palmar I: On the injuries to the ligaments of the knee joint. Acta Chir Scand 81(Suppl 53):2–282, 1938
25. Van Dijk R: The behaviour of the cruciate ligaments in the human knee. Doctoral Thesis, University of Nijmegen, Netherlands, 1983

16

Prevention of Cruciate Ligament Injuries

ROBERT J. JOHNSON

The primary thrust of this text to this point has concerned the biomechanics, diagnosis, and management of cruciate ligament injuries. There can be no doubt that the anterior cruciate ligament (ACL) is the most commonly totally disrupted ligament in the knee.[8,12,19] The majority of physicians confronting this problem concern themselves with "picking up the pieces" after an injury has occurred. An analogy that comes to mind is that of "closing the barn door after the horse has gone." Much controversy exists concerning the natural history of cruciate ligament injuries, as well as the "best" way to manage the problem after the injury has occurred. Few would dispute that the most appropriate management of the injury would be to prevent it. This enticing solution, however, appears to be unobtainable in today's fast-paced society. The ever-increasing popularity of physical fitness, often coupled with activities that place the cruciate ligaments at risk, appears to be producing an almost exponential increase in the numbers of major injuries of the cruciate ligaments. Efforts made to reduce the risk of injury in such sports as football and skiing have been disappointing. Rules changes and conditioning programs in football have apparently been partially successful in decreasing the severity and frequency of injury, but only to a small degree. In skiing, advances in boot and binding design have led to dramatic reductions in the production of ankle injuries and tibia fractures, but have been a total failure at protecting knee ligaments.[13] In fact, in recent years the frequency of ACL injuries has dramatically

risen.[11] Why can we not do better at devising methods to protect the cruciate ligaments?

The answers are many and surprisingly complex. The primary problem, however, is quite simple biomechanically. Two long bones are used to support a relatively heavy weight, and yet the articulation between these bones must be capable of great mobility and flexibility. This produces an "engineer's nightmare" in that the conflicting principles of stability and mobility are always at odds. Nature's means of stabilizing the knee articulation is ingenious and functional, as long as the loads applied to the long lever arms (tibia and femur) are relatively small and short-lived. However, when even moderate forces are applied to the long bones at a relatively large distance from the knee, the torques generated within the joint, and thus in the cruciates and other ligaments and capsular structures, can easily exceed these structures' material properties. One usually assumes that contact sports or high-energy trauma are necessary to generate these loads; however, many patients sustain these injuries by simply making rapid changes in direction or sudden decelerations, and are not affected by contact with another individual or object.

Probably the only means of preventing ACL injuries is to prevent exposure to those activities that require rapid changes in direction, jumping, rapid acceleration or deceleration, and contact. We realize that such an approach to the problem is totally impractical. Thus, the questions to be discussed in this chapter revolve around what has been done and what can be done to prevent injuries to the cruciate ligaments.[9] The models for this discussion will primarily involve the sports of skiing and football. Factors possibly related to changes in the incidence of cruciate injuries include conditioning, equipment, rules, foot fixation devices, and bracing. Let us consider the alarming increase in ACL injuries observed in the past 5 years in alpine skiing. In the 1970s, the incidence of cruciate ligament injuries among all ski injuries was 5 percent or less of the ski injuries we were observing, but since then the figure has risen to well above 10 percent.[11,12,14] Our observations of ski injury data gathered at Sugarbush North, Vermont, have revealed that the only adverse trend found to be statistically significant during the last 13 years involved the incidence of ACL injuries.[13] During this period, we have observed a dramatic improvement in the design and function of ski bindings. The rate of those injuries involving structures below the knee related to dysfunction of bindings has dropped dramatically.[13] Our statistics imply that the skiing industry has done something wrong in recent years that has produced an "epidemic" of knee ligament injuries. The problem has been in identifying the causes. There are obviously several variables involved, but our own evaluation of the situation has led us to believe that a combination of skiing style (lean-back technique), method of skill acquisition (modern equipment allows beginner skiers to advance much more rapidly than in the past), and, primarily, equipment design has resulted in the high number of ACL injuries we now observe. Undoubtedly other factors are involved as well, but their nature is not discernible.

We believe that the primary cause of ACL injuries in skiing can be divided into two categories. The first involves the classic method in which a forward fall allows the medial edge of the anterior portion of the ski to engage the snow (Fig. 16-1). As the skier's momentum propels him or her forward, the lower leg is externally rotated in relation to the thigh. This results in injury to the medial structures and the ACL if the adverse forces are not eliminated by release of the binding or disengagement of the ski edge from the snow. Often the only ligament injured in such falls is the medial collateral, but in approximately 20 percent of these cases the ACL also is destroyed.[11,13] Our previous investigations have shown that, in theory at least, properly adjusted and functioning modern bindings should protect the knee from such injuries.[14] In fact, we published data that revealed that a decrease in the number of grade 1 medial

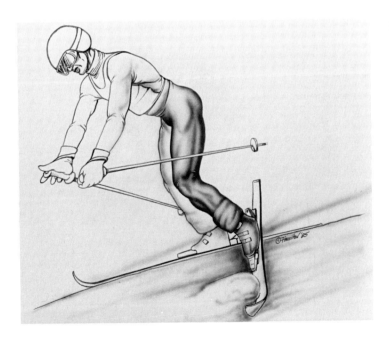

Fig. 16-1. A forward fall in which the inside edge of the left ski is caught in the snow, causing external rotation and valgus stress to the knee.

collateral ligament injuries had occurred in 1982.[13] However, our investigation of such accidents, including comprehensive testing of the boot binding system, has not always been able to explain why the knee ligaments were injured. We have also observed that forward falls that result in hyperextension or a combination of internal rotation and hyperextension may result in disruption of the ACL.[15]

In the second category of ACL injuries, it appears that the primary problem results from a backward fall, and in some cases only momentary loss of control in which the skier gets back too far. In such situations, the ACL may be damaged by the top of the boot driving the tibia forward, producing an "anterior Drawer maneuver" that results in "isolated" disruption of the ACL (Fig. 16-2). In an unpublished study, we observed videotapes of several such injuries as they happened to ski racers. Another mechanism we have evaluated on film occurs when a skier, often still in control, gets back on his or her skis, and then suddenly catches the inside edge of the tail of the ski, producing a sudden internal rotation of the hyperflexed knee, which again results in an appar-

ent isolated ACL injury (Fig. 16-3). In both of the injuries, the design of the boot (rigid shell posteriorly with a fixed forward-lean angle) directly contributes to the production of these injuries. In the past, when boot-tops were more flexible and allowed plantarflexion of the ankle, such injury mechanisms were less likely.

The inability of modern bindings to release in backward lean may also contribute to the production of ACL injury when the boot-top acts to drive the tibia forward (Fig. 16-2). Bindings designed to release upward at the toe and boots that in some way allow plantarflexion of the ankle when loads exceed the levels necessary for productive control may be able to eliminate these injuries. However, our pleas for these design changes have as yet been met by only a few of the binding manufacturers and by none of the boot manufacturers. We believe that only when the changes we have suggested are implemented in large numbers of the skiing population will we observe a decrease in the incidence of ACL injuries in skiing. Unfortunately, these changes will not occur in the foreseeable future, and thus those

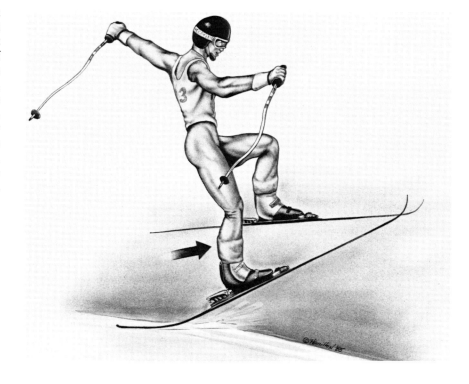

Fig. 16-2. Artist's recreation of the mechanism involved in several skiing accidents that resulted in complete tears of the ACL. The skier comes off a bump and lands on one ski, slightly off balance, with his upper body leaning backward. The tail of his ski hits the snow first, causing the ski to be driven into the snow quickly, allowing the boot-top to drive the tibia shaft forward. In each case that we have evaluated, the skier's involved knee is in almost full extension at the time of the accident, with the opposite arm thrown back in an attempt to regain balance. (Ettlinger C: How safe is racing gear? Skiing Magazine 37:92, 1985.© Wm. P. Hamilton 1986.)

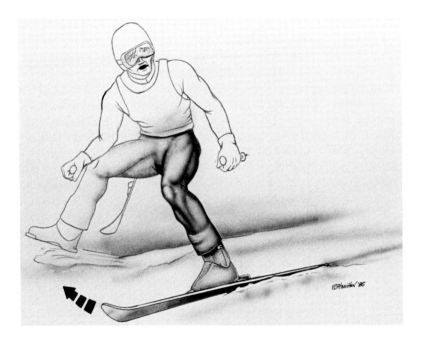

Fig. 16-3. This figure demonstrates a skier who has lost his balance, sat far backwards, and has caught the inside edge of the tail of his ski. In this situation, since no weight is borne on the portion of the ski in front of the boot, the knee is suddenly internally rotated, resulting in disruption of the ACL.

who are involved in the treatment of skiers' injuries probably will continue to observe this epidemic of ACL injuries.

For the present, we would advise those individuals interested in avoiding injury to knee ligaments, especially the anterior cruciate, to consider use of bindings with upward release capabilities at the toe. These include, at the time of this writing, only the Geze SE3 and the Look XM toe pieces among presently manufactured equipment.

RULES

For a long time we have accepted the notion that knee ligament injuries, including those of the ACL, are common in American football. Certain activities associated with the sport have been recognized as being most dangerous. Thus changes in the rules have been used to reduce these risks. Perhaps the most important of these has been the reduction of the incidence of severe neck injuries resulting from penalizing the use of the spearing maneuver. To reduce the incidence of lower extremity injuries, and especially those involving the knee ligament, several rules changes have been made. Clipping,

blocking below the waist on punts and downfield, and crack-back blocking have all been made illegal because they were identified as instrumental in the production of knee ligament and other lower extremity injuries. Although these rule changes have probably helped reduce the number of injuries, they have clearly not been as effective as we would like.

In any sport in which rules changes could result in a decrease in the number of injuries, they should be supported. However, in the cases where such changes may markedly affect the cost of continuing the sport from the standpoint of a team or an individual or cause great financial hardships for manufacturers of equipment necessary for the sport, care must be taken in proceeding to such changes too rapidly. An example of such a "rules change" may be given in the case of voluntary standards produced by the American Society of Testing and Materials (ASTM) as they affect the production of skiing equipment.[2] A standard approved by ASTM, although voluntary, is, in fact, essentially an edict to the industry to follow that standard. If equipment or practices that do not follow the standard are used and result in injury to a skier, the manufacturer would fare very poorly in a suit concerning the responsibility for the injury. Thus it is little wonder that the manufacturers resist vigorously the development of a standard that results in cost or inconvenience to themselves until it is absolutely proven that such a standard would improve safety. Since the standards process depends on agreement by representatives of many interested parties besides the manufacturers of equipment (skiers, safety experts, ski area owners, ski patrollers, physicians, engineers, and others), the production of meaningful standards that are practical and helpful in reducing injuries proceed at what appears to individuals interested in safety to be an agonizingly slow pace. Clearly, it is important for physicians and others who are expert in the problems surrounding knee ligament sprains to participate in the standards writing process, which has directly led to advances in the safety of skiing, football, and many other sports.

CONDITIONING

Innumerable authors have stated that conditioning programs will reduce the incidence of injuries in sports, but surprisingly few data are available to substantiate such contentions. It appears logical that the well-conditioned athlete would be less likely to sustain an injury by being not only stronger but also less likely to tire during the performance of a sport. Yet in the skiing injury literature, no convincing studies exist to prove this reasoning. In controlled studies of ski injuries, Young et al.[22] and Criqui[6] have demonstrated that injury rates in general do increase late in the day, and that fatigue is a likely factor.

We do know that in animal models the strength of knee ligaments has been demonstrated to increase with exercise, and that inactivity (immobilization) greatly weakens them.[3,16,18] We can assume that similar changes are probable in human knee ligaments as well. Our own research[17] has demonstrated that a single bout of exercise by athletes participating in hockey, soccer, basketball, and skiing all resulted in an increased compliance of the medial collateral ligament (MCL) immediately after the activity. We observed a return to normal ligament stiffness within 1 hour after the exercise. In vivo experiments utilizing the rat medial collateral ligament (MCL)

revealed that such an increase in compliance was associated with a reduction in the ligaments' tensile strength. This implies that athletes are more vulnerable to knee ligament injury as time passes during an episode of activity. We observed that individuals with little laxity in their MCLs appeared to be more susceptible to the effects of cyclic loading than those who had greater amounts of "normal" laxity.[21] This was also consistent with our observation that individuals with tight MCLs were more likely than those with relatively lax ligaments to sustain complete disruptions of the MCL in skiing accidents.[16] It appears likely that repeated bouts of exercise coupled with the increase in compliance observed in our experiments may stimulate the changes that resulted in increased ligament strength observed during prolonged training programs.

In 1978, Cahill and Griffith[4] published a study in which they demonstrated a decrease in the number and severity of knee ligament injuries in a group of high school football players who had undergone a preseason conditioning program compared to a similar group which had not. The preseason conditioning included a comprehensive program involving some weight training. Unfortunately, the authors did not provide specific details of the training program or the nature of the knee ligament injuries they considered that they had prevented. *Although no certain information proves beyond a doubt that conditioning programs directly strengthen human ACLs, or that this added strength significantly reduces the incidence of injury, it appears probable that some benefits accrue.*

BRACING

In recent years, a significant number of knee braces have become available that allegedly protect knee ligaments during physical activity. Two types of braces have been defined that are relevant to this discussion.

The first are termed *prophylactic* knee braces, designed to prevent or reduce the severity of knee ligament injuries in high-risk sports such as football.[1,10] They include designs with a single lateral bar hinged by single axis, dual axis, or polycentric hinges fitted with a hyperextension stop, or plastic cuffs with polycentric hinges. They are designed to protect the knee from contact loading, which could result in collateral ligament injuries. Some of their manufacturers claim that these braces have the potential to protect the ACL. However, I know of no substantiating evidence. Studies done at the Universities of Iowa, Iowa State, Notre Dame, North Carolina, and Southern California[1,10] demonstrated a trend toward the reduction of MCL injuries, while evaluations of such braces at the Universities of Arizona and Oregon demonstrated no beneficial effects in the reduction of MCL injuries.[1] None of these studies has shown any benefit from the use of these braces in the prevention or decrease in the incidence of ACL injuries and only one suggests a contribution to a decrease in meniscal injuries.[1,10]

The second group of braces includes those classified as *functional* knee braces.[1] These are designed to provide functional stability for unstable knees or to avoid reinjury to repaired or reconstructed ligaments when an individual is ready to return to high-risk activities. Functional stability was defined as "a dynamic condition in which the knee joint does not give way, thereby providing stability to the lower limb" in a recent publication of the American Academy of Orthopaedic Surgeons at a seminar on knee braces.[1] Examples of such braces include the CTI, Can-Am, Don Joy RKS, Feanny, and Lenox Hill braces, and a number of others. In spite of claims about the protection provided by these braces for repaired or reconstructed ACLs, or stability for joints lacking an ACL, there is little evidence available that they can effectively protect the knee from the high forces commonly generated in activities requiring jumping, turning, or cutting.[1] *Present information reveals that available functional braces provide little or no control of knee laxity in the anteroposterior direction.* Only during application of very low forces can these braces resist anterior motion of the tibia relative to the femur.[1] Thus, functional knee braces cannot be relied upon as the sole protection for injured or weakened anterior cruciate ligaments.

No clear explanation exists for why a significant number of individuals with functional instability due to absence of the ACL benefit from the use of these braces. However, there can be little doubt that some individuals either eliminate or diminish the severity of functional pivot shift episodes with their use. Unfortunately, it is not now known how to predict which individuals will benefit, and thus braces that appear to be of no help to many individuals continue to be prescribed. The suspected proprioceptive benefits of knee braces may be more important than their mechanical stabilizing potential.

FOOT FIXATION DEVICES

In skiing, it has long been recognized that the unnatural "elongation" of the foot by locking the boot to the ski results in a lever system that can easily overwhelm the knee ligaments if torques are applied through the ski to the leg. Ellison[7] observed that fixing of the ski edge to the snow was one component of the injury mechanism. A second necessary factor was termed "enhancement." For enhancement to occur, the rotation or bending moments imparted to the lower extremity must be augmented by inertia, causing the skier's upper body to be propelled inexorably into a position that prevents the ski edge from leaving its trapped position on the snow surface. If such conditions occur and the binding does not release, an injury to the leg or knee is likely. In other sports similar circumstances also result in loads that exceed the strength of the ACL. For instance, sudden changes in direction occurring simultaneously with acceleration or deceleration all too frequently result in a torn ACL. No contact with another individual or object is necessary. In this circumstance entrapment results from the "fixation" of the foot to the playing surface by cleats or high-friction shoe surfaces. The rotation imparted by the sudden change in direction acts to "enhance" the fixation, imparting moments that result in disruption of the ACL. Even when contact occurs in a clipping mechanism in football, or a similar accident in other sports, fixation of the foot to the playing surface contributes to production of the injury. If the foot can be freed from the surface at the time of contact, an injury may be avoided. In either case, high friction between the foot and the playing surface appears to be at least partially responsible for knee ligament and other lower extremity injuries. In most sports the ability of a player to quickly alter his or her direction of progress, avoid slipping when landing after a jump, or change speed rapidly is necessary to be competitive. This means that in almost all running sports a high-friction interface is essential between the shoe and the playing surface. Yet the higher the friction, the more likely are serious knee ligament injuries. Thus an apparently unsolvable dilemma faces the athlete, coach, and physician in sports in which high friction is necessary between the foot and playing surface. In football, efforts have been made to resolve the problem by changing the length and number of cleats, based on findings from several studies.[5,20] Torg et al.[20] revealed that a shoe/surface interface friction coefficient above 0.49 was unnecessary for playing performance and probably unsafe. The introduction of artificial playing surfaces during the past 20 years has added fuel to the problem. Many studies have indicated an increase in injury rates on these surfaces, but the exact causes and effects are still quite controversial and no certain advice can be advanced.

CONCLUSIONS

Prevention of all ACL injuries is impossible. The interaction of sports equipment and playing surfaces undoubtedly contributes to the production of these injuries, but surprisingly little is known about the multitude of variables that interact to cause each individual injury. Much more work is necessary to advance our understanding of these factors so that appropriate changes can be instituted to help reduce the number of injuries. Rules changes, improvements in protective equipment, and conditioning prescriptions will undoubtedly be altered in the future in efforts to protect knee ligaments. Efforts by individuals knowledgeable in physical education, biomechanics, epidemiology, and a multitude of related disciplines will be necessary to identify further the means of preventing ACL injuries. All of us interested in the treatment of anterior cruciate injuries should be encouraged to contribute to minimizing the problem by preventing as many of these injuries as possible.

REFERENCES

1. American Academy of Orthopaedic Surgeons: Knee braces: seminar report. D. Drez, Chairman. AAOS, Chicago, 1985
2. Bahniuk E, Hulse WF: ASTM Committee F-27 on Snow Skiing. Skiing Trauma and Safety. pp. 5–16. In Johnson RJ, Mote CD (eds): Fifth International Symposium, ASTM STP 860. American Society for Testing and Materials, Philadelphia, 1985
3. Cabaud HE, Chatty A, Gildengorin V, Feltman RJ: Exercise effects on the strength of the rat anterior cruciate ligament. Am J Sports Med 8:79–86, 1980
4. Cahill BR, Griffith EH: Effect of preseason conditioning on the incidence and severity of high school football injuries. Am J Sports Med 6:180–184, 1978
5. Cameron BM, Davis O: The swivel football shoe: a controlled study. J Sports Med 1:16–27, 1973
6. Criqui MH: The epidemiology of skiing injuries. Minn Med 60:877–880, 1977
7. Ellison AE: Skiing injuries. CIBA Symposium 29:2–40, 1977
8. Feagin JA, Curl WW: Isolated tear of the anterior cruciate ligament. 5-year follow-up study. Am J Sports Med 4:95–100, 1976
9. Feagin JA, Lambert KL: Mechanism of injury and pathology of anterior cruciate ligament injuries. Orthop Clin North Am 16:41–46, 1985
10. Hansen BL, Ward JC, Diehl RC: The preventive use of the Anderson knee stabler in football. Phys Sportsmed 13:75–76, 81 (Sep), 1985
11. Howe J, Johnson RJ: Knee injuries in skiing. Clin Sports Med 1:277–288, 1982
12. Johnson RJ: The anterior cruciate: a dilemma in sports medicine. Int J Sports Med 3:71–79, 1982
13. Johnson RJ, Ettlinger CF: Alpine ski injuries: changes through the years. Clin Sports Med 1:181–197, 1982
14. Johnson RJ, Pope MH, Weisman G, White BF: Knee injury in skiing: a multifaceted approach. Am J Sports Med 7:321–327, 1979
15. Marshall JL, Johnson RJ: Mechanisms of the most common ski injuries. Phys Sportsmed 5:49–51, 1977
16. Noyes FR, Torvik PJ, Hyde WB, DeLucas JL: Biomechanics of ligament failure: an analysis of immobilization, exercise, and reconditioning effects in primates. J Bone Joint Surg 56A:1406–1418, 1974
17. Pope MH, Johnson RJ, Weisman G, Johnson KH: Objective evaluation of the medical collateral ligament of the knee. Iowa Orthop J 1:32–38, 1981
18. Tipton CM, James SL, Mergner WA, Tcheng T: Influence of exercise on strength of medial collateral knee

ligaments of dogs. Am J Physiology 218:894–902, 1970

19. Torg JS, Conrad W, Kalen V: Clinical diagnosis of anterior cruciate ligament instability in the athlete. Am J Sports Med 4:84–93, 1976

20. Torg JS, Quedenfeld TC, Landau S: The shoe–surface interface and its relationship to football knee injuries. J Sports Med 2:261–269, 1974

21. Weisman G, Pope MH, Johnson RJ: Cyclic loading in knee ligament injuries. Am J Sports Med 8:24–30, 1980

22. Young LF, Oman CM, Crane H: The etiology of ski injury: an eight year study of the skier and his equipment. Orthop Clin North Am 7:13–29, 1976

17
Counseling Patients with Career-Ending Injuries

BRUCE C. OGILVIE

Reasons for an athlete's involuntarily terminating a career in sports may differ, but symptoms and maladaptive behaviors of such athletes appear to have a common pattern. This pattern, frequently simulating the sequence of grief reactions, is evident in athletes, from those sustaining multiple injuries to those sustaining severe disruption of the cruciate ligaments in only one knee. Treatment of the physical injury is an accepted practice. Treatment of the level of psychological trauma to the patient is a growing concern among physicians and other counselors (Presentations, Fifth World Congress of Sports Psychology, Ottawa, Canada, 1982).

In this chapter, I will present some of the background about athletes with career-ending injuries (particularly an injury to the cruciate ligaments). The first portion will be a defense of counseling these athletes. The next section will give the physician some insight into the pattern of emotional reactions he or she may expect in these athletes. The last section will offer some practical suggestions about how physicians may provide successful counseling to the athlete with a career-ending injury.

BACKGROUND: ATHLETES WITH CAREER-ENDING KNEE INJURIES

In preparing this chapter, I wondered about the frequency with which the surgeon and other medical personnel would be called upon to counsel athletes with career-ending cruciate injuries. In the absence of any substantial data, I queried sports medicine physicians. Martin Trieb, M.D., a university team physician and one of the pioneers in sports medicine in the United States, estimated in his subjective recollection, based on his and his colleague's experience, that approximately 30 percent of the athletes with cruciate ligament injuries either had to terminate participation in their sport while at university, or had only short careers in active playing after leaving university. He raised the issue of sports specificity in terms of the mechanical requirements of sports; for example, does the same cruciate ligament damage affect the future participation of a skier as it does the basketball player or the football player? We have no hard data with which to answer such a question.

Chandy and Grana,[1] in their comprehensive 3-year study of 42,774 athletes (ages 14 to 18), reported that knee injuries were the most frequent cause of terminating play. Whiteside et al.,[2] in their comprehensive 12-year study of university football players, also reported that knee injuries contributed to more time loss from competition than any other cause. If these demographic studies are representative of the incidence of knee injuries at both the secondary school and university levels, and if we project these data into the one and a half million players, we can anticipate that approximately 200,000 (20 percent) of the athletes will incur a time-loss knee injury during their sports participation in school. We have no data on the number of these players who will be forced to end their careers in sports because of the injury to the cruciate ligaments and the ligamentous complexes of the knee.

Some bias is inherently introduced into our clinical observations on the pattern of emotional and behavior reactions of the athlete with career-ending injury because our samples are based on elite athletes from professional, Olympic, and national teams, or participants in intercollegiate athletics who may be aiming towards a professional career in sport. Our attention was first drawn to the aberrant behavior of the elite athlete by the media's often lurid depiction of such behavior. In clinical practice, we see some dramatic episodes, but more frequently we see a gradual evolution of the trauma. This evolving of the sequence is what has shown us the pattern. Although the higher levels of athletic excellence seem related to some special problems of adaptation when competitive days are over, a sufficient number of athletes with lesser talent respond in an identically traumatic way. *My counseling experience with every age group of young people who have been forced out of every form of sports clearly documents that a significant number are subject to these same traumatic effects.* However, the level at which the athlete competes may influence the degree of emotional trauma and the length of time necessary to recover.

Counselors and physicians will have an impact upon a variety of the athlete's personal issues, such as financial implications and alterations in athletic status (particularly those athletes who have tied their personal worth and self-esteem to their sense of being an athletic hero). One example of such an athlete is the university scholarship holder in one of the major sports who may see his knee injury as not only costing him his scholarship and depriving him of an education but also costing him his dream of a professional contract. Another example is the 16-year-old figure skater, who has spent 9 years in dedicated sacrifice, sees her dream of the Olympic gold medal melt away when she can never again complete a triple toe loop. In my practice I have seen one patient population that challenges the counseling skills of the most experienced clinicians: athletes in the endurance sports, such as the distance runners, swimmers, and cross-country skiers.

The quest for excellence in any line of endeavor can produce a unidimensional personality. The time commitment and dedication necessary to meet performance criteria in sport have forced too many of our young athletes to sacrifice development in other areas. Patients at greatest risk are those who have limited their definition of self-worth to accomplishments within a particular sport. They have no alternatives for ego acclimation. The threatened loss of social and psychological rewards that accrue from the role of ''hero'' in the only field in which they have attained identity may make the relinquishing of such an identity emotionally untenable. Such an example was the 26-year-old hockey player whose injured knee ended his professional career. He paced back and forth while ranting about his inability to live without the roar of the crowd. Shortly afterwards he verbalized his preoccupation with his only means to escape from such a painful reality: suicide. Suicidal rumination has surfaced in some of our athletes participating at the elite level in sports of figure skating and gymnastics when they are as young as 14 years.

With the background provided above, I will expand upon the emotional reactions I have seen in athletes with career-ending injuries. The consequences may be more numerous or financially devastating in the elite athlete but the social and psychological trauma may be just as profound for the recreational athlete.

EMOTIONAL REACTIONS

Denial: The Primary Maladaptive Response

The patient will use every mental manipulation to deny the reality of medical judgment. Often we see the perversion of one of the fine characteristics of the successful athlete: persistence in the pursuit of a personal goal. Tenacity, perseverance, and the capacity to sustain effort over time are hallmarks of achieving athletes and certainly add to the joy in sports medicine practice. The newly injured athlete may translate these same strengths into unrealistic goals and extremely aberrant behavior. The suicidal professional hockey player may continue to dress for practice despite objective evidence that his days as a superior skater are over. Another athlete may seek a tryout in the minor leagues and honestly believe that one season at this lower level is all he needs to make it back into the big leagues. Another athlete, a National Basketball Association forward, may continue to come to practice and sit on the sidelines, fully believing that the coach will turn to him and invite him to play. The figure skater's mother may search for the magic surgeon, the special prosthesis, and possibly even the hypnotist who will reinforce some form of denial in her daughter. In a very real sense we are seeing patients who are employing elaborate obsessive defenses as a means to protect themselves against a reality that is painful emotionally and sometimes dangerous socially.

When denial takes this obsessive form it may be especially difficult for the physician not to be threatened by the rejection of sound medical judgment. It is best for the physician to keep in mind that this is a near-universal emotional smokescreen used whenever self-disclosure becomes more threatening than the confrontation with reality.

Projection: Anger, Resentment, Hostility

The maladaptive use of projection in any of its forms becomes evident as a phase of the career termination syndrome as the athlete becomes less able to deny the validity of the medical judgment. Projection may manifest itself during the early rehabilitation period or after an extended period of unusual commitment to the medically recommended program. Although the rehabilitation specialist may describe such patients' commitment and dedication to the program in glowing terms, we cannot infer that the patients have been realistic about the treatment goals the physician sets forth.

We begin to see anger, resentment, and sometimes hostility as the unbearable truth begins to emerge into consciousness. Those athletes who experience the loss of their skills as the loss of love object or something in life that can never be replaced may seek to displace any personal responsibility for their present unpleasant life situation.

In my correspondence I have a comment from an athlete in crisis that reflects eloquently the pain some athletes feel when the truth of reality hits home. This 19-year-old university basketball player was a scholarship athlete at one of our fine western universities. She wrote,

> Even though I had lost a lot of my game I was so happy to be playing again. I guess I was so happy I

did not realize I was favoring my knee, anyway, my good knee could not take the strain and I hurt it. It was ligament damage again which required surgery. Again I was crushed, I became so depressed and down, I felt like my life was ruined. I knew now that I could never play major college ball and that my dream was dead. I felt like a failure, I felt so helpless that I wanted to hide from everyone, finally I became angry.

At this point in the adaptation curve, angry feelings and resentment may be projected by placing the responsibility on another situation or another person: the team, the coach, athletic trainer, or team physician, and in some cases the sports governing body. If the scapegoating is directed toward the surgeon, it is certainly a burden no professional person can carry lightly. This will be a critical point in the relationship between the patient and the physician. How does one remain empathetic and supporting when one is being subjected to unwarranted resentment and hostility? As professional persons in human services, our security must rest upon the inner voice that says "I offered the best of my training and ability" and to feel comfort in this form of self-validation.

Grief: The Final Negative Phase

The final negative phase in the career termination process is comparable to grief and may continue for weeks or months, depending upon the extent the injured athlete's self esteem is threatened. Persons in this phase of the crisis reaction may manifest a constant mood of not caring, listlessness, decreased ambition, and feelings of helplessness. Some athletes slip into profound forms of depression. These are the athletes who seek to escape through the use of chemicals or engaging in some form of irrational risk taking. During this mourning phase they become highly vulnerable to suggestions from less than reliable sources, particularly those who offer quick cures or escapes.

Although grief may be the most painful period of the adaptation process, it seems that certain athletes must live through this reaction of total grief before they can move into the final stage of reintegration. I have no better way to reinforce this point than to quote again from the university basketball athlete: "I felt as if something inside me died, I knew I could never be the superior athlete I had always been. Yes, for me it was much like the death of a part of me." Although we may feel as medical professionals that her commitment to her sport was less than reasonable, we must still be prepared to meet her at her own level of need. *We need not accept her total behavior but we are duty-bound to honor her feelings.*

Reintegration: The Process of Exploring New Options

At this stage in the termination cycle, we sense that the athlete is beginning to take total responsibility for getting on with his or her life. Now the physician and therapists may begin the process of helping the athlete explore new options, particularly those athletes who must include some form of recreational or competitive sport in their lives. The program of rehabilitation may be reinforced. The treatment plan can be outlined with specific measurable goals that can act as incentives and provide motivation. The fine traits of the athlete's persistence and commitment can be revitalized in the pursuit of realistic and attainable goals.

Patient should avail themselves of recreational or athletic specialists at universities or community centers who will enable any interested person to explore all the reasonable options. The athlete may never again break down the lane and drive for the basket, but there may be no reasons why he or she cannot derive almost as much satisfaction from competitive cycling, swimming, or recreational skiing.

SUCCESSFUL COUNSELING

Crucial to effective counseling is the maxim "it is better to know the patient with the injury than to know the injury the patient has." Only through gentle exploration of meaning of the injury to the patient, the athlete's ego investment, and the relevant social factors can the physician elicit intelligent responses from the patient. Rarely is it possible to anticipate the level of trauma, the nature of the defensive reactions, or the potential for an injured athlete to slip into an aberrant pathologic escape pattern. However, successful counseling begins in

physicians' private moments when they retreat into their mental computers, review all the evidence both physical and behavioral, and formulate an estimate of the future mechanical integrity of the patient's injured knee. Then, counseling proceeds with physicians formulating a strategy, enlisting the patient's cooperation, seeking a support network, and being prepared with alternative programs in case the first plan is not effective.

Preparation

The true art/science of the skilled diagnostician becomes a statement of probabilities about anticipated future functioning of the patient: both the person and the injured knee. The weight of this judgment will vary greatly. For team physicians (particularly professional teams), the reliability of the physician's diagnostic skill has ramifications throughout the entire organization. Also, the considerations will vary with the elite athlete and the recreational athlete. The physician's skill in handling the counseling of each patient is crucial to the restoration of the person and his or her reintegration into living. The physician must mentally review all the evidence and relative factors influencing the patient's personality as well as activities.

Communication Strategy

A physician's skill as a counselor can be enhanced if he or she takes time to outline the communication strategy most appropriate for the patient. This will be contingent upon the physician's crystallizing an appraisal of the patient's potential for recovery and future participation. Based on considering all the relevant data and arriving at a probability statement, the physician knows that this is an athlete among the 20 to 30 percent who has a career-ending injury. The harsh reality must be faced by the physician and he or she must plan a strategy to help the patient face the reality, even if the patient must pass through the grieving sequence.

An excellent strategy is to rehearse mentally the content of subsequent counseling sessions wherein the physician reviews his or her insights about the patient. In a sense, the physician will try to anticipate the patient's responses to his or her inquiries.

Some insight could be gained by asking the patient to respond to a questionnaire (see Appendix). One set of questions (A) taps feelings of loss of control, helplessness, possible despair; another line of inquiry (B) identifies a patient who is expressing an intense ego involvement in sports participation and who needs to gain an objective view of other ways to reinforce self-esteem; a third set (C) taps the tendency for a patient to respond to injury by the use of psychosomatic defenses. From the patient's responses to the three sets of questions, the physician should be able to do the following:

Estimate the level of ego strength and the emotional components supporting the patient's commitment to sport

Examine the social and economic consequences of the injury's dramatically lowering the patient's athletic potential

Recognize the signs of "exercise addition" or other indications of an obsessive/compulsive commitment to the sport

Gather information about the patient's years of dedication, level of achievement, and age, which will help to predict the patient's response with greater objectivity

Attempt to formulate the degree to which the patient has a neurotic commitment to sport (i.e. proving self-worth through the sport)

Attempt to measure the extent to which misguided parental or family expectations pressure the athlete to the point that he or she cannot face reality. (Is the athlete seeing the injury as "letting others down"? Are parents, coaches, or others causing the injured athlete to feel guilty?)

Frequently the medical judgment will create a confrontation with the patient's dreams or fantasies about future participation. It would be unusual for the deeply committed athlete to exhibit complete resignation upon hearing the physician's professional opinion of the reality for the first time. Furthermore, to some athletes it becomes a contest or challenge to prove the physician wrong if they hear him or her say "I have seen only three patients with your degree of instability in the knee ever return to varsity play."

Contributions of the Support Group

In those cases where the physician anticipates that the patient will be excessively vulnerable, he or she should gather a support group and enlist their support for the patient. Such a support group may include the team trainer, team physician, team psychologist, the coach, and, in some cases, a member of the family. After the physician outlines what can be expected with respect to physical recovery, each person will be encouraged to discuss in an open manner how he or she can contribute to the treatment. The injured athlete is encouraged to play an active part in designing the rehabilitation program and setting specific goals to accomplish the best recovery. The more the patient feels a part of the decision-making process, the better the prognosis. Of the many possible contributions of the support group, the one that may be the most helpful to the athlete in crisis is the continuing reinforcement of reality. Of course, the patient's capacity to deal with the reality of the career-ending injury will be determined greatly by the degree to which his or her self-esteem is woven into identity with the sport and the dimensions of his or her personality and interests.

Alternative Plans

In addition to plans and programs to handle the possibilities for unexpected or extreme reactions by the patient, the physician should examine his or her own desire and skills at counseling the patient. Some physicians have a natural aversion to counseling. Patient counseling, like speaking on the telephone, account keeping, or public speaking may not be personally rewarding. If the physician finds that counseling is among the least meaningful aspects of his or her practice, he or she has the responsibility to select someone skilled in counseling who will provide this service to patients under his or her direction. This person may be the office nurse, rehabilitation specialist, team trainer, a colleague, or professional counselor.

The person counseling the patient must keep the physician informed about the patient, particularly the postoperative patient who slips into the depression phase and seems to be unable to find a way out.

Speaking from thirty years of clinical practice, I suggest that approximately 6 percent of such patients benefit from outpatient psychotherapy. Psychiatric or psychological referral may be the best option.

SUMMARY

Career-ending injuries involving the cruciate ligaments may produce in some athletes a maladaptive behavior pattern similar to a grief reaction. Elite athletes, professional athletes, and addicted recreational athletes are at greatest risk. Clinical experience documents that economic and psychosocial threats and lack of other interests have been underlying causes of maladaptive responses. Crisis reactions include denial, projection of responsibility (with anger and hostility), some form of depression, and finally reintegration. Counseling will be most effective when the physician has insight into the level of ego commitment and the degree to which the athlete's self-esteem is bound to achievement through sports. Counseling will proceed most successfully when the physician is able to honor the athlete's underlying feelings. Exploration of the greatest number of options available to the patient before offering final medical judgment will help the physician avoid the feeling of being trapped. Referring patients to resource persons can enlighten patients about alternative recreational sports after they recover sufficiently from the career-ending injury. In some cases serious depression is an underlying facade or is conspicuously verbalized by the patient. In such cases, the physician should refer the patient immediately to a counselor skilled in treating depression. We know that the earlier the treatment is instituted the better the prognosis. If the physician finds counseling unrewarding or too time-consuming, then his or her responsibility lies in referring the patient to those skilled and experienced in such services.

REFERENCES

1. Chandy TA, Grana WA: Secondary school athletic injury in boys and girls: a three-year comparison. Physician Sportsmed 13 (No. 3):106–111, 1985
2. Whiteside JA, Fleagle SB, Kalenak A, Weller HW: Manpower loss in football: a 12-year study at The Pennsylvania State University. Physician Sportsmed 13:103–114, 1985

Appendix

The patient is asked to respond to the three parts of the questionnaire and to return the pages to the physician so that together they may plan the rehabilitation program. There are no right or wrong answers. On (A), a score of 50 or above suggests a need for counseling; a score between 39 and 49 indicates that the surgeon should gently reinforce the reality of recovery possibilities; a score below 38 invites discussion of realities. On (B), a score above 50 is a strong indication for counseling; a score between 39 and 49 shows that the patient could benefit from exploring the degree to which he has allowed himself to be judged or valued upon only one limited aspect of his total nature as a person; a score below 38 suggests points that could be used to generate insights into negative feelings affecting recovery. On (C), a score over 50 shows a definite trend toward overuse of psychosomatic defenses; a score between 39 and 49 indicates that some type of rehabilitation program designed to help the patient take more responsibility for her recovery is needed; a score below 38 may serve as a cue for discussion during the recovery phase.

Please circle the number on the right-hand side of the page that represents your response to each statement

	ALWAYS TRUE		SOMEWHAT TRUE		NEVER TRUE
(A)					
1. I feel restless and can't seem to settle down.	5	4	3	2	1
2. I feel emotionally down and sad.	5	4	3	2	1
3. I don't know what to do with myself.	5	4	3	2	1
4. My moods seem to swing too high or too low.	5	4	3	2	1
5. I feel that something important has been taken away from me.	5	4	3	2	1
6. I need to find a new meaning to my life.	5	4	3	2	1
7. I feel helpless and out of control.	5	4	3	2	1
8. I am irritable and fly off the handle without a good reason.	5	4	3	2	1
9. I seem to have lost control over my life.	5	4	3	2	1
10. To apply myself at school or at work is difficult.	5	4	3	2	1
11. I wonder if I will ever regain my former level of competition.	5	4	3	2	1
12. I question why I keep trying to come back.	5	4	3	2	1
13. I doubt if I will return to my sport.	5	4	3	2	1
14. I am just kidding myself about being able to compete again.	5	4	3	2	1
15. I do not think it is worth the effort to try to regain my skills.	5	4	3	2	1

NOW ADD UP YOUR SCORE _____

	ALWAYS TRUE		SOMEWHAT TRUE		NEVER TRUE
(B)					
1. Without sport, I do not have other ways to feel good about myself.	5	4	3	2	1
2. My sport is the only way I could measure my self-worth.	5	4	3	2	1
3. Through my sport, I could show I was a better person.	5	4	3	2	1
4. I need to match my skills in sport against others.	5	4	3	2	1
5. I need to have others recognize my achievements in sports.	5	4	3	2	1
6. I miss the excitement that comes from competition.	5	4	3	2	1
7. I need to have others see me advance in my sport.	5	4	3	2	1
8. I am more comfortable with competitors like myself.	5	4	3	2	1
9. I miss the opportunity to place my athletic talent on the line.	5	4	3	2	1
10. The only time I feel alive is when I am expressing myself in my sport.	5	4	3	2	1
11. My life without sport is boring.	5	4	3	2	1
12. Through sport I gain a true sense of who I am.	5	4	3	2	1
13. When I am only a spectator, I do not feel good about myself.	5	4	3	2	1
14. Sport is the only way I have to prove myself to others.	5	4	3	2	1
15. If I cannot compete again, the biggest part of me has died.	5	4	3	2	1
NOW ADD UP YOUR SCORE					

	ALWAYS TRUE		SOMEWHAT TRUE		NEVER TRUE
(C)					
1. Without participating in my sport I do not sleep or rest well.	5	4	3	2	1
2. Without training, my eating habits are not good.	5	4	3	2	1
3. Without training, my body functions (e.g. elimination) are not regular.	5	4	3	2	1
4. Without training, my sexual energy has decreased.	5	4	3	2	1
5. Missing training has caused my body to feel heavy.	5	4	3	2	1
6. Without training, I have more muscular aches and pains.	5	4	3	2	1
7. Since my injury I am irritable and jumpy.	5	4	3	2	1
8. My body feels tense.	5	4	3	2	1
9. I feel my body wasting away.	5	4	3	2	1
10. I find it difficult to relax.	5	4	3	2	1
11. I find it difficult to think about other things than my inability to participate in my sport.	5	4	3	2	1
12. I daydream about the great plays I am going to make when I recover.	5	4	3	2	1
13. I will talk about my injury to anyone who will listen.	5	4	3	2	1
14. I enjoy the attention I get when someone hears about my injury.	5	4	3	2	1
15. I do not really believe I will fully recover from my injury/surgery.	5	4	3	2	1

NOW ADD UP YOUR SCORE

TOTALS (A) _____   (B) _____   (C) _____

SEQUELAE

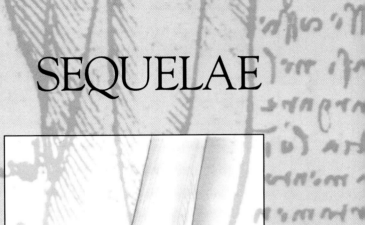

18

Knee Ligaments in Osteoarthritis of the Knee

FRANKLIN H. SIM
FRANK J. FRASSICA
KURT D. MERKEL
EDMUND Y. S. CHAO

Osteoarthritis is the most common human joint disease. The term *osteoarthritis* is used interchangeably with *degenerative joint disease* and *osteoarthrosis*.[8] The principal pathologic features of the disease include progressive focal disintegration of the articular cartilage and formation of new bone in the floor of the cartilage lesion and at the joint margins (osteophytes).[9] Synovial hypertrophy and reaction are usually secondary phenomena. A general classification is given in Table 18-1 and an outline of the clinical features of osteoarthritis is shown in Table 18-2.[8,9]

In this chapter we present a section on the natural history, with subsections on patterns of knee deformity, adaptive changes, and stress deprivation; and another section on surgical considerations for the osteoarthritic knee, with subsections focusing on the role of knee ligaments in osteotomy and the role of the knee's ligamentous structures in total joint replacement.

BIOLOGY AND NATURAL HISTORY OF OSTEOARTHRITIS OF THE KNEE

Overview

Primary osteoarthritis of the knee is common.[19] The medial or the lateral compartment or both may be involved, with or without destruction of the articular cartilage in the patellofemoral joint. As with osteoarthritis in other joints, pain is usually worsened by motion and relieved by rest. Localized tenderness may occur on direct palpation, and bony enlargement secondary to osteophytes may be visible as well as palpable. Effusions are usually not a prominent feature, and crepitus may occur with flexion of the knee. The criteria for radiologic diagnosis are shown in Table 18-3.[12]

Although the cause of osteoarthritis of the knee is multifactorial, one of the principal causative and accelerating factors is abnormal stress produced by biomechanical alteration of the mechanical axis of the hip, knee, and ankle.[16] Even minor varus or valgus deformity prevents equal medial and lateral tibial plateau loading and, with time, may result in degenerative changes. The initial pathologic changes involve destruction of the articular cartilage. When erosion of the cartilage is complete, the subchondral bone is liable to be affected next. Unfortunately, cartilage has essentially no capacity for self-repair. However, the underlying subchondral bone has a striking reparative ability and attempts to repair the destroyed cartilage by forming new bone (osteophytes). The abnormal pressures generated by the malaligned extremity produce subcortical cysts, further contributing to the loss of bone in the compromised compartment. A vicious cycle is often

Table 18-1. Classification of Osteoarthritis

Primary
  Idiopathic
  Generalized osteoarthritis
  Erosive osteoarthritis

Secondary
  Mechanical incongruity
    Congenital or developmental
    Posttraumatic

  Prior inflammatory joint disease
    Rheumatoid arthritis and variants
    Chronic gouty arthritis or pseudogout
    Infectious arthritis

  Endocrinopathies
    Diabetes mellitus
    Acromegaly
    Sex hormone abnormalities

  Metabolic disorders
    Hemochromatosis
    Ochronosis
    Wilson's disease
    Paget's disease

  Miscellaneous

    Avascular necrosis
    Hemarthrosis associated with chronic coagulopathy

Although much has been written on the biologic aspects of ligament repair, relatively little research has been done on the aging of ligaments and the adaptive changes that occur in osteoarthritis. Adaptive changes may include contracture or attenuation, "softening" of the ligament substance, and changes in the characteristics of the bone ligament insertions. These adaptive changes may be caused by repetitive overloading of the ligament (as in the lateral collateral ligament when there is severe varus deformity of the knee) or by stress deprivation

Table 18-2. Clinical Features of Osteoarthritis

Common joints involved
  Distal interphalangeal joints of the fingers
  Proximal interphalangeal joints of the fingers
  First carpometacarpal joint
  First metatarsophalangeal joint
  Hips
  Knees
  Cervical spine
  Lumbar spine

Joints spared include
  Metacarpophalangeal joints
  Wrists
  Elbows
  Shoulders
  Ankles

Characteristics of joint discomfort
  Worsened by use, relieved by rest
  Jelling phenomenon
  Morning stiffness absent, or present for less than 30 minutes

Signs on joint examination
  Local tenderness
  Bony or soft-tissue (or both) swelling (joint enlargement)
  Crepitus
  Effusions

Characteristics of synovial fluid
  High viscosity
  Normal mucin test
  Mild leukocytosis ($<$2,000 leukocytes/mm^3), predominantly mononuclear cells

established: the more varus deformity created by loss of articular cartilage and subchondral bone, the more overloading of these tissues, with resulting degeneration (Fig. 18-1).

Thus, in summary, osteoarthritis may be viewed as a focal mechanical disorder that first destroys the articular cartilage and thereafter the subchondral cortical and cancellous bone.[20] The subchondral bone attempts to repair the articular cartilage by forming reactive new bone. The involvement of the major knee ligaments (collateral, cruciate, and posterior capsule complex) is secondary to the cartilage and bony loss and is an adaptive feature. The various patterns of malalignment in the osteoarthritic knee (varus or valgus, with or without a fixed flexion contracture) place the knee ligaments in abnormal positions in reference to their function.

Table 18-3. Criteria for Radiologic Diagnosis of Osteoarthritis (OA)

Criteria

    Formation of osteophytes in the joint margins or at ligamentous attachments

    Periarticular ossicles, mainly at distal and proximal interphalangeal joints

    Narrowing of the joint space associated with sclerosis of subchondral bone

    Cystic areas with sclerotic walls situated in the subchondral bone

    Altered shape/contour

Grading (according to number of criteria)

    0 = No OA

    1 = Doubtful OA

    2 = Minimal OA

    3 = Moderate OA

    4 = Severe OA

(as might occur in the posterior capsule ligaments in a fixed flexion deformity).

Patterns of Knee Deformity

Neutral Knee

In the early stages of osteoarthritis with mild destruction of the articular cartilage, the alignment of the knee may be near normal. Radiographs taken during weightbearing may reveal mild misalignment with a loss of the normal 7° to 9° valgus angle (Fig. 18-2). In these early stages, the knee has not progressed into the common varus deformity (or the less common valgus deformity). The length and tension of the collateral ligaments may be subtly affected by osteophyte formation. Rarely, a neutral knee may be found with the symmetrical loss of bone and cartilage and soft tissue contracture.

Varus Deformity

In theory, varus deformity of the knee may be caused by either loss of cartilage and bone medially or rupture or elongation of the lateral soft tissues.[20] Disruption of the lateral ligament complex probably does not occur in osteoarthritis. Varus deformity is caused by loss of bone and cartilage medially and

by elongation of the lateral ligaments. As the varus deformity worsens, the mechanical axis of the resultant forces through the knee passes further medial to the most medial point of contact in the knee (Fig. 18-3). These forces tend to hinge the femorotibial articulation open laterally, subjecting the lateral and midline soft tissues to further tensile load. The result is elongation and attenuation of the lateral soft tissues. In general, 1 cm of medial bone and cartilage loss will result in 10° of varus misalign-

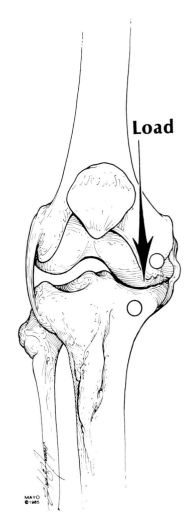

Fig. 18-1. Diagrammatic representation of loading forces in the unbalanced knee. (By permission of the Mayo Foundation.)

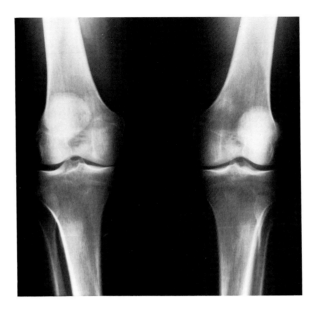

Fig. 18-2. Anteroposterior standing roentgenogram of a 55-year-old patient with early degenerative changes of the left knee (medial joint space narrowing with a valgus angle of 4°). The right knee has a greater loss of medial joint space with 3° varus deformity.

ment. However, this approximation is related to the width of the tibial plateau. For more accurate assessment, the angle must be measured in reference to the mechanical axes of the femur and tibia. Loss of a full 2 cm of bone and cartilage is common in the medial compartment, and this loss accounts for the 10° to 15° of varus deformity usually seen in osteoarthritis.

As bone and cartilage are lost on the medial side of the joint, the intercondylar eminence of the tibia moves upward relative to the femur and tilts so that its apex moves laterally. The combined effect is to produce a false midline articulation (a form of impingement) between the normally nonarticular central structures of the femur and tibia (Fig. 18-4). The formation of a false midline joint is encouraged by the development of osteophytes at the margins of the femoral intercondylar notch.

Fixed varus deformity is caused by contracture of the shortened medial soft tissues in addition to the loss of medial bone and cartilage and lateral elongation of soft tissue. The constricted tissues include the medial collateral ligament (MCL), the medial

half of the posterior capsule, and the muscles crossing the medial side of the knee. In addition, medial osteophytes may displace the medial collateral ligament, thus contributing to the maintenance of deformity by effectively shortening the ligament.

Valgus Deformity

The development of valgus deformity about the knee is similar to that of the more common varus deformity; however, in contrast, the bone and cartilage are lost over the lateral compartment and the

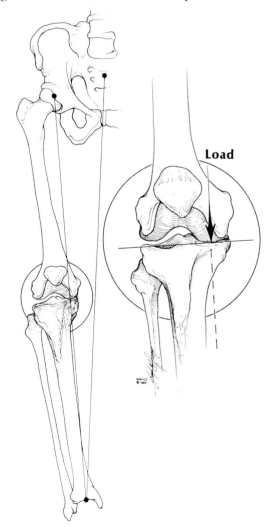

Fig. 18-3. Diagrammatic representation of the mechanical axis of the lower extremity, showing a varus deformity with the axis passing through the medial compartment of the knee. (By permission of the Mayo Foundation.)

Fig. 18-4. Anteroposterior standing roentgenogram of a 65-year-old patient with osteoarthritis of both knees. The right knee has a pronounced loss of medial joint space, a false midline articulation, and a 12° varus deformity. The changes in the left knee are similar but less advanced.

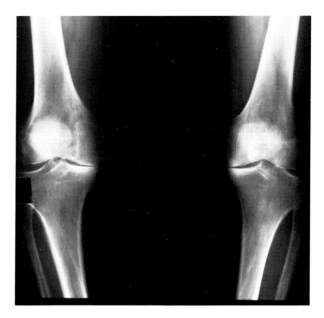

soft tissue changes involve the MCL (Fig. 18-5). Although valgus deformity may occur in osteoarthritis, it is much more common in rheumatoid arthritis. The tibial defect usually involves the posterior three quarters of the condyle while the anterior aspect is spared. The femoral condyle changes are usually more extensive than with medial gonarthrosis.

Fixed valgus deformities are caused by contractures of the lateral soft tissues. The contracted lateral structures include the iliotibial tract and biceps femoris. In addition, adhesions may form between the lateral femoral condyle and the posterior capsule.

Fixed Flexion Deformity

Flexion deformity is common in arthritic knees. The position of comfort in the knee (position of maximal intrasynovial volume) is between 15° and 25° of flexion. When pain prohibits full extension of the knee, contractures may develop in this position. Adhesions may form between the posterior capsule and the femoral condyle, hamstring muscles, and cruciate ligaments.

Adaptive Changes

In general, with joint deformities, muscle tendon units undergo contracture formation whereas ligaments form adhesions.[20] However, this concept, although well accepted, is oversimplified. Ligaments supply static support and guidance. They supplement bony geometry and the dynamic effects of muscle and tendon.[33,34] The function of the liga-

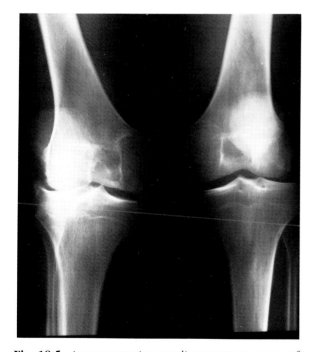

Fig. 18-5. Anteroposterior standing roentgenogram of a 30-year-old patient, showing lateral compartment degenerative changes with a 20° valgus deformity.

ments is closely related to that in normal biomechanical alignment. Ligaments should respond biologically to alterations in environment, according to Wolff's law, as bone so dramatically responds. Ligaments are composed mainly of a fine meshwork of fibrous elements (collagen, elastin, reticulin), ground substance, cells, and water. There is a complex interaction between the collagen and the surrounding ground substance, resulting in mechanical behavior considerably different from that of isolated fibrillar material. This interaction makes ligaments viscoelastic, having both time- and history-dependent properties. In addition, insertion sites of ligaments in bone are complex, with a gradual transition from collagen fibers to fibrocartilage to mineralized fibrocartilage to bone (Fig. 18-6).[13,29] Ligament fibers also directly insert into

bone without a transition site. The combination of insertion patterns may function to dissipate force and minimize insertional failures. Changes in environment (such as the fixed varus deformity of an osteoarthritic knee) may alter the ligament substance and the insertion site. No studies specifically address the biologic aspects of changes in ligaments of the knee in osteoarthritis. However, it is possible to speculate about changes based on studies of stress deprivation of insertion sites of ligament of bone.

Stress Deprivation

When immobilized, ligaments and periarticular connective tissues undergo substantial changes.[4] Although not exactly analogous, ligaments that are

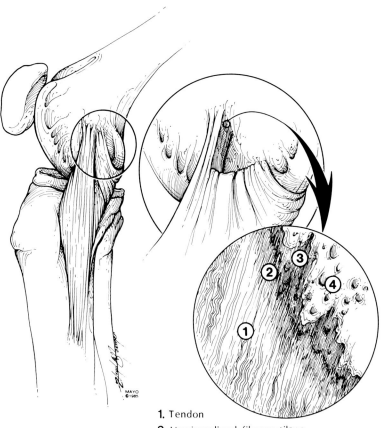

Fig. 18-6. Diagrammatic representation of the histologic features of the bone–ligament insertion site complex. (By permission of the Mayo Foundation.)

1. Tendon
2. Unmineralized fibrocartilage
3. Mineralized firbrocartilage
4. Lamellar bone

severely contracted, such as the medial soft tissues in the fixed varus deformity of an osteoarthritic knee, also may be stress-deprived.

Experimental studies have shown that stress-deprived ligaments have a dull appearance grossly and are more "woody" on palpation. Histologically, the pattern of orientation of collagen fibers is more random than the controls. The pattern of cellular alignment is also distorted, with a more random matrix orientation.[3] Other authors[39] have reported that "intercellular collagen fibers" may be decreased in thickness and numbers as the result of immobilization (collagen atrophy).

Biomechanical studies have demonstrated an increase in stiffness of the knee joint after immobilization. These changes may be due to adhesions, pannus, and decreased lubrication capacity.[42] However, the ligament substance is uniquely affected by immobility. Paradoxically, ligaments become less stiff after stress deprivation.[32,39,42] The ultimate load, stiffness, and energy-absorbing capacity are reduced to about one third of normal. These studies have suggested a qualitative "softening of the ligament substance."

The insertion sites of ligament in bone also are compromised with stress deprivation. Noyes et al.[32] reported a decrease of 39 percent in maximal failure load of the anterior cruciate ligament complex after 8 weeks of immobilization in the primate.

Many biochemical changes accompany stress deprivation, including decreased water content,[40] decreased total glycosaminoglycan content,[1,3] and increased collagen turnover.[5,10,35] These changes parallel increases in certain types of collagen cross-linking with increased synthesis.[2] There seems to be no change in collagen subtype in immobilized tissues and only a small alteration in total collagen content.[5,10,39]

Aging also may affect the properties and composition of the ligament, secondary to osteoarthritis. Many believe that periarticular tissue stiffening due to aging may alter joint motion and loading conditions, which could contribute to osteoarthritis. However, reduction of joint motion and load-bearing activities may induce ligament changes as a result of stress deprivation. Unfortunately, there are no scientific data to substantiate such hypotheses.

SURGICAL CONSIDERATIONS

Ligaments of the Knee in Osteotomy

Upper tibial osteotomy for varus and valgus deformities slows down or arrests the degenerative process by transferring weightbearing stresses to relatively normal articular cartilage. The role of the collateral ligaments in upper tibial osteotomy is important, particularly in more severe deformities.[14-16]

Varus Deformity

Because of the biomechanical alteration caused by varus deformity, the medial compartment continues to degenerate. The asymmetrical loading of the medial compartment leads to progressive loss of cartilage and bone, which results in increasing deformity. As the varus deformity increases, the lateral collateral ligament and lateral capsule are elongated, leading to progressive ligamentous instability. The increasing loss of substance of the medial bone and the resultant instability make it difficult or impossible for both condyles to articulate with the tibial plateau. This lack of dual plateau loading has been termed by Kettelkamp as the "teeter effect" and produces an unstable knee and a poor outcome.[28] The amount of ligamentous instability that contraindicates osteotomy has not been precisely defined; however, there is a correlation between instability and amount of deformity. Generally, if varus angulation is 10° or less while the patient is standing, the knee is reasonably stable and upper tibial osteotomy can be performed.[24] However, if the varus deformity exceeds 15° or if loss of medial bone exceeds about 1 cm, the resultant instability from ligamentous laxity and bone loss may preclude a satisfactory outcome after osteotomy.[24,27] Coventry[16] implies that patients with varus deformity greater than 10° should generally not undergo upper tibial osteotomy and that ligamentous laxity should be corrected by soft-tissue reefing. Slight overcorrection (3° to 5°) has been recommended for valgus osteotomy in varus knees because of the inherent varus moment (side thrust) during gait.[11,36]

In patients with severe varus deformity in whom upper tibial osteotomy cannot be performed, correction can be obtained by medial opening wedge osteotomy with iliac bone grafting or by Maquet's barrel-vault osteotomy above the tibial tubercle.[31] Another option suitable for less active patients is total knee arthroplasty.

Valgus Deformity

The development of deformity in the valgus knee is similar to that found in the varus knee: increased asymmetrical loading (this time on the lateral compartment) leading to progressive loss of cartilage and bone in the lateral compartment, which increases the valgus deformity. Secondary elongation of the MCL and soft tissues occurs with instability.

With relatively moderate valgus deformity (less than 10° to 15° excess valgus deformity), upper tibial osteotomy (with the wedge based medially) can provide adequate alignment and ligamentous stability, with an expectation of a satisfactory outcome. However, the superficial MCL and medial soft tissues are lengthened. In this situation, reefing of the medial soft-tissue structures may be required.[16]

In patients with more severe valgus, upper tibial osteotomy is less predictable.[14,16,38] Under these circumstances, the large medial wedge results in significant joint obliquity (greater than 10° to 15°). The mechanical effect will be to shift weight onto the lateral aspect of the tibial spine and not the medial compartment. Also, with the wedge based medially, the superficial collateral ligament is lengthened and thus is more unstable. During gait, the normal medial thrust of the femur during the stance phase tends to cause recurrence of the valgus deformity with weightbearing on the tibial spine. This recurrence leads to erosion of the lateral femoral condyle, followed by medial subluxation of the femur on the tibia, and finally may result in a varus deformity. For these reasons, supracondylar femoral osteotomy or total knee replacement should be considered.

In summary, upper tibial osteotomy can be performed with predictable results in mild to moderate valgus or varus deformity, because of the integrity of the soft tissues and ligamentous structures. However, with more severe deformities, results are often poor after upper tibial osteotomy. Thus, in patients with severe varus deformity, a barrel-vault osteotomy or a total knee arthroplasty may be considered, whereas supracondylar femoral osteotomy or total

knee arthroplasty is indicated in patients with severe valgus deformity.

Ligaments of the Knee in Total Joint Replacement

In patients selected for total joint replacement, ligamentous structures about the knee have an extremely important role. Early experiences with the constrained prosthesis, which does not require ligamentous support for stability, have shown unacceptable results from loosening, prosthetic breakage, and infection.[7,17,36] The results with semiconstrained surface replacement arthroplasties, which require existing ligamentous structures for stability, have been superior to those with totally constrained systems.[21,25,37] Thus, in most patients who require total knee arthroplasty, a semiconstrained prosthesis should be selected in which the existing soft-tissue structures of the knee are necessary for stability. In addition, the more anatomic the motion at the joint, the less the abnormal contact forces, which may predispose to loosening of the tibial component.

Not only are the knee ligaments essential for stability, but proper surgical management of the soft tissues around the knee also is required to attain correct alignment and ligamentous balance. Recent reports have suggested a relationship between postoperative alignment and surgical outcome. Lotke and Ecker[30] studied the relationship of knee alignment and component position to the final results in patients with geometric prostheses. They found a direct relationship between good clinical results and normal roentgenographic alignment. Johnson et al.[26] demonstrated asymmetrical loading of the knee with improper alignment, which implies that this may hasten loosening in total knee replacement. Insall et al.[23] reported the outcome of 100 condylar total knee replacements in patients with osteoarthritis after 5 to 9 years of follow-up. In that series, in both of the components that had loosened, loosening was due to the inadequate soft tissue correction of varus angulation. Ewald et al.,[18] reporting on 124 kinematic condylar total knee arthroplasties, found a direct relationship between postoperative varus angulation and roentgenographic evidence of radiolucency at the bone–cement interface 2 to 4 years after operation. Thus, reestablishing the normal anatomic alignment (defined as existing when a hypothetical straight line drawn from the center of the hip to the middle of the ankle bisects the knee joint while the patient is standing) by balancing the knee ligaments is vital to obtaining an acceptable long-lasting result.

Although most authorities acknowledge the critical role of the collateral ligamentous structures in total knee replacement, controversy exists concerning the role of the cruciate ligaments. Some authors advocate complete excision of both the anterior and the posterior cruciate ligaments (ACL and PCL) as necessary to reestablish knee alignment and to allow better visualization for placement of components.[22] Others disagree, citing the increased incidence of posterior subluxation,[18] increased stresses on the bone–cement interface,[42] and inferior range of motion in gait analysis studies[6] in knee arthroplasties with cruciate excision.

We attempt to preserve the posterior cruciate ligament if possible. The PCL is an important structure in preventing posterior subluxation. Furthermore, if the PCL is excised, forces normally absorbed and dissipated by the PCL are transmitted to the tibial component and may predispose to its loosening.[41] Although we recognize that the PCL can interfere with reestablishing normal ligamentous balance and anatomic alignment, we have found it necessary to excise completely the PCL only in knees with severe valgus or varus deformity. The ACL must be excised in most semiconstrained surface replacement procedures currently used. To date, little evidence exists to demonstrate any significant function of the anterior cruciate in semiconstrained total knee arthroplasties.

Varus Deformity

Patients with varus deformity have attenuation and lengthening of the lateral soft tissues, with the medial soft tissue structures being of normal length or contracted. Exerting a valgus stress often will demonstrate ligamentous pseudolaxity of the medial collateral ligament (the term *pseudolaxity* is used because the MCL is not lax but seems to be lax owing to loss of medial cartilage and bone). If, by valgus stressing of the knee in extension, the knee can be corrected to between 5° and 7° of valgus

during the preoperative examination, lengthening of the medial soft tissues will probably not be required. However, the deformity is more commonly fixed or only partially corrected. Under these circumstances, the surgeon must anticipate the need of medial soft tissue release to obtain anatomic alignment and balanced ligamentous tension.

To attain proper ligamentous balance, the medial soft tissues are progressively released until anatomic alignment can be obtained with similar tension on the medial and lateral ligamentous structures. Because the lateral structures are elongated, the medial soft tissues are lengthened beyond their present length. The release of the medial structures needed for realigning a varus knee is done in a sequential fashion; one must check to determine if adequate alignment and ligamentous balance have been produced after each step. The medial structures are released only enough to allow balanced ligamentous tension with the knee in anatomic alignment. To release more than necessary is not required and can lead to instability of the medial joint.

The first step to realigning the varus knee is to remove the medial osteophytes from the femoral condyle and tibial plateau; removal may include part of the medial tibial flare. After removal of the medial osteophytes, the MCL resumes a more normal position, rather than being tethered across the osteophytes of the medial joint line, and thus is effectively lengthened. This lengthening is often all that is required in knees with mild varus deformity (<10° varus).

If the knee is not properly aligned after removal of the medial osteophytes, a soft tissue sleeve is created from the medial aspect of the tibia. The soft tissue sleeve should begin anteriorly on the proximal tibia and initially include periosteum, tendons of the pes anserinus, and the deep portion of the medial collateral ligament (Fig. 18-7). In moderate varus deformities (i.e., approximately 15°), this usually will be all that is required. In more severe varus deformities, the soft tissue sleeve must be extended by subperiosteal dissection distally and posteriorly, with care taken to retain soft tissue continuity of the medial soft tissue structures. Thus, the superficial MCL and a portion of the posterior capsule will be released (Fig. 18-8). If alignment is still

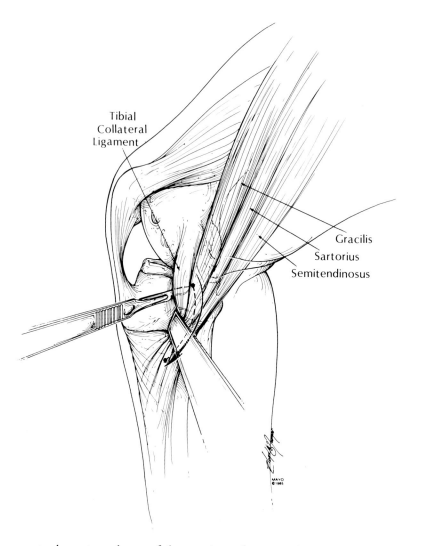

Tibial
Collateral
Ligament

Gracilis
Sartorius
Semitendinosus

Fig. 18-7. Diagrammatic representation of a medial soft tissue release, including periosteum, pes anserinus tendons, and the deep medial collateral ligament. (By permission of the Mayo Foundation.)

not adequate, release of the semimembranosus insertion and of the deep fascia that invests the soleus and popliteus muscles may be required. As mentioned earlier, the PCL should be preserved if possible. However, in severe varus deformity, partial or complete excision may be needed to achieve the necessary correction.

Stability of the collateral ligament depends on reestablishing a balanced length–tension ratio between the medial and lateral soft tissue structures. Either excessive or inadequate release of the soft tissue will result in malalignment with asymmetrical component loading, which may affect the long-term survivability of the prosthesis. Thus, at the end of medial soft-tissue release, the knee must be ana-

tomically aligned, which usually results in 5° to 7° of valgus alignment.

In some patients a 6-foot-long radiograph, including all joints of the lower extremity, is required to achieve desirable joint orientation and ligament alignment.

Valgus Deformity

Although the principles for correcting a valgus deformity are similar to those for correcting a varus deformity, for anatomic reasons the contracted lateral structures in valgus deformity are released proximally from the femur. Again, preoperative examination will give the surgeon an indication as to the amount of soft tissue release required. Deformi-

Fig. 18-8. Diagrammatic representation of an extensive release of the medial soft tissue, including the posterior capsule and the superficial medial collateral ligament. (By permission of the Mayo Foundation.)

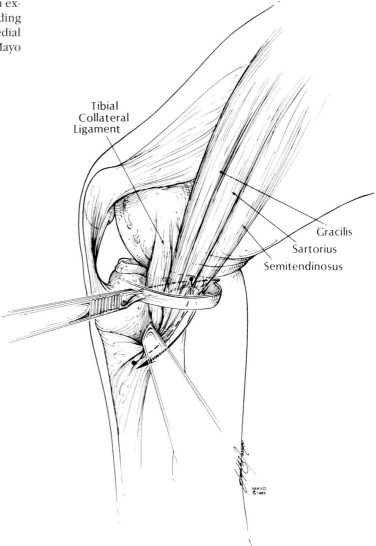

Tibial Collateral Ligament

Gracilis

Sartorius

Semitendinosus

ties that can be corrected with a varus stress when the knee is in extension will require little or no release (usually less than 5° to 7° valgus deformity), whereas those that are fixed or with severe deformity require extensive release.

As with the varus correction, the contracted soft tissues are progressively lengthened in a sequential stepwise fashion, with the alignment being checked after each step. The release is begun by removing the lateral osteophytes from the femoral condyle and lateral tibial plateau. In mild deformities, this may be all that is required. If complete correction is not attained, the iliotibial band is resected 6 to 10 cm above the joint line, which helps to correct any associated external rotation deformity in addition to valgus deformity (Fig. 18-9). At the level of the lateral femoral condyle, the lateral and posterolateral capsule is reflected, and the lateral collateral ligament and popliteus tendon elevated subperiosteally or with a small portion of bone. Usually, the knee can be corrected and balanced with this amount of lateral release. If sufficient alignment cannot be achieved, the lateral head of the gastrocnemius sometimes needs to be released. If more

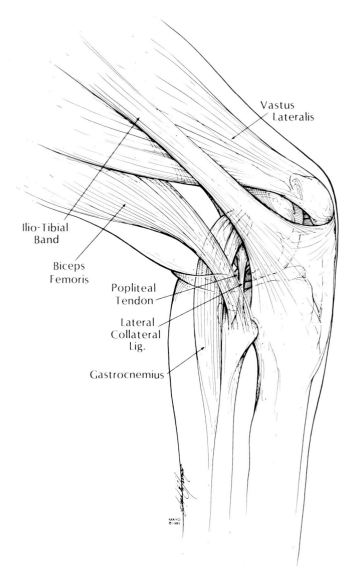

Fig. 18-9. Diagrammatic representation of the lateral aspect of the knee, showing the anatomic structures that may need to be released. (By permission of the Mayo Foundation.)

Vastus Lateralis

Ilio-Tibial Band

Biceps Femoris

Popliteal Tendon

Lateral Collateral Lig.

Gastrocnemius

correction is required, partial or complete division of the biceps femoris can be done.

Several points should be remembered with regard to the PCL in patients with valgus deformity. The PCL can inhibit correction and may need to be released or, in severe deformity, completely excised. When the cruciates are excised and the lateral soft tissues released, a tendency toward posterolateral rotatory instability exists. Although healing of the lateral capsule usually provides stability, one should never rely on scarring to provide stability. If

excision of the posterior cruciate is necessary at surgical correction with lateral release, a prosthesis that provides posterior stabilization should be utilized.

After lateral release, realignment of the patella is often necessary. This can be accomplished by releasing the lateral patellar retinaculum. However, in so doing, the inferior and superior lateral geniculate arteries are violated, which interferes with blood flow to the patella and may promote avascular necrosis. Also, after patellar realignment and lateral retinacular release, subcutaneous tissue and skin provide the only soft tissue coverage for the prosthesis. Thus, if a problem occurs with wound healing, the prosthesis is extremely vulnerable. For these reasons, we prefer to achieve patellar realignment by releasing the interval between the iliotibial band and the biceps femoris. This release allows for preservation of the inferior lateral genicular artery and for more adequate soft tissue coverage.

Flexion Contracture

Most flexion contractures will be corrected by resection of the distal femur and tibial plateau. However, with more severe contractures (generally 40° or more), posterior capsulotomy may be necessary. This can be performed by placing vertical incisions in the posterolateral and posteromedial corners, which can be done safely because there are no important structures nearby. A curved hemostat can be passed within the popliteal fat behind the posterior capsule and the posterior capsule can be cut transversely, thus protecting the posterior neurovascular structures. The posterior capsule is divided from one vertical incision to the other. Posterior capsulotomy should be carried out only after the distal femoral and proximal tibial cuts have been performed. To prevent the recurrence of flexion contractures after operation, early motion should begin immediately, with stress put on the importance of full extension, or the knee should be splinted in full extension.

In summary, constrained prostheses that substitute for ligamentous stability generally have been associated with unacceptable results and their use is rarely indicated. Semiconstrained surface replacement prostheses have given superior results and are indicated for most patients undergoing total knee replacement. However, semiconstrained surface replacement prostheses rely on preexisting ligamentous structures for stability, and the long-term functional result depends on reestablishing anatomic alignment, which requires ligamentous balance. Thus, in total knee arthroplasty the surgeon must have knowledge of the soft tissue techniques designed to correct angular deformities and attain ligamentous balance. Only by proper surgical management of the ligamentous and soft tissues about the knee will normal alignment and motion be restored

with sufficient stability to achieve optimal results in most total knee replacements.

CONCLUSION

The ligaments of the knee have an important role in deformity of the knee in osteoarthritis. The pathologic changes (contracture and attenuation) are secondary to changes in the bone and articular cartilage. If information on the biologic aspects of knee ligaments can be extrapolated from the work on stress deprivation of knee ligaments, histologic and biochemical alterations must occur in the knee ligaments in osteoarthritis because of the altered mechanics of the knee.

The importance of correcting the secondary imbalance of the major knee ligaments in reconstructive surgery of the knee cannot be overemphasized.

REFERENCES

1. Akeson WH, Amiel D, LaViolette D: The connective-tissue response to immobility: a study of the chondroitin-4 and 6-sulfate and dermatan sulfate changes in periarticular connective tissue of control and immobilized knees of dogs. Clin Orthop 51:183–197, 1967
2. Akeson WH, Amiel D, Mechanic GL: Collagen cross-linking alterations in joint contractures: changes in the reducible cross-links in periarticular connective tissue collagen after nine weeks of immobilization. Connect Tissue Res 5:15–19, 1977
3. Akeson WH, Woo SL-Y, Amiel D et al: The connective tissue response to immobility: biochemical changes in periarticular connective tissue of the immobilized rabbit knee. Clin Orthop 93:356–362, 1973
4. Akeson WH, Woo SL-Y, Amiel D, Frank CB: The biology of ligaments. pp. 93–148. In Hunter L, Funk FJ Jr. Rehabilitation of the Injured Knee. St Louis: CV Mosby, 1984
5. Amiel D, Woo SL-Y, Harwood FL, Akeson WH: The effect of immobilization on collagen turnover in connective tissue: a biochemical-biomechanical correlation. Acta Orthop Scand 53:325–332, 1982
6. Andriacchi TP, Galante JO, Fermier RW: The influence of total knee-replacement design on walking and stair-climbing. J Bone Joint Surg 64A:1328–1335, 1982

7. Bargar WL, Cracchiolo A, Amstutz HC: Results with the constrained total knee prosthesis in treating severely disabled patients and patients with failed total knee replacements. J Bone Joint Surg 62A:504–512, 1980

8. Brandt KD: Osteoarthritis: clinical patterns and pathology. pp. 1432–1448. In Kelley WN, Harris ED Jr, Rudy S, Sledge CB (eds): Textbook of Rheumatology, ed. 2. WB Saunders, Philadelphia, 1985

9. Brandt KD: Pathogenesis of osteoarthritis. pp. 1417–1431. In Kelley WN, Harris ED Jr, Rudy S, Sledge CB (eds): Textbook of Rheumatology, ed. 2. WB Saunders, Philadelphia, 1985

10. Brooke JW, Slack HGB: Metabolism of connective tissue in limb atrophy in the rabbit. Ann Rheum Dis 18:129–136, 1959

11. Chao EY: Biomechanics of high tibial osteotomy. pp. 143–160. In Reconstructive Surgery of the Knee. AAOS Symposium. CV Mosby, St Louis, 1978

12. CIOMS: The epidemiology of chronic rheumatism. p. 10. In Atlas of Standard Radiographs of Arthritis, vol. 2. Blackwell Press, Oxford, 1963

13. Cooper RR, Misol S: Tendon and ligament insertion: a light and electron microscopic study. J Bone Joint Surg 52A:1–20; 170, 1970

14. Coventry MB: Osteotomy of the upper portion of the tibia for degenerative arthritis of the knee: a preliminary report. J Bone Joint Surg 47A:984–990, 1965

15. Coventry MB: Stepped staple for upper tibial osteotomy. J Bone Joint Surg 51A:1011, 1969 (brief note)

16. Coventry MB: Osteotomy about the knee for degenerative and rheumatoid arthritis: indications, operative technique and results. J Bone Joint Surg 55A:23–48, 1973

17. Deburge A, Guepar: Guepar hinge prosthesis: complications and results with two years' follow-up. Clin Orthop 120:47–53, 1976

18. Ewald FC, Jacobs MA, Miegel RE et al: Kinematic total knee replacement. J Bone Joint Surg 66A:1032–1040, 1984

19. Forman MD, Malamet R, Kaplan D: A survey of osteoarthritis of the knee in the elderly. J Rheumatol 10:282–287, 1983

20. Freeman MAR: Surgical pathology of arthritis. p. 505. In Insall J (ed): Surgery of the Knee. Churchill Livingstone, New York, 1984

21. Hui FC, Fitzgerald RH Jr: Hinged total knee arthroplasty. J Bone Joint Surg 62A:513–519, 1980

22. Insall JN: Technique of total knee replacement. Instr Course Lect 30:324–341, 1981

23. Insall JN, Hood RW, Flawn LB, Sullivan DJ: The total condylar knee prosthesis in gonarthrosis. J Bone Joint Surg 65A:619–628, 1983

24. Insall JN, Joseph DM, Msika C: High tibial osteotomy for varus gonarthrosis. J Bone Joint Surg 66A:1040–1048, 1984

25. Insall J, Scott WN, Ranawat CS: The total condylar knee prosthesis: A report of two hundred and twenty cases. J Bone Joint Surg 61A:173–180, 1979

26. Johnson F, Leitl S, Waugh W: The distribution of load across the knee: a comparison of static and dynamic measurements. J Bone Joint Surg 62B:346–349, 1980

27. Kettelkamp DB: Tibial osteotomy. pp. 249–265. In Evarts CM (ed): Surgery of the Musculoskeletal System, vol. 3. Churchill Livingstone, New York, 1983

28. Kettelkamp DB, Leach RE, Nasca R: Pitfalls of proximal tibial osteotomy. Clin Orthop 106:232–241, 1975

29. Laros GS, Tipton CM, Cooper RR: Influence of physical activity on ligament insertions in the knees of dogs. J Bone Joint Surg 53A:275–286, 1971

30. Lotke PA, Ecker ML: Influence of positioning of prosthesis in total knee replacement. J Bone Joint Surg 59A:77–79, 1977

31. Maquet PGJ: Biomechanics of the Knee. Springer-Verlag, New York, 1976

32. Noyes FR, DeLucas, JL, Torvik PJ: Biomechanics of anterior cruciate ligament failure: an analysis of strain-rate sensitivity and mechanisms of failure in primates. J Bone Joint Surg 56A:236–253, 1974

33. Noyes FR, Grood ES, Butler DL, Paulos LE: Clinical biomechanics of the knee—ligament restraints and functional stability. pp. 1–35. In Funk FJ Jr (ed): American Academy of Orthopaedic Surgeons: Symposium on the Athlete's Knee: Surgical Repair and Reconstruction. CV Mosby, St Louis, 1980

34. Palmer I: On the injuries to the ligaments of the knee joint: A clinical study. Acta Chir Scand Suppl 53:1–282, 1938

35. Peacock EE Jr: Comparison of collagenous tissue surrounding normal and immobilized joints. Surg Forum 14:440–443, 1963

36. Prodromos CC, Andriacchi TP, Galante JO: A relationship between knee joint loads and clinical changes following high tibial osteotomy. Trans. 31st Orthop Res Soc Meeting, Las Vegas, 1985, p. 282

37. Scott WN (ed): Symposium on total knee arthroplasty. Orthop Clin North Am 13:1–252, 1982

38. Shoji H, Insall J: High tibial osteotomy for osteoarthritis of the knee with valgus deformity. J Bone Joint Surg 55A:963–973, 1973

39. Tipton CM, Matthes RD, Maynard JA, Carey RA: The influence of physical activity on ligaments and tendons. Med Sci Sports Exerc 7:165–175, 1975

40. Tipton CM, Tomanek RJ: Influence of physical activity on the strength of knee ligaments in rats. Am J Physiol 212:783–787, 1967
41. Walker PS, Greene D, Reilly D et al: Fixation of tibial components of knee prostheses. J Bone Joint Surg 63A:258–267, 1981
42. Woo SL-Y, Matthews JV, Akeson WH et al: Connective tissue response to immobility: correlative study of biomechanical and biochemical measurements of normal and immobilized rabbit knees. Arthritis Rheum 18:257–264, 1975

19

Osteoarthritis in the ACL-Deficient Knee

MARY A. LYNCH
CHARLES E. HENNING

The controversy continues over the relationship between osteoarthritis and the anterior cruciate ligament (ACL)-deficient knee. Cox[2] showed that the knee of dogs suffers deleterious effects after removal of the cartilage. Likewise, the Iowa series conducted by Johnson et al.[4] also showed roentgenographic evidence of osteoarthritis in patients with meniscectomy. However, the specific relationship of isolated tears of the anterior cruciate in a large group had not been examined until we conducted a retrospective study.[5] We compared the relationship of the chronic ACL-deficient knee, and its associated sequelae, to the incidence of osteoarthritis.

Our criteria for determining the presence of osteoarthritis were based on those set forth in 1948 by Fairbank.[3] These included flattening, narrowing, ridging, and combinations of these (Fig. 19-1).

The database was designed to provide demographic data (including previous surgical procedures to the knee), results of physical examination, standing roentgenographic findings, subjective and objective functional ratings, comparisons to the uninvolved side, and arthroscopic findings.

In this chapter we summarize our findings. The natural history is clear. *Degenerative osteoarthritis in the ACL-deficient knee is inevitable. The only real variable is the rate at which it will occur. The incidence correlates directly with the treatment of the meniscus.*

ANALYSIS OF DATABASE

Study Population

Between 1971 and 1985, a total of 1,081 patients with chronic ACL-deficient knees were evaluated using 198 comparative values. The data were collected and evaluated by multivariant statistical analyses.

The patients ranged in age from 14 to 65 years with an average age of 24.6 years (Table 19-1). Of these patients, 1,045 underwent surgery for reconstruction of the ACL. These procedures were done by the same surgeon (CEH). The data for analysis included the arthroscopic information as a part of the database.

The population incurred the primary ACL injury in sports-related incidents in 96 percent of cases. The time from injury to evaluation ranged from 3 months to 36 years with an average of 5 years and 2 months. Nineteen percent (205 knees) had histories of undergoing one or more surgical procedures (Table 19-2).

Demographic Data

Demographically there were 53 percent (573) men and 47 percent (508) women, with a larger proportion of the women in the 30 to 34-year age group (Table 19-1). Patients with an average body weight greater than 20 percent above the ideal (compared

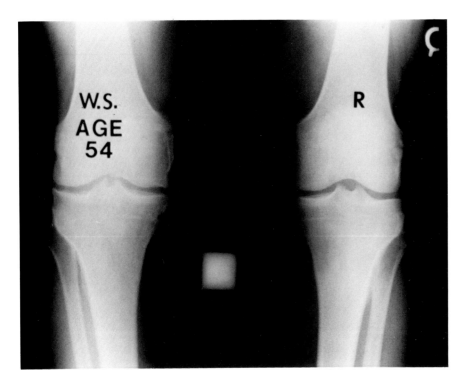

Fig. 19-1. A 54-year-old man 36 years from the time of injury to his left ACL-deficient knee, with no prior surgery. He shows ridging, flattening, and narrowing as well as hypertrophic lipping.

to the Metropolitan Life tables, January 1985) showed an increased incidence of Fairbank changes regardless of age or sex (Fig. 19-2, Table 19-3). The number of years they had been overweight and the level of activity likewise correlated with an increased incidence of Fairbank changes (Fig. 19-3, Table 19-3).

Physical Examination

We measured stability objectively by the Lachman test, pivot shift, anterior Drawer, including medial and lateral as well as straight medial and lateral sta-

bility (Table 19-4). No correlation was detected between laxity and the number of Fairbank changes, nor was a significant correlation found between laxity and associated meniscus damage (Table 19-4).

The mechanism of injury predominantly involved one or several forms of deceleration: one-step, vertical, and often an associated rotational component (Table 19-5). We found no significant correlation between mechanism of injury and the presence or absence of osteoarthritis. Patients with a history of locking (195 patients [23 percent] with documented tear) showed a higher correlation with the presence of osteoarthritis than those who did not have a history of locking.

Table 19-1. Summary of Patient Population[a]

	Age (years) at Time of Injury						Total No.	%
	<15	15–19	20–24	25–29	30–34	>35		
Male	45	358	113	76	40	9	641	59
Female	20	193	98	32	90	7	440	40
Total	65	551	211	108	130	16	1081	100
%	6	51	19.5	10	12	1.5	100	100

[a] Patients ranged in age from 14 to 65 years (average age, 24.6 years). All were treated 3 months or more after the time of injury.

Table 19-2. Summary of Previous Surgical Procedures[a]

Procedures	No.
Medial meniscectomy	28
Lateral meniscectomy	24
Medial and lateral meniscectomy	11
Medial collateral ligament repair	17
ACL repair	9
ACL debridement	14
PCL repair	3
Shaving articular surfaces	2
Combination of above	97
Total	205

[a] Procedures performed before this evaluation.

Roentgenographic Findings

Roentgenographically, 35.2 percent of the ACL-deficient knees had two or more Fairbank changes. These include the group who had undergone meniscectomies. Of those ACL-deficient knees that had no previous surgery and had both menisci intact, only 3 percent had two or more Fairbank changes. In those knees with one or more meniscal tears but no removal of meniscal substance, 7 percent had two or more Fairbank changes (Fig. 19-4, Table 19-6).

Standing roentgenograms showed a statistically significant correlation between the incidence of Fairbank changes and the presence or absence of the meniscus. However, no correlation existed between those with an absent ACL and those with a nonfunctional band. The type of meniscus tear, likewise, did not correlate well with the incidence of osteoarthritis except in those patients with longitudinal tears with broken handles, with marked degenerative tears in which pieces were absent, or with partial or total meniscectomy. Those patients with osteoarthritis evident on the tibial and femoral surfaces had a high incidence of chondromalacia. The presence of chondromalacia directly correlated with the state of the meniscus and did not correlate with stability or the presence or absence of a nonfunctional ACL.

Subjective and Objective Functional Ratings

Ninety-two percent of those patients with objective and subjective ratings of two or fewer Fairbank changes rated their knees worse than those with

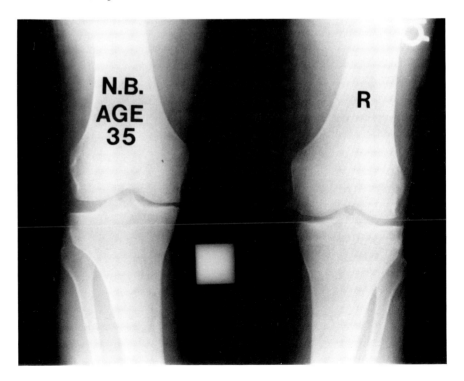

Fig. 19-2. This 35-year-old man was 7 years from injury (no prior surgery) but was 10 percent overweight. He was sedentary with an activity level of 0, and had had no giving way events after his initial injury.

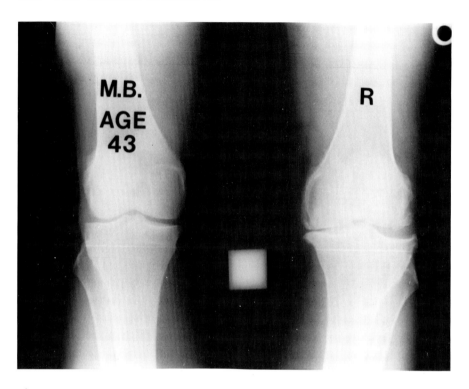

Fig. 19-3. This 43-year-old man had previously had a right medial meniscectomy and was 14 years from the time of injury. He had continued level 3 to 4 activity for 7 years after injury. His present activity level is 0. He had been at ideal weight for all 14 years, but finds it difficult to maintain.

three or more changes. When these data were analyzed for activity level, patients with three or more changes showed an activity rating of 80 percent less than those with two or fewer Fairbank changes. The latter group of patients were still attempting activities at a lower athletic level than the level at which they had been previously participating. The use of a brace did not correlate statistically with the degree of osteoarthritis. Braces did, however, correlate with fewer episodes of giving way. Of all the chronic ACL-deficient knees we evaluated, 26 percent had associated contralateral ACL deficiencies. Forty of those persons wearing braces, including derotation

braces, who returned to sports participation showed an increase in bilateral knee involvement (from 26 to 43 percent) (Fig. 19-5).

The type of associated meniscus tear was not as relevant as the surgical intervention for partial or total meniscectomy. Ninety-three percent of patients with partial meniscectomy and 97 percent of those with total meniscectomy had some chondromalacia. These values were only slightly affected by stability and activity level. Those knees with meniscus tears but no history of meniscectomy or arthroscopic procedure had one-third the incidence of chondromalacia and only one-sixth the incidence of

Table 19-3.   Weight and Level of Activity: Correlation with Fairbank Changes[a]

Weight Distribution	Population		Fairbank Changes			Activity Level 0–4
	% (no.)	Years	None	1	≥2	
Ideal weight	27% (292)	7	98% (286)	0	2% (6)	Average 2 (range 0–4)
<10% overweight	49% (530)	3	62% (329)	9% (48)	29% (153)	Average 2 (range 0–4)
≥20% overweight	24% (259)	7.7	7% (18)	36% (93)	57% (148)	Average 1 (Range 0–3)

[a] Weight distribution and the average number of years at that weight was calculated for each patient. The results were compared to the Metropolitan Life tables, 1985. Activity level was 0–4, with 0 being no activity, 1 minimal activity, 2 average activity, 3 moderate activity including recreational sports, and 4 very active.

Table 19-4. Evaluation of Stability (Percentage of Population)[a]

Positive	Activity Levels 2–4	Fairbank Changes		
		None	1	≥ 2
Lachman	99	99	99	99
Pivot shift	77	28	81	88
Anterior Drawer	84	2	24	89
Anteromedial rotatory	78	4	24	84
Anterolateral rotatory	57	0	12	67
Posterior Drawer	1	0	0.5	0.5

[a] Stability was measured in terms of the following tests: Lachman, pivot shift, anterior Drawer, anteromedial and lateral rotatory instability.

Table 19-5. Mechanism of Injury[a]

Mechanism	Percentage of Population
Valgus	14.0
Deceleration cut-from	12.5
Vertical deceleration–hyperextension	7.7
Valgus external rotation	7.3
Hyperextension	9.3
Unknown	4.4
Deceleration–external rotation	4.0
Combination—deceleration or extension	64.1

[a] Mechanism of injury was predominantly deceleration combined with a rotational component.

osteoarthritis. The values were actually less than in those with no meniscus tears but with a deficient cruciate. When activity and weight were evaluated, those without meniscus tears were less active but had slightly higher weight compared to those who weighed less and were more active. The latter group also had a larger number of meniscus tears and episodes of giving way.

Arthroscopic Findings

At arthroscopy, 81 percent (847) of all patients had tears or a history of treatment for one or more menisci in conjunction with the ACL deficiency. Of the 1,045 knees viewed arthroscopically, 79 percent (826) had an absent ACL while the remainder had only a fibrous band that would not tighten on loading.

Fig. 19-4. This 27-year-old woman was 14 years from the time of her ACL/MCL tear. At surgery she had double bucket handle tears and some degenerative tears of both menisci. No Fairbank changes were noted. She has had a 0 activity level.

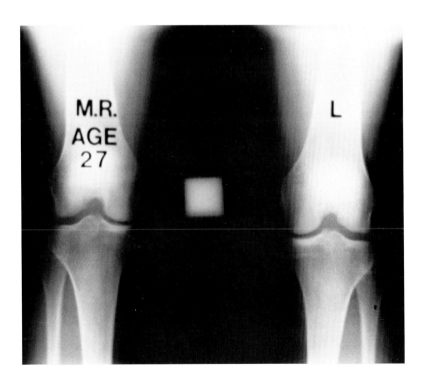

Table 19-6. Meniscus Damage at Time of Arthroscopy[a]

Prior Treatment of Menisci	No. of Patients	Fairbank Changes		
		None	1	≥2
Prior surgery with removal of meniscal tissue	157	0	1% (16)	99% (141)
No prior surgery; meniscal tears present	847	77% (620)	16% (167)	7% (60)
No prior surgery; no meniscal tears	198	97% (172)	1% (20)	3% (6)

[a] The state of meniscus damage at time of surgery. This is based on 1,045 who underwent arthroscopy.

PERSPECTIVE ON FACTORS ASSOCIATED WITH OSTEOARTHRITIS

Menisci

McDaniel and Dameron[6] noted that more than 80 percent of the patients they studied had been treated by meniscectomy. These patients were unable to pursue lateral sports. Those in this series[6] who were unable to alter their lifestyles by limiting activity dramatically ultimately faced the prospect of surgical reconstruction. *Besides providing the obvious stability, the purpose of reconstruction must be primarily to restore the ability of the ACL to preserve the meniscus.* Failure to provide functional menisci is failure to prevent osteoarthritis despite reestablishment of stability.

Casscells[1] demonstrated that degenerative menisci did not cause degeneration of the joint surfaces. Even with a chronic ACL-deficient knee, the degenerating menisci still distribute some load. These knees are far better than those treated with partial or total meniscectomy. It is better to repair and create a stable degenerative meniscus out of an unstable degenerative meniscus than to do even a partial meniscectomy. The results are improved stability and longevity of the knee.

The appearance of osteoarthritis was directly related to the inability of the ACL-deficient knee to protect the meniscus, which is directly responsible for the protection of the joint surfaces.

Weight, Level of Activity, Time

We were not able to correlate symptoms of osteoarthritis with the number or degree of Fairbank changes. The importance of Fairbank changes is that

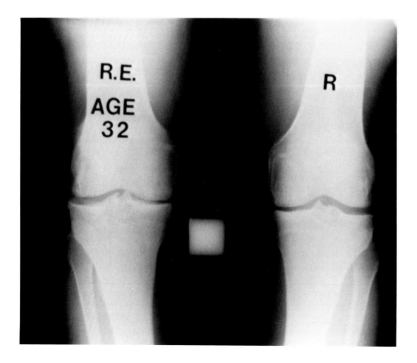

Fig. 19-5. This 32-year-old man had had a deficient right ACL for 9 years but continued running and playing vigorous sports with a right derotation brace. It is 4 years since he tore his left ACL, which shows a greater degree of Fairbank changes. His weight is ideal and he had, through activity, performed his own automeniscectomy on the left.

they are the hallmark of a unidirectional process that ultimately leads to osteoarthritis. The rate of these changes is affected by weight, level of activity, and the number of years of instability. With time, patients seem to be able to decrease episodes of giving way by altering their mechanics and lifestyle. The progression of meniscus damage appears to be relentless. It is affected by all of these factors — weight, activity, and years of instability — regardless of the number of episodes of giving way. Controlling instability with a brace did nothing to change the natural history. All the tears significant enough to lock the knee, regardless of type of tear, would have had more significant chondromalacia and Fairbank changes if locking episodes had recurred with any frequency.

Bracing the knees improved the patient's sense of well-being but seemed to give a false sense of confidence. The evidence showed that the incidence of bilateral knee involvement doubled. This observation generates sincere concern in those individuals returning to sport with a brace. An individual with an ACL-deficient knee must know his or her limitations and abide by them.

COMMENTS

Although the time range in our studies (from time of injury to diagnosis) was 36 years, the average time was only slightly over 5 years. Even with this relatively brief time of instability, more than one-third of this young population had Fairbank changes. These changes did not correlate with the degree of instability-associated secondary ligament damage or the presence or absence of the nonfunctional ACL band.

The natural history of osteoarthritis in the ACL-deficient knee is clear. The only real variable is the rate at which degenerative osteoarthritis occurs. *Although 19 percent of the patients had no damage to their menisci, without an exception this was the group who restricted their lifestyle, kept an ideal weight, and pursued no other sports or recreational activity.* When symptoms in this group did appear, they were as often associated with the unaffected knee as with the ACL-deficient knee.

The development of osteoarthritis in the ACL-deficient knee is an insidious event that directly corre-

lates with the treatment of the meniscus. In the ACL-deficient knee, *no* surgical procedure is usually better than partial meniscectomy, either as an open procedure or an arthroscopic procedure. Repair of the meniscus along with a well-performed isometric ACL reconstruction offers the only chance to redirect and, in fact, to change the natural history.[5] The meniscus must be salvaged whenever possible. Meniscal transplantation may become a key surgical procedure in the next decade.

SUMMARY

We have summarized our analysis of the data base of accumulated findings from 1,081 patients with chronic ACL-deficient knees. The patients ranged in age from 14 to 65 years (average, 24.6 years). The demographic data, physical examination and roentgenographic findings, and arthroscopic studies revealed that osteoarthritis was directly related to the inability of the ACL-deficient knee to protect the meniscus. The progression of meniscal damage appears to be directly related to weight, activity, and years of instability. Repair of the meniscus, along with a well-performed isometric ACL reconstruction, offers the only chance to redirect and change the natural history.[5]

REFERENCES

1. Casscells SW: Arthroscopic and cadaver knee investigations. pp. 122–141. In Symposium on Arthroscopy and Arthrography of the Knee. American Academy of Orthopaedic Surgeons. CV Mosby, St. Louis, 1978
2. Cox JS: The degenerative effects of medial meniscus tears in dogs' knees. Clin Orthop 125:236–242, 1977
3. Fairbank TJ: Knee joint changes after meniscectomy. J Bone Joint Surg 30B:664–670, 1948
4. Johnson RJ, Kettelcamp DB, Clark W, Leaverton P: Factors affecting late results after meniscectomy. J Bone Joint Surg 56A:719–729, 1974
5. Lynch MA, Henning CE, Glick KR: Knee joint surface changes. Long-term follow-up meniscus tear treatment in stable anterior cruciate ligament reconstruction. Clin Orthop 172:148–153, 1983
6. McDaniel WJ, Dameron TB: Untreated ruptures of the anterior cruciate ligament. J Bone Joint Surg 62A:696–705, 1980

SURGICAL
TREATMENT

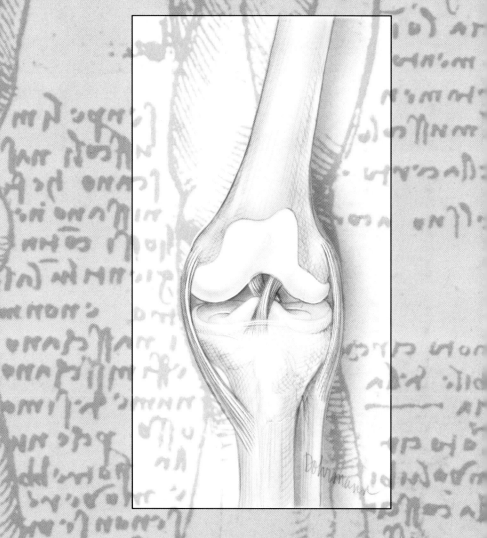

20

Surgical Treatment of Cruciate Ligament Injuries: Present Techniques, Future Technology

The Unstable Knee

KENNETH G. JONES

The knee of an active patient that has a deficiency of one or both cruciate ligaments is, and will remain, an unstable knee until surgically corrected.

The instruments, materials, and techniques today's knee surgeon can apply to solving his or her patient's problem have increased exponentially during the past two decades. Expanding technology augurs for developments in this area that will continue beyond our limited perspective. Though we have welcomed this augmentation of our accoutrements for repair and for salvage, surgeons have been presented with few cogent arguments for modification of their concepts of the pathomechanics affecting the abnormal knee joint and of the treatment. Total replacement for the advanced arthritic knee and acceptance of the superiority of a partial meniscectomy to total meniscectomy which has been too often performed as a reflex, are the most significant of the recently altered concepts in management of the disabled knee. The contribution of the menisci (even a partial meniscus) to the total stability of the knee is now, happily, more widely appreciated. Although those structures, like all tissues that constitute the knee, must make some contribution to its

stability, in the presence of normal osseous structures, the ligaments are, of course, recognized as the primary contributors to its stability. The performing surgeons and their trappings have changed, but the scenario of "the unstable knee" continues to be unchanged.

Selective systematic transection of the capsule, collateral, cruciate, and patellar knee ligaments by an investigator will demonstrate varied patterns of instability (as many as 16 patterns have been described!) when that knee is stressed by hand or by a machine. The application of various stresses by the examiner to a patient's injured knee may convince the surgeon that one or more of the supporting ligaments are functionally deficient. Though specific knowledge is helpful, when correct, it is much more imperative that the evaluating surgeon appreciate the presence of "true" (pathologic) instability, irrespective of which ligament or ligaments may be torn. How the taxonomist may choose to classify "instability patterns" has considerably less importance. Furthermore, the surgeon must possess the dedication to initiate totally corrective measures. Anything less will not serve the best interest of his or her active patient. Physicians need to recognize and respond to the truism that in active patients, only limited ligamentous sprains in "stable knees" can be managed successfully nonsurgically. If the surgeon cannot be satisfied (by clinical evaluation and the other diagnostic means available) of the soundness of the knee ligaments, surgery for purposes of investigation and correction of the demonstrated pathology is indicated for the recently injured knee in active patients. Seldom, if ever, will the concerned, knowledgeable, capable surgeon have reason to regret this approach. That same surgeon should experience little difficulty reconstructing a recently torn capsule or damaged collateral ligaments. Results from these undertakings should be successful routinely.

Recently torn cruciate ligaments present a greater challenge, but repair of these structures is also technically feasible for the adequately prepared surgeon. In the presence of continuing instability, degenerative changes of that knee are inescapable as a consequence of it having acquired the abnormal motion of "grinding." The unstable knee physiologically functions as a mortar and pestle. The inevitable results will, in time, be devastating. Menisci (which may have been undamaged initially), articular cartilage, synovia, capsule, ligaments, and even bone all become "grist" for the "mill of the unstable knee." Again, the initial surgeon will command the best opportunity to alter this preprogrammed sequential pattern of destruction of the significantly injured knee. He may prevent tragedy, or he will become a participant in it. Unfortunately, the reconstructive surgeon who may in time see an incompletely surgically treated or a surgically failed unstable knee is never privileged to the opportunity of repair. She is presented only with an opportunity to obtain *maximum salvage*. Salvage cannot be as rewarding for the patient or for the surgeon as an adequate initial repair.

Sutured tendons isolated within a synthetic membrane to prevent potential cellular ingrowth and then placed in the knee joint of laboratory animals where they are nourished only by the synovial fluid have shown that they routinely heal soundly. This investigative information, added to our clinical experience, should permanently lay to rest the curious/spurious assumption that tendons and ligaments within joints do not heal. Also, as has ever been obvious, torn intraarticular ligaments that are repaired are much more likely to heal and to provide stability than intraarticular ligaments left unrepaired.

Failure to repair an acutely torn cruciate ligament is no longer an acceptable alternative. Repair of all acutely torn knee ligaments for an active patient must be the surgeon's objective. Even though, in some knees, best efforts may achieve less than total (preinjury) stability, the surgeon remains obligated to pursue that goal, since many extensively damaged knees, having torn cruciate ligaments in addition to torn collateral ligaments, can obtain an excellent result following an adequate total repair. While we seem destined to be denied the luxury of absolute predictability of the final result in an individual patient, prognosticating guidelines do exist. As observed, adequately repaired collateral ligaments do well as a group as do cruciate ligaments that have been avulsed with an attached bone fragment from the femur or from the tibia if the block is resecured within the bed from which it was avulsed.

It is true that mop-head tears through the substance of the cruciate ligaments do less well, but meticulous suture that does not compromise the diameter of the ligament can, in many instances, yield good and even excellent results. These repairs can be initially supplemented by an overlay of fibroelastic tissue derived from the posterior aspect of the patellar ligament, or from any convenient fascial donor site if the surgeon is less than totally satisfied with the suture. Recognition of a deficient cruciate ligament by an operating physician and acceptance of that deficiency should be considered an option only under unusual circumstances. The active patient deserves better. Surgical treatment of the acutely injured knee must be instituted with total repair as the objective. The fact that we may never secure absolute stability for every patient with torn cruciate ligaments is not a logical argument against initial repair of those structures. Patients whose torn ligaments are repaired initially are given the maximum opportunity for recovery of knee stability. This is not true for those patients whose torn cruciate ligaments are left unrepaired. Methods and techniques of repair, old and new, are options for the operating surgeon.

We need to take cognizance that the arthroscope has not changed the patient's needs, although regrettably it seems to have altered some surgeons' concept of the problem. Before the advent of the arthroscope, a sound clinical approach to the situation was initiated when the surgeon recognized "an internal derangement" of the knee and then entered the knee, usually through a medial utility incision to effect a total repair, including all damaged ligaments. This still remains an acceptable approach to management when the surgeon is confronted with an unequivocal ligamentous deficiency. With the arthroscope, however, he or she can gain additional knowledge through limited surgery and, in some instances, complete surgical correction may be possible by this limited surgical approach. However, surgeons who would prefer to restrict their exertions to procedures that can be done conveniently through the arthroscope are not relieved of their obligation of early repair of all torn knee ligaments, collateral and cruciate. Diagnosis only establishes the imperative for proper treatment. A confirmed diagnosis followed by failure to repair will be little solace to the unhappy patient left with a "mortar and pestle knee."

To inform the patient that she or he has a torn cruciate ligament and that, since not all cruciate ligament repairs are successful, a repair was not attempted, does not fulfill the surgeon's obligation as physician for an active patient. As observed, techniques and methods are options for the surgeon, but failure to repair is not! Each patient deserves a chance for repair by way of the arthroscope, should this become technically feasible for the surgeon, or through a more extensive exposure that is still feasible and that may remain the most practical means for most surgeons. No matter how our techniques may change, a knee with a deficient cruciate ligament will continue to be an unstable knee! The dynamics of the abnormal grinding motion will destroy that knee by attrition. The athlete who continues to perform expedites this destruction. For that reason (not because this is my opinion), failure to repair acutely torn ligaments of the knee in active patients cannot be an acceptable option for the arthroscopic operator. The surgeon who elects that escape route may no longer be acceptable as a surgeon. He or she is obligated to learn how to repair all of the knee ligaments and to perform these exertions routinely or to withdraw from the arena. It seems superfluous to observe that in addition he or she must be prepared to and willing to supervise an adequate program of rehabilitation.

For those patients who have been neglected and for those who failed to obtain a satisfactory result from their initial repair, substitution procedures have been demonstrated to be valuable adjuncts to the problem of management of "the unstable knee." Substitution for the deficient stabilizing ligament would seem to be the most reasonable approach if that knee is still salvageable.

The need to provide stability for the pathologic unstable knee remains unchanged notwithstanding recent great technical progress.

The Knee: Joint of Necessity

JOHN A. FEAGIN, JR.

Problems left unattended within the knee do not become easier with the passage of time . . . Technology is an essential adjunct to our surgical management of the knee. Today we are appropriately selective in our choice of techniques; tomorrow we must be prepared to be precisely selective in our use of technological advances. We are in the dawn of greatly improved treatment of the knee.

The focus of this book has been the surgical treatment of the knee-injured patient. Judgment, or patient selectivity, is the basic element in carrying out the skills outlined in the case studies and in the chapters that follow in this section. This selectivity is especially important as we entertain more complex surgical treatments. Our current surgical techniques are imperfect and future technology is uncertain. This chapter, in the heart of *The Crucial Ligaments,* is written to help you integrate the basic science of knee care with the surgical skills available in an appropriately selective fashion for each patient.

Evolution of the knee is not a factor that will change your career. Indeed, as outlined by Dr. Dye (Chap. 2), we have had 350 million years of obviously satisfactory tetrapod function without significant evolutionary change. The knee is a "joint of necessity." The change in our discipline has been thrust upon us, not by evolution of the joint, but by evolutions in sports and sports equipment. These will continue to be dynamic and of immediate concern to us.

NATURAL HISTORY OF THE ACL-DEFICIENT KNEE

We could have established, early on in this epidemiologic revolution, a registry that could have defined the natural history of the anterior cruciate ligament (ACL)-deficient knee. In the short term perhaps it would have been better for our patients. In the long run, though, would that have constrained the remarkable development of arthroscopy as exemplified by Dr. Jackson, kinematics as exemplified by Dr. Müller, and pathophysiology as contributed by Drs. Noyes and Grood? I hope that orderliness will come to our craft through peer review, through the foundations laid by our international contributors, and through the quest of young orthopaedic practitioners. I believe that this lack of natural history will be circumvented by the emergence of an operation so simple and so reliable that it will resolve the problem, much as the total hip replacement intervened to change the natural history of the osteoarthritic hip.

SURGICAL METHODS

In our current state of the art, surgery of the knee is either acute or reconstructive and either intraarticular or extraarticular. To say that all knees should be treated one way or the other would deny the complexity and challenge that knee problems present. Indeed, this complexity that makes the surgical treatment of the knee a life-long discipline.

In 1950, O'Donoghue gave us the dictum that results of acute repair will be better than those of reconstruction. None have come forward to challenge this. Indeed, as we have gained understanding of the kinematics of the knee and acquired new skills and materials, it seems that we are leaning more toward acute repair, thereby satisfying Dr. O'Donoghue's dictum. This I believe will be most favorable for the course of the patient and the craft of knee surgery.

The choice of intraarticular or extraarticular reconstruction is a major dilemma in the minds of the practitioner doing daily knee surgery. Our scientific programs have not resolved the uncertainty and confusion centering on this choice. I perceive, however, a heartening trend toward restoration of the central pivot. This does not mean that the merits of the extraarticular tenodeses are to be ignored. It merely means that many are seeing the reliable results of accurately placed intraarticular grafts that protect the secondary restraints from further surgery. I hope this trend will continue. To this end, four surgical chapters follow:

Drs. Lambert and Cunningham's, with a well-illustrated, concise contribution on the anatomic substitution of the ruptured ACL using a vascularized patellar tendon graft with inference fit fixation

Drs. Rosenberg, Paulos, and Abbott's experience with arthroscopic repair and reconstruction

Drs. Andrews, Baker, Curl, and Gidumal's discussion of the surgical treatment of the secondary supporting structures

Dr. DeLee's chapter on ACL insufficiency, both nontraumatic and posttraumatic, in children

Each of these authors brings to this volume a maturity and judgment that is to be respected. Their chapters are meant to be complementary: a broad spectrum of the highest quality knee care is represented. Certainly more surgical chapters could have been included, but I believe surgeons will find that these chapters represent the essence of cruciate ligament surgery today and will prepare them well for tomorrow.

ANTICIPATED RESULTS

Many surgeons are dismayed that long-term surgical results are not available. They forget how new is our understanding of knee ligament anatomy and kinematics. They forget how recently this epidemic of knee injuries has been thrust upon us. They forget that a public previously concerned with depression and war has so recently turned to sport. It is the choice, thrust upon us by the multiplicity of new and emergent disciplines, that creates confusion. Let us analyze briefly some of the factors that have created this confusion.

One could easily say that with the contributions of Hey Groves, Ivar Palmer, and Brantigan and Voshell it was "all there." These men made enormous contributions but their works were isolated events, coming from different perspectives and different cultures. The contributions were founded on individual genius and not on a body corporate of scientific knowledge. Nevertheless, they produced the foundations that give us today significant insight as well as scientific knowledge. This history deserves review, because it is certain that those who choose to ignore history are doomed to repeat it.

ARTHROSCOPY

The advent of arthroscopy has been likened to the epic of flight. From Icarus to the Wright brothers was a long time. From the Wright brothers to the moon was ever so brief. Thanks to the leadership of such giants as Drs. Richard O'Connor, Robert Jackson, Robert Metcalf, and a host of others, arthroscopic surgery is already into the Space Age. Where will it go from here? Onward and upward, as a tool that is absolutely essential to you, the knee surgeon. Arthroscopy is a discipline that demands your utmost attention to develop the skills necessary to perform the newer techniques that are and will be available for your patients. Using arthroscopy as an essential adjunct, we will be replacing ligaments, menisci, and joint surfaces during our lifetimes as surgeons.

SELECTIVITY IN CARE OF THE CRUCIATE-DEFICIENT KNEE

Selectivity is difficult now because there is such a broad range between acute and reconstructive surgery, and between the intraarticular and extraarticular implementation of these procedures. The only tragedy would be if one discipline suggested that we ignore the other disciplines. There must be selectivity and, after evaluation of the information, our patients deserve the opportunity to participate in "selectivity" as it relates to their problems. What will become of this selectivity, given the creative and exciting advances that are upon the horizon? The breadth of selectivity will decrease, provided that practitioners equip themselves with the appropriate technical skills. This is a profound responsibility and demands the highest quality of content and efficiency of instruction in our educational courses. It also demands liaison between the disciplines. I am confident that, in light of today's knowledge, we are appropriately selective and will be precisely selective as we prepare for future obligations imposed by technological advances.

ADVANCING REHABILITATION TECHNIQUES

To impose our "old empiric rehabilitation" on newer technology is truly a disadvantage to the patient. Already it is exciting to shorten morbidity, based on advanced rehabilitation techniques, such as outlined by Drs. Arvidsson and Eriksson, Steadman, Hamilton, Stanish, and their coauthors in this text. More is yet to come. The quantification of our rehabilitation techniques through measurement of muscle function has just begun. More needs to come from our scientific community in this area. I anticipate that those who direct our orthopaedic research efforts will give stimulus to this development. A broad core of knowledge is just around the corner and waiting to be applied in a practical fashion to rehabilitation. The challenge to the clinician is to apply the appropriate rehabilitation practices to complement the surgery he or she currently performs.

OUR SURGICAL FUTURE

I did not initiate this book with a feeling of despair; rather it was with a feeling that we are in the dawn of greatly improved surgical treatment of the knee. This treatment will consist of the implantation of ligaments, menisci, and joint surfaces to fill defects or restore weight-bearing surfaces. Our responsibility is clear: to acquire the basic science knowledge and the technical arthroscopic skills necessary to accomplish these tasks as they become available. It is not what skills must be acquired but how these skills can be acquired by the busy practitioner that is our concern. The socioeconomic climate must be such that teachers continue to step to the forefront as they have done in the past. Psychomotor laboratories must be readily available for self-paced learning. There must be a partnership between the orthopaedic surgeon and the commercial interests that develop new products, which must be endorsed and enhanced by the appropriate regulatory bodies and patient advocates. These are the imponderables of progress.

This chapter is the link between the case studies of Section 1, supported by the theory of the subsequent sections, and the surgical considerations. These surgical considerations are the essence of our discipline; therefore, if surgery is the only alternative, the following chapters can be used as recommendations.

21

Anatomic Substitution of the Ruptured ACL Using a Vascularized Patellar Tendon Graft with Interference Fit Fixation

KENNETH L. LAMBERT
R. RAYMOND CUNNINGHAM

The intraarticular anatomic reconstruction of the anterior cruciate ligament (ACL) is necessary to reconstitute the central pivot of the knee. It is implicit that this reconstruction protects the knee from laxity that causes degeneration of other structures in and about the knee (Fig. 21-1).

Embryologically, the intercondylar notch may develop secondary to the volume and motion of the ACL. A relatively small-volume ligament may well result in a narrow intercondylar notch. Abnormal rotation or extreme extension may cause impingement of the femoral condyle on the ligament and may even result in its rupture.[7] The graft and its vascularized pedicle, because of its greater volume or mass, will need more room to avoid the fate of the original ligament.[5]

The objective of the surgical procedure to be described is to reconstitute anatomically a strong and correctly placed ACL with an enlarged intercondylar notch. If this objective is met, early motion, full weightbearing, and a fully functioning knee will be the result.

CHOICE OF REPLACEMENT STRUCTURE

One-third of the patellar tendon is chosen as the replacement structure because it offers

Strength
Bone-to-bone fixation and subsequent union
The option of maintaining the blood supply to the graft
Ease of surgical exposure to graft and ACL

Strength

One third of the patellar tendon is stronger than any other available tendon about the knee.[1] Although all transplanted ligaments seem to weaken for a time, the patellar tendon retains a strength close to that of the ACL.[2]

Bone-to-Bone Fixation

The strongest form of healing is bone-to-bone.

401

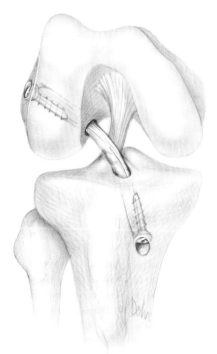

Fig. 21-1. An anatomically placed patellar tendon graft with interference fit of bone plugs in an enlarged intercondylar notch to reconstitute the central pivot of the knee.

Donor bone plug to femur or tibia, with a cancellous screw as a wedge, allows solid fixation until bone union occurs. This technique is termed *interference fit fixation.*

Vascular Supply

The blood supply may be maintained to the tendon graft through the medial and/or lateral geniculate arteries if the infrapatellar fat pad is not detached.

Ease of Exposure

The location of the infrapatellar tendon donor site allows intraarticular access to the knee, especially the intercondylar notch. The parapatellar incision is not needed for ACL reconstruction. The midline surgical approach is ideal for the complete procedure.

TECHNIQUE

Arthroscopy precedes the open reconstruction to confirm the ACL's status, and to evaluate the articular cartilage and menisci. Repair and/or limited excision of meniscus can usually be accomplished arthroscopically.

The midline surgical approach avoids patellar dislocation, which may be the cause of patellofemoral problems.

Other advantages of the midline approach include less likelihood of hematoma formation, improved healing, and a lessened incidence of infrapatellar neuroma formation.

Cosmesis is enhanced with meticulous intracuticular closure. Even though the incision is midline, when necessary the medial and lateral flaps can be raised to reach the posteromedial and posterolateral corners of the knee without danger of skin loss.

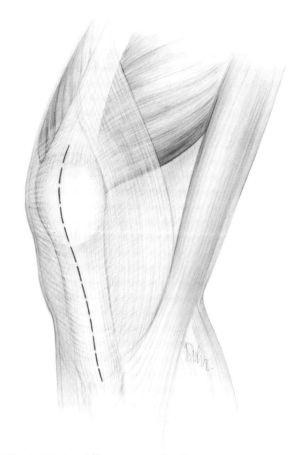

Fig. 21-2. A midline approach offers wide exposure to the knee. A less noticeable scar may be obtained with a meticulous intracuticular closure.

Graft Selection and Preparation

There seems to be a proportional width and length relationship for the patellar tendon to the ACL. One third of the patellar tendon, rather than a set linear dimension, is chosen as the size of the graft. This prevents one from harvesting too large a segment of a narrow patellar tendon.

Parallel incisions are made through the patellar tendon after elevating the prepatellar bursa and paratenon (Fig. 21-2). If the surgeon elects, the tendon–bone complex may be harvested as a free graft, but, if the blood supply is to be maintained to the graft, one of the incisions must be carried

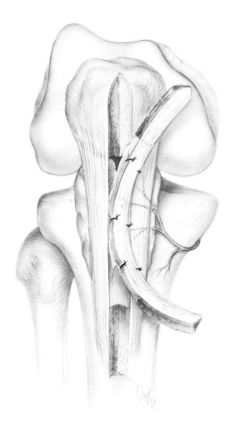

Fig. 21-4. Exposure to the intercondylar notch is accomplished by making a complete incision through the fat pad laterally, carefully avoiding damage to the lateral meniscus. The blood supply to the graft is thereby maintained from the medial inferior genicular artery.

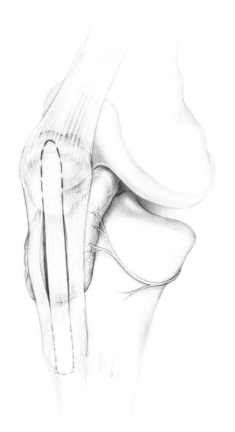

Fig. 21-3. Marking incisions for the saw cuts are made in the patella and tibial tuberosity projecting from the tendon incisions.

through the fat pad (usually laterally) leaving the tendon attached to one of the genicular arteries. Then parallel marking incisions are extended onto the patella and tibial tuberosity (Fig. 21-3). The depth of the incisions in the patella is gauged to avoid overcutting and possible fracture. Anchoring sutures of absorbable material are placed from fat pad to tendon to prevent avulsion of the blood supply as the graft is placed into the notch (Fig. 21-4). Release of the fat pad from the inferior pole of the patella and from the anterior tibia at the base of the tendon is often necessary. Bone plugs, triangular in cross section, are made with an oscillating saw using a fine blade. The average length of the bone plugs is 2.0 to 2.5 cm. They are shaped to pass through a sizer hole 9.5 mm in diameter. The bone plugs must be as large as possible to ensure interference fit fixation with a 6.5 mm screw used as a wedge.

The 2 mm drill holes are placed near the ends of the plugs for traction sutures to pass the plugs through the femoral and tibial canals (Fig. 21-5).

Remodeling the Intercondylar Notch

The anterior notch is routinely enlarged with the use of osteotomes, gouges, and curettes, to avoid impingement on the graft by the lateral femoral condyle, and provide adequate exposure of the posterior inlet, which is not enlarged (Fig. 21-6). The notch remodeling allows precise placement of the femoral canal, avoiding lateralization of the graft, and thereby places the graft in an anatomic position for isotonic function.

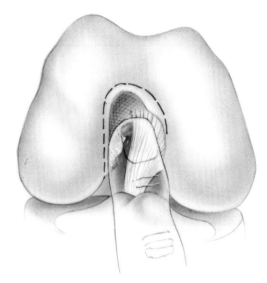

Fig. 21-6. An adequate notchplasty should allow the surgeon's index or fifth finger to palpate the posterior inlet at its osteochondral junction. A properly placed thigh holder allows the popliteal structures to fall away from the posterior inlet.

Anatomic Location of Drill Holes

Anatomic location of the drill holes that will accept the bone plugs is the most important step of this or any procedure that purports to treat ACL insufficiency. Fibers of both the femoral and tibial attachments of the ACL are usually present as a reference (except in long-term chronic cases). It is imperative to achieve a position that coincides with the original structure.

With today's instrumentation, it is impossible to achieve this location except by drilling from the lateral aspect of femoral condyle toward the interior of the notch, that is, from the outside in. A drill guide may improve the accuracy of canal placement (Fig. 21-7). It is critical that the femoral canal be at the osteochondral junction. The femoral canal is placed laterally on the vertical wall, 4 to 5 mm inferior to the arch of the posterior inlet. A guidewire is placed using the drill guide. An 8.5 mm AO reamer is then drilled over the guide wire to form the canal. The AO countersink is passed down the canal to remove bone possibly damaged by the reamer. The edge of the canal is chamfered with a curette to provide a smooth, rounded surface to minimize abrasion of the graft during knee motion (Fig. 21-8).

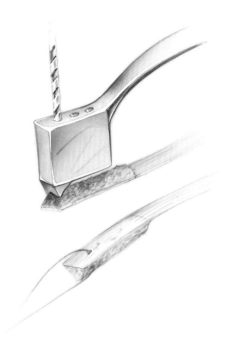

Fig. 21-5. The 2 mm drill holes are placed near the ends of the plugs for traction sutures, which should be of a strong, nonabsorbable material.

Fig. 21-7. A drill guide is used for precise placement of the femoral drill hole.

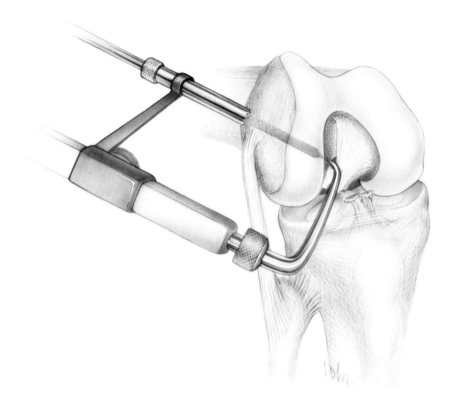

Inserting the Bone Plugs

The patellar plug is placed in the femur. We do not invert the graft. This avoids the possibility of torsion of the vascular supply to the graft. The isodensity of patellar bone plug and femoral canal enhances the screw/bone interference fit.

A suture passer is used to bring the traction suture through the canal to which the bone plug is attached. The bone/tendon graft is passed first through the femoral canal since it is difficult to visualize.

One may choose to suture the remnants of the tibial stump to the ACL. In the chronic case, the tibial stump is often attached to the posterior cruciate synovium by scar. Dissection of the stump may be necessary to facilitate passage of the femoral graft.

Graft Fixation

The screw is driven between bone plug and the bone wall. When the screw engages, it advances equally between canal and plug (Fig. 21-9). It is

impossible for the screw to push the bone plug ahead of it, nor is there a "lag effect" on the plug that can increase graft tension. It is mandatory that the screw not be deflected into the cancellous bone out of the canal away from the bone plug. Absence of fixation will result (Fig. 21-10). After screw fixation, the graft should be rigidly fixed, and there should be no movement of the bone plug, even with firm manual traction on the tendon or the traction sutures.

The graft should be tested for anatomic position before fixing the tibial side. Since the femoral side is solidly fixed, any piston-like motion of the graft can be palpated if the traction suture is wrapped around the surgeon's finger under tension, and the knee is placed through a range of motion. If there is more than 4 mm of pistoning of the graft, small changes can be achieved by twisting the graft or changing the position of the screw in relation to the plug. A larger variation would require new placement of the holes.

Twisting of the graft about its longitudinal axis can be done to simulate the helicoid course of the ACL. Graft placement and fixation are visualized

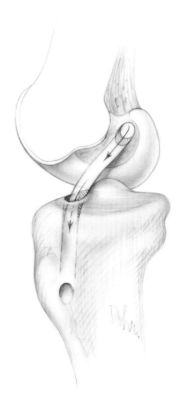

Fig. 21-8. The edges of the canals are chamfered to avoid chafing the graft.

through a range of motion to make certain there is no impingement (Fig. 21-11).

The closure is done over two suction drains. Gelfoam is placed in the donor sites of the patella and tibia. The paratenon and prepatellar bursae are closed with a single running 2-0 absorbable suture that extends onto the patellar tendon defect and closes the area in from proximal to distal. The lateral release is cauterized to avoid excessive bleeding. One of the drains is placed in the lateral gutter, the other in the knee joint. The subcuticular tissue is closed with interrupted 2-0 absorbable suture and the incision is closed with a running 4-0 intracuticular closure.

DISCUSSION

It seems logical to repair what is injured if the surgeon possesses the necessary skill. The primary goal remains replacement of the central pivot structure. Extraarticular procedures are not physiologic and seem to be based on the concept of the knee as a rotating box rather than as complex sliding surfaces about the pivoting helicoid axis.

The posterior horns of the menisci are the most important secondary stabilizers of the knee. Every effort should be made to save meniscal tissue if it is damaged. Arthroscopic or open repair is indicated whenever possible.

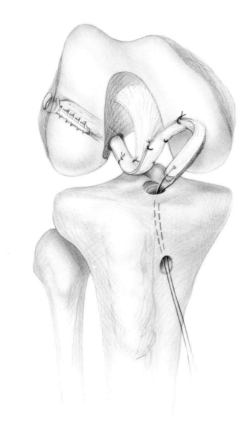

Fig. 21-9. The femoral side is passed first. A 6.5 mm cancellous screw is driven down the gap between the plug and wall, engages both equally as a threaded wedge, and gives interference fit of plug to hole.

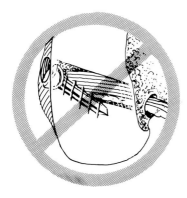

Fig. 21-10. Deflection of the screw occurs if the surgeon does not allow the screw to self-seek the interface between plug and hole.

POSTOPERATIVE CARE AND REHABILITATION

Pressure dressing is applied, and the knee is placed in a 15° Universal Velcro knee immobilizer. (Richards; 26 inches or 22 inches for the smaller patient).

Prophylactic cephalosporin is infused intravenously for the first 24 to 48 hours, usually until the suction drain has been removed. The suction drain is allowed to stay in place until the drainage level drops to 30 to 40 ml during a 12-hour period.

The patient is discharged from the hospital 3 to 4 days after the operation.

Depending on pain tolerance, the patient may walk with full weightbearing, although it is not un-

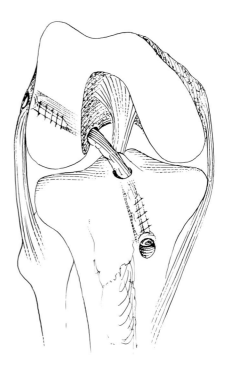

Fig. 21-11. Graft placement and fixation are visualized through a range of motion to make certain there is no impingement on the graft, especially in extension. Manual testing (i.e., Lachman test and pivot shift) is performed at this time.

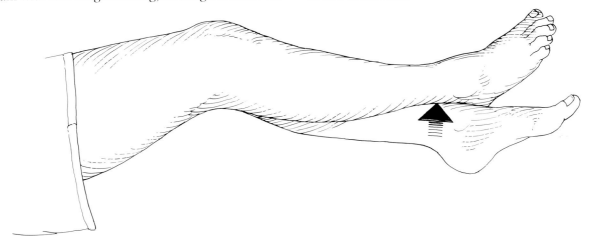

Fig. 21-12. The well leg is used for support during motion exercises to prevent possible graft stress by quadriceps contraction.

common for the patient to use crutches for a week, until the first reevaluation in the outpatient clinic. The exercise program includes active hamstring exercises while standing with the thigh braced against a table, in addition to passive flexion and extension of the operated knee using the support and muscles of the normal leg to flex and extend the knee (Fig. 21-12). We expect the patient to have 90° of flexion of the operated knee by 3 weeks and 110° to 120° of flexion by 6 weeks postoperatively.

The patient wears a knee immobilizer for protection for 6 weeks, and removes it several times daily to perform exercises. At the end of 6 weeks the patient begins exercising on a stationary bicycle, if he or she has an appropriate 110° to 120° of flexion of the knee.[4] At 10 weeks postoperatively, the patient is generally started on a low-weight, high-repetition lifting program, with isolated quadriceps exercise withheld until 12 weeks. The patient is generally discouraged from participating in any sort of high-risk activity such as skiing, football, basketball, or racquetball, for approximately 1 year.

If the patient does not have adequate range of motion by 12 weeks after operation (i.e., 90° of flexion), we recommend that the knee be manipulated with the patient under general anesthesia. Following manipulation, and with the knee iced after manipulation, the patient is taken to the physical therapy department within 2 to 3 hours and started on a range of motion program.

We do not see any need for the patient to wear a protective brace. The patient will continue to use the stationary bicycle for 1 year, for 30 to 45 minutes per day.

COMPLICATIONS AND COMPLAINTS

We have treated over 600 patients with the vascularized patellar tendon graft and interference fit fixation.[6] In 8 years, less than a dozen patients have had complications. One patient fell 2 days after removal of the knee immobilizer, struck his patella, and sustained a transverse fracture of the patella. Two patients developed a subcutaneous hematoma in spite of suction drainage, necessitating their return to the operating room. We found bleeding from the lateral retinacular release in both patients' knees. Several patients have not obtained adequate motion at 12 weeks (i.e., 6 weeks out of splints), and have required manipulation under anesthesia. They have all gained normal range of motion of the knee.

Within 1 year of surgery, we expect patients to be back to their previous level of activity in sports and daily living, and with adequate rehabilitation and quadriceps development.[3]

SUMMARY

A technique has been described for the reconstruction of the ACL using a vascularized patellar tendon graft and bone plug, using interference fit fixation and bone union. Its results have proven reproducible and predictable over an 8-year period.

REFERENCES

1. Butler DL, Noyes FR, Grood ES et al: Mechanical properties of transplants for the anterior cruciate ligament. Trans Orthop Res Soc 4:81, 1979
2. Cabaud HE, Chatty A, Gildengorin V et al: Exercise effects on the strength of the rat anterior cruciate ligament. Am J Sports Med 8:79–86, 1980
3. Daniel D, Malcom LL, Stone ML et al: Quantification of knee stability and function. Contemp Orthop 5:83–91, 1982
4. Henning CE: An in vivo strain gauge study of elongation of the anterior cruciate ligament. Presented at the American Orthopaedic Society for Sports Medicine (Interim Meeting), New Orleans, LA, January 20–21, 1982
5. Kieffer DA, Curnow RJ, Southwell RB et al: Anterior cruciate ligament arthroplasty. Am J Sports Med 12:301–312, 1984
6. Lambert KL: Vascularized patella graft with rigid internal fixation for anterior cruciate ligament insufficiency. Clin Orthop 172:85–89, 1983
7. Norwood LA, Cross MJ: The intercondylar shelf and the anterior cruciate ligament. Am J Sports Med 5:171–176, 1977

22
Arthroscopic Cruciate Repair and Reconstruction: An Overview and Descriptions of Technique

THOMAS D. ROSENBERG
LONNIE E. PAULOS
PAUL J. ABBOTT, JR.

Arthroscopy has evolved from a purely diagnostic procedure to a surgical technique. Now synovectomies and meniscal repair are performed. Recently, cruciate ligament surgery has moved into the arthroscopic realm. Arthroscopic surgery reduces morbidity, compared to many open procedures, and contributes to our understanding of joint pathology and anatomy.

Arthroscopic surgery is a specialized technique — not a separate discipline — and must remain subordinate to fundamental orthopaedic principles. Concepts of isometricity, proper graft selection, tissue remodeling, and appropriate rehabilitation must be practiced. Open techniques are proven and will be the standard by which all new techniques are judged. A well-executed open procedure will obviously produce superior results than a less rigidly controlled arthroscopic procedure. Arthroscopic techniques of cruciate ligament surgery, however, offer a number of potential advantages.

In this chapter we present some of the advantages of arthroscopic cruciate ligament repair over open procedures, an overview of arthroscopic techniques, and a section on the techniques we prefer for reconstructing the anterior (ACL) and posterior cruciate ligaments (PCL).

ADVANTAGES OF ARTHROSCOPIC SURGERY

Arthroscopic cruciate surgery avoids the need for an arthrotomy. In arthroscopic surgery, there is no need to divide the vastus medialis obliquus (VMO) tendon or capsule. Arms et al.[1] demonstrated the importance of the anteromedial capsule in strain protection of the ACL. The capsule may be compromised with arthrotomy; capsular laxity may develop later. Grimby et al.[12] evaluated patients isokinetically 2 years after ligament reconstruction and rehabilitation. They found an average of 20 percent difference in strength between the operated limbs and nonoperated limbs.

No published studies compare rehabilitation of patients after open cruciate surgery to rehabilitation of those after arthroscopic procedures. Several studies[3,14,19] comparing open meniscectomy to arthroscopic meniscectomy are available. For example, one study[14] comparing isokinetic strength of the quadriceps at 1 week after surgery showed a 40 percent decrease of isokinetic strength of the quadriceps in patients treated arthroscopically compared with a 70 percent reduction at 1 week after open total meniscectomy.

Cruciate ligament surgery requires some delays in rehabilitation, such as the obligatory periods for graft revascularization, remodeling when biologic tissues are used, and other aspects of healing, which confuse the interpretation of positive or negative effects of arthrotomy compared with arthroscopy.

Arthroscopic cruciate ligament surgery, as opposed to conventional cruciate surgery, results in less pain and edema, which produce muscle inhibition[7,13] and contribute to muscle atrophy.[18] Arthroscopic procedures minimize disturbance in proprioceptive feedback causing permanent muscle atrophy,[8,11] which is a hazard of open procedures. Reduction of the kinesthetic sense of the knee and loss of sensory afferents involved in the muscle stretch reflex[17] may hamper rehabilitation efforts aimed at regaining neuromuscular coordination. Limitation in neuromuscular perceptiveness can affect the reinjury rate. Requirements for bracing the knees of some (open) surgically treated patients may be secondary to diminished proprioceptive feedback as a result of injury or surgery.[17]

With arthroscopically controlled cruciate ligament surgery, there is relatively minimal disturbance of the extensor mechanism and little chance of altering patellar tracking. This is critically important in chronic posterior cruciate ligament (PCL)-deficient knees where there is an increased incidence of patellofemoral disorders. In our experience (T.D. Rosenberg, M.D. and D. Coward, M.D., unpublished data), 17 of the 50 patients had patellofemoral signs and symptoms, including radiographic changes, when we evaluated their cases 5 to 10 years after cruciate ligament repair or reconstruction (performed by a variety of surgeons). Paulos and Noyes (in presentation, 1984) reported that 30 percent of their patients had mild to moderate patellofemoral crepitation after ACL reconstruction by vascularized patellar tendon graft. While arthrotomy may play a role in the development of patellofemoral problems after cruciate ligament surgery, other factors may be implicated including preexisting articular pathology and postoperative immobilization.

Injury to the infrapatellar or sartorial branches of the saphenous nerve occurs frequently with arthro-tomy. Johnson et al.[16] reported that, in a series of 99 patients whose knees had been treated by open meniscectomy, 23.2 percent had sensory loss around the tibial tubercle that was not irritating while 28 percent complained of hypersensitivity or paresthesias. With closed techniques, hyaline cartilage desiccation is avoided and cosmesis is improved.

ACL surgery allows for precise graft placement with its excellent illumination and magnification. The femoral anatomic attachment site is easily identified. The intercondylar "notchplasty" can be assessed dynamically to avoid impingement and also to avoid excessive removal of bone from the intercondylar region.

Hospital time and sick time are shortened with arthroscopic meniscal surgery.[6] In our experience, cruciate ligament surgery performed arthroscopically allows the patient to leave the hospital after 1 day (average). In certain circumstances, arthroscopic cruciate surgery may be performed as an ambulatory surgical procedure.

ARTHROSCOPIC TECHNIQUES

Repair of cruciate ligament ruptures without augmentation is generally associated with a high failure rate.[9] Arthroscopic techniques would not be likely to improve upon these results. Arthroscopic ACL repair is more difficult than comparable open techniques because of the technical factors associated with the liquid medium of arthroscopy. These include additional edema of the ligament secondary to the distention/irrigation fluid. Arthroscopic suture placement is particularly difficult because of the "floating" nature of the disrupted fiber bundles. Appropriate tension adjustment may not be achievable. Instrument confinement inherent in the use of arthroscopic portals can impair surgical efficiency. Also, time restraints and difficulty controlling the infrapatellar fat pad make arthroscopic ACL repair impractical with the present state of our art.

Currently, proposed arthroscopic techniques of repair include stapling of the distal anterior cruciate ligament stump to the femur.[15] Problems inherent in this technique include the violation of isometricity, concern over the biomechanical integrity of the injured ACL, ligament necrosis under the staple resulting in loss of fixation, and loosening of a metal staple within the knee.

An experimental approach, described by Bartlett[2] and performed in cadavers only, involved the use of a fish hook arthroscopically placed to provide fixation and repair of the ligament in conjunction with ligament augmentation. Some surgeons use special holders or meniscal repair cannulae to perform arthroscopic repairs. All methods are subject to technical constraints. Fox et al.[10] reported preliminary results of arthroscopic repair of the ACL. At follow-up evaluations (average 9.2 months), none of the patients had a satisfactory result.[10] The authors[10] expressed concerns about the feasibility of arthroscopic repair of the ACL. In acute cases when repair and augmentation are indicated, we recommend open procedures until techniques improve or better instrumentation becomes available.

In 1980, Drez (personal communication) demonstrated an ACL reconstruction by using fascia lata pulled through tibial and femoral drill holes under arthroscopic control. In 1981, Dandy et al.[5] described his arthroscopic technique for the placement of a carbon fiber ligament substitute for reconstruction of the ACL. His technique involved "free-hand" placement of a bone awl through the lateral femoral condyle to enter the notch at the former attachment site of the ACL. The bone awl was withdrawn and the hole enlarged with a drill. The tibial tunnel was likewise drilled free-hand.* Because of problems with this prosthesis, including synovitis, sinus tract formation, and results often inferior to those cases using iliotibial band, Dandy et al.[5] discontinued its use after a small series pending review of the long-term results. Johnson[15] has described an arthroscopic technique of ACL reconstruction using semitendinosus tendon with staple fixation.

Surgical reconstruction of the PCL historically has

had a low success rate for a number of reasons. First, the PCL is more commonly damaged by severe trauma resulting in extensive damage to other structures including nerves, vessels, ligaments, and cartilage surfaces. Second, the PCL has few secondary restraints to help prevent posterior tibial sag. Therefore, tissues selected for reconstruction of the PCL must maintain exceptional strength during and after healing. Third, large posterior Drawer forces occur constantly during daily living activities. The result is cyclic loading of the reconstruction. Fourth, because of the posterior tibial sag, a "functional" patella baja is created with leads to progressive patellofemoral arthrosis. For these reasons, a knee that demonstrates posterior cruciate insufficiency presents a formidable challenge.

Another factor associated with the low success rate and high morbidity of the PCL surgery is that open surgery requires extensive dissection near the posterior neurovascular structures and musculature. Arthroscopic techniques may allow for reduction of surgical morbidity and improvement of surgical results. This impression has been reinforced by our recent short-term review of both open and arthroscopic PCL reconstructions. Reconstruction of the PCL, as we emphasize with the ACL, must adhere to principles of isometricity, proper graft selection, tissue remodeling, and appropriate rehabilitation, whether surgery is performed open or under arthroscopic control.

TECHNIQUE FOR ACL AND PCL REPAIR AND RECONSTRUCTION

From 1981 to 1985, we (Rosenberg and Paulos, Salt Lake City) developed a technique for arthroscopic reconstruction of the ACL and, in the last 2 years, we developed a technique for reconstruction of the PCL. We use arthroscopically controlled drill guides for placement of a ligament graft or synthetic substitute.

ACL Reconstruction

After routine diagnostic arthroscopy through anteromedial and anterolateral portals, arthroscopic meniscal repair or partial meniscectomy is com-

---

*Present techniques of arthroscopic ACL and PCL reconstruction generally involve the use of arthroscopically controlled drill guides. Guide design allows for the drilling of femoral and tibial tunnels that enter the joint at the anatomic attachment sites of the respective cruciate ligaments.

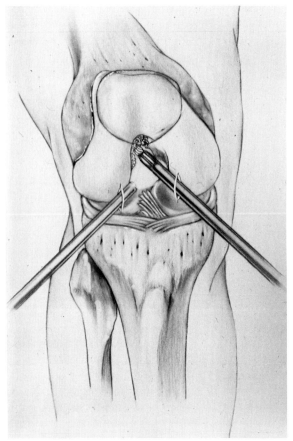

Fig. 22-1. A motorized suction cutter and abrader are used to smooth and adjust finely the contour of the notchplasty.

pleted, if necessary. If a repair is performed, sutures are not tied until completion of the ligament reconstruction. Partial excision of the contracted ACL stumps may be performed to facilitate exposure. We attempt to preserve vascular tissue in the intercondylar notch and take care to avoid injury to the PCL and its synovium. Then we evaluate the dimensions of the notch.

Patients with a so-called "A-frame" notch require a "notchplasty" to prevent impingement of the substitute anteriorly and laterally during terminal extension. Notch impingement is believed to be a frequent cause of graft failure in cases in which notchplasty has not been performed. More frequently, a notchplasty is required because of nar-

rowing of the notch due to osteophyte formation in chronic ACL-deficient knees. At times, adequate identification of the femoral anatomic attachment site is not possible until a notchplasty has been completed. The notchplasty can be performed by using a gouge or curved osteotome inserted through the anteromedial portal. An adequate notchplasty requires removal of bone over the superior and lateral portions of the notch extending to the femoral attachment of the PCL. The anterior area is decompressed with the knee at 30° to 45° of flexion while the inferior and posterior portions may be reached with the knee flexed 90°. Osteochondral fragments of the notchplasty remain attached to soft tissue in the notch until grasped and removed through the anteromedial portal. A motorized suc-

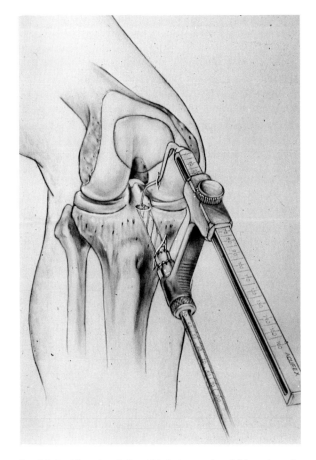

Fig. 22-2. The tip of the tibial aimer should be placed at the tibial anatomic attachment site of the ACL.

Fig. 22-3. The tip of the femoral aimer is placed on the femoral anatomic attachment site of the ACL.

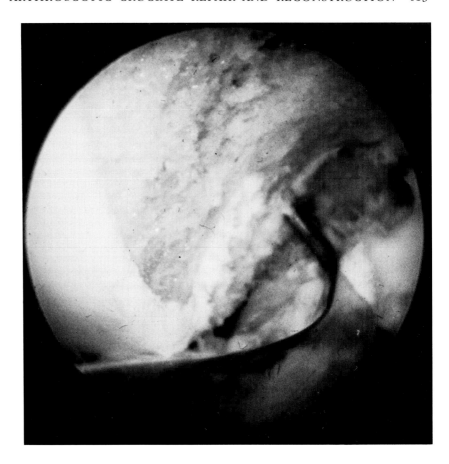

Fig. 22-4. The tunnel should be directed to minimize tunnel divergence.

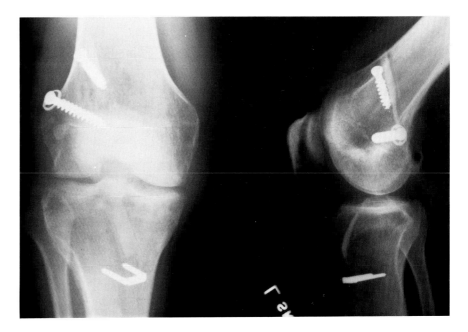

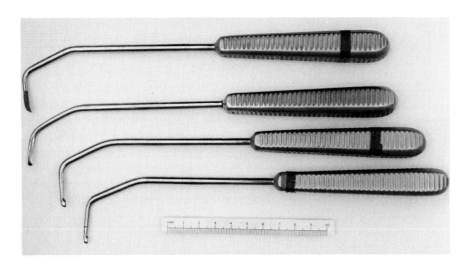

Fig. 22-5. The posterior tibial attachment site is prepared with specially designed reverse cutting knives, curettes, and rasps through the anteromedial portal.

tion cutter and abrader are used to smooth and finely adjust the contour of the notch (Fig. 22-1). The femoral anatomic attachment site of the ACL is identified and marked with a small curette.

A vertical incision, approximately 3 cm long and 3 cm distal to the joint line on the anteromedial surface of the tibia, is then made and carried down to the periosteum, which is elevated. The distal aspect of this incision should be above the superior margin of the pes anserinus. The tip of the tibial aimer should be placed at the tibial anatomic attachment site of the ACL (Fig. 22-2). The residual ACL stump, if present, can be used as a landmark. Otherwise the anterior slope of the medial intercondylar eminence can be used (with the surgeon extrapolating from other anatomic reference points as well). If the surgeon is unsure of exact placement, it is better to err anteriorly. This may have negligible effects on isometricity (M. Siegel, M.D., in presentation, 1983) but may require that one expand the notchplasty. As an alternative, the posterior lip of the internal tibial aperture can be chamfered to achieve correct placement.

After the tibial anatomic attachment site is chosen, the drilling outrigger is advanced along the tibial aimer until its teeth engage the tibial cortex. The set screw is then tightened. The appropriate size of drill sleeve and bit are chosen by sizing the intended graft. It is desirable to match closely the tunnel size with the graft diameter. Tunnels 10 to 12 mm are usually drilled for patellar tendon grafts,

and slightly smaller tunnels are used for fascia lata grafts, semitendinosus tendon, or prosthetic ligaments. Importance is placed on keeping the drill bit sharp to prevent thermal necrosis in the tunnel wall which, in turn, may affect the ultimate graft fixation. Once the drilling is completed and the drill guide removed, the soft tissue at the posterior rim of the tunnel within the joint is removed with a motorized suction cutter inserted through the anteromedial portal. The appropriate margins of each tunnel opening are chamfered to avoid any sharp edges that may erode through the graft or resorb focally and cause relaxation of the substitute. The tibial tunnel is then sealed with a conical rubber plug and attention is directed toward drilling the femoral tunnel.

A lateral longitudinal incision is made over the distal femur, centered over the iliotibial band. A limited lateral release is performed, extending to the joint line. The lateral release remains extrasynovial and continues proximally into the fascia, superficial to the vastus lateralis muscle. This allows the iliotibial band to drop posteriorly. The periosteum is incised on the lateral aspect of the femoral metaphysis and elevated. The femoral aimer is placed through the anterolateral portal with the scope in the anteromedial portal. The tip of the femoral aimer is placed on the femoral anatomic attachment site of the ACL (Fig. 22-3). The drilling outrigger is placed on the femoral aimer and advanced until the teeth engage the cortex and the set screw is tightened. The tunnel should be directed to minimize tunnel divergence (Fig. 22-4). The previously chosen drill bit and sleeve are used. Both tunnel openings are chamfered, using either a motorized back-cutting abrader or a chamfering rasp. The graft is then pulled into place. The tension is preliminarily adjusted and the substitute is fixed to cortical bone, proximal to the femoral tunnel.

The knee should now be taken through a range of motion and the graft observed for excursion. With anatomic placement of the graft, there should be no more than 1 to 2 mm of excursion. The knee is then flexed 10° to 30°, depending on the specific ACL substitute, and the final tension is adjusted as the substitute is fixed to the tibia, distal to the tibial tunnel. After the graft is fixed at both ends, the arthroscope is reinserted into the joint. Dynamic behavior of the graft is observed to determine whether further decompression of the intercondylar notch is necessary and to ensure that proper tension has been achieved. Any areas of impingement should be decompressed. Extraarticular surgery, if indicated, is completed. The postoperative care is determined by the nature of the substitution placed in the joint.

PCL Reconstruction

Routine arthroscopy is performed with the arthroscope in the anterolateral portal. Correction of meniscal pathologic conditions is addressed as necessary. Overhanging osteophytes from both the medial and lateral femoral condyles are removed using small osteotomes or motorized abraders. If a biologic substitute is used, care is taken to preserve synovial tissues in the area of the normal PCL.

Using specially designed reverse cutting knives, curettes, and rasps through the anteromedial portal (Fig. 22-5) with the 30° arthroscope in the anterolateral portal, we prepared the posterior tibial attachment site by removing all soft tissue between the tibial condyle and the posterior attachment site of the PCL replacement. Usually the remaining stump of the PCL on the tibia can be visualized. This remaining stump is used as a guide for preparing the attachment site.

The posterior joint capsule attaches to a posterior tibial shelf distal to the PCL attachment. This area must be prepared properly because it serves as a consistent bony landmark for placement of the tibial drill guide (Fig. 22-6).

Preparation of the tibial attachment site may be performed in a similar manner but under direct vision with the 30° arthroscope in the posteromedial portal. This may be difficult at times because of extravasation of fluid and subsequent loss of distention. A small posteromedial arthrotomy may sometimes aid in preparation of the tibial attachment site; one can use a finger for placement of instruments.

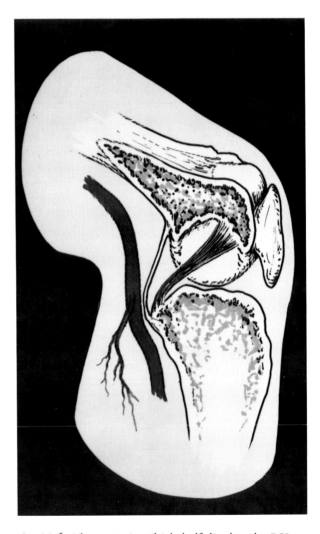

Fig. 22-6. The posterior tibial shelf distal to the PCL attachment serves as a consistent bony landmark for placement of the tibial drill guide.

These maneuvers are helpful when the surgeon is first learning to use arthroscopy but may become unnecessary as the surgeon gains experience.

The tibial drill guide is passed through the anteromedial portal while one is viewing the joint anterolaterally. The guide is rotated 90° to the long axis of the leg to facilitate passage through the intercondylar notch. It is then rotated back in line with the leg as soon as the tip of the guide reaches the posterior aspect of the plateau. The guide follows the normal contour of the posterior tibial plateau and fits snugly into the posterior tibial fovea to allow correct mediolateral positioning. A small hook on the tip of the tibial guide is designed to hook se-

curely over the posterior tibial shelf. To aid in the placement of the tibial guide, it is sometimes necessary to extend the leg to 30° to allow the tibial guide to descend further down the back of the tibia. After the tibial guide is secured over the posterior shelf, the tibia is brought back to the 90° position.

The drill guide is positioned to allow drilling from an anteromedial exposure, inferior and medial to the tibial tubercle. When positioning the tibial drill guide, it is important that the tunnel begin 1 to 2 cm below the tibial tubercle (Fig. 22-7). A more proximal drilling position may leave insufficient bone between the proximal tunnel aperture and the tibial plateau, thus permitting tunnel drift. In addi-

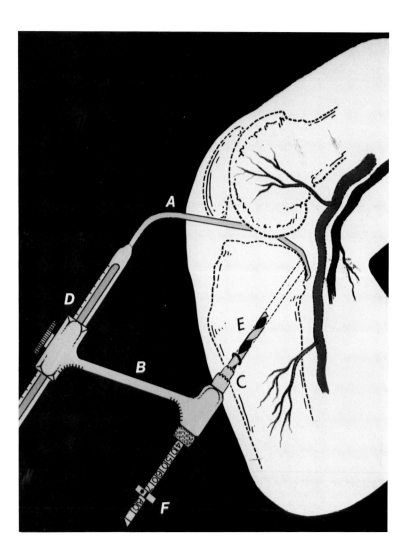

Fig. 22-7. When positioning the tibial drill guide, it is important that the tunnel begin 1 to 2 cm below the tibial tubercle.

Fig. 22-8. To ensure that the drill bit does not penetrate beyond the tibial guide, the guide must be freely positioned without bending and a drill point stop must be used to avoid double penetration of the posterior tibial cortex. A lateral radiograph of the knee should be obtained if there is any question about the location of the tibial drill guide or drill bit.

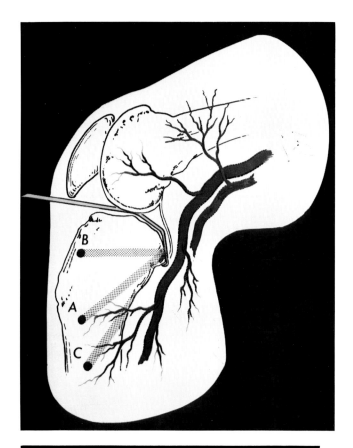

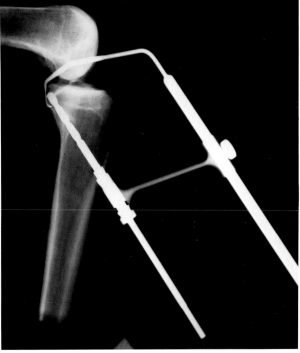

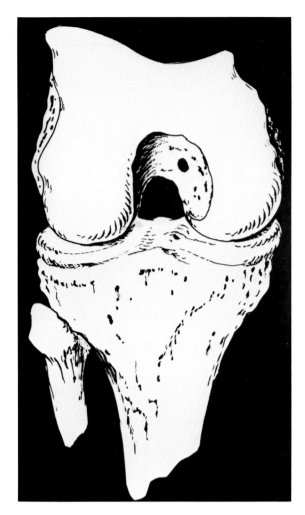

Fig. 22-9. The femoral attachment of the PCL is determined at 90° of knee flexion. This position is located approximately 8 mm proximal to the margin of the articular surface of the medial femoral condyle at the 2 o'clock (10 o'clock) position of the intercondylar notch.

tion, a more acute tunnel angle could possibly lead to graft attenuation. In contrast, drilling from a site too distal on the anterior tibial cortex will cause a double penetration of the posterior tibial cortex, which is undesirable (Fig. 22-8A).

After placement of the tibial drill guide through the anteromedial portal, the drilling outrigger is passed up the guide and a small incision is made in the skin at the point of contact. The periosteum is elevated and the drill guide sleeve held in contact to

the bone. The appropriately sized drill bit is selected based on the ligament replacement used. The smaller size, which permits passage of the substitute, should be selected to avoid tunnel dead space. A drill point stop is placed on the drill bit. Its position is determined by the length of the tunnel as measured from the drill guide before drilling. This prevents penetration of the drill point beyond the

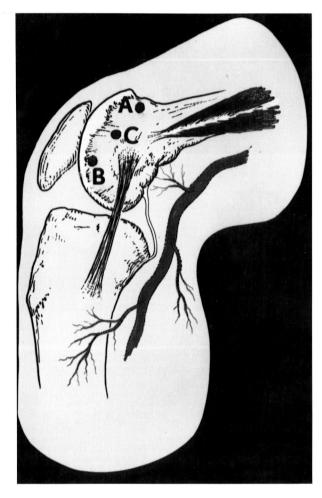

Fig. 22-10. Point A results in minimal tunnel divergence in full extension and in maximal tunnel divergence in flexion. Point B, conversely, results in maximal tunnel divergence in full extension and minimal tunnel divergence in flexion. Point C represents the "ideal" extraarticular opening of the femoral tunnel to minimize tunnel divergence through the complete range of motion, as illustrated in Figure 22-11, 22-12, and 22-13.

posterior tibial cortex into the neurovascular structures.

Because of the location of the posterior tibial drill hole, the emergence of the tibial drill point must be felt rather than seen. To ensure that the drill bit does not penetrate beyond the tibial guide, the guide must be freely positioned without bending and the drill point stop must be used. If any question exists about the location of the tibial drill guide or drill bit, a lateral radiograph of the knee should be obtained (Fig. 22-8B).

After the tibial tunnel is made, the guide and drill bit are removed and chamfering rasps or curettes are used to bevel and smooth the margins of the tibial tunnel. The tibial tunnel is sealed with a conical rubber plug.

Now the femoral attachment of the posterior cruciate ligament is determined. The position is determined at 90° of knee flexion. Using a calibrated curette, the surgeon can mark the medial wall of the intercondylar notch at the center of the normal attachment of the posterior cruciate ligament. This position is located approximately 8 mm proximal to the margin of the articular surface of the medial femoral condyle at the 2 o'clock (10 o'clock) position of the intercondylar notch (Fig. 22-9). Previous

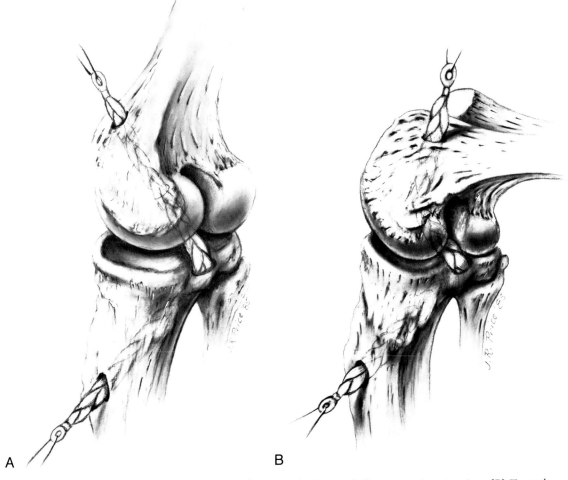

A   B

Fig. 22-11. **(A)** Point A, Figure 22-10, results in minimal tunnel divergence in extension. **(B)** Tunnel divergence is increased in flexion.

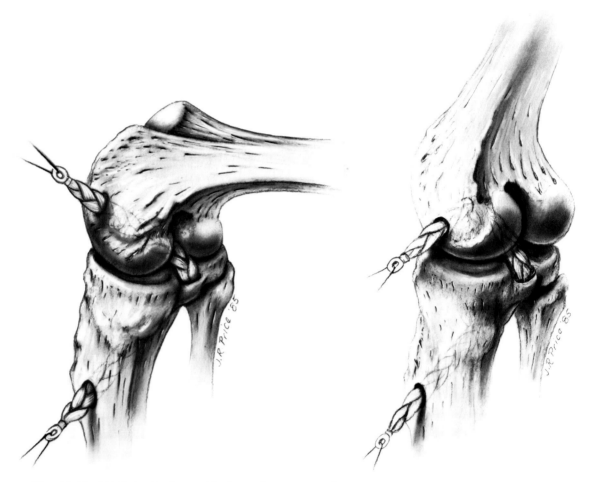

Fig. 22-12. (A) Point B, Figure 22-10, results in minimal tunnel divergence in flexion. **(B)** Tunnel divergence is increased at full extension.

recommendations of a more anterior position for the femoral attachment site do not apply when close conformity of the graft and tunnel diameter is preferred. A strong substitute will indeed restrict knee flexion if an excessively anterior site is chosen.

While viewing from the anterolateral portal, the surgeon passes the PCL femoral guide through the anteromedial portal and impales the point of the guide at the center of the desired attachment site. The surgeon then passes the drilling outrigger along the guide and makes a small incision in the skin to allow its contact to the medial femoral cortex. This site is selected with the knee at 90° of flexion. The preferred site is midway between the

medial femoral epicondyle and the medial articular margin of the femoral sulcus on a line between the medial epicondyle and the upper third of the patella (point C, Fig. 22-10). After the skin incision is made in this area, the vastus medialis obliquus muscle can be seen and is retracted superiorly to expose the medial femoral condyle. An appropriate sized drill bit is used to drill the femoral tunnel. Care must be taken not to torque or bend the drill guide. After the tunnel is created, the drill guide and drill point are removed and the tunnel edges are beveled.

The direction of the femoral tunnel, described in the previous paragraph, was chosen because it reduces stress on the ligament substitute at its entrance into the joint. *Tunnel divergence* is the angulation or change in direction the graft or substitute must take as it leaves the joint and enters the bony tunnel. This tunnel divergence changes with flexion and extension and is more pronounced with the femoral tunnel than with the tibial tunnel, since the femoral tunnel is nearer the center of rotation.

In full extension, tunnel divergence is minimized if the tunnel entrance is located proximally (point A, Fig. 22-10; Fig. 22-11A). This will result, however, in marked tunnel divergence in full flexion (Fig. 22-11B). In full flexion, tunnel divergence is minimized if the tunnel entrance is located more distally (point B, Fig. 22-10; Fig. 22-12A). This will result in marked tunnel divergence in full extension of the

knee joint (Fig. 22-12B). Consequently, the preferred tunnel entry site (point C, Fig. 22-10) is a compromise between the proximal and distal sites to avoid the extremes in tunnel divergence (Fig. 22-13).

With the tunnels prepared, a double 18-gauge wire or another suitable suture passer is directed through the tibial tunnel from below. It can be hooked arthroscopically and pulled into the intercondylar notch near the intraarticular opening of the femoral tunnel where it can be pulled through the femoral tunnel in a second step. A Dacron tape or other passing device is then pulled back through the tunnels. The passing tape can be calibrated to measure the required graft length before the graft is placed. The graft or its leader is then fastened to the

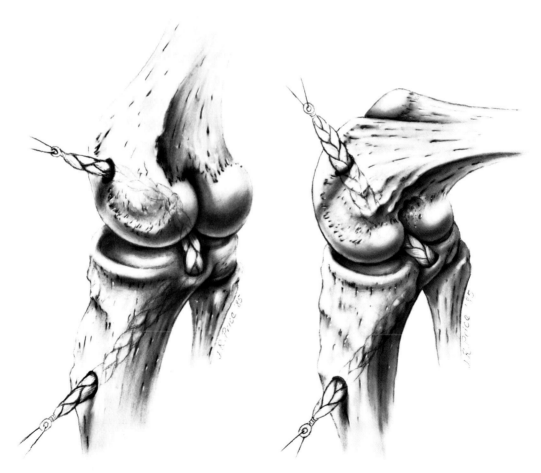

Fig. 22-13. (A,B) Point C, Figure 22-10, minimizes tunnel divergence over the full range of motion.

passing tape and pulled into the joint through the tibial tunnel and out the femoral tunnel. To facilitate pulling the substitute into position, the knee is flexed to 90° as the new ligament passes through the intercondylar notch and is then extended to approximately 30° as it enters the femoral tunnel.

With the substitute held under tension but not yet secured it can be studied through a range of motion. The replacement should be observed to tighten slightly as the knee proceeds from 20° to 100° of flexion. There should be no impingement at the intercondylar notch, and the proximal and the posterior margins of the femoral tunnel opening should be beveled to prevent stress concentration.

The femoral end of the posterior cruciate substitute is pulled proximally 2 cm and secured proximal to the medial epicondyle to prevent soft tissue impingement. The distal portion is held on tension as the knee is taken through a full range of motion. Isometric placement of the graft is present if ligament tension is maintained through the range of motion and flexion is not impeded. If the femoral attachment site has been placed too far distally, the new ligament will tighten and impede motion as the knee is taken into flexion. If the femoral attachment is placed too far proximally, the substitute will tighten excessively as the knee is extended.

With the knee in 30° to 45° of flexion, an anterior Drawer force is applied to the tibia and the substitute is pulled under tension and fixed to the tibia. Proper tension will prevent tibial sag and, at the same time, allow full range of motion.

Postoperative immobilization and rehabilitation after PCL reconstruction must be individualized according to the material selected for reconstruction, the size of the patient, and concomitant surgery performed. A femoral–tibial transfixion pin can be used for fixation of the joint; however, in our experience, this has resulted in increased morbidity. In general, if posterolateral rotary stability is present or has been achieved surgically, the knee can simply be immobilized in 20° to 30° of flexion.

SUMMARY

Interest in arthroscopically controlled ACL reconstruction has increased in recent years. Although achievement of stability has been well-documented in open ACL reconstructive procedures,[4] truly excellent results may depend on avoiding operative morbidity. Arthroscopically controlled cruciate ligament reconstruction appears to offer significantly diminished morbidity due to lower incidence of neuromuscular impairment relative to the procedure and by more predictable rehabilitation following surgery.

Proper graft selection is another important factor. Autogenous grafts, allografts, xenografts, and synthetic ligaments are all being used. The theoretical advantages of using nonautogenous materials are readily apparent: normal tissue is not sacrificed and grafts may be taken of sufficient size and strength without fear of compromising function at the donor site. The use of nonautogenous grafts may complement arthroscopic reconstruction by allowing further reduction in surgical morbidity.

In this chapter we have expanded on some of the advantages of arthroscopic cruciate ligament repair in contrast to open procedures, given an overview of arthroscopic techniques for cruciate ligament surgery, and described the techniques we prefer for repair of the ACL and PCL.

Arthroscopic surgery is a specialized technique that must incorporate fundamental orthopaedic principles, such as concepts of isometricity, proper graft selection, tissue remodeling, and appropriate rehabilitation.

REFERENCES

1. Arms SW, Pope MH, Johnson RJ et al: The biomechanics of anterior cruciate ligament rehabilitation and reconstruction. Am J Sports Med 12:8–17, 1984
2. Bartlett EC: Arthroscopic repair and augmentation of the anterior cruciate ligament in cadaver knees. Clin Orthop 172:107–111, 1983
3. Campbell DE, Glenn W: Foot-pounds of torque of the normal knee and the rehabilitated post-meniscectomy knee. J Am Phys Ther Assoc 59:418–421, 1979
4. Clancy WG, Nelson DA, Reider B, Narechania RG: Anterior cruciate ligament reconstruction using one-third of the patella ligament augmented by extra-articular tendon transfers. J Bone Joint Surg 64A:353–359, 1982
5. Dandy DJ, Flanagan JP, Steenmeyer V: Arthroscopy and the management of the ruptured anterior cruciate ligament. Clin Orthop 167:43–49, 1982

6. Dandy DJ, Hodge GJ: Closed partial meniscectomy. Physiotherapy 64:367–368, 1978

7. deAndrade JR, Grant C, Dixon SJ: Joint distension and reflex muscle inhibition in the knee. J Bone Joint Surg 47A:313–322, 1965

8. Eriksson E: Rehabilitation of muscle function after sport injury. Major problems in sport medicine. Int J Sports Med 2:1–6, 1981

9. Feagin JA, Curl WW: Isolated tears of the anterior cruciate ligament. 5-year follow-up study. Am J Sports Med 4:95–100, 1976

10. Fox JM, Sherman OH, Markoff K: Arthroscopic anterior cruciate ligament repair. Preliminary results and instrumented testing for anterior stability. Arthroscopy 1:175–181, 1985

11. Gardener ED: The innervation of the knee joint. Anat Rec 101:109–130, 1948

12. Grimby G, Gustafsson E, Peterson L et al: Quadriceps function and training. Med Sci Sports Exerc 12:70–75, 1980

13. Gydikov A: Patterns of discharge of different types of alpha motor neurons and motor units during voluntary and reflex activities under normal physiologic conditions. In Komi PV (ed): Biomechanics VAB. University Park Press, Baltimore, 1976

14. Hamburg P, Gilquist J, Lysholm J, Oberg B: The effect of diagnostic and operative arthroscopy and open meniscectomy on muscle strength in the thigh. Am J Sports Med 11:289–292, 1983

15. Johnson L: The LCR system videotape. Surgi-Series Instrument Maker, Inc, 1983

16. Johnson RJ, Kettelkamp DB, Clark W, Leaverton P: Factors affecting late results after meniscectomy. J Bone Joint Surg 45A:719–729, 1974

17. Markey KL: Rehabilitation of the anterior cruciate ligament deficient knee. Clin Sports Med 1:513–526, 1985

18. Sherman WM, Pearson DR, Plyley MJ et al: Isokinetic rehabilitation after surgery. A review of factors which are important for developing physiotherapeutic techniques after knee surgery. Am J Sports Med 10:155–161, 1982

19. Sherman WM, Plyley MJ, Pearson DR et al: Isokinetic rehabilitation after meniscectomy. A comparison of two methods of training. Physician Sportsmed 11:121, 1983

23

Surgical Repair of Acute and Chronic Lesions of the Lateral Capsular Ligamentous Complex of the Knee

JAMES R. ANDREWS
CHAMP L. BAKER
WALTON W. CURL
RAMESH GIDUMAL

The surgical repair and reconstruction of injuries to the lateral compartment of the knee is fundamentally based on the functional anatomy of the anterolateral and posterolateral compartments of the knee.[13] Injury patterns are determined by the mechanism of injury and the clinical entities of anterolateral and posterolateral rotatory instability can be diagnosed by specific clinical tests. We will review these diagnostic tests and the lateral anatomy and demonstrate means of surgical repair and reconstruction of the anterolateral and posterolateral corners of the knee.

ANATOMY

The ligaments of the lateral compartment of the knee may be classified into three parts: the anterior, middle, and posterior thirds. The anterior third is composed of a capsular ligament extending posteriorly from the lateral borders of the patellar tendon and the patella to the anterior border of the iliotibial band. It is reinforced by the lateral extension of the quadriceps retinaculum. The anterior third of the lateral capsular ligament has no actual attachment to the femur.

The middle third of the lateral ligament is composed of the iliotibial band and the capsular ligament deep to it, extending posteriorly to the fibular collateral ligament. The middle third capsular ligament is partially reinforced by the iliotibial tract, which provides static support, and by the iliotibial band, which functions dynamically. Often the middle-third capsular ligament is thought to be merely areolar tissue because of its close association with the lateral extension of the fat pad, but it is technically strong and is a major lateral static support for the knee at 30° of flexion. The middle third of the lateral capsular ligament attaches proximally to the lateral epicondyle of the femur and distally at the tibial joint margin.

The posterior third includes both capsular and noncapsular ligaments, which form a single functional unit called the arcuate complex. The components of this complex are the fibular collateral ligament, the arcuate ligament, and the tendoaponeurotic unit formed by the popliteus muscle. The posterior third receives dynamic reinforcement from the biceps femoris and the popliteal muscles as well as from the lateral head of the gastrocnemius. Of these the biceps femoris is considered the most important of the dynamic stabilizers as it pulls on its insertion into the posterolateral capsule, thus providing dynamic stability.

Terry et al.[31] have investigated the role of the iliotibial tract, iliopatellar band, and the iliotibial band as both dynamic and static stabilizers, of the lateral side of the knee. The iliotibial tract extends from the greater trochanter down the lateral side of the leg and attaches to the linea aspera through the lateral intermuscular septum. At the knee it separates into the iliotibial band and the iliotibial tract (Fig. 23-1). The iliotibial band is anatomically divided into the aponeurotic, superficial, middle, deep, and capsuloosseous layers. The aponeurotic layer crosses the patellar tendon and makes up the fascia overlying the patella and patellar tendon area. Directly beneath the aponeurotic layer is the superficial layer, which consists of the vastus lateralis, the iliopatellar band, the lateral patellar band, the lateral patellar ligament, the iliotibial tract, and the biceps femoris. The middle layer is composed of fibers in a different orientation from the superficial layer, thus forming a cross-weave that strengthens the iliotibial tract. The deep layer consists of fibers that begin at the termination of the lateral intermuscular septum approximately 6 cm proximal to the lateral epicondyle and cover roughly a triangular area on the lateral

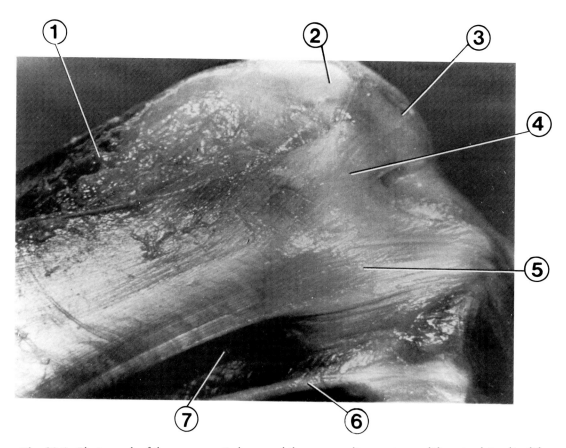

Fig. 23-1. Photograph of the aponeurotic layer and the surrounding anatomy: (1) vastus lateralis; (2) patella; (3) arciform fibers; (4) iliopatellar band; (5) iliotibial tract; (6) long head, biceps femoris; (7) short head, biceps femoris. (Terry GC, Hughston JC, Norwood LA: The anatomy of the iliopatellar band and iliotibial tract. Am J Sports Med 14:39–45, 1986. © 1986 American Orthopaedic Society for Sports Medicine.)

supracondylar face of the femur. The layer then extends laterally in the coronal plane and curves distally following the lateral femoral condyle to blend with the superficial layer in the sagittal plane (Fig. 23-2). The deep layer serves to thicken and strengthen the superficial layer of the iliotibial tract and iliopatellar band. The capsuloosseous layer functions as a medial retaining wall for the deep layer. It acts as the anterolateral ligament of the knee. The short head of the biceps inserts into it along its course. The iliopatellar band anatomically connects the posterior aspect of the iliotibial tract and the femur to the patella (Fig. 23-3).

PATHOLOGY

Anterolateral rotatory instability is a spectrum of injuries occurring to the anterior cruciate ligament, the middle third capsular ligament, and the deep and capsuloosseous layers of the iliotibial tract. Depending on the exact position in rotation of the knee at the time of injury, any of these three structures may be injured alone or in combination. The most common presentation is an injury to the anterior cruciate ligament (ACL), the middle third capsular ligament, and the iliotibial tract. This is gener-

ally a significant injury causing moderate to severe anterolateral rotatory instability. Isolated injuries to the middle third capsular ligament, as well as to the deep and capsuloosseous layers of the iliotibial tract, have been documented as the cause of a milder form of anterolateral rotatory instability.

Posterolateral rotatory instability occurs when the arcuate complex in the posterolateral aspect of the knee is injured. The ACL may or may not be torn. If it is torn, the severity of the posterolateral rotatory instability is increased. When both the posterior cruciate ligament (PCL) and the arcuate ligament complex are injured, the result is a combined posterior cruciate and posterolateral instability.

BIOMECHANICS

Biomechanically, anterolateral rotatory instability (ALRI) has been documented by the "pivot shift test"[10,14] and the "jerk test,"[12,14,29] among others. The jerk test is elicited when the flexed, internally rotated tibia, under valgus stress, is brought from flexion to extension. If the test is positive, subluxation of the lateral femoral–tibial articulation becomes maximum with 30° of flexion. As the knee extends further, spontaneous relocation occurs.

Fig. 23-2. The three-dimensional relationships of the iliotibial tract to the femur and vastus lateralis. **(A)** Artist's depiction of the plane of section used to display the anatomy shown in **B.** Note that this plane of section is not a straight anteroposterior coronal view; the femur and tibia are cut on a "bias." **(B)** Artist's rendering of the anatomic relationships as they appear when the femur is cut at the oblique angle shown in **A.** (Terry GC, Hughston JC, Norwood LA: The anatomy of the iliopatellar band and iliotibial tract. Am J Sports Med 14:39–45, 1986. © 1986 American Orthopaedic Society for Sports Medicine.)

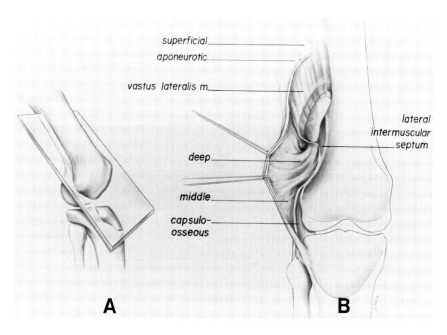

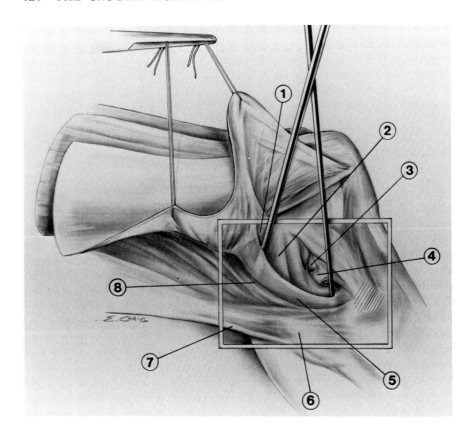

Fig. 23-3. Further dissection of the lateral knee demonstrates the capsuloosseous layer of the iliotibial tract and its relation to other anatomic structures: (1) plantaris tendon; (2) tendon, lateral head, gastrocnemius; (3) midlateral incision exposing lateral femoral condyle; (4) lateral meniscus; (5) capsuloosseous layer of iliotibial tract; (6) head of fibula; (7) long head of biceps; (8) area where short head of biceps is intimate with capsuloosseous layer. (Hughston JC, Terry GC, Norwood LA: The anatomy of the iliopatellar band and the iliotibial tract. Am J Sports Med 14:39–45, 1986. © 1986 American Orthopaedic Society for Sports Medicine.)

The relocation takes the form of a sudden change in the relative velocities of the tibia and the femur; there is a sudden change in the rate of acceleration of the two surfaces, which in engineering terminology is called a "jerk." The pivot shift test is the same maneuver performed in reverse from extension to flexion with subsequent location to subluxation taking place.

DIAGNOSIS

Anterolateral Rotatory Instability

ALRI is usually evident by history and the diagnosis is confirmed by physical examination. Only rarely is examination under anesthesia necessary for a diagnosis, although it is quite helpful in quantifying the degree of instability present.[32] The event causing the ACL tear is usually quite traumatic and the pa-

tient can frequently recall its exact nature. The most common mechanisms of injury are a clipping injury, an internal rotation injury, a hyperextension, or varus stress to the knee. The patient is rarely able to continue to play after the injury. Noyes et al.[26] found that 67 percent of their patients noticed swelling within 1 hour. Other studies report that from 34 to 65 percent of patients recalled either hearing or feeling a pop in their knee at the time of injury.

As mentioned previously, the diagnosis of instability is made on physical examination by a positive pivot shift test,[10,14] jerk test,[12,14,29] or flexion–rotation test.[25] Other findings commonly associated with ALRI are those suggestive of anteromedial rotatory instability (AMRI).[12] They include a positive abduction test at 30° of flexion and a positive anterior Drawer sign with the tibia externally rotated.

Radiographically, Segond's fracture,[24,28] or the lateral capsular sign, is frequently seen in cases of ALRI. The fracture is caused by an avulsion of the lateral tibia by the lateral capsule or, perhaps, by the iliotibial tract.

Posterolateral Rotatory Instability

This usually occurs by one of two mechanisms of injury: noncontact varus hyperextension injury or a blow to the anteromedial aspect of the tibia while the knee is in extension. Less commonly, pure hyperextension will produce clinical posterolateral rotatory instability.

A positive adduction stress test[12] at 30° of knee flexion arouses clinical suspicion and denotes an injury to the lateral complex, but is not specific for posterolateral rotatory instability. A positive posterolateral Drawer test[16] at 30° of flexion is most indicative of posterolateral instability. When positive at 90° of flexion, this test denotes injury to the posterolateral corner as well as a common injury to the PCL. The external rotation-recurvatum test[16] usually can be a subtle indicator of injury to the posterolateral corner when the injury is more directed to the tibial side. The reverse pivot shift test denotes a more serious injury and confirms posterolateral rotatory instability.

SURGICAL REPAIR AND RECONSTRUCTION IN ANTEROLATERAL ROTATORY INSTABILITY

Before treatment, a complete assessment of the patient should be made. What are his or her expectations from surgery, goals, and financial and job constraints? As Smillie[30] said, "No treatment known can restore perfection of function." An accurate sports profile should also be included. Is the patient a red shirt senior with no eligibility left after the present year or a freshman with four to five years of college still ahead?

Treatment of the torn ACL remains controversial. Some orthopaedic surgeons recommend conservative care in selected patients,[5,11,26] others, intraarticular stabilization,[6,8,20] and others, extraarticular repairs.[7,19,33] The ideal treatment and its effectiveness remains to be determined.

Acute Injuries

Some agreement exists, however, among surgeons that acute ACL tears should be arthroscopically evaluated in patients when there is a question about the extent of the damage. The associated meniscal pathology should be addressed and appropriate meniscal repair or partial excision should be done.

In cases of acute moderate to severe ALRI we perform an extraarticular reconstruction[1] or a primary reconstruction, arthroscopically aided, using a patella tendon graft. Noyes et al.[27] found that 35 percent of knees with torn ACLs had severe reinjury by 6 months and 51 percent within 1 year. Other authors[2,9,23] report that nonsurgically treated patients noticed increasing disability with time due to their instability. We believe that this steady deterioration in function can be prevented by an early intervention.

As mentioned previously, intraarticular repairs, augmentations, or reconstructions were all choices for the acute situation in the past. We avoided intraarticular augmentation or reconstruction for fear of postoperative arthrofibrosis, but with newer techniques and quicker rehabilitation, we are now doing acute primary reconstructions. We prefer the extraarticular repair. When patients do not want a surgical procedure, we treat them with a brace that limits flexion and extension to the 30° to 90° range for 4 weeks. A slowly progressive rehabilitation program is followed, stressing hamstring redevelopment and limiting quadriceps work from 90° to 45° of flexion for 3 months. We then place the patient in a derotation brace and restrict activities to allow the capsular ligaments to heal for approximately 7 months. This represents a conservative nonoperative treatment protocol for an acutely torn ACL.

The goal of the lateral extraarticular procedure is to prevent anterior subluxation of the lateral tibial plateau by maintaining the iliotibial tract posterior to the center of rotation of the knee joint. In this position, the tract parallels the course of the anterior cruciate ligament. Because it is farther from the center of rotation, its lever arm is better suited to resist rotation and anterior translation from the lateral side of the knee. Most of the lateral extraarticular procedures function in a similar manner. Some are theorized to function in a dynamic fashion, as does the biceps tendon transfer. However, electromyographic studies have shown that the muscle reaction time is too slow to function in a dynamic method.

Chronic Injuries

In chronic cases of ALRI, the disability experienced is secondary to the anterior subluxation that causes the patient to feel insecure about the injured knee. Since the patient's disability is related to the degree of subluxation, the choice of procedure should be based on the degree of the pivot shift and not the amount of anterior Drawer. In cases of 1+ or 2+ pivot shift, an extraarticular repair can be appropriate. In cases of 3+ pivot shift phenomenon or global instability, an intraarticular repair reinforced by an extraarticular repair is preferred. The extraarticular repair can reinforce and protect the intraarticular repair while vascularization and maturation progress. When anteromedial rotatory instability is also present, a reefing of the posteromedial capsule, with or without advancement of the semimembranosus, is needed.

A patient needing surgery must have access to adequate follow-up and rehabilitation. The rehabilitation must be specific for the procedure performed and is most important to the ultimate success of the procedure.

The Mini-Reconstruction (Andrews)

The lateral extraarticular procedure described by Andrews et al[1] is a tenodesis of the iliotibial tract to the lateral femoral condyle. Two bundles are created along the fibers of the posterior part of the iliotibial tract. The tenodesis to the femur maintains these two bundles posterior to the center of rotation of the knee joint as the knee goes into extension. By not detaching the iliotibial tract either proximally or distally, its neurovascular supply is not jeopardized.

Under tourniquet control, a 9 to 10 cm incision is made laterally, starting just distal to the lateral femoral condyle and extending proximally (Fig. 23-4). The incision exposes the iliotibial band and tract. The anterior and posterior skin flaps are raised in a manner that allows visualization of the lateral intermuscular septum posteriorly. The iliotibial tract is then incised, in the course of its fibers, 4 cm anterior to its posterior border, allowing for visualization of the vastus lateralis. The vastus lateralis is retracted anteriorly to expose the area of the linea aspera of the femur. Hemostasis is achieved and the lateral femoral condyle is cleaned of all soft tissue and periosteum and is roughened with an osteotome. The posterior edge of the lateral femur in the area where the shaft meets with the metaphyseal flare is dissected free. In this region the origin of the lateral head of the gastrocnemius muscle is identified and protected. A second 4 cm longitudinal incision is made medially, centered over the adductor tubercle and carried down through the fascia. At this time, an interval is dissected beneath the distal edge of the vastus medialis obliquus and the adductor magnus tendon is identified deep to it. The subcutaneous tissue is cleaned off the femur in this region so that the metaphysis is evident.

Two Beath needles are used to place drill holes from the area of the linea aspera of the lateral femur through the femur medially. Through these holes the sutures placed in the iliotibial tract will be tied over a 1 cm bone bridge medially. The first hole is placed at the distal portion of the linea aspera at the junction of the femoral shaft and the lateral condyle just anterior to the most posterior border of the cortex. The second drill hole is placed approximately 1 cm anterior and 0.5 cm distal to the first hole. These two drill holes are within the isometric point of the femur relative to tenodesing of the iliotibial tract. Two #5 Ti-cron sutures are woven through the iliotibial tract using a criss-cross stitch. The sutures are then drawn medially by threading the suture ends through the eyes of the Beath needles. Tension is applied to the sutures and they are tied over a 1 cm bone bridge (Fig. 23-5). The iliotibial tract is inspected and care is taken to see that it has been advanced to approximate the lateral cortex of the knee at the isometric point. When the knee is put through a complete range of motion the anterior bundle will be relatively tight in flexion and the posterior bundle will be relatively tight in extension. However, both bundles are predominantly tight in flexion (Fig. 23-6). If the iliotibial tract has not been advanced to the bone, or if the patient

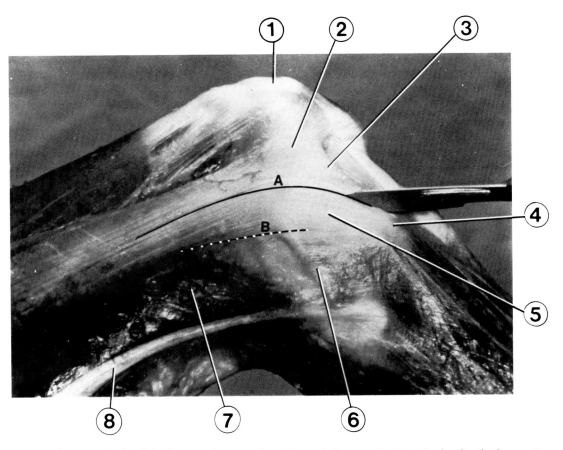

Fig. 23-4. Lateral side of the knee with surgical incisions. *A* shows an incision in the iliotibial tract; *B* shows a second incision between the iliotibial tract and the short head of the biceps femoris. (1) Lateral border of the patella; (2) iliopatellar band; (3) lateral patellotibial ligament; (4) Gerdy's tubercle; (5) iliotibial tract; (6) fibular collateral ligament; (7) short head, biceps femoris; (8) long head, biceps femoris. (Terry GC, Hughston JC, Norwood LA: The anatomy of the iliopatellar band and the iliotibial tract. Am J Sports Med 14:39–45, 1986. © 1986 American Society for Sports Medicine.)

lacks either complete extension or flexion, the drill holes should be redirected. After proper placement has been verified, the sutures are buried beneath the vastus medialis medially. The fiber-splitting incision in the iliotibial tract is then closed and the two skin incisions are closed over Hemovac drains after the tourniquet is released and adequate hemostasis has been obtained.

In the chronic case, the patient is placed in a cylinder cast with 30° of flexion. At 4 weeks the cast is replaced with a Watco rehabilitation knee brace (range of motion 15° to 90°) for an additional 4 weeks. In the acute case, the patient is placed in a

rehabilitation brace (range of motion 15° to 90°) at the time of operation. Four weeks later the range of motion is increased to 0° to 90°, which is maintained for an additional 2 weeks.

This exact procedure has been used for acute and chronic ALRI since 1977. In a review[1] of 62 knees that underwent this procedure, 31 for acute and 31 for chronic anterolateral rotatory instability, satisfactory objective results were obtained in 94 percent of the patients and subjective improvement was noted in 92 percent of the patients with a followup of greater than 2 years. Ninety-three percent of the patients returned to athletic activities that involved

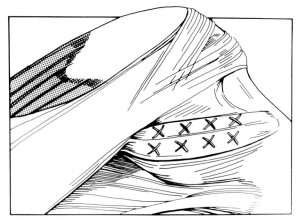

Fig. 23-5. Andrews' iliotibial band tenodesis. The iliotibial tract is attached to the distal femur by two parallel rows of Bunnell sutures that are tied to each other on the medial side of the femur.

rapid change in momentum or pivoting movement. This procedure offers multiple advantages, including a simple longitudinal incision, lack of intraarticular or patellofemoral complications, and ease of rehabilitation.

Hughston Procedure

This procedure also uses a section of iliotibial tract in the form of a tenodesis. After the subcutaneous tissues is dissected, the iliotibial band is identified using a lateral incision. A fiber-splitting incision is made in the band approximately 1 cm above the junction with the lateral intermuscular septum. The posterior half of the iliotibial tract is then separated from the anterior half to allow a pants-over-vest closure. Next, the peroneal nerve is dissected free of the surrounding tissues to preserve it. The long head of the biceps is freed from its attachment to the fibular collateral ligament on the fibula. A vertical incision is then made anterior to the fibular collateral ligament through the lateral capsule, to allow visualization of the lateral joint. After the joint is inspected, the lateral capsule is plicated using a vest-over-pants reefing technique. With the tibia held at 60° of flexion in maximal external rotation, the superior edge of the lower half of the iliotibial band is sutured snugly along the interosseous septum to the linea aspera. Hughston recommends advancement of the biceps tendon to the iliotibial tract

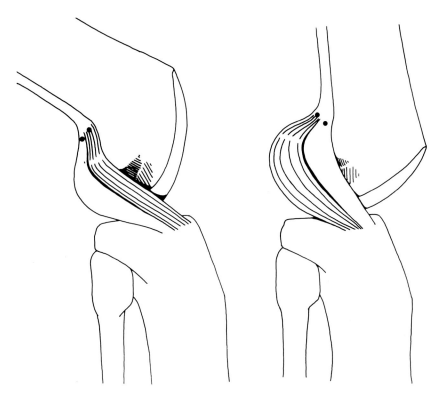

Fig. 23-6. During range of motion of the knee, the anterior bundle will be relatively tight in flexion and the posterior bundle will be relatively tight in extension, if the sutures are correctly placed.

at the region of Gerdy's tubercle (Fig. 23-7). The lower and posterior edge of the long head of the biceps is resutured to the posterior aspect of the fascia at the fibular collateral ligament to restore its dynamic input to this ligament. This procedure, as with the Andrews procedure, causes minimal disruption of the iliotibial tract's blood supply. It has been done at the Hughston Clinic since approximately 1970 with good results.

MacIntosh and Similar Procedures

The MacIntosh procedure for control of anterolateral rotatory instability uses a 1.5 cm wide strip of iliotibial band taken from its midportion for approximately a 16 cm length and left attached distally. The strip is passed beneath a tunnel deep to the fibular collateral ligament and through a hiatus created in the distal end of the intermuscular septum of the lateral femoral condyle. It is then looped back and sutured to the region near Gerdy's tubercle. MacIntosh and Darby[22] initially described this procedure in 1976 and reported good results with 100 patients.

The Losee procedure,[21] modified MacIntosh procedure,[17] and lateral tenodesis procedure (James)[18] are similar to the MacIntosh procedure. They use the distally based iliotibial tract routed beneath the fibular collateral ligament to maintain static stability. The lateral capsule in these procedures is reefed also to provide additional support.

Ellison Procedure

This procedure[7] to control anterolateral rotatory instability uses a proximally based transfer of the iliotibial tract routed beneath the fibular collateral ligament. The proximal attachment is preserved and, theoretically, so is its blood supply. Under tourniquet control the incision is begun just proximal to the lateral femoral condyle and is carried distal in a gentle S shape across the anterolateral aspect of the knee to the lateral margin of the patella tendon. The iliotibial tract is then dissected free from the surrounding subcutaneous tissue. An incision is made along the superior aspect of the tract in the course of its fibers down to the level of Gerdy's tubercle. Gerdy's tubercle is osteotomized and a proximally based flap of iliotibial tract is raised. The tract is approximately 1.5 cm wide. The fascial strip is broadened superiorly and inferiorly to create a broader blood supply. The iliotibial tract is then

Fig. 23-7. The Hughston procedure for chronic anterolateral rotatory instability.

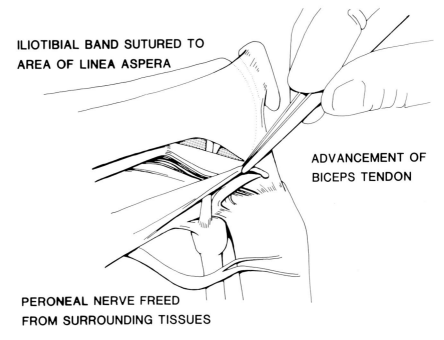

ILIOTIBIAL BAND SUTURED TO
AREA OF LINEA ASPERA

ADVANCEMENT OF
BICEPS TENDON

PERONEAL NERVE FREED
FROM SURROUNDING TISSUES

dissected superiorly and inferiorly and released from the patella and intermuscular septum respectively. This allows some relaxation of the band and closure. The fibular collateral ligament near its insertion onto the femoral condyle is dissected from the surrounding tissue to allow passage of the iliotibial band with its attached bone. At this time the lateral capsule and arcuate complex may be reefed, if necessary. The tract is then advanced anteriorly and distally and fixed using a staple or screw. With the knee in 90° of flexion, a straight line of pull should exist from the staple along the transferred iliotibial band with no kinking as it passes beneath the lateral collateral ligament. If the knee can be extended completely, the transfer is too loose and should be readjusted to allow for only 30° of extension.

All of these lateral extraarticular reconstructions have been used by their various authors with success. We recommend a lateral extraarticular reconstruction as the procedure of choice in ACL-deficient knees with moderate or severe acute anterolateral rotatory instability and mild to moderate chronic anterolateral instability. These extraarticular procedures may be used to supplement intraarticular repairs performed for the more severe form of anterolateral instability with a severe pivot shift phenomenon. The major advantage of an extraarticular procedure is that it is less invasive.

SURGICAL REPAIR AND RECONSTRUCTION IN POSTEROLATERAL ROTATORY INSTABILITY

Injury mechanisms that damage the structure of the posterolateral corner in the knee are quite poorly understood, and a myriad of injury patterns exists. Therefore, classifications of these injuries can include isolated posterolateral as well as combined instabilities. PCL is often injured at the same time as lateral capsular structures, although the damage to the PCL is often not severe enough to cause a demonstrable laxity.[3]

Surgical repair of acute ligamentous damage to the lateral complex of the knee can be accomplished through a lateral hockey-stick incision, which allows for evaluation of the lateral capsular and extracapsular structures.[4] Tears of the capsular structure of the posterolateral corner seldom occur in combination with bony avulsion, although the so-called "arcuate sign" can represent a ligamentous avulsion of the arcuate ligament off the head of the fibula or the posterolateral corner of the tibia. Injuries to posterolateral structures usually occur due to an overstretching phenomenon with interstitial hemorrhage and loss of normal tendinous consistency. When bony avulsions occur, they should be reattached to the donor site using accepted ligament-to-bone repair techniques such as direct suturing, tension banding, and screw fixation if the fragment is of sufficient size.

Injuries to the popliteus usually occur at or about the musculotendinous junction. When the tendinous portion is pulled from the femur, it usually can be reattached to the femur with a nonabsorbable Bunnell-type suture placed through the tendinous insertion and attached directly to the femur through drill holes. When the tear is in the pure muscle belly structure at the posteromedial corner, it can be tenodesed to the posterolateral corner of the tibia through drill holes passed from the anteromedial or anterolateral aspect of the tibia to the posterior corner. Sutures are brought forward and tied anteriorly over bony bridge. Midportion substance tears can be reapproximated using a pants-over-vest mattress advancing suture. In cases of severe total disruption without repairable substance, the tendinous portion of the lateral head of the gastrocnemius muscle can be advanced anteriorly and superiorly with a bone block onto the lateral gastrocnemius and act as an anchor for direct repair of the popliteus or arcuate ligament to this.

The arcuate ligament is, likewise, more commonly injured in its midportion and similar repairs can be accomplished.

The fibular collateral ligament is often torn from the styloid process of the fibula itself and can be reapproximated to its bony insertion. Care should be taken to maintain its normal relationship to both the short head of the biceps and the popliteus tendon. Both the long and short heads of the biceps femoris can be avulsed from either the tibial or fibular attachment. The surgeon should pay careful attention to this tendinous structure insertion and seek out and repair any damage.

Reconstruction of *chronic instability of the posterolateral corner* largely depends on the site of the initial injury.[15] If the injury is known to be distal (from the tibia or fibular head determined at the time of exploration or by radiographic evidence of avulsion of the bone fragments from this area), the repair needs to be distal. The repair should be made through drill holes to reestablish the continuity of the posterior corner to the tibia.

When the initial site of injury is not known or is interstitial or proximal, an anterosuperior displacement of the entire arcuate ligament complex of the bone block is presently the surgical procedure of choice.

A lateral hockey-stick incision is made and the entire lateral structure is identified. An arthrotomy is made anterior to the popliteus and fibular collateral ligament, exposing the insertion of these two structures on the lateral femoral condyle. The iliotibial band has previously been incised in line with its fibers, and when the inferior portion is retracted the entire arcuate ligament complex (popliteus, fibular collateral ligament, arcuate ligament, and tendinous head of the lateral gastrocnemius) can be identified and isolated. Using an osteotome, the entire insertion is removed with a flap of bone and used as a bone block. The surgeon must carefully divide the posterior aspect of the gastrocnemius from the remainder of the posterior capsule and advance it anteriorly and superiorly (Fig. 23-8). Sutures should be placed in this division so that the posterolateral corner can be reapproximated and no deficit is left.

After the completion of other indicated procedures, such as medial repair or intraarticular surgery, the leg is acutely flexed and internally rotated. Using a staple, the bone block is advanced anteriorly and superiorly and twisted on itself to afford greater length and is secured to an area of the lateral

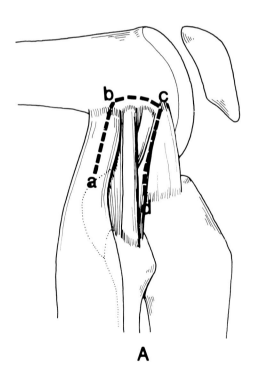

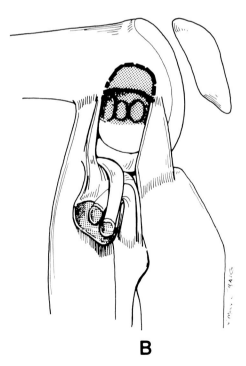

A   **B**

Fig. 23-8. Surgical repair for posterolateral rotatory instability. Line *ab* in **A** is the incision along the medial border of the lateral gastrocnemius tendon. Line *bc* is the edge of the osteotomized area. Line *cd* is the lateral capsular incision.

femoral condyle in an area that has been denuded. Nonabsorbable sutures are then used to attach the soft tissues to periosteum around the lateral capsule, and the remainder of the soft tissues are closed in a routine manner (Fig. 23-9).

Postoperative immobilization is accomplished with the foot in internal rotation in a long-leg cast. A pelvic band is applied to prevent the leg from externally rotating and putting an adduction strain on the knee, causing the repair to stretch. The cast is removed at 6 weeks. The patient remains non-weight-bearing in a double upright long-leg brace that slowly allows the return to extension. When the patient is within 15° of full extension, toe-touch weightbearing is begun. The brace is worn for 2 to 3 months to allow gradual return of extension to prevent recurvatum.

COMMENTS

The diagnosis of acute or chronic lesions of the lateral capsular ligamentous complex depends on a precise understanding of the functional anatomy of the lateral compartment. The classification of the laxity depends on specific clinical tests and the associated anatomic lesions.

Once the clinical diagnosis has been established, the proper repair or reconstruction is dictated by the severity of the clinical laxity. In acute cases, surgery is based on direct anatomic repair. Caution must be used in applying reconstructive procedures to the lateral compartment in acute injuries lest increased surgical morbidity result.

In chronic cases, surgical reconstructive procedures are still based on applied functional anatomic

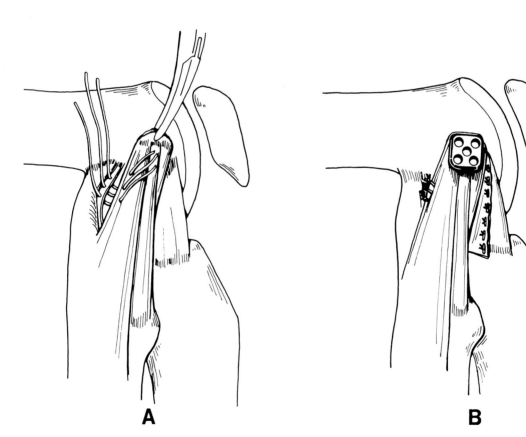

A

B

Fig. 23-9. (A) The arcuate complex is advanced and held at a point farther proximal than its original position. **(B)** The bone plug is secured to the previously prepared raw surface of the condyle with a staple.

principles. It is imperative to recognize the combined clinical laxities and other associated ligamentous injuries, such as injury to the ACL, PCL, or both, or to the medial capsuloligamentous complex.

Proper recognition and early treatment of acute ligamentous lesions of the knee give a much better clinical result than the reconstruction of a chronic ligamentous instability.

The lateral side of the knee should no longer be considered the dark side of the moon. When it is injured, it should be approached systematically and anatomically and repaired or reconstructed accordingly.

ACKNOWLEDGMENT

This work was supported in part by the Hughston Sports Medicine Foundation, Columbus, Georgia.

REFERENCES

1. Andrews JR, Sanders RA, Morin B: Surgical treatment of anterolateral rotatory instability. A follow-up study. Am J Sports Med 13:112–119, 1985

2. Arnold JA, Coker TP, Heaton LM et al: Natural history of anterior cruciate tears. Am J Sports Med 7:305–313, 1979

3. Baker CL, Norwood LA, Hughston JC: Acute combined posterior cruciate and posterolateral instability of the knee. Am J Sports Med 12:204–208, 1984

4. Baker CL, Norwood LA, Hughston JC: Acute posterolateral rotatory instability of the knee. J Bone Joint Surg 65A:614–618, 1983

5. Chick RR, Jackson DW: Tears of the anterior cruciate ligament in young athletes. J Bone Joint Surg 60A:970–973, 1978

6. Clancy WG, Nelson DA, Reider B, Narechania RG: Anterior cruciate ligament reconstruction using one-third of the patellar ligament, augmented by extra-articular tendon transfers. J Bone Joint Surg 64A:352–359, 1982

7. Ellison AE: Distal iliotibial band transfer for anterolateral rotatory instability of the knee. J Bone Joint Surg 61A:330–337, 1979

8. Ficat P, Duzacq JP, Ricci A: Chirurgie repartrice des laxities chroniques des ligaments croises du genou. Rev Chir Orthop 61(2):89–100, 1975

9. Fetto JF, Marshall JL: The natural history and diagnosis of anterior cruciate ligament insufficiency. Clin Orthop 147:29–38, 1980

10. Galway HR, MacIntosh DL: The lateral pivot shift: a symptom and sign of anterior cruciate ligament insufficiency. Clin Orthop 147:45–50, 1980

11. Giove TP, Miller SJ, Kent BE et al: Nonoperative treatment of the torn anterior cruciate ligament. J Bone Joint Surg 65A:184–192, 1983

12. Hughston JC, Andrews JR, Cross MJ, Moschi A: Classification of knee ligament instabilities. Part I. The medial compartment and cruciate ligament. J Bone Joint Surg 58A:159–172, 1976

13. Hughston JC, Andrews JR, Cross MJ, Moschi A: Classification of knee ligament instabilities. Part II. The lateral compartment. J Bone Joint Surg 58A:173–179, 1976

14. Hughston JC, as cited in Edmondson AS, Crenshaw AH (eds): Campbell's Operative Orthopaedics. CV Mosby, St. Louis, 1980, p. 923

15. Hughston JC, Jacobson KE: Chronic posterolateral rotatory instability of the knee. J Bone Joint Surg 67A:351–359, 1985

16. Hughston JC, Norwood LA: The posterolateral drawer test and external rotation recurvatum test for posterolateral rotatory instability of the knee. Clin Orthop 147:82–87, 1980

17. Ireland J, Trickey EL: MacIntosh tenodesis for anterolateral instability of the knee. J Bone Joint Surg 62B:340–345, 1980

18. James SL: Knee ligament reconstruction. pp. 31–104. In Evarts CM (ed): Surgery of the Musculoskeletal System. Churchill Livingstone, New York, 1983

19. Johnson LL: Lateral capsular ligament complex: anatomical and surgical considerations. Am J Sports Med 7:156–160, 1979

20. Jones JG: Reconstruction of anterior cruciate ligament: a technique using the central one-third of the patellar ligament. J Bone Joint Surg 45A:9–25, 1963

21. Losee RE, Johnson TR, Southwick WD: Anterior subluxation of the lateral tibial plateau. A diagnostic test and operative repair. J Bone Joint Surg 60A:1015–1030, 1978

22. MacIntosh DL, Darby TA: Lateral substitution reconstruction. J Bone Joint Surg 58B:142, 1976

23. McDaniel WJ, Dameron TB: Untreated ruptures of the anterior cruciate ligament. A follow-up study. J Bone Joint Surg 62A:696–705, 1980

24. Milch H: Cortical avulsion fracture of the lateral tibial condyle. J Bone Joint Surg 18:159–164, 1936

25. Noyes FR, Bassett RW, Grood ES, Butler DL: Arthroscopy in acute traumatic hemarthrosis of the knee.

Incidence of anterior cruciate tears and other injuries. J Bone Joint Surg 62A:687–695, 1980

26. Noyes FR, Matthews DS, Mooar PA, Grood ES: The symptomatic anterior cruciate-deficient knee. Part II: The results of rehabilitation, activity modification, and counseling in functional disability. J Bone Joint Surg 65A:163–173, 1983

27. Noyes FR, Mooar PA, Matthews DS, Butler DL: The symptomatic anterior cruciate-deficient knee. Part I: The long-term functional disability in athletically active individuals. J Bone Joint Surg 65A:154–162, 1983

28. Segond P: Récherches cliniques et experimentales sur les épanchements sanguines du genou par entorse. Prog Med 7:279, 1879

29. Slocum DB, James SL, Larson RL, Singer KM: Clinical test for anterolateral rotatory instability of the knee. Clin Orthop 118:63–69, 1976

30. Smillie IS: Injuries of the Knee Joint. Churchill Livingstone, Edinburgh, 1946

31. Terry GC, Hughston JC, Norwood LA: The anatomy of the iliopatellar band and iliotibial tract. Am J Sports Med 14:39–45, 1986

32. Torg JS, Conrad W, Kalen V: Clinical diagnosis of anterior cruciate ligament instability in the athlete. Am J Sports Med 4:84–93, 1976

33. Unverferth LJ, Bagenstose JE: Extra-articular reconstructive surgery for combined anterolateral-anteromedial rotatory instability. Am J Sports Med 7:34–39, 1979

24
ACL Insufficiency in Children

JESSE C. DELEE

Acute or chronic anterior cruciate ligament (ACL) insufficiency is extremely unusual in children younger than 14 years of age with open physes.[3,7,29,33] Furthermore, reports of knee ligament injuries of any type in children younger than 14 years of age are extremely uncommon.[2,3,6] Practitioners therefore have few guidelines in their approach to the cruciate-deficient knee in a child.

The marked increased participation in sporting activities and the accompanying awareness of knee ligament injuries and their disabilities in adults have stimulated interest in these problems in children.[2,3,29,34] Certainly, the increased participation of children in soccer, snow skiing, and other sporting activities has resulted in a higher incidence of ACL injuries than a review of the current literature would indicate.

Orthopaedic injuries in children, particularly fractures, classically have been reported to do better than the corresponding injuries in adults.[27,29,32] This finding, however, does not apply to all soft tissue injuries, and specifically not to ligamentous injuries in children. The natural conservatism that pervades fracture management in children has not produced acceptable results when used in the treatment of knee ligament injuries. Clanton et al.[3] and Delee and Curtis[6] have both emphasized the importance of treating these injuries using the guidelines accepted for adults. Even with the use of aggressive surgical treatment, these authors[3,6] reported residual ligamentous laxities comparable to those found in adults after similar injuries. These studies lend support to the surgical treatment of these ligamentous injuries in children.

CATEGORIES OF PATIENTS

ACL insufficiency in children is found in two broad groups: nontraumatic ACL insufficiency and posttraumatic ACL insufficiency.

ACL Insufficiency In Children

1. Nontraumatic ACL insufficiency
   Generalized nonpathologic joint laxity
   Congenital absence of the ACL
2. Posttraumatic ACL insufficiency[14,33]
   Avulsion of the intercondylar eminence of the tibia[10,19,21,22,28,30,35]
   Midsubstance tears of the ACL[6]
   Avulsion of the femoral attachment of the ACL[7]

Nontraumatic ACL Insufficiency

Generalized Nonpathologic Joint Laxity

Children with generalized joint laxity, may have a 1/3 to 2/3 anterior Drawer (bilaterally) with the foot in neutral rotation without any associated symptoms.[18] The flexion–rotation Drawer and pivot shift test may also be positive, and hyperextension of both knees is often noted. These patients may also have a positive reverse pivot shift test. It is extremely important to recognize such generalized ligamentous laxity when evaluating a child with an acute injury to the knee. Therefore, it is even more important in children than in adults to examine the opposite un-injured knee to establish a baseline of ligamentous laxity.

Congenital Absence of the ACL

Those children who present with ACL insufficiency without a history of significant trauma may have congenital absence or attenuation of the ACL. Such absence or attenuation is often associated with other congenital anomalies of the involved limb. These anomalies should suggest the diagnosis.[2] Congenital absence or attenuation of the ACL has been reported in association with congenital dislocation of the knee,[5,15] proximal focal femoral deficiency, and in patients with a valgus knee and leg length discrepancy.[14] I have seen this entity in a patient with a ball-and-socket ankle joint and absence of the fibular two rays of the foot. The associated congenital anomalies often limit participation in sports and hence these patients may not present with the usual athletics-related symptoms of ACL insufficiency. However, these are patients in whom the insufficiency may become symptomatic in the activities of daily living.

Additionally, the ACL may be totally absent in an otherwise normal knee.[11] Giorgi[11] presented a radiographic analysis of the appearance of the intercondylar eminence in 2,500 normal knees. He reported several variations in the radiographic appearance of the intercondylar eminence (Fig. 24-1). Total aplasia of the intercondylar eminence suggests congenital absence of the ACL that may occur in an otherwise normal extremity. Giorgi sug-

gested that development of the intercondylar eminence may be arrested if the traction supplied by the ACL is absent.[11,14] Although isolated congenital absence is distinctly unusual, it should be considered when a chronically lax ACL is evaluated. Radiographic absence of the intercondylar eminence in conjunction with the cruciate-deficient knee suggests this diagnosis.

Posttraumatic ACL Insufficiency

The limited number of reports of injuries to the ACL in children is probably due to two factors. The first is that in children, the knee ligaments are stronger than the adjacent physeal plate.[7,24,29,31] Therefore, physeal plate disruption or long bone fractures occur before ligament failure.[2,3,31,32] In addition, the anatomic location of all knee ligament origins and insertions in relation to the physeal plates of the distal femur and proximal tibia is responsible for the fact that physeal separations are more common than ligament disruptions (Fig. 24-2). Only the tibial collateral ligament has an origin or insertion distal to either the femoral or tibial physeal plate, and hence stress applied to the knee joint is concentrated at these two physeal plates in preference to the collateral or central pivot ligaments.[3] The second reason is that in the past, children have not been engaged in the same traumatic activities that produce ligament disruptions in the adolescent and adult.[8,23] Eilert[8] reported that most knee problems in children younger than 12 years of age are congenital while those in children older than 12 years of age are more

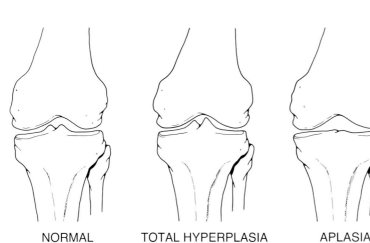

NORMAL   TOTAL HYPERPLASIA   APLASIA

Fig. 24-1. Variations in the morphologic appearance of the intercondylar eminence of the tibia. Total aplasia of the eminence suggests congenital absence of the ACL.

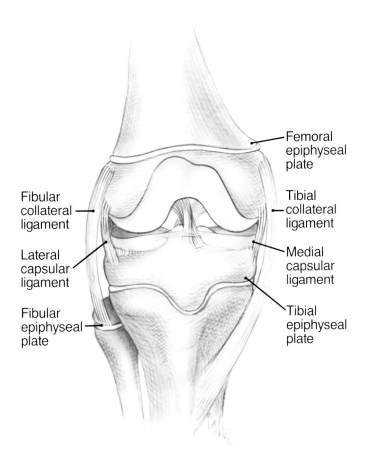

Fig. 24-2. Neither the capsular nor the cruciate ligaments cross the physeal plates. Due to this peculiarity of their origin and insertion and the relative strength of the ligaments, stress concentrates at the physeal plates, producing physeal separation rather than ligament failure.

often related to trauma. In a series of children who underwent knee arthroscopy, Morrissy et al.[23] found that only 36 percent of the patients related a history of significant trauma. It is important to emphasize, however, that changing participation in sports in younger children will alter this and increase the incidence of recognized knee ligament injuries in children.

Avulsion of the Intercondylar Eminence of the Tibia

The ACL is attached to the tibia in a depressed area in front of and lateral to the anterior tibial spine. There is also a fibrous attachment to the base of the anterior spine and a slip to the anterior horn of the lateral meniscus.[12,35] (Fig. 24-3). This anatomic arrangement and the relative strength of the ligament itself compared to that of the adjacent bone and physeal plate explain why most ACL injuries in children are avulsions of the ligament insertion into bone at the tibial eminence.[9,11,24,29,35] Rinaldi and Mazzarella[28] report that, in young patients before the growth plate is fused, the intercondylar eminence offers less resistance to traction forces than does the ACL itself. Therefore, anterior, posterior, and rotatory stresses in children result in avulsions of the tibial eminence while in the adult they result in stretching or disruption of the cruciate ligament.[2,3,16,17,21,22]

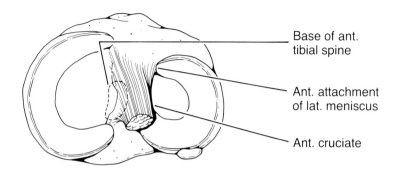

Base of ant. tibial spine

Ant. attachment of lat. meniscus

Ant. cruciate

Fig. 24-3. The ACL inserts anterior and slightly lateral to the anterior tibial spine.

The diagnosis of tibial spine avulsion is suggested by the history of a knee injury associated with an acute hemarthrosis.[28] A lateral radiograph will demonstrate elevation of the tibial eminence and is diagnostic. Rinaldi and Mazzarella[28] recommend surgical fixation only in cases of obvious separation of the fracture fragment. They report that although displaced fractures not treated by anatomic reduction will heal, this will result in an effective lengthening of the anterior cruciate ligament and excessive anterior–posterior laxity.[28] The ACL avulsions treated by open reduction in their series were stable and without roentgenographic evidence of arthrosis at follow-up examination.[28] Clanton et al[3] have reported that there is often collateral ligament damage associated with tibial spine fractures and that a careful evaluation must be done to rule out secondary capsular injuries.

Garcia and Neer[10] recommend treating displaced intercondylar eminence fractures by aspiration and closed reduction with hyperextension of the knee. Their criterion for acceptable reduction was simply the ability to straighten the knee; no radiographic criteria of reduction were presented. These authors reported no anterior instability in patients with isolated avulsion of the intercondylar eminence (i.e., without associated collateral ligament injury). They concluded, therefore, that if the anterior Drawer sign in these patients is positive, there must be an associated injury to a collateral ligament.[10]

Rang[27] emphasized that in addition to avulsion of the bony eminence noted radiographically, wings of articular cartilage are lifted from the weightbearing surface of the medial and lateral aspects of the tibial plateau when the intercondylar eminence is avulsed. In his opinion, the femoral condyles "ram" these wings of articular cartilage into position as the knee is extended, which would explain the hyperextension mechanism of reduction reported by Garcia and Neer.[10] Rang[27] emphasized, however, that failure of closed reduction is usually secondary to an interposed meniscus or to abnormal rotation of the eminence fragment. In these cases, he recommends open reduction.

Myers and McKeever,[21,22] in a series of isolated fractures of the intercondylar eminence, found that avulsion of the ACL at the intercondylar eminence was usually present without severe damage to other supporting knee structures. Only four of their patients had clinically detectable anterior instability of the knee and all four had associated medial collateral ligament (MCL) injuries.

Myers and McKeever[21,22] classified tibial eminence fractures into four groups: type I avulsions have only slight anterior elevation of the eminence, while in type II the anterior elevation is more marked. They recommend treating these two types by aspiration and immobilization in a long leg cast with the knee in 20° of flexion. Type III injuries are those in which the entire eminence is elevated and displaced. Type III+ injuries are those in which there is rotation in addition to complete displacement. They recommend that types III and III+ be treated by open reduction and fixation by suturing with absorbable suture. More elaborate means of fixation that require secondary arthrotomy for removal are not indicated.[19,21,22] Myers and McKeever[21,22] do not recommend an attempt at closed reduction in types III and III+ fractures. Their results indicated that all patients undergoing open reduction and internal fixation have good to excellent results. By comparison, four of five type III fractures treated by closed means had poor results.

Zaricznyj[35] reported 10 children younger than 15 years of age with avulsion fractures of the tibial eminence. In 9 of these 10 patients the avulsion was the only injury. He warns against permitting residual displacement of the tibial eminence following closed reduction, because a displaced eminence can mechanically block full knee extension and cause relative lengthening of the ACL.[35] He emphasized that if this displacement is allowed to persist, atrophy, shortening, and laxity of the ligament will result. All the patients he reported in whom an anatomic reduction was obtained by open or closed means returned to their preinjury level of activity.

Recently the association of avulsion of the intercondylar eminence with other ligamentous injuries to the knee in children has been stressed.[2,3,13] Injuries to the collateral ligaments in conjunction with tibial spine avulsion produce a degree of ligamentous laxity greater than that following either injury occurring as an isolated entity.[2,3] Hyndman and Brown[13] reported seven cases of avulsion of the tibial spine, all of which were associated with other ligamentous disruptions of the knee. Bradley et al.[2] reported six cases of MCL disruption in children younger than 12 years of age, and three of these six patients had associated ACL injuries. Two had spine avulsions and one had a midsubstance tear. Clanton et al.[3] reported nine cases of collateral ligament injury in children less than 14 years of age. Five of these nine had associated intercondylar eminence fractures. It is significant that four of these five also had evidence of insubstance damage to the ACL. These reports emphasize the need for a complete evaluation of all knee ligaments in children in whom a tibial spine avulsion is diagnosed.

Midsubstance Tear of the ACL

Midsubstance tears of the ACL alone or associated with other knee ligament injuries in children are distinctly unusual.[2,3,13] Clanton et al.[3] reported a single patient with a midstance ACL tear. This patient had symptomatic ACL insufficiency at follow-up. Bradley et al.[2] also reported one patient with a mid-substance ACL tear associated with a MCL injury. This was the only patient in their series with a poor result secondary to marked residual instability. DeLee and Curtis[6] reported three patients under the age of 14 with a midsubstance ACL injury without associated collateral ligament injuries. All three patients underwent a primary repair of the ACL after a method modified from the technique of Marshall et al.[20] Two years postoperatively, all three patients had returned to their preinjury activity levels including sports. However, two of the three complained of episodes of giving way when they attempted to cut on the involved knee. It was more important that clinical examination of these two patients revealed grade II anterior Drawer laxity with the foot in neutral rotation, a positive pivot shift test, and a positive flexion–rotation Drawer test. Although the third patient had no complaints of instability, he did have a grade I anterior Drawer test with the foot in neutral rotation. His flexion–rotation Drawer and pivot shift tests were negative. The authors[6] were careful, however, to state that this patient was less athletically active than the other two patients in whom the repair had not resulted in a stable knee. The authors concluded that the laxity demonstrated by their patients warns of future difficulty. This finding is in agreement with that of Clanton et al., who reported the return of children to preinjury activity levels in spite of significant ligament laxities following primary ligament repair. These two studies suggest that primary repair of these injuries, although it permits the children to return to their preinjury activities, results in pathological clinical laxity and strongly suggests that the ACL functions no better after primary repair in children than in adults.

Avulsion of the ACL from the Femur

Avulsion of the ACL from the femur in a child was reported by Eady et al.[7] in 1982. The patient, a 7-year-old girl, had an avulsion of the femoral attachment of the ACL. The patient had a 3+ anterior Drawer but a negative pivot shift. After reattachment of the femoral insertion, the knee was stable. Thus the reattachment of the ACL origin (or insertion) in the child can result in a stable knee, if it is diagnosed and treated by anatomic reduction.

DIAGNOSIS

The criteria for the diagnosis of an ACL injury in a child, with few exceptions, are little different than that in an adult. A careful physical examination and specific radiographs point to the diagnosis in most cases.

The history, like that in an adult, is that of a twisting or hyperextending injury. The patient often hears or feels a pop in the knee and there is subsequent "slipping of the knee." Often, the patient will describe pivot shifting associated with the injury. The rapid onset of swelling, suggesting a hemarthrosis, usually is noted in the "isolated" ACL injury.

Isolated ACL injuries are usually noncontact injuries that occur with the rapid change of position or hyperextension. Accompanying varus or valgus stress on the knee may result in injury to the medial or lateral collateral ligament systems.

PHYSICAL EXAMINATION

After an acute injury there is a tense hemarthrosis. Careful palpation at the joint line may reveal tenderness at the medial and/or posterolateral corners, suggesting associated meniscal injury. The examiner should carefully palpate the origins and insertions of the medial and lateral collateral ligaments to detect associated ligamentous instabilities. An area of tenderness just above the lateral femoral condyle in the area of insertion of Kaplan's fibers of the iliotibial band may be present.

The size of a child's leg makes the Lachman test relatively easy to perform, even in the presence of a hemarthrosis. The pivot shift test is also easy to elicit in a child because of the size of the limb. In my experience, the positive Lachman, flexion–rotation Drawer, and pivot shift tests are easy to elicit and uniformly present in this injury. A positive anterior Drawer test should suggest associated collateral ligament damage.

In the evaluation of a patient with a suspected ACL tear, it is critical to obtain both routine and stress radiographs. Since the most frequent injury to the ACL in a child is an avulsion of the tibial spine, radiographs to evaluate this area are essential. Additionally, because of the location of the insertions of the medial and lateral collateral ligaments in reference to the physes of the tibia and femur, varus and valgus stress radiographs are important to detect associated physeal plate disruption or ligamentous injuries.

The place of arthroscopy in diagnosing an injury to the ACL in children, in my opinion, is no different than in the adult. In most patients the diagnosis should be perfectly obvious from the physical examination. The finding of a positive flexion–rotation Drawer test, Lachman test, and pivot shift test accompanied by a compatible history, should lead the examiner to the correct diagnosis. The role of arthroscopy is not in diagnosing a torn ACL, but in evaluating the menisci before ligament repair and/or reconstruction.

Children with a chronic ACL deficiency present with a classic history of giving way with associated episodes of swelling. On physical examination it is easy to elicit a positive Lachman, pivot shift, and flexion-rotation Drawer test. These patients usually have a grossly positive anterior Drawer test with the foot in neutral rotation, indicating combined anteromedial and anterolateral rotatory instability secondary to stretching of the collateral ligaments. Meniscal lesions are also usually present.

TREATMENT

Just as treatment of the ACL injury in an adult is in a state of controversy, so is its treatment in the child. In children, long-term follow-up of a congrol group to delineate clearly the natural history of the injury is not available. DeLee and Curtis[6] report that children with a cruciate-deficient knee and concomitant episodes of instability are not functionally limited. However, the fact that episodes of pivot shifting occur portend a poor long-term prognosis, at least from a theoretical standpoint. The fact that tears of the menisci occur with these giving way episodes, and that meniscectomy in a child is known to produce a bad result, I approach the ACL injury in a child with the goal of stabilizing the knee. I reemphasize, however, that the diagnosis must be accurate, and a nontraumatic ACL insufficiency not be present.

The Acute ACL Injury

After a thorough clinical examination and radiographs that show no evidence of a fracture or physeal injury, patients with the clinical findings of an ACL injury are taken to the operating room to be examined under anesthesia. A thorough arthroscopic examination of the knee is performed, with specific attention being paid to the location of the ACL tear and the status of the medial and lateral menisci. Peripheral detachments of the posterior horns of the menisci, which are present in these injuries, are carefully evaluated. If the detachment is in a region with vascularity, meniscal repair is performed. Unstable tears within the body of the meniscus that do not have a vascular supply are treated by limited partial meniscectomy. The ACL is carefully evaluated to determine its point of disruption.

At this point, the ACL disruption is addressed. In the acute injury with no associated collateral ligament injuries, I prefer to perform a primary repair of any avulsion of the ACL insertion off the femur or tibia.

In a midsubstance tear, an open repair of the ACL using a method modified from that of Marshall is performed.[20] Three sutures are placed in the distal portion of the ligament and are brought out through the femoral epiphysis using two small Kirschner wires for drill holes. The proximal end of the ligament is then sutured to the distal portion using simple interrupted sutures. No sutures cross the phy-

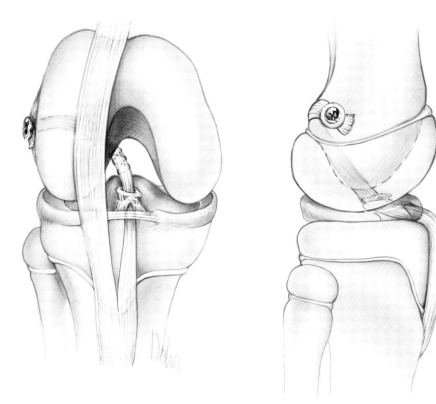

Fig. 24-4. The patellar tendon is left attached to the tibial tubercle and passed over the front of the tibia. It is fixed to the femoral origin using one suture which enters and exits through the distal femoral epiphysis and one that goes "over the top." The stump of the ACL is used to "augment" the graft. An extra-articular reconstruction may be added to this procedure.

seal plates. The fat pad is then sutured to the cruciate ligament repair. An extraarticular augmentation is then performed. A strip of the iliotibial band 2.5 cm wide and 15 cm long is detached proximally and left attached at Gerdy's tubercle. This strip of fascia is passed beneath the fibular collateral ligament, and brought out above the fibular collateral ligament. It is fixed to the femur above the physis with a 4-0 cancellous screw and spiked washer. It is then brought back over the fibular collateral ligament and put down to bone below Gerdy's tubercle. Fixation is obtained with a 4-0 cancellous screw and spiked washer. Great care is taken in positioning the screws so that they do not cross the physes. Preliminary location of screw direction using a small smooth K-wire is recommended. The defect in the iliotibial band is closed with interrupted suture. The patients are placed in a long leg brace with knee motion from 30° to 70° of flexion for 4 weeks. Progressive mobilization is then begun.

The Chronic ACL-Deficient Knee

In the patient with symptomatic chronic ACL laxity, reconstruction is considered only if instability occurs during activities of daily living. Participation in athletics is not considered an indication for reconstruction. Also, the age of the patient is critical. If the patient is nearing the time of physeal closure, surgical treatment is delayed.

Careful evaluation of the secondary capsular restraints is undertaken. Posteromedial and posterolateral corner laxity are corrected by ligamentous plication. The anterior cruciate ligament deficiency is approached with a combined intraarticular and extraarticular reconstruction. The remnant of the anterior cruciate ligament is exposed surgically. The ACL remnants proximally and distally are carefully teased away from the scar tissue and left intact. A strip of the patellar tendon is left attached to the tibial tubercle, allowed to ride over the anterior border of the tibia, and is sutured to the area of the femoral insertion of the ACL. I learned this technique from Dr. John Bergfeld; it is called the "tomato steak" approach[1] (Fig. 24-4). The remainder of the scar tissue is sutured around the graft. The sutures in the graft are brought out through two drill holes in the femoral epiphysis. Again, drill holes do not cross the physeal plates. The extraarticular reconstruction described earlier is performed just as described in the acute injury. The patient is placed in a brace with knee motion from 30° to 70° of flexion for 4 weeks. Mobilization and rehabilitation are then instituted and followed, as in the adult, with a combined intraarticular/extraarticular reconstruction.

COMMENTS

It is important to recognize that there is not enough experience with either acute or chronic ACL deficiency in children to warrant recommending principles without hesitation. I consider the principles of significance to be (1) meniscal preservation; (2) stabilization of the knee using techniques that do not involve drill holes or sutures across the physeal plate; and (3) limited activities for a minimum of 9 to 12 months until the range of motion and muscle strength in the knee have been restored.

ACKNOWLEDGMENT

John A. Bergfeld, M.D., in a personal communication, suggested the "tomato stake" techique for ACL reconstruction in children.

REFERENCES

1. Blount WP: Fractures in Children. Williams & Wilkins, Baltimore, 1954
2. Bradley GW, Shives, TC, Samuelson KM: Ligament injuries in the knees of children. J Bone Joint Surg 61A:588–591, 1979
3. Clanton TO, DeLee JC, Sanders B, Neidre A: Knee ligament injuries in children. J Bone Joint Surg 61A:1195–1201, 1979
4. Crowninshield RD, Pope MH: The strength and failure characteristics of rat medial collateral ligaments. J Trauma 16:99, 1976
5. Curtis BH, Fisher RL: Congenital hyperextension with anterior subluxation of the knee. J Bone Joint Surg 51A:255–269, 1969
6. DeLee JC, Curtis R: Anterior cruciate ligament insufficiency in children. Clin Orthop 172:112–119, 1983

7. Eady JL, Cardenas CD, Sopa D: Avulsion of the femoral attachment of the anterior cruciate ligament in a seven year-old child. A case report. J Bone Joint Surg 64A:1376–1378, 1982

8. Eilert RE: Arthroscopy of the knee joint in children. Orthop Rev 5:61–65, 1976

9. Furman W, Marshall JL, Girgis FG: The anterior cruciate ligament—a functional analysis based on post-mortem studies. J Bone Joint Surg 58A:179–185, 1976

10. Garcia A, Neer CS: Isolated fractures of the intercondylar eminence of the tibia. Am J Surg 95:593–598, 1958

11. Giorgi B: Morphologic variations of the intercondylar eminence of the knee. Clin Orthop 8:209–217, 1956

12. Girgis FG, Marshall JL, Al Monajem RS: The cruciate ligaments of the knee joint: anatomical, functional and experimental analysis. Clin Orthop 106:216–231, 1975

13. Hyndman JC, Brown DC: Major ligament injuries of the knee in children. Read at the Annual Meeting of the Canadian Orthopaedic Association, British Columbia, June 1978

14. Johansson E, Aparisi T: Congenital absence of the cruciate ligaments. A report of a case and review of the literature. Clin Orthop 162:108–111, 1982

15. Katz MP, Grogono BJS, Soper KC: The etiology and treatment of congenital dislocation of the knee. J Bone Joint Surg 49B:112–120, 1967

16. Kennedy JC, Hawkins RJ, Willis RB, Danylchuk KD: Tension studies of human knee ligaments. Yield point, ultimate failure and disruption of the cruciate and tibial collateral ligaments. J Bone Joint Surg 58A:350–355, 1976

17. Kennedy JC, Weinberg HW, Wilson AS: The anatomy and function of the anterior cruciate ligament—as determined by clinical and morphological studies. J Bone Joint Surg 56A:223–235, 1974

18. Larson RL, Jones DC: Dislocations and ligamentous injuries of the knee. p 1480. In Rockwood CA, Green DP (eds): Fractures in Adults. JB Lippincott, Philadelphia, 1984

19. Lee HG: Avulsion fracture of the tibial attachments of the cruciate ligaments. Treatment by operative reduction. J Bone Joint Surg 19A:460–468, 1937

20. Marshall JL, Warren RF, Wickiewicz TL, Reider B: The anterior cruciate ligament: a technique of repair and reconstruction. Clin Orthop 143:97–106, 1979

21. Meyers MH, McKeever FM: Fracture of the intercondylar eminence of the tibia. J Bone Joint Surg 41A:209–222, 1959

22. Meyers MH, McKeever FM: Fracture of the intercondylar eminence of the tibia. J Bone Joint Surg 52A:1677–1684, 1970

23. Morrissy RT, Eubanks RG, Park JP, Thompson SB: Arthroscopy of the knee in children. Clin Orthop 162:103–107, 1982

24. Noyes FR, DeLucas JC, Torvick PJ: Biomechanics of anterior cruciate ligament failure: an analysis of strain-rate sensitivity and mechanics of failure in primates. J Bone Joint Surg 56A:236–253, 1974

25. Noyes FR, Grood ES: The strength of the anterior cruciate ligament in humans and rhesus monkeys. Age-related and species-related changes. J Bone Joint Surg 58A:1074–1082, 1976

26. Palmer I: On the injuries to the ligaments of the knee joint. A clinical study. Acta Chir Scand Suppl 53:1–282, 1938

27. Rang M: Children's Fractures. JB Lippincott, Philadelphia, 1974

28. Rinaldi E, Mazzarella F: Isolated fracture–avulsions of the tibial insertions of the cruciate ligaments of the knee. Ital J Orthop Traumatol 6:77–83, 1980

29. Roberts JM: Fractures and dislocations of the knee. p. 891. In Rockwood CA, Wilkins KE, King RE (eds): Fractures In Children. JB Lippincott, Philadelphia, 1984

30. Robinson SC, Driscoll SE: Simultaneous osteochondral avulsion of the femoral and tibial insertions of the anterior cruciate ligament. Report of a case in a thirteen year-old boy. J Bone Joint Surg 63A:1342–1343, 1981

31. Salter RB: Textbook of Disorders and Injuries of the Musculoskeletal System. Williams & Wilkins, Baltimore, 1970

32. Tipton CM, Matthes RD, Martin RK: Influence of age and sex on the strength of bone–ligament junctions in knee joints of rats. J Bone Joint Surg 60A:230–234, 1978

33. Tolo VT: Congenital absence of the menisci and cruciate ligaments. J Bone Joint Surg 63A:1022–1025, 1981

34. Waldrop JI, Broussard TS: Disruption of the anterior cruciate ligament in a three year-old child. A case report. J Bone Joint Surg 66A:1113–1114, 1984

35. Zaricznyj B: Avulsion fracture of the tibial eminence: treatment by open reduction and pinning. J Bone Joint Surg 59A:1111–1115, 1977

REHABILITATION

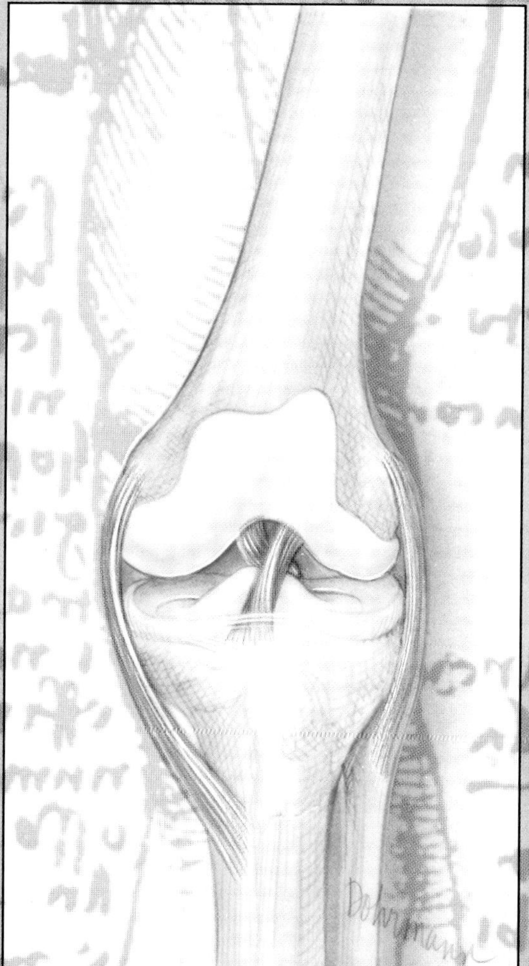

25

Counteracting Muscle Atrophy after ACL Injury: Scientific Bases for a Rehabilitation Program

INGA ARVIDSSON
EJNAR ERIKSSON

Few areas of rehabilitation are debated as much as rehabilitation programs for an anterior cruciate ligament (ACL) injury.[11,18,21,22] The pronounced muscle atrophy of the thigh muscles[26,31] seems inevitable following most open knee operations. Atrophy is one of the great problems in rehabilitation after a knee ligament injury. This atrophy occurs rapidly and is pronounced within a week after arthrotomy.[12,13]

Over the years, the attitude towards postoperative rehabilitation after ACL surgery has changed from a reliance on long immobilization periods[27] with isometric muscle training to a more active postoperative program with early mobilization and more dynamic treatment.[7,19] Our group at the Karolinska Hospital in Stockholm has been particularly interested in optimal rehabilitation for patients with knee injuries for more than 15 years. We have published a number of papers on the subject.

We will summarize here some of our studies and describe some of the findings that have determined how we conduct postoperative care and rehabilitation program for knee surgery patients. Our goal has been to counteract muscle atrophy and to determine the factors involved in its rapid onset. We will discuss the studies that led us to determine the optimal degree of knee flexion during immobilization,

the advantages of epidural analgesics, optimal degrees of range of motion during continuous passive motion immediately postoperatively and during the first 9 weeks, the advantages of muscle stimulation, and the suggested activity plan for 12 months after surgery. We caution physicians about muscle strength testing on an isokinetic dynamometer before the patient has regained stability and proprioceptive control of the leg (about 10 months postoperatively).

MUSCLE ATROPHY: CLINICAL OBSERVATIONS AND RESEARCH FINDINGS

Häggmark in our group[12,13] used percutaneous muscle biopsies to study the postoperative changes in the quadriceps after ACL surgery. Atrophy is significant already within a week. It seemed as if the type 1 fibers (slow twitch or red muscle fibers) were more sensitive to immobilization in a standard cast at 10° to 15° of flexion than the type 2 (short twitch or white muscle fibers). In a similar study with the knee immobilized at 40° to 45°, Arvidsson et al.[5] found no difference in the degree of atrophy between type 1 and type 2 fibers. Also, the atrophy was less than in knees immobilized in a greater degree of extension.[16] This makes sense since maintaining a muscle under some tension does prevent atrophy in studies performed on animals.[6,30] Studies by Häggmark et al.[12,13] showed that a cast brace resulted in a faster rehabilitation than a standard cast. In a small pilot study Eriksson and Häggmark[10] used transcutaneous muscle stimulation in an attempt to improve muscle rehabilitation. They found that electrical stimulation together with isometric muscle training was better than isometric training alone. The investigation was based on the activity of an oxidative enzyme succinate dehydrogenase (SDH). Häggmark et al.[14,15] also found that the circumference of an extremity is a poor measurement of the degree of atrophy when the circumference was compared with the actual area of the muscle as measured by computed tomographic (CT) scanning. Similar results have been reported by other authors.[25,26] At the same time as the muscle bellies atrophy, the subcutaneous tissues increase so that simple measurements of the circumference of the thigh do not reveal the real degree of atrophy.

Arvidsson et al.[2,3] found that pain after an ACL reconstruction leads to a significant decrease in maximal voluntary muscle activation. This pain-induced muscle inhibition is the most probable cause of the early advanced muscle hypotrophy. Another possible explanation is the postoperative catabolism that follows all surgical procedures.[25] In the studies of Arvidsson et al,[2] we also found that an epidural block with a dilute local anesthetic solution (0.25 percent lidocaine with epinephrine) could block this muscle inhibition and allow an increase of muscle activation. Therefore, we use this treatment for 2 to 3 days after open knee ligament surgery. Our group has also compared the possible beneficial effect of other pain treatments postoperatively. Transcutaneous nerve stimulation (TNS) relieves pain and allows a better muscle activation, although the relief is not as dramatic as produced by epidural analgesia.[3] In a study of the possible beneficial effect of a nonsteroidal anti-inflammatory drug (NSAID), Arvidsson and Eriksson[4] found that piroxicam given for 10 days postoperatively improved rehabilitation after partial meniscectomies performed with an open standardized miniarthrotomy. We used objective measurements such as iso-

kinetic torque recordings and range of motion before and after surgery and found that piroxicam did improve the rehabilitation.

In our further studies (unpublished observations), we have also shown that patients treated with epidural analgesia and early muscle activation for 2 to 3 days, compared with another group of patients treated similarly but without epidural analgesia, had a higher activity of the oxidative enzyme SDH than the group not receiving this postoperative pain treatment. The positive effect of epidural analgesia may not only be by blocking pain and thus allowing earlier muscle activation. It may also be, as has been shown by Kehlet et al.,[23] that the epidural analgesia also inhibits the information from the operative wound to the adrenals so that the shock reaction, evidenced by high blood cortisol levels, is reduced. Continuous epidural analgesia may thus also prevent some postoperative muscle catabolism and allow patients to become anabolic earlier. We have been using continuous postoperative analgesia for 2 to 3 days following anterior cruciate surgery for more than 10 years and found that this enables the patient to participate in early muscle training.

RANGE OF MOTION STUDIES

From several studies including those of Salter et al.,[28] it is obvious that immediate postoperative passive motion will reduce cartilage damage in the knee joint. Other studies have also indicated that early motion improves healing of ligament insertions, which leads to stronger ligaments than if the joint is immobilized.[24,29] Although many studies have shown that active quadriceps contractions put strain on the ACL in the range from at least 0° to 20°, passive motion of the knee joint[17,27] does not lead to quite as much load on the ACL. We therefore studied the effect of simulated quadriceps activity on autopsy knees and also measured the actual strain on the ACL on living patients after anterior cruciate reconstructions. *In the autopsy studies,[1] we found that simulated quadriceps contractions significantly increased the stress on the ACL from 0° to 60° of flexion.*

In recent, hitherto unpublished, studies we applied a Hall effect transducer on the reconstructed

Fig. 25-1. (A) Hall effect transducer attached to the ACL. **(B)** Measurements from patient with implanted Hall device. These measurements were made 4 hours after reconstruction of the ACL in a 27-year-old athlete. A Hall effect transducer was implanted on the cruciate reconstruction. When the motor block of the epidural had worn off and the patient could move his knee, these recordings were made. They show that a Lachman test puts strain on the reconstructed ligament. They also show that an active extension of the knee causes a very high load on the ACL. We stopped at 30° because we were afraid that the sutures in the ligament might break if we continued to straighten the knee.

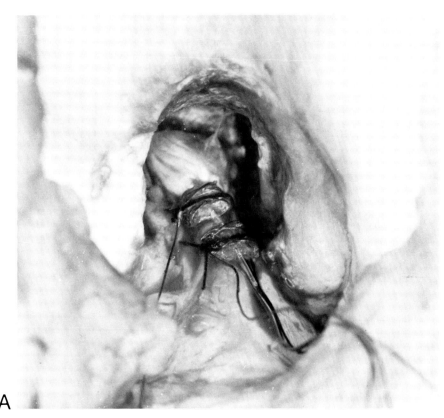

A

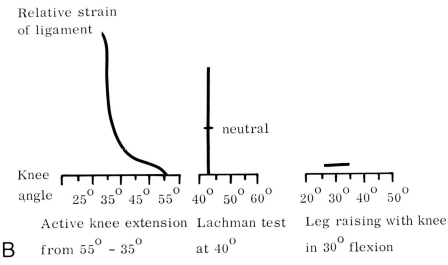

B

Relative strain of ligament

neutral

Knee angle

$25°$ $35°$ $45°$ $55°$ $40°$ $50°$ $60°$ $20°$ $30°$ $40°$ $50°$

Active knee extension
from $55°$ – $35°$

Lachman test
at $40°$

Leg raising with knee
in $30°$ flexion

ACL in the operating room. Five hours after surgery, when the motor block of the epidural analgesia subsided so that the patients could contract their quadriceps and move their knee joints, we recorded the stress of their reconstructed ACL with the Hall effect transducer (Fig. 25-1). Extension of the knee caused such increased stress on the ACL that we had to stop the extension at 30° of flexion. When the patient lifted the leg with the knee in 40° flexion there was no stress on the ACL. A possible explanation for this observation is a simultaneous contraction of the hamstrings and the quadriceps muscles. We also found that a Lachman test puts considerable stress on the reconstructed ACL.

Whatever technique of anchoring a ligament flap is used to reconstruct the ACL, autogenous or heterologous, it is advisable to respect the fact that early active motion should only be allowed in the range of 30° to 60° of flexion since otherwise there is a risk of rupturing the sutures in the repaired or reconstructed ligament. *If one prefers to use a standard cast without motion, it is advisable to cast in 40° to 45° of flexion, to avoid loading ACL cruciate and also to prevent muscle atrophy.* The reason for this is that several studies[6,30] have shown that a muscle kept under some tension does not atrophy as much as when kept relaxed. In a study of transcutaneous electrical stimulation,[5] in which we immobilized our control cases in 45° of flexion, we found less muscle atrophy than that reported by Halkjaer-Christensen and Ingemann-Hansen, who immobilized their knees in 5° to 10° of flexion.[16]

ELECTRICAL MUSCLE STIMULATION

In a recent extended series we have studied transcutaneous muscle stimulation in an attempt to prevent muscle atrophy in 38 patients immobilized in standard cast at 45° of flexion. In this study,[5] we found that electrical stimulation given with a battery operated stimulator with a pulse rate of 40 Hz (Respond II) led to a significant reduction of muscle atrophy in female patients and to somewhat less atrophy in male patients. We also found a significantly more pronounced postoperative muscle atrophy in female than in male patients undergoing ACL reconstruction. In this study we corroborated our earlier findings that measurement of the circumference of the thigh is a poor measurement of the degree of muscle atrophy[14,19,20] since the fat layer augments during immobilization. We furthermore found, by measurement of the CT attenuation pre- and postoperatively, that the fat content of the immobilized vastus medialis and vastus lateralis increased while the fat content of the rectus femoris (which for anatomic reasons is not immobilized by a knee cast), decreased somewhat.

Based on all these reported studies we therefore recommend the following postoperative rehabilitation after ACL surgery.

REHABILITATION PROGRAM

The rehabilitation schedule is summarized in Table 25-1.

Table 25-1. Rehabilitation Schedule

Postoperative Period	Program
Day of operation → 2–3 days	Epidural analgesia Passive motion machine (e.g., Ortomatic)
Day 3–4 → 6 weeks	Electrical muscle stimulation
1 week	Cast brace 30–60° flexion
1–6 weeks	Walk with crutches; increased load on operated leg: leg muscle training (e.g. with elastic band)
6 weeks	Cast brace 30–90° flexion
8 weeks	Cast brace 20–90° flexion
9 weeks	Removal of cast brace; temporary brace *If* ROM is >110° flexion, begin training on bicycle
3–4 months	Pool training
4–4-1/2 months	Cautious jogging on soft surface Proprioception training
4-1/2–5 months	Cautious trampoline training
6 months	Increased amount of jogging
8–9 months	Cautious sports training
10 months	Cybex testing of strength
12 months	Sports training and competition

Immediate Postoperative Treatment

Whether the ACL is reconstructed with a synthetic ligament (resulting in an immediate stability of the knee) or a ligament flap, such as a piece of the patellar tendon, all patients should be given continuous postoperative epidural analgesia for 3 days. During the first postoperative week the patient is placed in a passive motion machine (Fig. 25-2) in which we recommend a range of motion between 20° and 80°. The device should be used every second hour during the daytime for about 30 minutes and for the rest of the time the knee is kept in 40° to 45° of flexion. The patient is stimulated to perform active muscle work consisting of:

Isometric hamstring contractions
Lifting of the leg with the knee kept at 45° of flexion
Dynamic foot movements to train the calf muscles and improve the blood circulation of the leg

The patient is instructed to do these active muscle exercises for 15 minutes every other hour. From day 3 or 4 electrical muscle stimulation is given with one electrode in the groin and one electrode placed distally over the medial side of the quadriceps about 10 cm above the patella. The patient is taught how to use a battery-operated stimulator such as the Respond II (Fig. 25-3). Electrical stimulation is given at a frequency of about 40 Hz three times daily for 20 to 25 min each time. The patient is also asked to contract the quadriceps simultaneously with the electrical stimulation.

One to Six Weeks Postoperatively

If a synthetic ligament that is well-anchored at both ends has been placed in the knee, the patient is allowed a relatively dynamic training starting on the fourth day after operation. The patients are given a semisoft orthosis that prevents the last 20° of extension. The patients are allowed to put weight on the

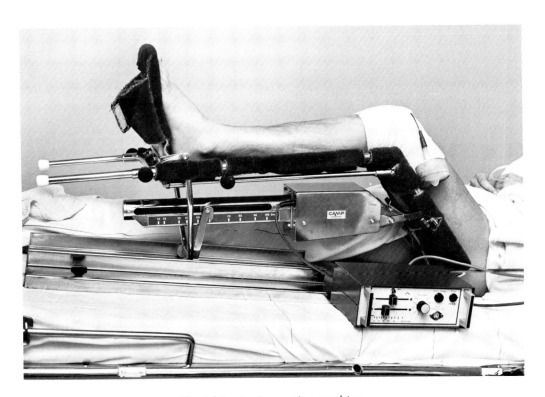

Fig. 25-2. Passive motion machine.

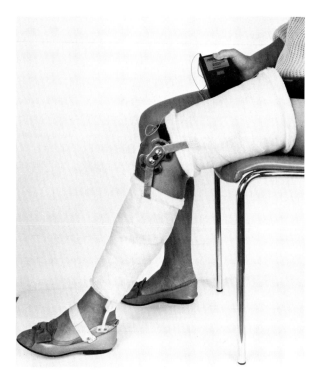

Fig. 25-3. Electrical stimulation of quadriceps.

operated leg, but use crutches as support. Progressive resistance exercises are applied as well as training for balance and proprioception. The patients should wear their orthosis for 12 weeks.

Patients with patellar tendon reconstructions or a similar procedure are given a cast brace with the hinges adjusted to allow motion of 30° to 60° (Fig. 25-4). The patients are given crutches and are informed that they are allowed to put some weight on the leg but should avoid walking too much for the first couple of weeks. They are given a training program consisting of exercises for all muscle groups of the leg. The program is outlined in the Appendix.

The electrical stimulation is continued during the cast brace period. The distal electrode of the electrical stimulator is pushed in under the cast brace to reach an area about 10 cm above the patella. The proximal electrode is applied in the groin as mentioned earlier. The patient uses the electrical stimulation three times daily for 25 to 30 minutes (Fig. 25-3).

When patients are activating their quadriceps with the electrical stimulator, they are told to keep their knee at 60° of flexion, since ACL strain due to quadriceps contraction will be minimal in this position. The patient is urged to train the hamstrings dynamically from 30° to 60° of flexion during this period.

Six to Nine Weeks

At 6 weeks we usually allow some more flexion of the knee and open the hinges up to 90° of flexion but keep the 30° limit for extension. Hamstring training is still emphasized; quadriceps training is performed isometrically and by electrical stimulation at 60° of flexion. At the end of this period we allow more extension to 20° or later 10° of flexion in the cast brace, which is removed 9 weeks postoperatively. When the patients are taken out of their cast brace they are given a temporary brace with a range from 20° to 90°. It is too early to prescribe a Lennox-Hill or a similar protective brace, since the patient will usually still have some muscle atrophy. As soon as normal (more) muscle volume is regained we refer our patients to a brace shop to receive a permanent brace (Fig. 25-5), which we want them to use for 3 to 12 months after surgery and preferably in the future while they participate in games such as soccer, ice hockey, and basketball.

Three to Six Months

When patients attain 110° of flexion we allow cycling and also urge them to train on both an ordinary bicycle and an ergometer bicycle at home. From 4 to 4½ months, depending on how well the patients have regained their muscles, we allow jogging on a soft surface, but only straight ahead. They are not allowed to change direction abruptly or cut. At the same time they are urged to train on a balance-board to improve proprioception. At 4 to 5 months we also start trampoline training. This should be done very carefully, however, since the trampoline may be hazardous. We allow swimming training relatively early. Slight jogging on the bottom of a pool may be allowed during the cast brace period since it is an excellent way of training the muscles. Studies by Cabaud et al.[8] and Clancy et al.[9] have shown that it takes about 1 year for the reconstructed ligament to

Fig. 25-4. Cast brace with hinges set at 30° to 60° of flexion.

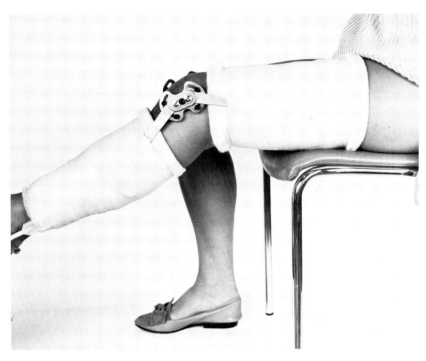

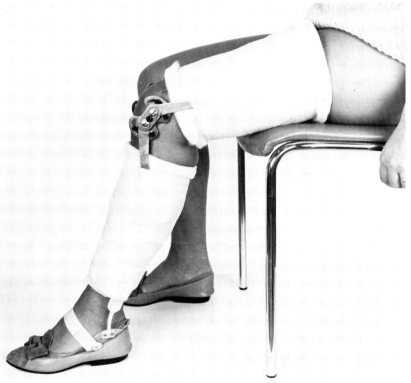

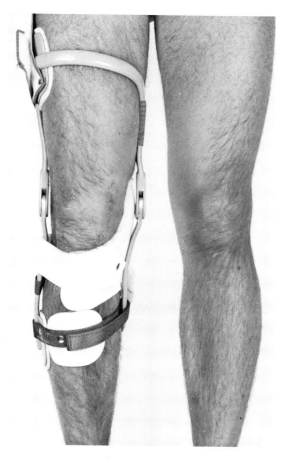

Fig. 25-5. Protective knee brace.

get good blood supply and to regain its original strength. Before surgery the patients are informed that the rehabilitation after an ACL reconstruction with a tendon flap usually takes about a year, even if the muscles are strong earlier. The risk of reinjuring the ligament is so high that they definitely should refrain from sports for at least 8 and preferably 12 months.

Six to Twelve Months (24 to 52 Weeks)

We now allow patients to increase the amount of jogging. We recommend that they always use their protective brace when they are training so that they will not sustain any injuries to the knee. They are also carefully instructed that if the training leads to effusion or pain, they should reduce it.

TESTING MUSCLE STRENGTH

When should the muscle strength be checked on an isokinetic dynamometer? Since many sports medicine centers today have a Cybex II or similar equipment, it is tempting to test the patient's muscle strength early on such a device. We warn against early tests of muscle strength on a Cybex unit, since, especially at low angular velocities, full extension may put too much stress on the newly reconstructed ACL. We therefore refrain from using Cybex testing until 10 months after the operation. The goal of our treatment is that 1 year after surgery the quadriceps and hamstring strength of the operated leg should be the same or greater than that of the control leg, that the knee should be stable, and that the patient should have regained full proprioceptive control of the leg.

It has been claimed by Jaeger in West Germany (personal communication) that it is impossible to obtain so good an end result after a late ACL reconstruction that a top athlete can reach the same performance as before injury. We disagree; many of our patients have returned to peak sports activity after surgery. One of them, 29 years old, who underwent a patellar tendon reconstruction of his ACL combined with reefing of his PCL insufficiency, returned to his elite soccer team 1 year after surgery and played so well the first year that he scored the highest number of goals of all players of the Swedish elite division.

SUMMARY

Recognizing that muscle atrophy inevitably follows most open knee operations, we directed our research toward counteracting this problem. Our studies showed that some tension on muscle fibers prevents some atrophy; hence we immobilize the knee at 40° to 45° of flexion. Our studies also showed that epidural analgesics, transcutaneous electrical stimulation, and continuous passive motion were advantageous in the first postoperative week. A cast brace seemed preferable to a standard cast. Motion is limited (30° to 80°). After the patient regains flexion to about 110°, he or she can begin training on the bicycle, in the pool, and progress to proprioceptive training with cautious jogging on soft surfaces and activity on the trampoline. The patient should be sufficiently rehabilitated, with a stable knee and proprioceptive sense, by 10 months. Not until that time should patients be tested on the isokinetic dynamometer. By 12 months postoperatively, they should be able to return to sports activity of their choice. Even top athletes who have participated in this rehabilitation program, designed based on the findings of our scientific analyses, have been able to return to sports activity at their preinjury performance levels.

REFERENCES

1. Arms SW, Pope MH, Johnson RJ et al: The biomechanics of anterior cruciate ligament rehabilitation and reconstruction. Am J Sports Med 12:8–18, 1984

2. Arvidsson I, Eriksson E, Knutsson E, Arnér S: Reduction of pain inhibition on voluntary muscle activation by epidural analgesia. Orthopedics 9:1415–1419, 1986

3. Arvidsson I, Eriksson E: Postoperative TENS pain relief after knee surgery: Objective evaluation. Orthopedics 9:1346–1351, 1986

4. Arvidsson I, Eriksson E: A double blind trial of piroxicam. Orthopedics (in press, 1987)

5. Arvidsson I, Arvidsson H, Eriksson E, Jansson E: Prevention of quadriceps wasting after immobilization—an evaluation of the effect of electrical stimulation. Orthopedics 9:1519–1528, 1986

6. Booth FW, Gollnick PD: Effects of disuse of the structure and function of skeletal muscle. Med Sci Sports Exerc 15:415–420, 1983

7. Burri C, Hutzscehnreuler P, Pässler HH et al: Functional postoperative care after reconstruction of knee ligaments: an experimental study. p. 108. In: The Knee Joint. Recent Advances in Basic Research and Clinical Aspects. Amsterdam, Excerpta Medica 1974

8. Cabaud HE, Rodkey WG, Feagin JA: Experimental studies of acute anterior cruciate ligament and repair. Am J Sports Med 7:18–22, 1979

9. Clancy WG, Narechania RG, Rosenberg TD et al: An-

terior and posterior cruciate ligament reconstruction in rhesus monkeys. J Bone Joint Surg 63A:1270–1284, 1981

10. Eriksson E, Häggmark T: Comparison of isometric muscle training and electrical stimulation supplementing isometric muscle training in the recovery after major knee ligament surgery. Am J Sports Med 7:169–171, 1979

11. Giove TP, Miller SJ, Kent BE et al: Non-operative treatment of the torn anterior cruciate ligament. J Bone Joint Surg 65A:184–192, 1983

12. Häggmark T, Eriksson E: Cylinder or mobile cast brace after knee ligament surgery. Am J Sports Med 7:48–56, 1979

13. Häggmark T, Jansson E, Eriksson E: Fiber type area and metabolic potential of the thigh muscle in man after knee surgery and immobilization. Int J Sports Med 2:12–17, 1981

14. Häggmark T, Jansson E, Svane B: Cross-sectional areas of the thigh muscle in man measured by computed tomography. Scand J Clin Lab Invest 38:355–360, 1978

15. Häggmark T, Eriksson E: Hypotrophy of the soleus muscle in man after Achilles tendon rupture. Am J Sports Med 7:121–126, 1979

16. Halkjaer-Kristensen J, Ingemann-Hansen T: Wasting of human quadriceps muscle after knee ligament injuries. Scand J Rehab Med Suppl. 13:5–20, 1985

17. Henning CE, Lynch MA, Glick KR: An in vivo strain gage study of elongation of the anterior cruciate ligament. Am J Sports Med 13:22–26, 1985

18. Hughston JC, Barrett GR: Acute anteromedial rotatory instability. J Bone Joint Surg 65A:145–153, 1983

19. Ingemann-Hansen T, Halkjaer-Kristensen J: Lean and fat component of the human thigh. Scand J Rehab Med 9:67–72, 1977

20. Ingemann-Hansen T, Halkjaer-Kristensen J: Computerized tomographic determination of human thigh components. Scand J Rehab Med 12:27–31, 1980

21. Johnson RJ: The anterior cruciate: a dilemma in sports medicine. Int J Sports Med 3:71–79, 1982

22. Johnson RJ, Eriksson E: Rehabilitation of the unstable knee. p. 114. In Frankel V (ed): Instructional Course Lectures 31. CV Mosby, St. Louis, 1982

23. Kehlet H: Epidural analgesia and the endocrine-metabolic response to surgery. Update and perspectives. Acta Anaesthesiol Scand 28:125–127, 1984

24. Laros GS, Tipton CM, Cooper RR: Influence of physical activity on ligament insertions in the knee of dogs. J Bone Joint Surg 53A:275–286, 1971

25. Moore FD: Endocrine changes after anesthesia, sur-

gery and unanesthesized trauma in man. Recent Prog Horm Res 13:511–572, 1957

26. Nicholas JA, Strizak AM, Veras G: A study of thigh weakness in different pathological states of the lower extremity. Am J Sports Med 6:241–248, 1976

27. Paulos L, Noyes FR, Grood E et al: Knee rehabilitation after ACL reconstruction and repair. Am J Sports Med 9:140–149, 1981

28. Salter RB, Simmonds DF, Malcolm BW et al: The biological effect of continuous passive motion on the healing of full-thickness defects in articular cartilage. An experimental investigation in the rabbit. J Bone Joint Surg 62A:1232–1251, 1980

29. Tipton CM, James SL, Mergner W, Tscheng TK: Influence of exercise on the strength of the medial collateral ligament of dogs. Am J Physiol 218:894–901, 1970

30. Wåhlby L: Achilles tendon injury. Aspects of muscle structure and strength. Umeå University Medical Dissertation, 38, 1978

31. Watson-Jones R: Fractures and Joint Injuries, 5th ed. Churchill Livingstone, Edinburgh, 1976

Appendix

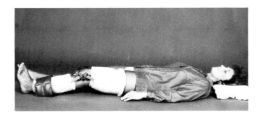 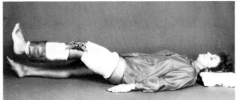

Leg Lifting

Lie flat on your back.
Contract your thigh muscles.
Lift up the leg—hold for 6 seconds.
When you feel stronger, put a weight on the cast.

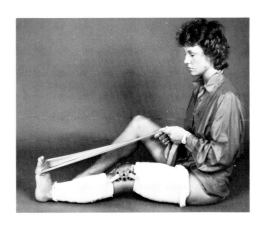 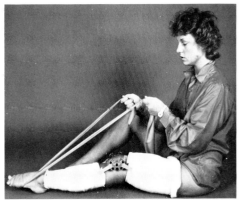

Calf Muscle Training

Put the elastic around your forefoot.

Plantarflex your foot; give resistance with your hands/arms.

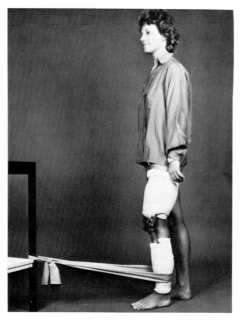 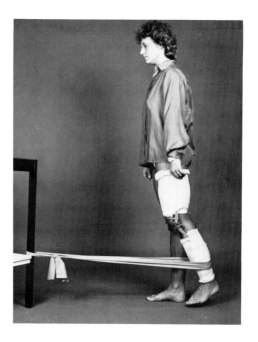

Hip Extension

Stand on your unoperated leg with a rubber tube around the ankle of the operated leg.

Extend your leg backwards — hold for 6 seconds.

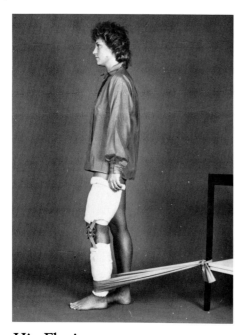 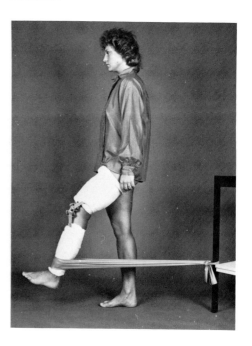

Hip Flexion

Stand on your unoperated leg with a rubber tube around the ankle of the operated leg.

Flex your leg forwards — hold for 6 seconds.

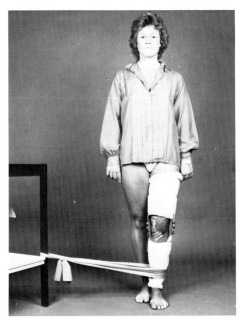
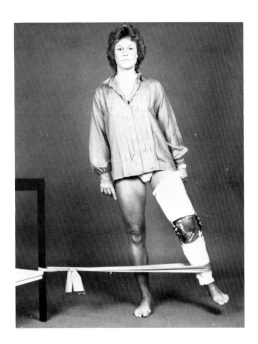

Hip Abduction

Stand on your unoperated leg with a rubber tube around the ankle of the operated leg.

Move the operated leg away from the other leg — hold for 6 seconds.

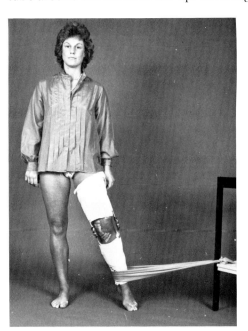
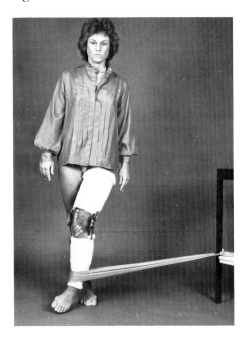

Hip Adduction

Stand on your unoperated leg with a rubber tube around the ankle of the operated leg.

Pull the leg back towards the other leg — hold for 6 seconds.

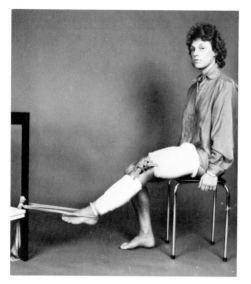 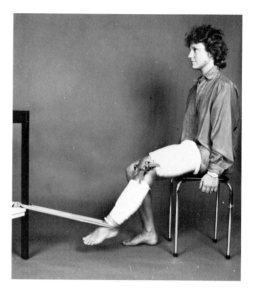

Knee Flexion

Sit with a rubber tube around your ankle (rubber tube attached in front).

Flex your knee about 30° — hold for 6 seconds.

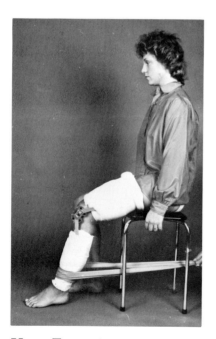 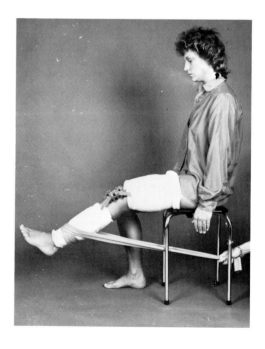

Knee Extension

Sit with rubber tube around your ankle (rubber tube attached behind).

Extend your knee about 30° — hold for 6 seconds.

26
Continuous Passive Motion in Postoperative Knee Rehabilitation

HENRY W. HAMILTON
DAVID V. HOFFMAN
JEFFREY S. MORRIS
JOHN S. PORTER

The philosophies of one age have become the absurdities of the next.

Sir William Osler

"Motion Versus Rest. Why Immobilize Joints?" was the challenging title of Robert Salter's presidential address to the Canadian Orthopaedic Association in 1981.[16] Salter[16] reviewed 26 centuries of struggle between "movers" and "resters" and concluded that "since immobilization of joints has been proven to be harmful and since joints are designed to move, we should keep them moving whenever it is feasible to do so."

The first "mover" is said to have been Herodicus, who used gymnastic exercises in the cure of disease.[3] It has been somewhat dubiously suggested that Hippocrates was exposed to these methods in the temple of Aesculapius in Cos.[3] Judging from the Hippocratic aphorisms "in every movement of the body, whenever one begins to endure pain, it will be relieved by rest," and perhaps humorously, "sailing the sea shows that motion disorders the body," the Father of Medicine was not unduly impressed by these methods and must be considered a "rester." The vigorous methods of the priests of Aesculapius were, however, still in vogue in the second century A.D. when Aristides, a hypochondriac, was ordered "to rub himself over with mud, to wash well, and to run three times around the temple."

Through the succeeding centuries the "resters" dominated the "movers." Percival Potts (1769) believed that "a short splint, which only extends a little above and a little below the fracture, and does not take in the two joints, is an absurdity; and what is worse, it is a mischievous absurdity." John Hilton (1860) delivered a course of lectures to the Royal College of Surgeons in England entitled "Rest and Pain" on the influence of mechanical and physiologic rest in the treatment of accidents and surgical diseases. Sir Arthur Keith commented, "never again shall anyone preach the gospel of rest so freshly, so practically, and so persuasively." Hugh Owen Thomas (1876) was chiefly concerned with treating joint tuberculosis when he condemned, among other things, "passive motion as only a mode of prolonging inflammation" and recommended that rest should be "complete, prolonged, uninterrupted and enforced." The Father of British orthopaedic surgery was just as much a "rester" when it came to the treatment of fractures, stating "we do not expect union if motion is permitted." Richard von Volkmann, in Germany, was an equally dedicated "rester," teaching that "the speed of reunion of bone is in direct ratio to the rigidity with which the two pieces are placed together."

In Britain the tradition of rest was carried on by

Thomas's nephew, Sir Robert Jones, who is remembered by the bulky bandage still used to immobilize knees, and his successor Sir Reginald Watson-Jones who held that "the cause of nonunion is inadequate immobilization." Meanwhile in Austria, Lorenz Bohler considered "all mistakes are made by taking the plaster off too soon, never leaving it on too long."

Only a few questioned the conservative inertia of the "resters." Lucas Champonnière, a French contemporary of Thomas, challenged the "resters," maintaining that "the return of the limb to the maximum possible muscular strength, and the maximum joint mobility is a hundred times more important than the exact form of the skeleton." Champonnière believed that "a certain amount of movement between the fracture fragments ensures the best bony repair."

John Dowden (1924), in Edinburgh, stressed that "massage and passive movement are better than immobilization, but active movement is far superior to passive." He was confident that "the principle of early active movement in the treatment of practically all injuries and in most inflammations will assuredly be adopted before long." Dowden[4] stressed that "movements should always be carried out just short of pain, and always advancing on the heels of pain." George Perkins, in London, in spite of having Jones as a teacher and Watson-Jones as a colleague, was another iconoclastic "mover." He advocated traction combined with early active movement for fractures of the femoral shaft and for fractures involving the knee joint. He stated "my condemnation of plaster is not absolute. By all means use plaster, provided that it does not immobilize a joint."[1]

The restoration of function in the injured limb, rather than the restoration of anatomy, was the guiding principle of the "movers." The introduction of modern fracture bracing techniques was the logical extension of this philosophy. The vastly improved methods of internal and external fixation of fractures, however, make it possible to restore both the anatomy and the function. All of these newer methods of treatment emphasize the importance of the soft tissues and joint function and provide a practical means of avoiding immobilization and encouraging movement.

CONCEPT OF CONTINUOUS PASSIVE MOTION

The stage was thus set for Robert Salter (1970), in Canada, to originate the concept of continuous passive motion (CPM). Salter's first published report[21] did not appear until January 1975. It was based on meticulous laboratory studies of the effects of CPM, cage activity, and immobilization on the healing of full-thickness defects in the articular cartilage of the rabbit knee. The apparent ability of CPM to induce cartilage healing in the rabbit stimulated the principal author of this chapter to construct a CPM knee device for the treatment of excised chondromalacic lesions of the human patella.

The design of this CPM device (Fig. 26-1) was extremely simple and has required no major modification. The machine was constructed in a community hospital workshop from materials that can be found in most hospital basements. The power is provided by a gear-reduction electric motor mounted on a Balkan beam above the patient's bed. The motor crank shaft rotates very slowly (about one revolution every 2 minutes), developing a torque of about 100 inch-pounds. A universal joint attached to the crank arm converts the rotatory movement of the shaft to an up-and-down movement (James Watt's "sun and planet" gear system in reverse). A steel rod links the universal joint to the proximal end of a padded aluminum splint in which the leg rests. No bandages or other attachments are required. The distal end of the splint is counterbalanced by a weight of about 1 pound to allow the heel of the splint to slide easily over the bedding. The excursion of the up-and-down movement, or range of knee movement, is controlled by varying the position of the universal joint on the crank arm.

Our first patient was subjected to CPM in March 1975. It was immediately apparent that the CPM was well tolerated by the human knee. Clinical results were often good and, on the basis of arthroscopic inspection, it appeared that CPM facilitated articular cartilage healing in the human.

Other applications of CPM were tried. CPM proved most beneficial in situations where the articular cartilage was damaged, such as stable or stabilized intraarticular fractures and osteochondritis

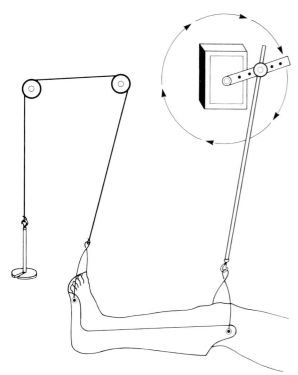

Fig. 26-1. Continuous passive motion machine. Electric motor above the bed powers a motor crank to revolve once every 2 minutes, producing a torque of approximately 100 inch-pounds.

dissecans. It also proved useful in situations where postoperative stiffness was a particular problem, such as synovectomy and quadricepsplasty. CPM was of no value in treating established contractures and, in our hands, did not enhance the results of total knee replacements. Some time later the indications were extended to include the treatment of septic arthritis.[18] The original CPM knee device was then modified so that CPM could be used in the treatment of similar problems in other synovial joints.

The initial favorable results of use of the CPM knee device were reported to the Ontario Orthopaedic Association in November, 1978, and the first 5 years' experience with CPM was presented to the Canadian Orthopaedic Association in June, 1981.[8]

SCIENTIFIC BASIS FOR CPM IN POSTOPERATIVE MANAGEMENT OF THE KNEE

The cruciate ligaments function by constraining motion; without motion a knee has no need for ligaments. The aim of cruciate ligament repair is to restore the integrity of the ligament without sacrificing that of the knee joint. Though the details of various ligament repairs are rightfully emphasized, the operation will fail if the subsequent management results in a stiff joint. In deciding what postoperative management policy to adopt, one can learn from the numerous animal experiments and clinical observations reported in the literature. The effects of immobilization and motion on normal and injured joints and soft connective tissues will be outlined.

Immobilization of Normal Joints and Soft Connective Tissues

In the normal rat knee joint, immobilization causes the intracapsular connective tissue to proliferate. The tissue gradually fills the joint cavity and becomes adherent to the articular cartilage. Progressive degeneration of the cartilage occurs and lesions develop in the subchondral bone. Contractures develop in the capsule and surrounding muscles. After a few weeks the damage becomes irreversible. Attempts to remobilize the joint, whether by forced manipulation followed by active motion, daily passive motion, or active motion only, cause tearing of the connective tissues that have proliferated in the joint, and the plane of the tear does not always follow the original joint cleft.[6]

In apparently normal human knees immobilized for a prolonged period of time, similar changes are found. Manipulation of these "frozen" knees creates a new plane of cleavage, pieces of articular cartilage being avulsed in some places and fibrofatty tissue remaining adherent to the joint surface in others.[5]

Normal monkey bone–anterior cruciate–bone units immobilized for 8 weeks have a decreased ability to resist load and elongation, which may take a year to recover fully.[12]

Immobilization of Injured Joints and Soft Connective Tissues

Full-thickness defects in the articular cartilage of the monkey,[9] rat,[10] or rabbit[22] knee cause dense adhesions to form between the defect and the synovial membrane or fat pad after a few weeks of immobilization. In the dog, repairs of complete lacerations of the medial collateral (MCL) and anterior cruciate (ACL) ligaments are associated with considerable damage to the articular cartilage when the joint is immobilized for 6 weeks.[14] A chicken tendon, when partially lacerated, progressively loses its tensile strength when immobilized for 3 weeks.[24]

Motion of Normal Joints and Soft Connective Tissues

Normal synovial joint function depends on some motion to prevent prolonged pressure on opposing articular surfaces and to permit the synovial fluid to supply nutrition to all of the articular surfaces. The normal rat exercised on a treadmill develops a stronger ACL.[2] The ACL, like bone, thus appears to be subject to Wolff's law.[23]

Motion of Injured Joints and Soft Connective Tissues

With cage activity, full-thickness defects in the articular cartilage of the rabbit knee do not cause adhesions and the defects fill with fibrous tissue and poorly differentiated cartilage. With immediate CPM many of the defects heal with what appears to be hyaline articular cartilage. This phenomenon has been termed "chondroneogenesis."[22]

In the human, articular cartilage lesions excised down to the subchondral bone and subjected to immediate CPM often appear on arthroscopic inspection to have undergone similar chondroneogenesis.

In the dog, repaired complete lacerations of the MCL are stronger and more resistant to elongation with motion. Repaired midsubstance lacerations of the ACL fail whether or not the knee is immobilized.[15] A chicken tendon, when partially lacerated, loses its tensile strength less rapidly and is restored sooner if motion is allowed.[24] In the rabbit, partial lacerations of the patellar tendon heal with increased tendon callus thickness and better alignment of collagen bundles in animals treated with immediate CPM than in animals treated with cage activity or immobilization.[17] Also in the rabbit, semitendinosus tenodesis used to replace the MCL and subjected to immediate CPM is stronger than with cage activity or immobilization.[20]

In soft connective tissue healing, wound strength is initially achieved by the formation of a myofibroblast–reticulin network, which subsequently disappears with scar maturation. This network is equipped with a "sensory apparatus" that has the ability to monitor the physical and chemical environment in which the healing is taking place.[7] It is thus able to direct the numerous aspects of connective tissue synthesis appropriately. Controlled motion appears to be one of the physical factors that influences this network, increasing the strength and resistance to elongation of the healing tissue.

Clinical Relevance

Therefore, evidence indicates that immobilization following ligamentous repair is harmful to both the joint and to the healing soft connective tissues. Early uncontrolled mobilization may disrupt the repair and cause recurrent instability and ultimately joint degeneration. Immediate controlled CPM, however, enhances soft connective tissue healing and ensures that joint integrity is preserved.

CPM FOLLOWING ACL REPAIR

Our former management of ACL repairs by simple suture and prolonged cast immobilization had evolved over a number of years. Augmentation of the repaired ligament or, when necessary, substituting the torn ligament with biologic or synthetic material has greatly improved the stability of the joints in the immediate postoperative period. This has made prolonged cast immobilization unnecessary and has allowed the use of immediate postoperative CPM.

At operation, before closing the wound, the tourniquet is deflated and bleeding points are cauterized. A single small Hemovac drain and a tensor bandage, applied for the first 48 hours, prevent the accumulation of a hemarthrosis. The traditional Jones compression bandage is not used because it prevents movement and because the pressure it exerts on the knee joint falls rapidly after the first few hours. It should be noted that a hemarthrosis is absorbed twice as fast from a joint subjected to CPM as from one that is immobilized.[13]

CPM is started immediately postoperatively in the recovery room. Patients react well psychologically to waking up from their operation with their repaired knee moving. It has been a common experience for patients to volunteer that their knee is more comfortable moving than when immobilized. Analgesic use is often reduced and we have not found femoral nerve blocks necessary. A plausible explanation of the apparent analgesic effect of CPM is that the continuous proprioceptive impulses reaching the spinal cord "close the gate" to painful impulses, in accordance with the "gate theory" of pain proposed by Melzak and Wall.[11] Another important benefit of immediate postoperative CPM is that quadriceps inhibition, which is so commonly encountered after knee surgery when the joint is immobilized, is eliminated.

The knee is flexed from 30° to 60° and back again every 2 minutes. This limited range of movement ensures that the repair is protected from undue stress. The ideal speed for CPM, if there is such a thing, has not been established. We have found that one revolution every 2 minutes is satisfactory and is so gentle that the patient is usually unconscious of the movement. Salter et al.[19] favor a faster speed of one revolution every 45 seconds.

The repaired knee is subjected to CPM day and night for up to 10 days after the operation. Patients are allowed up to go to the bathroom, bearing weight as tolerated on crutches, a few days after the operation. Crutches are used for several weeks. Formal physiotherapy does not start until after discharge and may be required for several months. Progress is assessed at intervals on a Kin-Com unit and therapy continued until the eccentric and concentric strength of the muscles of the repaired knee reaches 85 percent of that of the uninjured knee. Athletes returning to pivot sports are fitted with a brace.

With appropriate augmentation or substitution and immediate postoperative CPM, the results of our ACL repairs have improved and return the athlete to his or her chosen sport at an earlier date and in better condition than by previously practiced regimens. Our enthusiasm is shared by Johnson of Ottawa (Donald H. Johnson, M.D., personal communication), who has one of the largest series of knee ligamentous repairs managed by immediate postoperative CPM. He too has noted a reduction in the patients' postoperative pain, stiffness, and chondromalacia patellae and has reduced the overall rehabilitation time by one-half.

SUMMARY

. . ."Since immobilization of joints has been proven to be harmful and since joints are designed to move, we should keep them moving whenever it is feasible to do so," Salter[16] concluded after a review of 26 centuries of struggle between "movers" and "resters." Thus the stage was set for him (1970) to originate the concept of "continuous passive motion."

Immobilization is harmful to joints and related soft connective tissues. Postoperative stiffness after ligament repair is not due to the operation; it is due to the surgeon's failure to ensure that the joint moves. Forceful manipulation of a stiff joint causes further damage.

Early movement and, in particular, immediate postoperative CPM preserve the articular cartilage, prevent the development of adhesions and contractures, and accelerate the absorption of hemarthrosis.

CPM increases the strength and minimizes the elongation of healing soft connective tissues.

CPM reduces knee pain in the postoperative period, eliminates quadriceps inhibition, facilitates rapid rehabilitation, and returns the patient to normal function in the shortest possible time.

REFERENCES

1. Apley AG: Twenty-five years. [Editorials and Annotations]. J Bone Joint Surg 55B:3–6, 1973
2. Cabaud HE, Chatty A, Gildengorin V, Feltman RJ: Exercise effects on the strength of the rat anterior cruciate ligament. Am J Sports Med 8:79–86, 1980

3. Chance B: On Hippocrates and the *Aphorisms.* Ann Med Hist 2:31–46, 1930
4. Dowden JW: The principle of early active movement in treating fractures of the upper extremity. Clin Orthop 146:4–8, 1980
5. Enneking WF, Horowitz M: The intra-articular effects of immobilization on the human knee. J Bone Joint Surg 54A:973–985, 1972
6. Evans EB, Eggers GWN, Butler JK, Blumel J: Experimental immobilization and remobilization of rat knee joints. J Bone Joint Surg 42A:737–758, 1960
7. Forrest L: Current concepts in soft connective tissue wound healing. Br J Surg 70:133–140, 1973
8. Hamilton HW: Five years' experience with continuous passive motion. J Bone Joint Surg 64B:259, 1982
9. Hohl M, Luck JV: Fractures of the tibial condyles. A clinical and experimental study. J Bone Joint Surg 38A:1001–1018, 1956
10. Kettunen K: Effect of articular function on the repair of a full-thickness defect of the joint cartilage. An experimental study of mature rats. Ann Chir Gynaecol 52:627–642, 1963
11. Melzack R, Wall PD: Pain mechanisms. A new theory. Science 150:971–979, 1965
12. Noyes FR: Functional properties of knee ligaments and alterations induced by immobilization. A correlative biomechanical and histological study in primates. Clin Orthop 123:210–242, 1977
13. O'Driscoll SW, Kumar A, Salter RB: The effect of continuous passive motion on the clearance of a hemarthrosis from a synovial joint. Clin Orthop 176:305–311, 1983
14. Ogata K, Whiteside LA, Andersen DA: The intra-articular effect of various postoperative managements following knee ligament repair. Clin Orthop 150:271–276, 1980
15. Piper, TL, Whiteside LA: Early mobilization after knee ligament repair in dogs. Clin Orthop 150:277–282, 1980
16. Salter RB: Canadian Orthopaedic Association. Presidential address. J Bone Joint Surg 64B:251–254, 1982
17. Salter RB, Bell S: The effect of continuous passive motion on the realing of partial thickness lacerations of the patellar tendon of the rabbit. Orthop Trans 5:209, 1981
18. Salter RB, Bell RS, Keeley FW: The protective effect of continuous passive motion on living articular carti-lage in acute septic arthritis. An experimental investigation in the rabbit. Clin Orthop 159:223–247, 1981
19. Salter RB, Hamilton HW, Wedge JH et al: Clinical application of basic research on continuous passive motion for disorders and injuries of synovial joints. A preliminary report of a feasibility study. J Orthop Res 1:325–342, 1984
20. Salter RB, Minster RR: The effect of continuous passive motion on a semitendinosus tenodesis in the rabbit knee. Orthop Trans 6:292, 1982
21. Salter RB, Simmonds DF, Malcolm BW et al: The effects of continuous passive motion on the healing of articular cartilage defects. An experimental investigation in rabbits. Ann R Coll Phys Surg Can 8:50–51, 1975
22. Salter RB, Simmonds DF, Malcolm BW et al: The biological effect of continuous passive motion on the healing of full thickness defects in articular cartilage. J Bone Joint Surg 62A:1232–1251, 1980
23. Woo SL-Y, Gomez MA, Woo Y-K, Akeson WH: Mechanical properties of tendons and ligaments. II. The relationships of immobilization and exercise on tissue remodeling. Biorheology 19:397–408, 1982
24. Wray RC Jr, Ollinger H, Weeks PM: Effects of immobilization on tensile strength of partial tendon lacerations. Surg Forum 26:557–558, 1975

SUGGESTED READINGS

Guthrie D: A History of Medicine. Thomas Nelson, London, 1945

Hilton J: On Rest and Pain. William Wood, New York, 1879

Hippocratic Aphorisms (Adams F, Transl.). William Benton, Chicago, 1952

Perkins G: The Ruminations of an Orthopaedic Surgeon. Butterworths, London, 1970

Rang M: Anthology of Orthopaedics. Churchill Livingstone, Edinburgh, 1968

Thomas HO: Diseases of the Hip, Knee and Ankle Joints with Their Deformities Treated by a New and Efficient Method. T. Dobb, Liverpool, 1876

Watson-Jones R: Fractures and Joint Injuries. Churchill Livingstone, Edinburgh, 1960

27
ACL Injuries in the Elite Skier

J. RICHARD STEADMAN
ROBERT W. HIGGINS

In alpine skiing changes in equipment, technique, and possibly terrain have been causative factors in bringing anterior cruciate ligament (ACL) injuries to epidemic proportions. Other factors, such as relatively high, stiff boots and tight bindings with no upward release on the toepiece have also added to the risk of injury to the ACL.[14,19,30,39] The competition among racers has intensified, often causing them to ski at a level just beyond their control. A disproportionate number of ACL injuries have been sustained by American and international elite skiers in the last decade.

In this chapter we describe an evolving philosophy of treatment that has been successful in providing both early return to activity and static stability. In addition, we provide findings on 27 elite skiers treated from 1979 to 1984.[17]

TRANSITION IN TREATMENT OF ACL INJURIES

In the early 1970s, the understanding of the ACL injury was not what it is today. The anterior drawer, abduction stress, and Slocum tests were the standard tests for rotational stability. The Lachman test had not been described and the high correlation between traumatic effusion and ACL rupture was not appreciated. The pivot shift was just becoming an entity of evaluation. Thus, a large number of ACL injuries were not recognized during this period.

Surgically, it was apparent that repair with a simple Bunnell or figure-eight suture through the ligament and notch was not adequate for fixation.[13] Al-though the repair was occasionally successful, the reason for the occasional success was not understood. This promoted increasing interest in reconstructive and extraarticular procedures to enhance stability.

During this earlier period, one opinion was that due to the maintenance of a flexed position, skiing did not require an ACL. This was true in some events such as the slalom and giant slalom. It was proven, however, that in downhill racing the long jump required static ACL stability for landing. In addition, professional skiing developed a new format using several jumps of variable height in each course. This was an unacceptable hazard for the ACL-deficient knee. Several skiers who previously had been able to ski successfully with no ACL while skiing slalom and giant slalom were then forced to ski courses with jumps that resulted often in meniscal tearing and degenerative joint disease. Furthermore, the ski racer's basic nature impels him or her to push all activity to the limit, and this has frequently resulted in meniscal injuries during dry-land training. Although it is true that normal skiing can be performed without an ACL if the knee is flexed, the loss of the meniscus places additional stresses on the knee, promoting development of degenerative joint disease.[18,22,38,43]

A dilemma was created: ACL repairs were not successful,[5,13,31,37] yet the static stability provided by the ACL was a necessity because of jumps. To complicate the situation more, it was just being proposed that ACL reconstructions required prolonged immobilization and protection.[8] This was not an attractive prospect in the treatment of an elite athlete.

Both the technique of repair and methods of rehabilitation have been developed in an effort to gain static stability with early return to activity. As a first approach to the problem, an attempt was made to improve the existing techniques of repair.[23] The technique that evolved includes several improvements over the standard Bunnell stitch through the notch.

As improvements in examination were being made,[25] arthroscopy became available. Diagnostic capabilities were much improved, as was the treatment of meniscal injuries. Evaluation of the specific meniscal tears was more thorough and the newer ideas of meniscal repair could be instituted arthroscopically. Meniscal repair is essential, particularly in skiers with a lateral meniscal injury.[22] Without a lateral meniscus, stability is compromised and the likelihood of degenerative joint disease approaches 100 percent in the competitive skier. This has been monitored arthroscopically in skiers and, when significant changes are present, the athlete is advised against continuing to ski competitively. We have seen two cases in which the skiers were forced to retire because of these problems, even though both were the best in the country in their separate events.

Several technical developments[6] laid the foundation for the proper treatment of the ACL injury.[32] Kieffer et al.[20] pointed out the importance of notch impingement in ACL injury and recognized the need to widen and deepen the notch in order to perform an intraarticular reconstruction or repair. Obviously, if the narrow notch had created a rupture, it needed to be widened in an attempted repair. Notchplasty allowed better assessment of the position for fixation of the repair and/or graft. Also, since most skiing injuries result in a significant amount of cruciate tissue being ruptured at or near the femoral attachment, it becomes necessary to identify a point not quite as proximal as the broad anatomic site for reattachment. A raw bone surface also seems to be beneficial for healing. This is all made easier after adequate notchplasty. We found that a 1 cm deep trough could be made just anterior and distal to the "over-the-top" position in the lateral femoral condyle to provide a bed for the repaired ACL. This approximates the attachment of the posterolateral band of the ACL.

Protection of the repaired ligament is accomplished through the use of multiple double loop sutures at various levels in the ligament (Fig. 27-1).[15] The bands of the ligament are bunched with multiple sutures in much the same way as is used for an Achilles' tendon repair. The sutures are then pulled through separate drill holes in the raw bone bed and tied over the lateral femur.

Marshall et al.[27] proposed that vascularization of the ACL is improved by providing proximity to the fat pad. This technique was used in early cases, but it became apparent that the attached fat pad could become an iatrogenic infrapatellar plica. In addition, those plicae can often rupture, simulating a rerupture of the repaired ligament. For these reasons, we have abandoned the use of the fat pad as vascular supply for the repaired ACL.

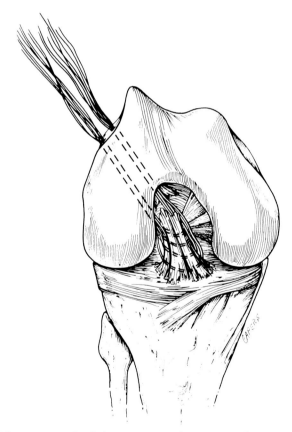

Fig. 27-1. Multiple loop suture technique. By placing sutures at different levels, tension will be maintained if one suture fails. The sutures are tied distal to proximal.

Another problem was the inability to assess intraligament stretch. As a solution to this problem, we chose a simple method to supply extraarticular stability — an iliotibial band tenodesis to act as an "internal device."

Procedures of MacIntosh, Losee et al.,[24] Andrews and Sanders,[4] and Ellison[12] were studied, and a similar procedure was elected. This evolved into a procedure slightly more complex than the original but also more effective.

Our technique consists of isolating a strip of iliotibial band 2 cm wide and approximately 10 cm long with the inferior border defined by the thickened area of the band. The strip is then divided again into an anterior and posterior band to mimic the two major bundles of the ACL, as in the Andrews procedure. Approximately 60 percent of the strip width is used for the posterior band, since these fibers seem to provide most of the stability in extension against the pivot shift. A 6.5 mm cancellous screw is placed

at the posterolateral edge of the femur just proximal to the condylar flare, which corresponds to the position recommended by Krackow and Brooks[21] (Fig. 27-2). After three sets of suture are used to reinforce the graft, the anterior band is released proximally and wrapped around the screw (Fig. 27-3). With tension held on the band, the screw and soft tissue washer are advanced. Because of the anterior angulation of the screw, the posterior band is caught under the washer and tightens with screw advancement. When the screw is tightened so that the washer is contacting bone, the proximal aspect of the posterior band is released. This was often accompanied by a loud "pop" because of the tension generated proximally. Without this step the pressure on the band may pop it over the washer, causing failure. Care should be taken to angle the screw and washer distally so that the inferior teeth of the washer will not amputate the graft. The range of motion should be tested at this point. There should

Fig. 27-2. This point of attachment of the anterior and posterior bands prevents significant loss of tension throughout a full range of motion.

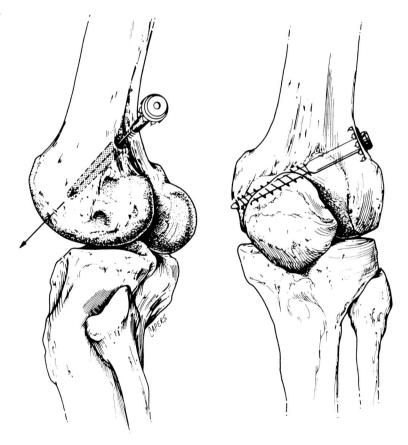

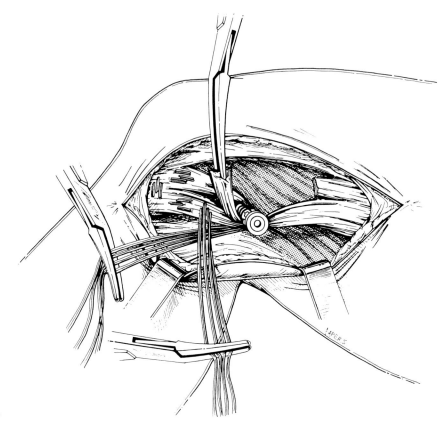

A

Fig. 27-3. (A) The anterior band is released proximally and wrapped around the screw. **(B)** The corresponding intraoperative appearance.

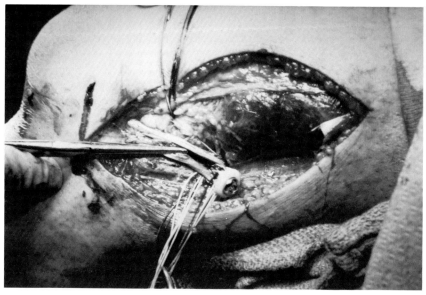

B

be a negative Lachman and anterior Drawer test, and the motion should be full.

Even with the combination of the repair and extraarticular reconstruction, the need for static stability occasionally requires other measures. If the Lachman is positive and the Drawer is negative, generally the posteromedial structures are intact. If the Drawer is positive and anteromedial laxity is noted, repair and reconstruction of the posteromedial corner are necessary.[15] The deep capsular portion of the medial collateral ligament (including the posterior oblique ligament) is usually torn from its femoral attachment with the superficial portion torn from the tibia.

An attempt was made to avoid, whenever possible, the use of the patellar tendon as an augmentation of repair in the skier's injuries, since revascularization of the graft might take longer than 6 months and thus prevent an early return to activity.[7] Our skier patient returns with a repaired ligament internally braced by the extraarticular iliotibial band tenodesis and externally braced as well. We rarely sacrifice the patellar tendon, and it is held in reserve in case reinjury should occur. Also, the reliance of the skier on the patellofemoral mechanism in a sport where victory margins are frequently measured by thousandths of a second makes a procedure that avoids the use of the patellar tendon quite appealing.

In combined ligament injury, we address each of the secondary restraints and repair each in a manner that allows motion. In knee dislocations with both cruciates ruptured, each is usually ruptured in a good position, allowing repair without intraarticular augmentation. In the high-level skier the tissues are usually quite strong and thick, allowing quality repairs.

If the cruciate is not repaired, a choice can be made about when and if reconstruction should be performed. In acute cases there is usually excellent tissue available for repair, which should be done within approximately 2 weeks. If the tissues are inadequate, the skier may possibly finish the season prior to having a reconstructive procedure. In only one case in our treatment of elite skiers was primary repair not accomplished. There were two reasons for this decision. First, the tear in the ligament did not lend itself to repair and; second, the skier

wished to postpone a reconstructive procedure so that she might return to competitive skiing in a relatively short time. In this case the rehabilitation after the initial injury was the same as for surgically treated injuries, except that the time to skiing was decreased. The secondary restraints were being treated rather than the primary restraint — the ACL. The knee later was reconstructed using an artificial substitute (Gore-Tex, W.L. Gore and Assoc., Inc. Flagstaff, AZ), since chondromalacia prevented the use of the patellar tendon as a graft.

EVALUATION OF ELITE SKIERS' KNEES AFTER TREATMENT FOR ACL INJURIES (1980s)

Clinical Findings

From 1979 to 1984, 27 patients (8 female and 19 male) who were either current or former members of the U.S. Ski Team or professional skiers sustained 30 ACL tears. The injuries were all caused by falls during skiing, except one which was a tennis injury. The average age of the patients was 22.4 years with the range from 14 to 33 years. There were 15 right and 15 left knee injuries. We were able to follow up 24 patients (27 knees), with an average objective follow-up of 57.6 months (range, 19 to 81). With phone conversations, we were able to extend the subjective follow-up to 59.3 months (range, 19 to 81).

Preoperatively, all patients had positive Lachman test and pivot shifts. Twenty-four patients had a combined anteromedial/anterolateral instability with six having just anterolateral. Of the ACL tears, 24 of 30 tore mainly off the femur with enough tissue to repair. Three of 30 were mainly torn from the tibia and were repaired to the tibia. Two of 30 were "midsubstance" tears requiring patellar tendon augmentations. One tear was observed to include an anteromedial band off the tibia and a posterolateral band off the femur and was repaired accordingly (Fig. 27-4).

Proximal ACL tears were the predominant type of ACL injury in our group. Our findings conflict with the findings of others.[15,28,29] We find that the literature is vague in this area. It is difficult to assess the

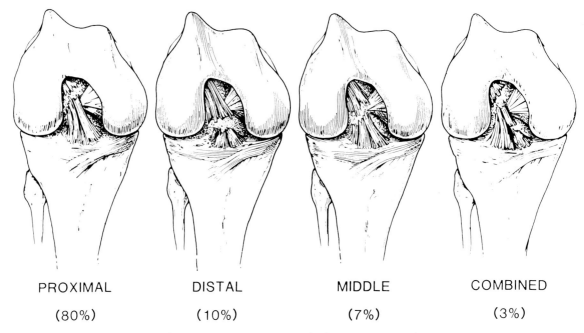

PROXIMAL   DISTAL   MIDDLE   COMBINED

(80%)   (10%)   (7%)   (3%)

Fig. 27-4. Most tears were proximal, allowing repair to bone.

exact type of ACL tear without careful dissection of the tissue.[15,28,29,44] Also, because we are positioning the repaired ligament at approximately the attachment of the posterolateral band, which is slightly distal and anterior to the "over-the-top" position, our method of repair may not require as much residual ligament tissue. Finally, a likely reason for our findings is that we are dealing with a very specific group of athletes experiencing similar mechanisms of injury.

Five patients had true knee dislocations with concomitant posterior cruciate ligament tears. Three of these five were femoral tears and two were tibial avulsions. All were repaired. Meniscal injuries totalled 24, with 16 medial and 8 lateral. The medial meniscus injuries were all peripheral and were all repaired. Of the eight lateral meniscus tears, three were repaired (one anterior flap, two peripheral). All the remaining patients had partial excision of the torn portion if the tear appeared unstable.

The medial collateral ligament complex (including the posterior oblique ligament) was injured in 24 of 30 knees, and all were repaired. In almost all cases the deep portion (meniscofemoral ligament) and the posterior oblique ligament were torn from

the femur and the superficial tibial collateral ligament was torn from the tibia distally. However, exact objective data regarding this could not be extracted from the charts. Sixteen of 30 had injuries to the lateral or posterolateral ligament complex and all complete tears were repaired. Nineteen patients had iliotibial band tenodesis at the initial procedure; two more patients experienced this after reinjuries.

Other knee injuries included two patellofemoral joint dislocations, one tear in the vastus medialis muscle, one lateral femoral condylar fracture, and two lateral femoral condylar articular cartilage defects.

Although they had difficulty remembering exact details of their injuries, most described either an external rotation, valgus injury, or some hyperextension injury. Almost all accidents occurred in downhill races.

Questions related to the knee injuries postoperatively centered around five areas: pain, swelling, "giving way," locking, and ability to climb or descend stairs (N = 27). For 21 of 27 (78 percent) knees, patients reported no pain and for 19 percent mild pain was reported, mostly related to vigorous activity. One patient ranked his pain as moderate, and again this was related to activity. Twenty-three of 27 (85 percent) had no swelling with 4 of 27 (15 percent) having mild swelling. For most knees (93 percent) there were no episodes of giving way. Two (7 percent) had previously experienced sensations of giving way. There were no reports of locking or problems with stairs (Table 27-1). All patients were able to return to pivoting activities. One patient was found to have a pivot shift on follow-up evaluation, but was able to return to active pivoting sports without episodes of giving way. It is noteworthy that this patient had exceptional muscle development.

Clinical examinations revealed 12 of 27 (44 percent) with a 1+ anterior Drawer. Twenty-six of 27 (96 percent) were without true pivot shifts, 1 of 27 (4 percent) had 1+ pivot shift, and 3 of 27 (11 percent) were found to have "glides," which we define as an increase in anterolateral laxity of the lateral tibial plateau without the dislocation or "clunk." Twelve of 27 (44 percent) had a negative Lachman test, 12 of 27 (44 percent) had a 1+, and 2 of 27 (7 percent) had 2+ (Table 27-2).

Only two patients lacked full extension with both failing to gain the last 5°. The average flexion recorded for the injured knee was 134°, representing a 10° loss compared to the uninjured knee.

Table 27-1. Subjective Results[a]

	None (%)	Mild (%)	Moderate (%)
Pain	78	19	4
Swelling	85	15	0
Giving way	93	7	0
Locking	100	0	0
Stair problems	100	0	0

[a] Average followup, 59.3 months for 27 knees

Table 27-2. Results of Clinical Examinations[a]

	0 (%)	Trace/1+ (%)	2+ (%)
Anterior Drawer	52	48	0
Lachman	41	52	7
Pivot shift	85	15	0
Abduction stress 30°	70	22	7
Adduction stress 30°	89	11	0

[a] Average follow-up 57.6 months for 27 knees.

The MEDmetric arthrometer model KT-1000 was used to test the injured and uninjured knees. Five tests were used to evaluate anterior laxity: anterior displacement with a 15 and 20 lb force (AD-15 and AD-20), anterior displacement between a 15 and 20 lb force (compliance index, CI), quadriceps active displacement (QAD), and a manual maximum displacement (MM). Right–left differences were also calculated in patients with only one injured knee, allowing the opposite knee to be used as control. (A "D" is added to the previously mentioned abbreviations to designate "difference.")

For the uninjured knee, the average AD-20 was 5.56 mm, as compared to the injured knee measurement with a repaired ACL of 7.17 mm (Figs. 27-5, 27-6). These measurements can be put into perspective because of previous studies by Daniel and associates,[9,10,26] whose team actually developed the KT-1000 arthrometer. Their group reported an average AD-20 of 11.4 mm for knees with an ACL injury. The AD-20 of 5.56 mm for the uninjured knee in our skier group is significantly less than the 7.1 mm reported by Daniel et al.[9] in the normal population, suggesting that the elite skier has less "normal laxity" than the average patient. We are aware of another similar study suggesting this in football players (G. Losse et al., personal communication, 1986).

The previous studies have emphasized that the most important measurement in distinguishing ACL deficiency is recording the difference between the injured and the uninjured leg. Most of the patients in the studies by Daniel et al.[9,10] with acute tears of the ACL had an ADD-20 of greater than or equal to 3 mm; the authors considered this diagnostic of an ACL injury. In their original study,[10] 92 percent of normal subjects had an ADD-20 less than or equal to 2 mm. Our finding of 1.53 mm in patients with repaired ACLs compares very favorably.

Similarly, compliance index differences (CID) were calculated. Previous reports revealed that 93 and 90 percent of normal subjects had right–left differences of less than or equal to 0.5 mm.[9,10] In those with acute ACL disruption, 79 percent had CIDs greater than or equal to 1 mm, with an average of 1.3.[10] In our patients with repaired ACLs, the average CID was 0.47 mm, with only 3 patients (12 percent) with CIDs measuring greater than 1 mm.

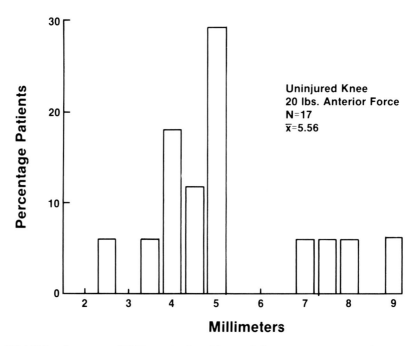

Fig. 27-5. KT-1000 arthrometer (MEDmetric, San Diego, CA) measurements on the uninjured knee, using 20 lb of anterior force (AD-20). (Patients with bilateral injuries were included as two reports.)

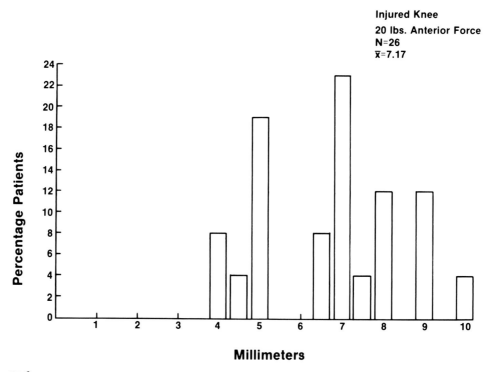

Fig. 27-6. KT-1000 arthrometer (MEDmetric, San Diego, CA) measurements on those knees having ACL repairs, using 20 lb of force (AD-20).

We encourage investigators to use objective testing devices[34] to report results because clinical examination reports are difficult to interpret.

Time Delay Until Skiing

Twenty-three patients were able to remember the length of time from original injury to when they skiied again. One patient with a knee dislocation did not return to competitive skiing for fear that the injury could happen again. For the other 22 patients, the average time to return to skiing was 5.4 months (range, 2 to 9). Twenty-one patients could remember when they were able to race or undergo full dry land training, the average being 9.1 months (range, 3.5 to 18). Two patients did not return to racing for psychological reasons.

Complications

Eighteen patients underwent 24 subsequent surgical procedures for several problems. In 18 of 30 knees, surgical hardware was removed, and in 13 of these knees arthroscopy was done concomitantly to observe the repaired ligament. No failures were evident on arthroscopic exam unless a reinjury had occurred.

Five patients had a reinjury to the ACL, with two of those five requiring repair again.

REHABILITATION

Rehabilitating these elite skiers has been an education. The opportunity to direct and observe their programs as they have adapted them has helped us design an active rehabilitation program which the long-term results have proven to be most effective.

The obvious advantage of weight-bearing in the rehabilitation of tibial fractures and functional treatment of fractures[35] suggested that the functional treatment of ligament injuries and reconstruction would also be successful. In 1975 the rehabilitation without surgery of the posterior cruciate ligament and medial collateral ligament injury in one skier, plus a personal rehabilitation, confirmed these ideas. The last time a cast was used other than the first week after cruciate ligament surgery in our practice was in 1977. Early motion has been used since then. Each skier seemed to be striving for a more effective method of rehabilitation and frequently added aggressive variations to their program. This was often helpful to the patient. In fact, it demonstrated to us that we could be more active with our rehabilitation program.

Multiple lessons were learned, including several that have become rules in rehabilitation. These rules include the following:

Ligaments should be set in position to allow full range of motion on the operating table.
All areas of instability should be corrected to allow for a balanced knee at the time of repair. Both primary and secondary restraints should be repaired and reinforced, if necessary, to allow this balanced motion.
Motion is desirable for ligament healing,[40–42] articular cartilage nutrition,[36] and to prevent capsular contractures.[1–3]
Stress without deformation is desirable for collagen make-up and formation of this collagen along the lines of stress.
Muscular contraction can deform ligaments due to the biomechanics of the joint. The quadriceps effect on the ACL begins as the knee is extended from about 60 to 30°.[33] Active quadriceps motion is safe if knee extension is not allowed beyond 45°.[16] A significant hamstring effect on the posterior cruciate ligament begins from about 80°
Resistive exercise hypertrophies healing tissue as long as there is no major deformation.
Some activities create subluxation while others are protective. Short knee bends and stationary biking seem to be the most protective and least deforming exercises.[16]
If the quality of the tissue or the stability is compromised for other reasons, (general pathologic laxity, posteromedial laxity, meniscectomy), progression to full activity should be delayed.

Our rehabilitation program is based on these principles. The program is dynamic and constantly being upgraded and, if a failure occurs, it is often because a principle has been misapplied.

Rehabilitation begins immediately postoperatively in either a surgically repaired or a nonoperatively treated cruciate injury. The knee is taken through a full range of motion on the operating table to ensure that full motion is available later. Immediately after closure, a hinged brace is applied with the hinges set for flexion to 90° and extension to 45° unless there is a meniscal repair, in which case it is set at 50 to 70°. Continuous passive motion is begun in this range in the brace and reciprocal electrical stimulation is begun at the same time. On the first day postoperatively knee bends are started in a 45 to 90° range and are continued for the duration of the treatment. In addition, the knee is removed from the hinged brace and allowed to extend passively and flex actively. Our goals are to obtain a range of 10° to 90° of passive motion out of the brace prior to the patient's discharge from the hospital. The well leg continues to exercise with knee bends and stationary biking. At 8 weeks the brace is released entirely so that the patient can use the stationary bike. From 8 to 16 weeks the patient continues knee bends, stationary biking, and works with a full range of motion of the hamstrings. Quadriceps exercises are allowed actively from 90 to 45°. No active isolated quadriceps extensions are used beyond 45° for at least 6 months, and if the knee is generally lax or if the tissues were of poor quality, the time may be extended from 6 to 12 months. The use of the stationary bike is continued with both legs during this period. In the later stages of rehabilitation, as strength improves, an elastic resistance cord is used to increase the difficulty of the exercises.

Early range of motion and no immobilization in the rehabilitation program undoubtedly account for the absence of flexion contracture problems. Only one patient had surgery for motion problems, and these were corrected with arthroscopic excision of adhesions.

By using this treatment program, we have been able to accomplish several goals. First, in cases where the ligament repair has been undertaken, we have avoided further meniscal tears. Second, we have avoided the use of patellar tendon in all but two cases. Since the patellofemoral mechanism may affect stability in ski racing, where fine tuning is important, we consider this an important principle. In addition, we have avoided the possibility of patellofemoral degenerative problems.

Functional bracing has been helpful in patients'

return to activity, and none of the functionally braced athletes have experienced a reinjury.

SUMMARY

Several improvements in examination, surgical technique, and rehabilitation have allowed us to obtain excellent results with anterior cruciate ligament problems in the elite skier. The notchplasty, multiple loop suture technique, and meniscal repair are key aspects. A more important consideration, however, is to provide the failsafe extraarticular procedure we have described. Early experiments in the laboratory have suggested that this procedure provides the most support against anterior subluxation in the postoperative period (P. Mandt, M.D., personal communication). The release of the "new ligament" proximally prevents early stretching and failure of the procedure.

The surgical technique is one contribution to success and it seems to be important that excellent tissues be present, although this is difficult to prove. Probably the most significant factor in the successful result is rehabilitation. The strong personality of the elite skier welcomes the most aggressive rehabilitation program as a challenge. We have proved that motion and some stresses on repaired ligaments are compatible with good functional and objective results. While it may be improper to apply these theories and principles to treating ACL injuries in other athletes, our general impression is that this is a safe approach. The area of tearing being proximal in a skier seems consistently to allow successful repair. Augmentation of nonrepairable lesions, however, must always be an option. Synthetic materials are presently being investigated and may not only provide a surgical option to repair but also an even earlier, safer return to activities. We will certainly continue to make progress in the areas of surgical technique and rehabilitation of the ACL injury.

REFERENCES

1. Akeson WH: An experimental study of joint stiffness. J Bone Joint Surg 43A:1022–1034, 1961
2. Akeson WH, Amiel GL, Mechanic GL et al: Collagen cross-linking alterations in joint contractures.

Changes in the reducible cross-links in periarticular connective tissue collagen after nine weeks of immobilization. Connective Tissue Res 5:15–19, 1977

3. Akeson WH, Amiel D, Woo SL: Immobility effects on synovial joints. The pathomechanics of joint contracture. Biorheology 17:95–110, 1980

4. Andrews JR, Sanders R: A "mini-reconstruction" technique in treating anterolateral rotatory instability (ALRI). Clin Orthop 172:93–96, 1983

5. Balkfors B: The course of the knee ligament injuries. Acta Orthop Scand Suppl 198, 1982

6. Butler DL, Noyes FR, Grood ES: Ligamentous restraints to anterior-posterior drawer in the human knee. A biomechanical study. J Bone Joint Surg 62A:259–270, 1980

7. Butler DL, Noyes FR, Grood ES: The effects of vascularity on the mechanical properties of primate anterior cruciate ligament replacements. Transactions of the 29th Annual Meeting of the Orthopaedic Research Society. 8:93, 1983 [abstr]

8. Cabaud HE, Rodkey WG, Faegin JA: Experimental studies of acute anterior cruciate ligament injury and repair. Am J Sports Med 7:18–22, 1979

9. Daniel DM, Malcom LL, Losse G et al: Instrumented measurement of anterior laxity of the knee. J Bone Joint Surg 67A:720–726, 1985

10. Daniel DM, Sachs R, Stone ML et al: Instrumented measurement of anterior laxity in patients with acute anterior cruciate ligament disruption. Am J Sports Med 13:401–407, 1985

11. Edmonson AS, Crenshaw AH (eds): Campbell's Operative Orthopaedics. 6th Ed. CV Mosby, St Louis, 1980, pp 933, 967–968

12. Ellison AE: Distal iliotibial-band transfer for anterolateral rotatory instability of the knee. J Bone Joint Surg 61A:330–337, 1979

13. Feagin JA, Curl WW: Isolated tear of the anterior cruciate ligament. Five-year follow-up study. Am J Sports Med 4:95–100, 1976

14. Garrick JG, Requa RK: Injury patterns in children and adolescent skiers. Am J Sports Med 7:245–248, 1979

15. Gollehon DI, Warren RF, Wickiewicz RT: Acute repairs of the anterior cruciate ligament. Past and present. Orthop Clin North Am 16:111–125, 1985

16. Henning CE, Lynch MA, Glick K: An in vivo strain gage study of elongation of the anterior cruciate ligament. Am J Sports Med 13:22–26, 1985

17. Higgins RW, Steadman JR: Anterior cruciate ligament repairs in elite skiers. Am J Sports Med (in press, 1987)

18. Johnson RJ, Kettlekamp DB, Clark W, Leverton P: Factors affecting late results after meniscectomy. J Bone Joint Surg 56A:719–729, 1974

19. Johnson RJ, Pope MH, Weisman G, White BF: Knee injury in skiing. Am J Sports Med 7:321–327, 1979

20. Kieffer DA, Curnow RJ, Southwell RB et al: Anterior cruciate ligament arthroplasty. Am J Sports Med 12:301–312, 1984

21. Krackow KA, Brooks RL: Optimization of knee ligament position for lateral extraarticular reconstruction. Am J Sports Med 11:293–302, 1983

22. Levy IM, Torzilli PA, Warren RF: The effect of medial meniscectomy on anterior–posterior motion of the knee. J Bone Joint Surg 64A:883–888, 1982

23. Liljedahl SO, Lindvall N, Wetterfors J: Early diagnosis and treatment of acute ruptures of the anterior cruciate ligament. A clinical and arthrographic study of forty-eight case. J Bone Joint Surg 47A:1503–1513, 1965

24. Losee RE, Johnson TR, Southwick WO: Anterior subluxation of the lateral tibial plateau. A diagnostic test and operative repair. J Bone Joint Surg 60A:1015–1030, 1978

25. McMaster JH, Weinert CR, Scranton P Jr: Diagnosis and management of isolated anterior cruciate ligament tears. A preliminary report on reconstruction with the gracilis tendon. J Trauma 14:230–235, 1974

26. Malcom LL, Daniel DM, Stone ML, Sachs R: The measurement of anterior knee laxity after ACL reconstructive surgery. Clin Orthop 196:35–41, 1985

27. Marshall JL, Arnoczky SP, Rubin RM, Wickiewicz TL: Microvasculature of the cruciate ligaments. Physician Sportsmed 7:87–91, 1979

28. Marshall JL, Warren RF, Wickiewicz TL: Primary surgical treatment of anterior cruciate ligament lesions. Am J Sports Med 10:103–107, 1982

29. Marshall JL, Warren RF, Wickierwicz TL, Reider B: The anterior cruciate ligament. A technique of repair and reconstruction. Clin Orthop 143:97–106, 1979

30. Marshall JL, Warren RF, Fleiss DJ: Ligamentous injuries of the knee in skiing. Clin Orthop 108:196–199, 1975

31. Odensten M, Lysholm J, Gillquist J: Suture of fresh ruptures of the anterior cruciate ligament. A 5-year follow-up. Acta Orthop Scand 55:270–272, 1984

32. O'Donoghue DH: An analysis of end results of surgical treatment of major injuries to the ligaments to the knee. J Bone Joint Surg 37A:1–13, 1955

33. Paulos L, Noyes FR, Grood E, Butler DL: Knee rehabilitation after anterior cruciate ligament reconstruction and repair. Am J Sports Med 9:140–149, 1981

34. Renstrom P, Arms SW, Stanwyck TS et al: Strain within the anterior cruciate ligament during hamstring and quadriceps activity. Am J Sports Med 14:83–87, 1986

35. Sarmiento A: Functional bracing of tibial fractures. Clin Orthop 105:202–219, 1974

36. Salter RB, Simmonds DF, Malcolm BW et al: The biologic effect of continuous passive motion on the healing of full thickness defects in articular cartilage. An experimental investigation in the rabbit. J Bone Joint Surg 62A:1232–1251, 1980

37. Solonen KA, Rokkanen P: Operative treatment of torn ligaments and injuries of the knee joint. Acta Orthop Scand 38:67–80, 1967

38. Tapper EM, Hoover NW: Late results after meniscectomy. J Bone Joint Surg 51A:517–526, 1969

39. Tapper EM, Moritz JR: Changing patterns in ski injuries. Physician Sportsmed 2:39–47, 1974

40. Tipton CM, Matthes RD, Maynard JA, Carey RA: The influence of physical activity on ligaments and tendons. Med Sci Sports 7:165–175, 1975

41. Tipton CM, James SL, Mergner WA, Tcheng T: Influence of exercise on strength of the medial collateral ligament of dogs. Am J Physiol 218:894–902, 1970

42. Vailas AC, Tipton CM, Matthes RD, Gart M: Physicial activity and its influence on the repair process of medial collateral ligaments. Connective Tiss Res 9:25–31, 1981

43. Walker PS, Erkman MJ: The role of the menisci in forced transmission across the knee. Clin Orthop 109:184–192, 1975

44. Warren RF: Primary repair of the anterior cruciate ligament. Clin Orthop 172:65–70, 1983

SUGGESTED READINGS

Arnoczky SP: Anatomy of the anterior cruciate ligament. Clin Orthop 172:19–25, 1983

Earle AS, Moritz JR: Ski injuries. JAMA 180:285–288, 1962

Hunter LY, Funk FJ: Rehabilitation of the Injured Knee. CV Mosby, St. Louis, 1984

Inglehart TK: Strength and motor task performance as affected by the carbon titanium knee brace in normal healthy males. Colorado State University, Department of Physical Education, Fort Collins, Colorado, Spring 1985

Johnson RJ, Pope MH, Ettlinger C: Ski injuries and equipment function. Am J Sports Med 2:292–307, 1974

Jurist KA, Otis JC: Anteroposterior tibial femoral displacements during isometric extension efforts. The roles of external load and knee flexion angle. Am J Sports Med 13:299–358, 1985

Laros GS, Tipton CM, Cooper RR: Influence of physical activity on ligament insertions in the knees of dogs. J Bone Joint Surg 53A:275–286, 1971

Lysholm J, Gillquist J, Liljedahl SO: Long-term results after early treatment of knee injuries. Acta Orthop Scand 53:109–118, 1982

Moritz JR: Ski injuries. Am J Surg 98:493–505, 1959

Norwood LA, Cross MF: The intercondylar shelf and the anterior cruciate ligament. Am J Sports Med 5:171–176, 1977

Noyes FR, Butler DL, Paulos LE, Grood ES: Intra-articular cruciate reconstruction. I. Perspectives on graft strength, vascularization and immediate motion after replacement. Clin Orthop 172:71–77, 1983

Noyes FR, DeLucas JL, Torvik PJ: Biomechanics of anterior cruciate ligament failure. An analysis of strain-rate sensitivity and mechanisms of failure in primates. J Bone Joint Surg 56A:236–253, 1974

Noyes FR, Keller CS, Grood ES, Butler DL: Advances in the understanding of knee ligament injury, repair, and rehabilitation. Med Sci Sports Exerc 16:427–443, 1984

Noyes FR, Torvik PJ, Hyde WB, DeLucas JL: Biomechanics of ligament failure. II. An analysis of immobilization, exercise, and reconditioning effects in primates. J Bone Joint Surg 56A:1406–1418, 1974

O'Donoghue DH: Surgical treatment of fresh injuries to the major ligaments of the knee. J Bone Joint Surg 32A:721–738, 1950

O'Donoghue DH, Frank GR, Jeter GL et al: Repair and reconstruction of the anterior cruciate ligament in dogs. Factors influencing long-term results. J Bone Joint Surg 53A:710–718, 1971

O'Donoghue DH, Rockwood CA, Frank GR et al: Repair of anterior cruciate ligaments in dogs. J Bone Joint Surg 48A:503–519, 1966

Palmer I: On the injuries to the ligaments of the knee joint. Acta Chir Scand Suppl 53:1–282, 1938

Robson M: Ruptured crucial ligaments and their repair by operation. Ann Surg 37:716–718, 1903

Steadman JR: Rehabilitation of athletic injuries. Am J Sports Med 7:147–149, 1979

Steadman JR: Rehabilitation of first-degree and second-degree sprains of the medial collateral ligament. Am J Sports Med 7:300–302, 1979

Steadman JR: Nonoperative measures for patellofemoral problems. Am J Sports Med 7:374–375, 1979

Steadman JR: Rehabilitation after knee surgery. Am J Sports Med 8:294–296, 1980

Steadman JR: Rehabilitation of tibial plafond fractures after stable internal fixation. Am J Sports Med 9:71–72, 1981

Steadman JR: Rehabilitation of skiing injuries. Clin Sports Med 1:289 294, 1982

Wang JB, Rubin RM, Marshall JL: A mechanism of isolated anterior cruciate rupture. Case report. J Bone Joint Surg 57A:411–413, 1975

28

Special Techniques in Rehabilitation

WILLIAM D. STANISH
SANDRA CURWIN

Rehabilitation means normalization. As part of the greater objective of returning the patient to normal function, rehabilitation after knee surgery has three major aims: (1) reduce pain, (2) increase range of motion (ROM), and (3) increase muscle strength. The reduction of pain is often a prerequisite for the latter two aims.

The objectives of anterior cruciate ligament (ACL) repair or reconstruction create the same postsurgical problems as other knee surgeries, but rehabilitation after such procedures is controversial. A dilemma exists for the patient, physician, and therapist in that the process of achieving these aims may compromise continuity and ultimate tensile strength of the healing tissue. This paradoxical situation has led to the examination of the mechanical interactions between quadriceps contraction, knee movement, and ACL stress/strain.[3,8,24,28,42] Meticulous rehabilitation programs have been designed based on the results of these mechanical studies.[7,43,44,55] Commonly these programs focus on anterior cruciate ligament kinematics alone, divorcing the mechanical aspects of rehabilitation from the objectives of function for the individual patient.

This chapter describes some special postoperative techniques that may not be part of the "routine" rehabilitation program, but can nevertheless be used to achieve the three major aims: pain relief, ROM, and muscle strength. These techniques still respect the time constraints of the healing process and, indeed, perhaps manipulate the latter to reduce the "paradox of exercise"[7] that accompanies

ACL rehabilitation. We can classify special techniques into two basic categories: those employed to control symptoms (pain relief) and those designed to increase the strength of healing tissues such as muscle or the repaired ligament itself. Some of these techniques are already well established and are in widespread clinical use for knee rehabilitation, while others are newer and more controversial. However, they are based on the principles of soft tissue healing.[23,56] The essential of ACL reconstruction, which is a high-strength, tension-free graft that remains isometric throughout most of the range of knee motion,[3] is assumed to exist before the application of the techniques to be described.

METHODS FOR PAIN RELIEF

After ligament repair and/or reconstruction the patient can experience considerable discomfort or pain in the immediate postoperative period or during the early stages of rehabilitation. Drugs can be used to control this pain but other methods, including electrical stimulation and cold therapy, can be equally successful.

Transcutaneous Electrical Neurologic Stimulation (TENS or TNS)

Electrical stimulation for pain relief appears to have been used as a therapeutic tool even in ancient times, but by the early 1900s this modality was regarded as a quack medicine. Interest was renewed by the Melzack and Wall[37] formulation of the gate theory of pain control. TNS was used after abdominal surgery and was found to decrease postoperative pain, atelectasis, ileus, and duration of intensive care.[30] Subsequent studies involving patients undergoing abdominal or thoracic surgery clearly showed that TNS was an effective means of reducing postoperative pain.[48,58] Placebo TNS units demonstrated little effect compared to active units.

TNS can also be effective after knee surgery. For example, Smith[49] described the use of TNS by 100 patients who had undergone either meniscectomies or total knee replacements. Those receiving TNS were able to perform a straight-leg raise earlier, received less narcotics, and had a shorter hospital stay. Jensen et al.[31] reported similar findings in 90 patients undergoing arthroscopic surgery of the knee. Those receiving TNS required 36 percent less pain medication than the control group during the first 3 postoperative days and had a greater range of motion at 3 weeks postsurgery. Our personal clinical experience parallels these findings and TNS is often used with our postsurgical knee patients.

The exact explanation for pain relief with TNS is unclear, however, there are two basic theories of the mechanism of function. One is based on the gate theory and holds that TNS overloads myelinated, faster conducting nerve fibers, thus preventing pain transmission to the spinal cord via small, unmyelinated, slow-conducting fibers. In effect, TNS "closes the gate" to pain transmission.[34,47] A second theory is that TNS stimulates the release of endogenous opiate peptides (endorphins).[22] This is supported by the fact that administration of opiate antagonists suppresses pain relief by TNS. Neither theory provides a complete explanation for the effects of TNS and it is likely that elements of both are involved. Although used for both chronic and acute pain, TNS seems to be most effective for acute pain situations, such as immediately after surgery. Electrodes can be applied flanking the painful region, or stimulation may be applied at trigger or acupuncture points.[38]

For TNS to be maximally effective, patient anxiety must be minimized by preoperative education. The pulse amplitude, pulse rate, and pulse duration (or width) should be explained to the patient and the appropriate settings for each determined. Each of the three settings, beginning with the amplitude, should be increased until a strong (but not unpleasant) sensation is felt. The purpose of TNS and the availability of pain medication if needed should be explained to the patient at the preoperative session.[46]

Following surgery, sterile electrodes are placed adjacent to the skin incision and the limb is wrapped in a compression bandage with the ends of the electrode leads free for insertion into the TNS unit (see Fig. 28-1). The TNS unit is adjusted to the preoperative settings while the patient is in the recovery room, since it appears that the best results are obtained if stimulation is begun while the patient is still under the effect of the general anesthetic.[12] Active quadriceps and hamstrings exercises commence immediately, since the knee is immobilized at 45° in a position that places minimal strain on the anterior cruciate ligament. Patients should be checked within 2 hours of application and settings adjusted if necessary.[46,49]

TNS is an effective means of pain relief, avoiding the use of analgesics or narcotics. There are few contraindications (pregnancy, pacemaker, allergy) and skin reactions occur infrequently. Strict documentation of electrode placement, type of unit, control settings, pain medications, patient activity levels, and the patient's subjective pain response should be kept to enable evaluation of treatment variables, at least until a sufficient number of patients have been treated to allow us to estimate common values.

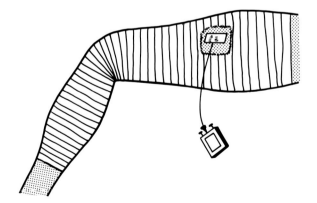

Fig. 28-1. TNS electrodes are placed adjacent to the surgical incision.

Cryotherapy

Similarly to cutaneous electrical stimulation, the use of cold in the treatment of soft tissue injuries originated in the time of the ancient Greeks.[35] Ice therapy has repeatedly been shown to reduce pain and disability after soft tissue injuries, especially if applied early. Thus it has become a cornerstone in the management of acute soft tissue injuries.[25,35,59] It is suggested that the reduction in temperature produced by cold application causes a decrease in the inflammatory response to trauma.[35]

The reduction of temperature accompanying cold therapy is of the order of 3 to 7° C, reducing peripheral tissue temperature to a minimum of 25° C. This temperature decrease has been demonstrated to reduce blood flow and histamine release following injury.[4] The drop in temperature of deeper tissues is smaller and less uniform. The duration of cryotherapy should be approximately 15 minutes if vasoconstriction is desired. Treatments longer than 30 minutes cause vasodilation and an increased inflammatory response may be evoked by long-duration cold application.

Superficial tissues are most affected by cryotherapy, thus this modality is very helpful in the early stages of rehabilitation after cast removal. Increases in knee joint movement and stresses on the joint capsule and ligaments, as well as the patellofemoral joint, can frequently lead to discomfort and slight swelling, which can be largely prevented by the application of cold immediately after therapy. Although many methods of cold application are available, crushed-ice packs, ice massage, and cold whirlpool are the most effective, so one of these methods should be used.[25,35]

A second use of cryotherapy is as a pretherapy analgesic. The local analgesia resulting from cold application is the result of decreases in nerve conduction velocity, particularly of the small sensory nerve fibers.[59] This skin analgesia occurs within about 5 minutes and decreases rapidly after removal of the ice, until no effect remains by 30 minutes. This pain-relieving effect may be used in much the same way as TNS, specifically to relieve discomfort prior to carrying out therapeutic exercises. The choice of cold or TNS would be determined by the response of the individual to each modality and the availability of each to the patient, since ice may be more practical for the client who is working independently of the therapist.

TECHNIQUES FOR INCREASING MECHANICAL STRENGTH

The dilemma in ACL reconstruction rehabilitation is to improve the mechanical function of the knee joint (ROM) and muscles (strength) without compromising the mechanical stability of the reconstruction. Although biologic grafts have comparable, or greater, tensile strength than the anterior cruciate ligament at the time of their insertion, necrosis and new collagen formation reduce the tensile strength to as little as 15 percent of this value at 4 weeks postoperatively.[42] The stages of soft tissue healing proceed through a period of decreased strength from 2 to 4 weeks postinjury, after which strength begins to increase.[56] There are differences, however, in the healing rates of different tissues; furthermore, the synovial fluid of the knee joint may inhibit fibroblast activity and growth.[2] The time sequence of healing (i.e., tensile strength of anterior cruciate reconstructions) is really unknown. It can be assumed, however, that the graft is most precarious during the early postoperative weeks, and during this time motion must be carefully restricted to 30° to 60°.[3] Isometric exercises are important, but simultaneous contraction of hamstrings and quadriceps should be encouraged.[7]

Although relative immobilization is needed to allow graft healing, the deleterious effects of immobilization on muscles, ligaments, tendons, and joints are well-known.[1,9,41] Conversely, exercise has been shown to increase soft tissue strength, including that of the normal anterior cruciate ligament.[10] The clinical problem becomes one of using the benefits of mechanical stress while avoiding excessive strain on the ACL.

Electrical Stimulation of Soft Tissue Healing

The piezoelectric effects of bone, tendon, and ligament are now well known and there has been a great deal of interest in this phenomenon.[5,6,11,19,20,29,32,40,45,50–52,60,61] These tissues respond to mechanical stress by producing an electric current, probably due to reorientation of dipoles in the polypeptide units of the collagen molecule, that ostensibly mediates the cellular effects. The mechanism of these effects, whether direct or via changes in membrane polarization or permeability, is unknown. Theoretically, however, one should be able to bypass the mechanical stress and get the same effects from electrical stimulation alone. Indeed, electrical stimulation has been shown to increase amino acid transport and protein synthesis,[11] to increase DNA synthesis and transcription, and to increase cell proliferation.[45] Electrical stimulation of bone growth is an accepted clinical method.[50]

Although Williams and Berger[60] demonstrated that bone and tendon have similar electrical properties, there is a great paucity of literature on the electrical stimulation of tendon or ligament healing. Since the piezoelectric effect is thought to be mediated by collagen, we might expect tissues such as ligament, skin, and tendon, which are composed largely of collagen, to respond even more dramatically to electrical stimulation. Indeed, various soft tissues have been shown to respond in a similar manner. Frank et al.[19] placed rabbit hindlimbs in an electromagnetic field and demonstrated increased histologic, biochemical, and biomechanical signs of healing of repaired medial collateral ligaments (MCL). These signs were evident at 21 days postoperatively, but by 42 days there were no significant differences between groups. Skin wounds have been shown to possess increased tensile strength as a result of electrical stimulation.[20,32] Articular cartilage chondrocytes respond to electrical stimulation with increased glycosaminoglycan (GAG) synthesis and cell proliferation.[40]

This apparently uniform response of connective tissues to electric current led us to develop several preliminary studies to assess the potential for electrical stimulation as a tool in ligament and tendon healing. One such study[52] involved the application of direct current to surgically repaired dog patellar tendons. Three groups were used: group I—control animals; group II—surgery only; group III—surgery plus electrical stimulation. The cathode of a DC electrical stimulator (Osteostim, BGS

Medical) was wrapped around the patellar tendon and the anode and body of the unit were placed subcutaneously in the medial thigh. A constant current (3 V, 20 μA) was applied. At 8 weeks postoperatively all dogs were sacrificed and the tendons inspected and mechanically tested with an Instron machine. The results are shown in Table 28-1. The stimulated group demonstrated increased tensile strength, even though the tendon callus of the three groups appeared similar in size on visual inspection. This suggests a qualitative change in the newly formed tissue, but further biochemical studies will be required to determine if this hypothesis is valid.

The results of this preliminary study have led us to propose cautiously that electrical stimulation will lead to a stronger tendon. The clinical implications of this are far-reaching. Electrical stimulation could be a tremendous adjunct in the surgical treatment of tendon ruptures or the nonsurgical treatment of chronic tendonitis. If we extrapolate the properties of tendon to ligament, electrical stimulation of ligament reconstructions could prove invaluable in preventing breakdown of these repairs, especially during the critical early postoperative period.

With these results in mind, a second clinical study was designed. Seventy cases of ACL reconstruction using an iliotibial band over-the-top procedure were evaluated.[51] During surgery, the cathode of a DC electrical stimulator was wrapped around the graft (anterior two-thirds of the iliotibial band), which was then passed through the joint capsule over the lateral femoral condyle, through the intercondylar notch, then over the anterior dome of the tibia, and attached to the patellar tendon adjacent to the tibial tubercle. The battery pack and anode were placed in a soft tissue cul-de-sac in the lateral thigh and constant current applied (3 V, 20 μA; Osteostim, BGS Medical) as shown in Figure 28-2. The electrical stimulator was removed under general anesthe-

Table 28-1. Ultimate Strength Values of Dog Patellar Tendons[a]

Group	Experimental (L Leg) (N)	Control (R Leg) (N)	Percent of Normal
I	941	426	47
II	960	454	49
III	627	582	92

[a] Experimental legs were stimulated, control legs were not.

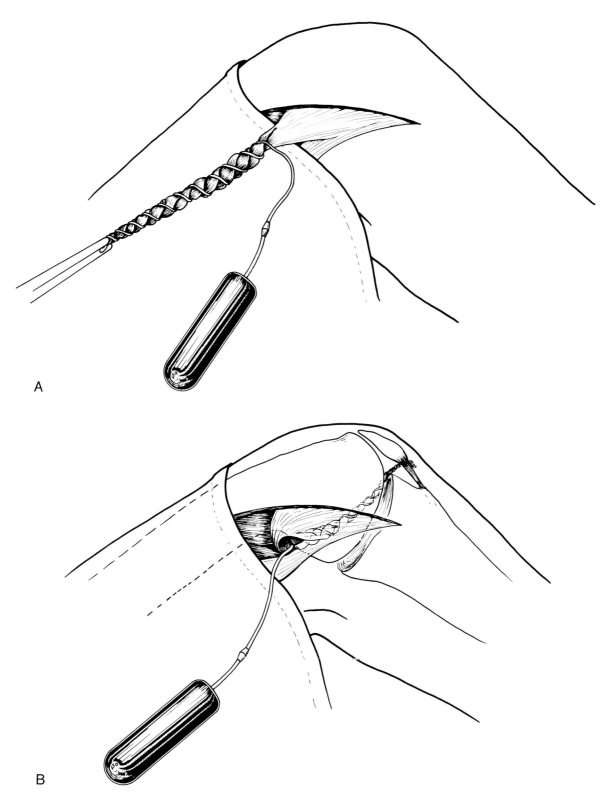

Fig. 28-2. (A) Cathode is wrapped around biologic graft, which is then passed through the knee joint. **(B)** The anode and battery are placed in the lateral thigh.

sia at 6 to 9 months, combined with arthroscopy and biopsy of the ligament. It is impossible, of course, to test the healed ligaments mechanically, but on visual inspection they were larger than usual. Since cross-sectional area has been shown to correlate directly with tensile strength,[9] this result suggests increased functional strength of the healed repair.

Although preliminary, these results and those of Frank et al.[19] have important implications for ACL reconstruction. Electrical or electromagnetic stimulation during the early stages of healing may augment the mechanical strength of the graft at precisely the time it is most needed. This feature would allow us to perform other therapies such as resisted exercise and range of motion exercise (to maintain joint surface integrity and muscle strength) without fear of disrupting the repair.

Electrical Muscle Stimulation (EMS)

The muscle atrophy and inhibition of muscle contraction that develop after knee surgery are well known,[17] and EMS has long been a clinical tool of therapists to overcome this inhibition and promote active contraction. Electrical stimulation has also been promoted as a muscle-strengthening tool.[34,36] When strength change is studied, the type of subject appears to influence the results. Subjects with knee injuries show a greater strength increase response to electrical stimulation than to isometric exercise,[17] whereas for normal subjects (without injury) there is little or no difference between the two treatment modalities.[13]

Immobilization has been shown to cause preferential atrophy of type I muscle fibers, which have a high oxidative capacity.[26] EMS during cast immobilization has been shown to prevent the fall in oxidative enzyme activity that occurs during lower limb immobilization. Eriksson and Häggmark[17] showed that succinate dehydrogenase activity (SDH) increased during intracast EMS but decreased in control subjects during 5 weeks of immobilization. Stanish et al.[53] showed an increase in myofibrillar ATPase in stimulated quadriceps muscle, compared to unstimulated controls. These results indicate that EMS can reverse at least some of the biochemical changes that accompany cast immobilization. EMS has also been shown to prevent the increase in sub-

maximal heart rate in response to exercise that usually occurs after immobilization.[18]

EMS has been shown to increase knee torque production in posttraumatic knee patients compared to isometric muscle contraction.[39] Six hours of EMS daily after ACL reconstruction restricted loss of quadriceps torque to 60 percent of normal values rather than the 80 percent loss that was observed in nonstimulated patients. These authors[39] began EMS after cast removal and observed a 7.2 cm decrease in thigh circumference during immobilization, while Eriksson and Häggmark[17] observed only a 2.0 cm decrease, pointing out the advantage of using EMS during cast immobilization rather than after cast removal. Since decreases in thigh circumference have been shown to be due to decreases in quadriceps bulk, in-cast EMS appears to preserve quadriceps strength. The time course for soft tissue healing when various postoperative techniques are used is shown in Fig. 28-3.

EMS is easy to apply both before and after cast removal. Electrodes may be applied at surgery in the same manner as those for TNS, or windows may be cut in the cast 7 to 10 days postoperatively. The former method is probably preferable with the smaller electrodes and stimulators that are now available. An advantage of electrical stimulation is that isometric quadriceps exercises are performed at a specific point in the knee's range of motion if used during cast immobilization, thus reducing the strain on the ACL, especially if done at 60° flexion.[3] A second advantage is that both type I and type II fibers are recruited, preventing the type I atrophy that accompanies immobilization. Third, if electrodes are placed on both the hamstrings and quadriceps, cocontraction is easily achieved in the early postoperative period. Resistance, however, is essential for the development of muscle strength using electrical stimulation as it is for other types of muscle contraction. This may explain the poor results sometimes obtained with normal subjects.[13,21]

Ultrasound

Ultrasonic therapy is widely used clinically to treat a variety of soft tissue injuries, yet little is known about the interaction between ultrasound and tissue. Ultrasound is a form of mechanical energy—

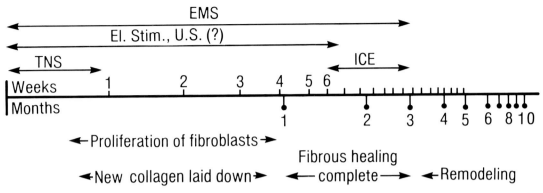

Fig. 28-3. Time course of soft tissue healing showing when special postoperative techniques are used.

sound waves (pressure waves) — with frequencies above 16 kHz, the limit of the audible frequency range. The sound waves are produced when a rapidly varying voltage is applied to a piezoelectric material, usually a circular ceramic disk.[57] When ultrasound is applied to tissue, two effects result: a mechanical action due to the pressure waves, and a thermal action due to dissipation of energy within the tissue. The biologic effects of ultrasound are attributed to these mechanical and thermal actions.

Therapeutic levels of ultrasound (0.25 to 3.0 W/cm²; 1.0 to 3.0 MHz) produce a wide range of biologic effects.[16] Tissue heating can be induced by ultrasound, and if the local temperature reaches 40°C, hyperemia results and the resolution of chronic inflammatory processes is assisted.[16] However, the thermal actions of ultrasound are considered secondary, and the mechanical actions are thought to have the most effect. These actions are highly dose-dependent. For example, low doses of ultrasound (0.5 W/cm²) increase blood flow while higher doses (3.0 W/cm²) actually causes red blood cell stasis.[33] These mechanical actions may be the direct result of piezoelectric effects or they may be due to streaming potentials that arise at the cell membrane as a result of the mechanical waves.[16,57] This may alter the permeability of the cell membrane, thus accounting for the increased cell synthetic activity known to result from ultrasound treatment.[27] Much more research is necessary, however, before the explanation of the effect of ultrasound on soft tissues can be determined exactly.

Although the mechanisms are unknown, experimental work on tissue repair in animals has shown that ultrasound can increase the rate of growth of replacement tissue at sites of injury.[15] Similar exposure levels can increase the rate of protein synthesis in fibroblasts.[27] Chronic varicose ulcers of the lower limb have been shown to heal much more rapidly with ultrasound therapy, becoming completely epithelialized after 21 treatments.[15] More recently, ultrasound has been used to promote bone healing. Duarte[14] reported increased callus area after ultrasound treatment of osteotomized rabbit fibulae, and a qualitative change in callus type. Our clinical experience with the same animal model, however, does not support these results.[54]

While there are no data available on the effects of ultrasound on ligament or tendon healing, the literature suggests that ultrasound may have a role to play in promoting the healing of soft tissue injuries. There are, however, many variables to control: frequency (and hence depth of penetration), pulsed vs. continuous ultrasound, intensity, treatment time, etc. Thus, although this technique appears to hold some promise, further research is needed to define its effects and their mechanism.

CONCLUSIONS

The objective of any surgery is to resolve the problem at hand and restore homeostasis. In the face of knee instability secondary to disruption of a knee ligament, achieving *static* stability is but the first step in solving the total problem. In the process of gaining an optimal *functional* result, pain control and muscle rehabilitation are paramount.

The clinical potential for deployment of electricity in rehabilitation after knee ligament surgery is most exciting. Our research has demonstrated consistently the ability of electrical energy to facilitate the recovery of muscle (and the cardiovascular system) after major knee ligament construction. Transcutaneous electrical stimulation may successfully control the postoperative pain while accomplishing simultaneous isometric contraction, both of which are essential ingredients in the restoration of function.

Frequently the preoperative training program includes electrical muscle stimulation (combined with active specific exercises), which may achieve such significant functional stabilization of the knee that surgery becomes unnecessary.

Finally, divorcing the technical surgery from the rehabilitation process must be deemed shortsighted and unacceptable in contemporary knee surgery. The thrust must be towards controlling the total healing environment to maximize the functional surgical product.

REFERENCES

1. Amiel D, Akeson WH, Harwood FL, Frank CB: Stress deprivation effect on metabolic turnover of the medial collateral ligament collagen. Clin Orthop 172:265–270, 1983
2. Andrish J, Holmes R: Effects of synovial fluid on fibroblasts in tissue culture. Clin Orthop 138:279–283, 1979
3. Arms SW, Pope MH, Johnson RJ et al: The biomechanics of anterior cruciate ligament rehabilitation and reconstruction. Am J Sports Med 12:8–18, 1984
4. Barcroft H, Edholm K: The effects of temperature on blood flow and deep temperature on the human forearm. J Physiol 102:5–20, 1943
5. Bentall R: Healing by electromagnetism — fact or fiction? New Scientist 70:166–167, 1976
6. Binder A, Parr G, Hazelman B, Fitton-Jackson S: Pulsed electromagnetic field therapy of persistent rotator cuff tendonitis. Lancet 1:695–698, 1984
7. Blackburn TA: Rehabilitation of anterior cruciate ligament injuries. Orthop Clin North Am 16:241–269, 1985
8. Burks R, Daniel D, Losse G: The effect of continuous passive motion on anterior cruciate ligament reconstruction stability. Am J Sports Med 12:323–327, 1984
9. Butler DL, Grood ES, Noyes FR, Zernicke RF: Biomechanics of ligaments and tendons. Exercise Sports Sci Rev 6:125–182, 1978
10. Cabaud HE, Chatty A, Gildengorin V, Feltman RJ: Exercise effects on the strength of the rat anterior cruciate ligament. Am J Sports Med 8:79–86, 1980
11. Cheng N, Van Hoof H, Bockx E et al: The effects of electric currents on ATP generation, protein synthesis, and membrane transport in rat skin. Clin Orthop 171:264–272, 1982
12. Cooperman A, Hall B, Mikalacki K et al: Use of transcutaneous electrical stimulation in the control of postoperative pain. Am J Surg 133:185–187, 1977
13. Currier DP, Lehman J, Lightfoot P: Electrical stimulation in exercise of the quadriceps femoris muscle. Phys Ther 59:1508–1512, 1979
14. Duarte LR: The stimulation of bone growth by ultrasound. Acta Orthop Trauma Surg 101:153–159, 1983
15. Dyson M, Pond JB: The effect of pulsed ultrasound on tissue regeneration. Physiotherapy 56:136–142, 1970
16. Dyson M, Suckling J: Stimulation of tissue repair by ultrasound: a survey of the mechanisms involved. Physiotherapy 64:105–108, 1978
17. Eriksson E, Häggmark T: Comparison of isometric muscle training and electrical stimulation supplementing isometric muscle training in the recovery after major knee ligament surgery. Am J Sports Med 7:169–171, 1979
18. Evans RT, Stanish WD: Transcutaneous faradic stimulation in the prevention of submaximal heart rate elevations at immobilized limbs: a preliminary report. Aust J Sports Med 14:27–34, 1982
19. Frank CB, Schacher D, Shrive N et al: Electromagnetic stimulation of ligament healing in rabbits. Clin Orthop 175:263–272, 1983
20. Frank CB, Szeto AYJ: A review of electromagnetically enhanced soft tissue healing. IEEE Eng Med Biol 2:27–32, 1983
21. Godfrey CM, Jayawardena H, Quance TA, Welsh P: Comparison of electrostimulation and isometric exercise in strengthening the quadriceps muscle. Physiotherapy Can 31:265–267, 1979
22. Goldstein A: Opioid peptides (endorphins) in pituitary and brain. Science 193:1081–1086, 1976
23. Goldstein WM, Barmada R: Early mobilization of rabbit medial collateral ligament repairs: biomechanic and histologic study. Arch Phys Med Rehab 65:239–242, 1984
24. Grood ES, Suntay WJ, Noyes FR, Butler DL: Biome-

chanics of the knee extension exercise. Effect of cutting the anterior cruciate ligament. J Bone Joint Surg 66A:725–734, 1984

25. Haines J: A survey of recent developments in cold therapy. Physiotherapy 53:222–229, 1967

26. Halkjaer-Kristensen J, Ingemann-Hansen T: Effect of immobilization on fiber composition in the human quadriceps muscle. Scand J Rheum 7:139–141, 1978

27. Harvey W, Dyson M, Pond JB, Grahame R: The in vitro stimulation of protein synthesis in human fibroblasts by therapeutic levels of ultrasound. Proceedings of the 2nd European Congress on Ultrasonics in Medicine. Excerpta Medica Int Congr Ser 363:10–21, 1975

28. Hofmann AA, Wyatt RWB, Bourne MH, Daniels AU: Knee stability in orthotic knee braces. Am J Sports Med 12:371–374, 1984

29. Honnart F, Patel A: The effect of high frequency electromagnetic energy following orthopaedic and traumatological surgery. A review of 65 cases (trans). Gaz Med France 87:2196–2198, 1980

30. Hymes AC, Yonehiro EG, Raab OE et al: Electrical stimulation for treatment and prevention of atelectasis and ileus. Surg Forum 25:222–227, 1974

31. Jensen JE, Conn RR, Hazelrigg G, Hewitt JE: The use of transcutaneous neural stimulation and isokinetic testing in arthroscopic knee surgery. Am J Sports Med 13:27–33, 1985

32. Konikoff JJ: Electrical promotion of soft tissue repairs. Ann Biomed Eng 4:1–5, 1976

33. Kramer JF: Ultrasound: evaluation of its mechanical and thermal effects. Arch Phys Med Rehab 65:223–227, 1984

34. Massey BH, Nelson RC, Sharkey BC et al: Effects of high frequency electrical stimulation on the size and strength of skeletal muscle. J Sports Med 11:136–144, 1965

35. McMaster WC: Cryotherapy. Physician Sportsmed 10:112–119, 1982

36. McMiken DF, Todd-Smith M, Thompson C: Strengthening of human quadriceps muscles by cutaneous electrical stimulation. Scand J Rehab Med 15:25–28, 1983

37. Melzack R, Wall PD: Pain mechanisms: a new theory. Science 150:971–978, 1965

38. Melzack R: Prolonged relief of pain by brief, intense transcutaneous somatic stimulation. Pain 1:357–373, 1975

39. Morrissey MC, Brewster CE, Shields CL, Brown M: The effects of electrical stimulation on the quadriceps during postoperative knee immobilization. Am J Sports Med 13:40–45, 1985

40. Nogami H, Aoki H, Okagawa T, Mimatsu K: Effects of electric current on chondrogenesis in vitro. Clin Orthop 163:243–247, 1982

41. Noyes FR: Functional properties of knee ligaments and alterations induced by immobilization. Clin Orthop 123:210–242, 1977

42. Noyes FR, Butler DL, Paulos LE, Grood ES: Intra-articular cruciate reconstruction. I: Perspectives on graft strength, vascularization and immediate motion after replacement. Clin Orthop 172:71–77, 1983

43. Noyes FR, Keller CS, Grood ES, Butler DL: Advances in the understanding of knee ligament injury, repair and rehabilitation. Med Sci Sports Exerc 18:427–443, 1984

44. Paulos L, Noyes FR, Grood E, Butler DL: Knee rehabilitation after anterior cruciate ligament reconstruction and repair. Am J Sports Med 9:140–149, 1981

45. Rodan GA, Bourret LA, Norton LA: DNA synthesis in cartilage cells is stimulated by oscillating electric fields. Science 199:690–692, 1978

46. Santiesteban AJ, Sanders BR: Establishing a postsurgical TENS program. Phys Ther 60:789–791, 1980

47. Serrato JC: Pain control by transcutaneous nerve stimulation. South Med J 72:67–71, 1979

48. Shealy CN: Transcutaneous electroanalgesia. Sur Forum 23:419–425, 1972

49. Smith MJ: Electrical stimulation for relief of musculoskeletal pain. Physician Sportsmed 11:47–55, 1983

50. Spadar JA: Electrically stimulated bone growth in animals and man. Clin Orthop 122:325–332, 1977

51. Stanish WD, Kozey J: The effect of electrical stimulation on iliotibial band reconstruction for the anterior cruciate deficient knee: an early report. Presented at the American Orthopaedic Society for Sports Medicine, Atlanta, February 1984

52. Stanish WD, Macgillvary G, Rubinovich M, Kozey J: The effects of electrical stimulation on tendon healing. Presented at the American Orthopaedic Society for Sports Medicine, Anaheim, CA, March 1983

53. Stanish WD, Valiant GA, Bonen A, Belcastro AN: The effects of immobilization and of electrical stimulation on muscle glycogen and myofibrillar ATPase. Can J Appl Sports Sci 7:267–271, 1982

54. Stanish WD, Woods E, Kozey J: The effects of ultrasound therapy on fracture healing in rabbits. Presented at the Canadian Orthopaedic Association, Hamilton Ontario, June 1985

55. Steadman JR: Rehabilitation of acute injuries of the anterior cruciate ligament. Clin Orthop 172:129–132, 1983

56. Steiner M: Biomechanics of tendon healing. J Biomech 15:951–957, 1982

57. Ter Haar G: Basic physics of therapeutic ultrasound. Physiotherapy 64:100–104, 1978

58. VanderArk GD, McGrath KA: Transcutaneous electrical stimulation in treatment of postoperative pain. Am J Surg 130:338–340, 1975

59. Waylonis GW: The physiological effects of ice massage. Arch Phys Med Rehab 48:47–52, 1967

60. Williams WS, Berger L: Piezoelectricity in tendon and bone. J Biomech 8:397–413, 1975

61. Wilson DH: Treatment of soft-tissue injuries by pulsed electrical energy. Br Med J 2:269–270, 1972

PROSTHETIC LIGAMENTS

29
Prosthetic Replacement of Knee Ligaments: Overview

ROBERT L. LARSON

The cruciate ligaments have a blood supply, provide proprioceptive response to stretching, have considerable tensile strength, have elasticity, have the ability to survive the action of the proteolytic enzymes of the synovial fluid, and have broad and precise attachment sites that allow normal motion while protecting against abnormal laxity. Their anatomic design and physiologic function guide the knee through a normal helicoid of motion, protect the menisci from injury, and restrain the tibia from being displaced too far anteriorly or too far posteriorly. They function in harmony with the other ligaments about the knee. The collateral and capsular ligaments and the cruciate ligaments contribute in some part to the major stabilizing function of the other.

When attempting, therefore, to replace the cruciate ligaments with a prosthesis, whether of biologic or synthetic material, deficiencies are immediately present.* The surgeon must also be aware that when the original ligament tore, a first failure had already occurred. The surgeon then becomes the second to try and construct a ligament that will withstand the stresses to which the knee joint is put. Matching our surgical ability with the original Creator should at least imbue us with a sense of humility and respect for such an exercise.

*References are not cited by number in the text, but the reader is invited to gain further insight into prosthetic replacement of knee ligaments by consulting the sources provided in the Suggested Readings.

The attention that knee injury and surgery have generated has yielded a better understanding of ligament pathology and the instability it produces. Improved and more exact evaluation has heightened our awareness and diagnosis of cruciate ligament injuries. Surgical techniques have incorporated isometric positioning and more exact and secure attachment sites. Rehabilitation has been directed toward earlier motion after injury and exercises that improve strength but do not excessively stress repair or reconstruction. The discipline of knee ligament surgery has therefore seen a modernization of procedures to improve results. Paralleling these more recent procedures has been the introduction of prosthetic materials, particularly for the anterior cruciate ligament (ACL).

HISTORICAL REVIEW

Attention to the need to replace or substitute for the ACL is not new. Although repair of the ACL was first attempted in the late 1890s by both Robson and Battle, by 1906 the first report of "artificial material" for stabilization of a flail joint was made by Herz in the German literature. In 1917 Hey Groves published a method for intraarticular reconstruction using fascia lata. Alwyn Smith, in 1918, modified Hey Groves' operative procedure after apparently trying silk as an artificial replacement. He reported that this failed in the 11th week after operation. Criticism of the use of autoplastic substitutes was voiced by Bischer in 1929 when he recommended the use of kangaroo tendon.

Kennedy, in an article written in 1983, mentioned Professor von Mironova, writing in the German literature, as having had a 25-year experience using Lavsan—a form of polyester. Satisfactory results after a 15-year follow-up were reported in 91 percent of 262 patients. Kennedy also reported on the work of Arai of Japan who had, since 1963, explored the possibility of suitable artificial materials without any major progress up to 1980.

In early 1974, a prosthetic ligament made of polyethlene (Polyflex) was marketed and used for a 2-year clinical period. Breakage and elongation occurred 2 years postoperatively and the clinical trials have since been discontinued.

Proplast was granted approval by the Food and Drug Administration for implantation as a ligament substitute in 1973. At least three modifications were used during its clinical trial. Average time to breakage was 13.2 months when used as an anterior cruciate ligament replacement and 16.2 months when used for posterior cruciate ligament (PCL) replacement. Its primary use was as a stent to protect the knee to allow healing of additional procedures done to improve stability. At an average follow-up of 33 months, Kellam reported that 52 percent of the ACL group and 77 percent of the posterior cruciate group had satisfactory results.

Because of the importance of the ACL in dogs and the frequency of its rupture, the veterinary literature includes many articles on uses for ACL replacement in dogs.

CHARACTERISTICS OF CRUCIATE LIGAMENT TISSUE vs. PROSTHETIC MATERIALS*

Two requirements become immediately apparent when discussing the use of prosthetics for cruciate replacement: biomechanical efficiency and biocompatibility.

---

*This section was prepared with the help of Stephen A. Cord, M.D., B.S., M.E., an orthopedist who now practices in Georgetown, Texas.

When comparing material properties of prostheses or ligaments, the terms, units, and testing methods should be consistent with accepted engineering standards. Terms used in describing material properties will be discussed later. The units used should be metric: newtons (N) to measure force, square meters (m²) to measure area, and pascals (1 N/m²) to measure stress. The rate of strain (elongation of the specimen) should approach 100 percent of its original length per second. This high rate is required to simulate ligament failure. Slower rates in anatomic specimens have resulted in bone failure instead of ligament failure.

Force or Load

The maximum *force* or *load* is the maximum that a material can absorb prior to failure and is measured in Newtons. This is, obviously, an important factor. The normal ACL of a young adult absorbs a maximum force of 475 to 1,730 N based on separate studies of Kennedy et al., Noyes et al., and Tremblay et al. The maximum load of the PCL is 560 to 1,710 N. Differences in these results appear to occur due to many factors, including age of the donor, length and method of postmortem storage, and methods employed for testing. For example, test speeds given above may vary from a strain rate of 50 mm to 1,500 mm/min. The higher values were measured as bone–tendon–bone specimens at high strain rates, approaching or equal to 100 percent/second.

Stress and Strength

Maximum stress and *tensile strength* are equivalent terms used to describe the force absorbed by material per unit of cross-sectional area. Its units are pascals. Strength and stress are synonymous, but are often confused with the terms *force* and *load*. Stress is useful in comparing different sizes of the same or different materials because dividing by the cross-sectional area eliminates the bias caused by changing sizes of the materials being tested.

Strain

Strength is only one aspect of the mechanical behavior of ligaments and prostheses. They also exhibit complex viscoelastic properties that can be shown pictorially with two curves (Fig. 29-1). Stress can be plotted against strain or force can be plotted against strain. *Strain* is the change in length divided by the original length of the material being tested. It is a dimensionless term given as a percentage or as meters per meter. The two curves produced are similar. Each shows an initial relationship that is concave upward, with a low slope, demonstrating an initial, highly elastic behavior of the ligament as it deforms easily with low stress. The typical stress vs. strain or load vs. strain curves of ligaments exhibit this initial "toe" region (flat or low slope) characteristic of low stiffness and high elasticity. As more and more fibers are recruited, virtually all fibers become loaded and the curve becomes increasingly more vertical: less change in length but increasing stress or load. With additional strain or force, the slopes of the curves (slope = stiffness) begins to increase rapidly, presumably due to the recruitment and straightening of the fibers. In the case of a biologic ligament, this would involve progressive straightening (loss of crimp) of the collagen fibers and stretching of an increased number of fibers (recruitment). Additional strain results in progressive rupture of the collagen fibers (plastic deformation) until the structure undergoes catastrophic failure.

Deformation

The ACL will elongate 15 to 25 percent of its original length before plastic deformation occurs. Elastic *deformation* of a material is its ability to return to the original resting length after stress is removed. Plastic deformation is the inability of a material to return to the original resting length after stress is removed. Studies by Tremblay et al. revealed that in flexion and extension the ACL elongated 17 percent of its resting length, while the PCL elongated 10 percent of its resting length. Therefore, an artificial or prosthetic ligament would need to have an initial elastic capability ("toe" region of stress vs. strain curve) in order to perform routine knee flexion and extension.

Yield Point

The *yield point* is the amount of stress applied when plastic deformation occurs. In the normal anterior cruciate ligament, this occurs at a strain of 25 percent with a stress of 25 ± 14 MPa.

Stiffness and Modulus of Elasticity

These terms are used to describe the characteristics of a material to resist deformation. *Stiffness* is measured in force per unit change in length (strain)

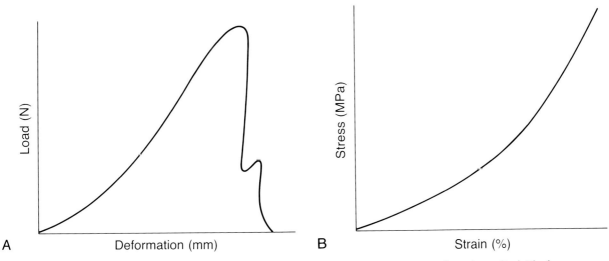

Fig. 29-1. **(A)** Load or force–strain curve depicts the elongation that occurs as force is applied. The low slope at the beginning of the curve is the "toe" and indicates the elasticity of the substance. As the slope becomes more vertical, the material becomes more stiff until eventual failure occurs. **(B)** Similar curve indicating a stress (strength)–strain curve showing the stretching that occurs to the material as stress is applied.

units (kN/m) and represents the slope of the curve on a force vs. strain diagram. The *modulus of elasticity* is the stress divided by the strain and represents the slope of the stress vs. strain curve in pascals. For each a horizontal slope and low number represent low resistance to deformation and a more vertical slope and higher number represent an increased resistance to deformation.

An ideal prosthetic substitute would need to have the ability to stiffen after the elastic region, exhibiting an increased modulus of elasticity, changing less in length as increasing forces are applied.

Creep

Artificial substances exhibit cumulative unrecoverable (plastic) elongation (deformation) after multiple cyclic loads. This phenomenon is called *creep*. In contrast, the living tissues of the cruciate ligaments (not withstanding their ability to have elongation memory with stretching exercises or "warming up") do not exhibit permanent elongation from cyclic loading during normal use. Materials, artificial or living, are tested for creep during a cyclic creep test. Minimal elongation after cyclic loading comparable to physiologic conditions for human cruciate ligaments is a further prerequisite for satisfactory function by an artificial substance. We can only estimate the proper testing conditions and cycles required to simulate the daily stresses applied to cruciate ligaments over a human life expectancy. It has been estimated that to be properly tested, a cruciate ligament or prosthesis must be tested from 500 to 1,400 N for 1 to 30×10^6 cycles. Typical values for creep after such cyclic loading range from 1 to 5 percent change in length in the synthetic material.

Fatigue

Fatigue is associated with creep. Living tissues have the ability to adapt and strengthen. Therefore, material fatigue is usually not a factor. However, artificial materials do not have the ability to strengthen and can fail, deform plastically, lose some of their ultimate strength, or fail completely when subjected to cyclic loading. Ideally, artificial ligaments should

be able to sustain a load approaching the maximum load of a natural ligament after undergoing a number of force cycles comparable to the number estimated for the lifetime of a human cruciate ligament. Prosthetic devices must be able to withstand these repetitive forces for at least a reasonable number of years and still maintain a high percentage of the maximum stress exhibited by a normal anterior cruciate ligament in order to be adequate for functional use as cruciate substitutes. Reproducing the forces and cyclic loading produced by normal human activity by mechanical testing is somewhat difficult. This is further compounded by the variability in patients' size and activity levels (Table 29-1).

Biocompatibility is ascertained in the laboratory and in the laboratory animal. Fluids that simulate the body environment are used to immerse the devices in and mechanically test them. Spectophotometric analysis is used to determine if any chemical agents are released. Tissue culture of the fluid is made and cell explants are used to determine if any untoward response develops. A laboratory animal is then used to determine the histologic response in the anatomic position for which the device is intended. Concurrent with this is the mechanical testing that attempts to mimic in vivo conditions. Laboratory animals are sacrificed to determine if any toxicity has been produced and if any mechanical deficiency of the device occurs.

The Food and Drug Administration (FDA) is the watchdog of devices used in the human body. Their charge is to obtain documented evidence of safety and efficacy of new devices used for human implantation. Clinical trials are allowed only after an investigational device exemption application has been approved. Such an application must show documented evidence of safety in animal models as well as a description of the clinical evaluation program. Monitoring by the developer, hospital investigational review board, and the FDA is maintained until enough data are accumulated to determine biocompatibility, safety, and efficacy by the FDA panel.

Efficacy is a term for which a precise definition is wanting. The intent is to determine if the device performs efficiently in the manner proposed by the investigator, not its effectiveness compared with other methods of treatment. The overall and long-term benefit of such devices with regard to anterior

Table 29-1. Biomechanical Characteristics of Prosthetic Material or Device

	Strain Rate (%/sec)	Maximum Force or Load (N)	Yield Load (N)	Strain at Yielding (%)	Creep (%Δl)	Fatigue Force (N) and No. cycles	Stiffness (kN/m)
ACL Butler et al., 1985 Noyes and Grood, 1976	100	1,730 ± 660	1,170 ± 750	25.5 ± 8		^{a}	182 ± 56
Carbon Cloes and Neugebauer, 1985	NA	2,461 ± 238	F 300 N	1.14	NA	60 @ 1×10^6	NA
Stryker-Meadox— Dacron Park et al., 1985	117	3,045 ± 15	NA	15	1% 1×10^6	2,850 @ 1×10^6	42 ± 1
Leeds-Keio	50	2,000	NA	NA	3–5% 1,400 N 30×10^6	830 @ 30×10^6	NA
Proplast James et al., 1979	2	1,565.6	671	2.4	NA	NA	NA
LAD (8 mm) McPherson et al., 1985	4	1,730 ± 660	NA	20	3% 500 N 1×10^6	1,560 @ 1×10^6	330
Gore-Tex Bolton and Bruchman, 1985	2.6	4,830 ± 280	1,000	2–5	4% 285 N 300×10^6	1,495 @ 10×10^6	322
Xenograft Xenotech Labs, 1983 Freeman, personal communication	100	2,210 ± 210	NA	4	0.2% 534 N 2×10^4	2,200 @ 10×10^6	56.9

NA, values not published in commonly available literature.

^{a} Mean load in the human ACL is estimated to be 300 N at 4.2×10^6 cycles per year.

cruciate replacement is difficult to measure because of the many variables and the prolonged follow-up.

After the presentation of data to the FDA advisory panel, a recommendation for premarket approval (PMA) is made to the FDA. The latter application, in addition to containing the information on clinical data, must also ensure that commercial production will contain the same safeguards used in the clinical investigational trials. If the advisory panel recommends approval and the FDA accepts this recommendation, the device is released for general use.

CATEGORIES OF ARTIFICIAL AND PROSTHETIC LIGAMENTS

A synthetic substance may function in one or all of the categories described below (as a scaffold, stent, or augmentation) and may be temporary or permanent.

The primary objective of a synthetic or biologic tissue as a scaffold is to provide support for the soft tissue to allow ingrowth of host tissue. The inducement of collagen ingrowth and orientation has also been claimed with the use of some of the synthetics. Any increase in the initial tensile strength of the repair or reconstruction also adds to the benefit of its use.

Scaffolding

Scaffolding may be temporary or permanent. Temporary scaffolding would include those substances that undergo degradation either chemically or mechanically or whose use would be interrupted by surgical removal. Though the intent of scaffolding is to develop host tissues that provide the tensile strength necessary for joint function, its initial strength should be sufficient to stabilize the joint while the host tissue is maturing fully to withstand the stress of joint activity. Too early degradation (as occurs with Dexon) allows stresses to the tissue that has not matured enough to withstand them.

Stents

Stents protect the joint from excessive stress while autogenous tissues are going through degradation, revascularization, and collagen deposition and maturation. Their function parallels that of a scaffold or prosthesis. They will eventually degrade, break, or be removed.

A problem in using stents is that they stress-shield the biologic tissue. When this occurs, the natural response of developing tensile strength comparable to the stresses placed upon the tissue is lost. When the stents break or are removed, the new tissue lacks the qualities necessary for functional use. A gradual degradation of the stent to allow increasing stress to the autogenous tissue as it matures would theoretically allow for the development of physiologic tensile strength.

Augmentation

A third use of synthetic materials is as an augmentation of autologous grafts used to replace a deficient cruciate ligament. The materials used for augmentation impart a greater tensile strength and help protect the graft from stress during the period of revascularization and collagen maturation necessary for functional efficiency. The material used for augmentation may produce stress shielding as noted above. Methods used to avoid stress shielding include fixation of the synthetic material at one end only. This allows the stresses to pass through the autogenous tissue, which has both femoral and tibial fixation. The strength contributed by the augmentation then depends on the strength of attachment of the synthetic material to the biologic tissue. Another proposed method is to fix the synthetic material at both ends initially. After the biologic tissue has had time to revascularize and develop ingrowth with the synthetic material, the synthetic device is then released at one end so that stresses will be transmitted to the biologic tissue. The device may also add to the overall tensile strength of the reconstruction of the ligament.

True Prosthesis

A final category is the *true prosthesis*. A device used in this manner is an artificial replacement of the cruciate ligament. It is meant to be permanent and to provide the function of the ligament it replaces. Although this is the ultimate goal, the restoration of the intrically designed cruciate ligament with its broad attachment sites, proprioceptive quality, multiaxial function, and biologic healing has not been achieved in the prostheses presently used.

Although host tissue may or may not invade the prosthesis, it is the ultimate strength and durability of the artificial substance that provide stability to the joint. The biomechanical characteristics of the synthetic will determine its long-term efficiency.

Many other terms to classify synthetics are used including temporary, permanent, or combinations; degradable, partially degradable, or nondegradable; type of material such as carbon-based, polymer fiber, porous polymers, biologic, allografts. Many categories overlap, so that an artificial or biologic substance could be classified in more than one category.

DEVICES CURRENTLY UNDER INVESTIGATION

The following devices have been or are currently being used in investigational studies. Their placement in a certain category is arbitrary and many overlap in their objectives and capabilities from one category to another.

Devices Currently Under Investigation

Scaffolds
  Carbon (Lafil, Plastifil, Integraft)
  Stryker-Meadox Dacron velour graft
  Leeds-Keio (Dacron)
  Dacron Velour fascia lata composite
  High-strength Dacron
  Allografts
Stents
  Proplast
  LAD (polypropylene)
  Dacron materials

Augmentation
  LAD
  (Other)
Prostheses
  Gore-Tex (polytetrafluoroethylene)
  Xenograft (bovine ligament and tendon)
  Dacron-Hytrel fiber
  Swiss polyethylene ligament

New synthetic devices are continuing to be developed both in this country and abroad.

Ideally, a comparison of the biomechanical characteristics of all of the devices would be useful. This is not possible because of the varied manner of testing used by the different investigators. Some comparisons are possible though not exact. The following section presents the data that can be gleaned by review of the literature available on the biomechanical characteristics of the material or device.

Definitions

Load = force

Maximum load = maximum force at failure in newtons (N)

Tensile strength = the highest stress on the stress–strain curve in N/m^2 or pascals (Pa)

Stress = load or force per unit area in N/m^2 or psi

Strain = change in length per original length (dimensionless): percent, m/m

Fatigue load = force at which failure occurs after a given number of cycles in units of Newtons

Fatigue strength = force per unit area at which failure occurs after a given number of cycles, units, N/m^2 or Pa

Ductility = percent elongation at failure or 100 times the strain at failure

Creep = elongation over time after multiple cyclic loads; units: percent change in length at a given number of cycles and given load

Creep is a form of plastic (permanent) deformation

Modulus of elasticity is the resistance to elastic strain and equals the slope of the stress-strain curve. It is given in units of Pa or N/m^2

Stiffness is similar to modulus of elasticity except it is derived from the slope of the force vs. strain curve and its units are N/m.

Units/Equivalents

One Newton (N) = 0.2248 pounds force
= the force required to give 1 kg mass an acceleration of 1 m/sec²

1 kilogram (kg) force = 9.8 N

1 lb force = 4.448 N

1 N/m^2 = 1 pascal (Pa)
= 0.145×10^{-3} lb force/inch² (psi)

14 megapascals (MPa) approximately = 2000 psi

OVERVIEW OF RESULTS OF VARIOUS DEVICES

Many of the synthetic materials and devices have been used in investigational studies for long enough periods to provide some data on their effectiveness. A major drawback in attempting to analyze results is the difficulty in comparing data from various studies. The many variables inherent in knee injury — severity of injury, type of surgery done, periods of immobilization or mobilization, rehabilitation, activity level on return, and constitutional factors relating to muscles, ligaments, and articular cartilage — compound the problems associated with the various methods of assessing results.

Comparison of the synthetic materials as augmentation of autogenous tissue or as true prostheses to present methods of autogenous reconstruction must be considered in the proper perspective. Many of the procedures were done because of failure of previous surgery. In some, the prosthesis was used as a salvage procedure when all others had failed. There are, therefore, significant differences in patient population types in the various investigational studies.

A brief note about various materials and devices will be made but only those that have had at least a 24-month follow-up will be evaluated for their effectiveness. Such comparison will be done using the values of objective stability as given in the various studies published or presented. Even the so-called objective measurements require subjective interpretation by the examiner. Although bias is, it is hoped, minimized by the use of objective tests, it cannot be completely eliminated. There remain variations: one examiner may interpret a test result as a "1+" while another may interpret the same test as a "0" or another as a "2+."

Complications are also difficult to compare among the various devices. The types of complications that occur vary. The way different devices are used makes their mechanical function different.

Carbon (Integraft)

A series of 155 patients who had ACL surgery alone or in combination with other ligamentous surgery around the knee were available for a 24-month (or longer) follow-up. The objective data are shown in Table 29-2. The incidence of some of the complications relating to carbon are: instability 7.3 percent, effusion 3.7 percent, resurgery 8.1 percent, and infections (deep) 1 percent.

Stryker-Meadox

A report of 300 patients in Europe who received this implant yielded 91 percent good results. Further information about this device has not been reported.

Table 29-2. Results (%) of Testing Carbon Prostheses

Test	Preoperative Results 2+ to 3+	Postoperative Results	
		2+ to 3+	0 to 1+
Lachman	90	12	88
Pivot shift	68	4.5	95
Anterior Drawer	93	11	89

Leeds-Keio

A report by Fujikawa of Keio University in Tokyo included 20 patients who received this scaffold since February 1982. Stability as determined by the Lachman test, pivot shift test, and anterior drawer was provided in 85 percent. Arthroscopy of 30 patients showed satisfactory tissue induction around the artificial ligament. Biopsy 10 months postoperatively showed collagen running longitudinally and parallel with more cells than in the natural tissue.

Fujikawa reported no problems with joint effusion and gave no indication of other complications.

Dacron Velour – Fascia Lata and Dexon – Dacron

These materials have been used in animal studies. Studies by Bassett using baboons showed that at 1 year success would depend on the use of an ample width of fascia lata. A report on Dexon – Dacron with fascia lata as the autogenous tissue used to reconstruct the anterior cruciate in dogs concluded that even with such tissue no fibrous ingrowth occurred and there was fraying and ultimate failure of the permanent Dacron portions of the prosthesis.

Allografts

Shino reported on 56 patients in whom free tendon allografts were used as anterior cruciate replacements along with extraarticular reconstructions with an 18 month follow-up on 18 patients. Excellent or good results were obtained in 89 percent. No rejections or infections occurred.

An experimental study by Nickolaou et al. used cadaveric deep frozen anterior cruciate ligaments from one dog to another. There was no significant difference between homografts and allografts. From the 8th to the 36th week, strength increased to 90 percent of the control level. No evidence of infection was seen. They concluded that deep frozen anterior cruciate ligaments obtained from a donor knee provided suitable material for anterior cruciate reconstruction.

Proplast

In 110 reconstructions using Proplast for stents for the ACL or PCL, the data showed the average lifetime of the ACL to be 13.2 months and 16.2 months for the PCL. This study, with an average follow-up of 33 months, showed satisfactory results in 52 percent of the anterior cruciate group and 77 percent in the PCL group based on a 200-point rating scale. Complications occurred in 16 percent.

Polypropylene-LAD

A series of 144 patients operated on by Kennedy and reported by Roth showed superior results with the use of the polypropylene braid as an augmentation of the middle third of the patellar tendon with the expansion of the quadriceps fascia over the patella compared with use of the same tissue without the synthetic braid. This type of reconstruction, as described by MacIntosh, takes the tissue through a bony tibial tunnel and over the top of the lateral femoral condyle.

An investigational study done in the United States reports on the objective testing results after 24 months (Table 29-3).

Review of 148 patients revealed a complication rate of 7 percent. Effusion requiring aspirations in 4.1 percent, infection in 0.7 percent, LAD breakage in 1.3 percent, and giving way in 7.4 percent are some of the complications reported. A life table analysis to 27 months reveals an 84 percent probability of success.

Gore-Tex

The report on 187 patients with greater than a 24-month follow-up revealed that 76 percent had undergone previous surgical procedures (Table 29-4).

A 14.3 percent complication rate is reported. The device failure rate of the total population group of 954 patients is reported to be 1.8 percent.

Xenograft

Abbink of the Netherlands presented a paper at the AAOS meeting in 1986 on 201 patients with an average follow-up of 3 years. Eighty-seven percent were said to have good or excellent results. Synovitis occurred in 20 percent, and 10 percent required second grafts.

Rojas and Teitge reported on 18 patients with a minimum follow-up of 1 year. Fifty percent of the

Table 29-3. Results (%) of Testing Polypropylene-LAD Prostheses

Test	Preoperative Results 2+ to 3+	Postoperative Results 2+ to 3+	0 to 1+
Lachman	94	5	95
Pivot shift	83	19	91
Anterior Drawer	100	10	90

Table 29-4. Results (%) of Testing Gore-Tex Prostheses

Test	Preoperative Results 2+ to 3+	Postoperative Results 2+ to 3+	0 to 1+
Lachman	85	11	89
Pivot shift	81	5	95
Anterior Drawer	85	15	85

grafts had to be surgically removed, usually due to recurrent effusion.

Abbink et al., in a later report of the series, discussed one group of 50 patients with 60 percent good to excellent results and synovitis in 40 percent. A second group of 89 patients had as part of their surgery notchplasty, chamfering of bone tunnel edges, and a lateral reconstruction (Lemaire type). This group had 95 percent good to excellent result with only 3.4 percent synovitis. The explanation given for the marked difference in the two groups relative to the synovitis was that fraying or rupture of the xenograft produced collagen particles that induced an inflammatory response. The better techniques used in the second group lessened this occurrence.

The learning curve necessary for successful surgical technique is evident in these studies.

Swiss Polyethylene Ligament

This was presented at an anterior cruciate ligament study group meeting in Zermatt, Switzerland, in 1986. This device has a tensile strength of 4,500 N, and an elasticity of 11 percent at 1,000 N. It is stapled at both ends to act as a true prosthesis. Preliminary results on 100 patients showed a reduction or elimination of the Lachman and pivot shift in over 90 percent of the patients.

Assessment of Devices

Although arthroscopic visualization and histologic evaluation have been carried out on many of the patients, neither is a reliable method of assessing the true value of the artificial reconstruction. Only by a reliable test of tensile strength and fixation strength, as well as an assurance of normal physiologic motion that protects articular cartilage and the menisci, can such an assessment be valid. This, of course, is not possible in the clinical evaluation of human subjects with such devices. The use of retrospective analysis remains the usual, albeit inadequate, method of appraising results.

ARTHROSCOPIC PLACEMENT OF SYNTHETIC BIOLOGIC ALTERED DEVICES

The ability to pass material through the knee joint, whether autogenous tissue or prosthetics, in the alignment of the ACL has provided a new avenue for cruciate reconstruction. Synthetic materials in particular lend themselves to this approach. A true prosthesis inserted in this manner eliminates the morbidity of harvesting autogenous tissue. Autogenous tissue augmented with a synthetic material inserted under arthroscopic control avoids a capsular incision and allows shorter incisions at fixation sites. This preserves some proprioceptive sensation around the joint and decreases the reflex inhibition that incisions into the quadriceps mechanism sometimes produce.

THE FUTURE OF SYNTHETIC AND PROSTHETIC DEVICES

The results after use of various synthetic or biologically altered tissue to replace, supplement, or augment autogenous tissue for anterior cruciate ligaments have indicated that there is a definite learning curve in achieving the proficiency necessary for reliable results. Materials will continue to improve, surgical techniques and the instrumentation to achieve better placement and fixation will continue to be devised, and the skill of the surgeon will increase with time.

Improvements in surgical techniques, such as more precise attachment sites, notchplasty to avoid any impingement or excess stress to the replaced material, chamfering of edges to reduce abrasion, attention to proper tension, and other nuances of technique, have provided better stabilization with a decrease in such problems as limitation of joint motion, prolonged immobilization, and prolonged rehabilitation.

The more widespread use of arthroscopic procedures will promote a more frequent use of synthetic and biologically altered tissue.

The question of long-term efficiency requires continued monitoring of valid results. The present advantages of artificial materials for cruciate replacement lie in the decreased morbidity and potentially quicker rehabilitation. Whether long-term stabilization will be maintained, whether the joint will be protected from further injury or degeneration, or whether as yet unrecognized or unforeseen problems will occur can only be determined as the devices are used. As new materials are developed, the continuation of appropriate safety checks and the use of investigational protocols that develop proper techniques are necessary to provide guidelines that allow the practitioner to utilize such devices with some confidence as to their value.

Still to be developed is standardized biomechanical testing of the synthetics to allow comparison with each other as well as with the characteristics of the normal anterior cruciate ligament. A uniform system of evaluation and rating of results is also lacking. Although a completely objective assessment of results is impossible, the use of a standard system would minimize the interpretive differences present in the many methods of recording results presently in use.

As with any developing product, the original designs and materials may be seen as crude as technologic advancement provides newer "models." *A cautionary note in the case of the ACL is that this is the most demanding of the clinical applications of synthetic implants.* The theoretical advantages proposed often do not conform to the clinical demands required. The scrutiny of time is a demanding arbitrator of clinical results. The long-term results of our present methods of autogenous reconstruction remain suspect when compared to the nonreconstructed deficient knees.

The short-term benefit would allow a more functional use of an unstable knee. It is hoped that the use of synthetic materials or allografts will allow a more rapid return to functional activity. The second benefit to be determined is the long-term function of the material or device. Will the joint maintain its normal function "in spite of " a synthetic or artificial substance being used instead of the host's biologic tissue? The fact that joints without a history of injury or ligamentous disruption deteriorate over the years clouds the issue.

Wise analysis should not be intimidated by the exuberance of discovery. Each step leading to a "solution" to the complex problem of the cruciate-deficient knee must be judged and compared to the previous "solutions." At present, there is no "ideal ligament replacement." No substitute is better than the original.

SUGGESTED READINGS

Abbink EP, Kramer F, Bom P: Assessing bovine xenograft knee ligament reconstructions. Presented at American Academy of Orthopaedic Surgeons 53rd Annual Meeting, New Orleans, 1986

Abbink EP: Surgical technique for correction of chronic anterior cruciate ligament deficiency with bovine xenografts. Prosthetic Ligament Reconstruction of the Knee, 3rd Annual Symposium, Scottsdale, AZ, 1986

Alexander H, Weiss AB, Parsons JR: Ligament repair and reconstruction with an absorbable polymer coated fiber stent. Prosthetic Ligament Reconstruction of the Knee, 3rd Annual Symposium, Scottsdale, AZ, 1986

Alwyn Smith S: The diagnosis and treatment of injuries to the crucial ligaments. Br J Surg 6:176, 1918

Arnoczky SP, Warren RF, Minei JP: Replacement of the anterior cruciate ligament using a synthetic prosthesis. An evaluation of graft biology in the dog. Am J Sports Med 14:1-6, 1986

Arnoczky SP, Warren RF, Minei JP: Replacement of the anterior cruciate ligament using.a patellar tendon allograft. An experimental study. J Bone Joint Surg 68A:376-385, 1986

Balduini FC, Clemow AJT, Lehman RC: Synthetic Ligaments. Scaffolds, Stents, and Prostheses. Slack, Thorofare, NJ, 1986

Bassett FH III: Quoted in Whipple TL: The role of exogenous materials in arthroscopic management of cruciate-deficient knees. p 148. In McGinty JB (ed); Arthroscopic Surgery Update. Aspen Sytems, Rockville, MD, 1985

Battle WH: A case after open section of the knee joint for irreducible traumatic dislocation. Clin Soc London Trans 33:232, 1900

Bischer: Die binnenverletzangen des kneiegelenkes. Schweiz Med Wochensehr, 1929

Bolton CW: Three years of clinical experience with the Gore-Tex cruciate ligament prosthesis. Prosthetic Ligament Reconstruction of the Knee, 3rd Annual Symposium, Scottsdale, AZ, 1986

Bolton CW, Bruchman WC: The Gore-Tex expanded polytetrafluoroethylene prosthetic ligament. An in-vitro and in-vivo evaluation. Clin Orthop 196:202-213, 1985

Butler DL, Grood ES, Noyes FR, Todd AN: On the interpretation of our anterior cruciate ligament data. Clin Orthop 196:26-34, 1985

Cloes L, Neugebauer R: In-vivo and in-vitro investigation of the long-term behavior and fatigue strength of carbon fiber ligament replacement. Clin Orthop 196:99-111, 1985

Collins HR: The Gore-Tex artificial anterior cruciate ligament. Results. Prosthetic Ligament Reconstruction of the Knee, 3rd Annual Symposium, Scottsdale, AZ, 1986

Fujikawa K: Clinical studies of the Leeds-Keio artificial ligament. Prosthetic Ligament Reconstruction of the Knee, 3rd Annual Symposium, Scottsdale, AZ, 1986

Grood CS, Noyes FR: Cruciate ligament prosthesis: strength, creep and fatigue properties. J Bone Joint Surg 58A:1083-1088, 1976

Hey Groves EW: Operation for the repair of the crucial ligaments. Lancet 2:674, 1917

Hoffman H: Development and evaluation of a synthetic ligament prosthesis. Prosthetic Ligament Reconstruction of the Knee, 3rd Annual Symposium, Scottsdale, AZ, 1986

James SL, Woods GW, Homsy CA et al: Cruciate ligament stents in reconstruction of the unstable knee. A preliminary report. Clin Orthop 143:90-96, 1979

Jensen JE, Slocum DB, Larson RL et al: Reconstruction procedures for anterior cruciate ligament insufficiency: a computer analysis of clinical results. Am J Sports Med 11:240-248, 1983

Kellam JF, Larson RL, James SL et al: Proplastic cruciate stents in reconstruction of the unstable knee. Presented at the American Academy of Orthopaedic Surgeons 50th Annual Meeting, Anaheim, CA, 1983

Kennedy JC: Application of prosthetics to anterior cruciate ligament reconstruction and repair. Clin Orthop 1972:125-128, 1983

Kennedy JC, Hawkins RJ, Wallis RB, Danylchuk KD: Tension studies of the human knee ligaments. J Bone Joint Surg 58A:350-355, 1976

Markolf KL, Kochan K, Amstutz HC: Measurement of knee stiffness and laxity in patients with documented absence of the anterior cruciate ligament. J Bone Joint Surg 66A:242–253, 1984

McPherson GK, Mendenhall HV, Gibbons DF et al: Experimental mechanical and histologic evaluation of the Kennedy ligament augmentation device. Clin Orthop 196:186–195, 1985

Nikolaou PK, Seaber AV, Bassett FH: Experimental anterior cruciate ligament transplantation. Presented at American Orthopaedic Society for Sports Medicine, New Orleans, 1986

Noyes FR, Grood ES: Strength of the anterior cruciate ligament in humans and Rhesus monkeys. Age and species-related changes. J Bone Joint Surg 58A:1074–1082, 1976

Park JP, Grana WA, Chitwood JS: A high strength dacron augmentation for cruciate ligament reconstruction. A two-year canine study. Clin Orthop 196:175–185, 1985

Robson AWM: Ruptured crucial ligaments and their repair by operation. Ann Surg 37:716, 1903

Rojas F, Teitge RA: Anterior cruciate ligament reconstruction using bovine xenograft prosthesis. Presented at American Orthopaedic Society for Sports Medicine, Atlanta, 1984

Roth JH: Polypropylene braid augmented and nonaugmented intra-articular anterior cruciate ligament reconstruction. Prosthetic Ligament Reconstruction of the Knee, 3rd Annual Symposium, Scottsdale, AZ, 1986

Seedhom BB: The Leeds-Keio ligament. Concepts and mechanical aspects of the device. Prosthetic Ligament Reconstruction of the Knee, 3rd Annual Symposium, Scottsdale, AZ, 1986

Shino K, Hirose H, Kimura T et al: Anterior cruciate ligament reconstruction using free tendon allograft. Presented at American Academy of Orthopaedic Surgeons, 51st Annual Meeting, San Francisco, 1984

Snook GA: A short history of the anterior cruciate ligament and the treatment of tears. Clin Orthop 172:11, 1983

Strum GM, Larson RL: Clinical experience and early results of carbon fiber augmentation of anterior cruciate reconstruction of the knee. Clin Orthop 196:124–138, 1985

Tremblay GR, Laurin CA, Drovin G: The challenge of prosthetic cruciate ligament replacement. Clin Orthop 147:88–92, 1980

Whipple TL: The role of exogenous materials in arthroscopic management of cruciate-deficient knees. p. 139. In McGinty JB (ed): Arthroscopic Surgery Update. Aspen Systems Corp., Rockville, MD, 1985

Whipple TL: Arthroscopic cruciate reconstructions: xenograft anterior cruciate ligament. Prosthetic Ligament Reconstruction of the Knee, 3rd Annual Symposium, Scottsdale, AZ, 1986

30

Prosthetic Replacement of the Cruciate Ligaments with Expanded Polytetrafluoroethylene

WILLIAM C. BRUCHMAN
JAMES R. BAIN
C. WILLIAM BOLTON

The numerous and varied attempts to develop cruciate ligament replacements can be reduced to two categories: those requiring intraarticular healing for long-term strength and true prostheses.

The first category includes:

Repairs effected with autologous or homologous tissues

Degradable devices intended to elicit the formation of a new ligament

Augmentation devices that provide protection or added length and a practical means of surgical fixation to transplanted host tissues

With each of these options, the strength of the reconstruction ultimately depends on the viability and mechanical properties of the transplanted or "regenerated" host tissues. Autologous tissue transplants undergo early degeneration when placed in the synovial environment. Butler et al.[4] have shown that patellar tendon grafts in primates fall to 15 percent of their original strength within 6 weeks after surgery. Strength of the implant thus depends upon subsequent healing. Kennedy et al.[13] suggested that there is a minimal likelihood of regaining the full original strength.

Augmentation devices implanted in conjunction with autologous tissue grafts are useful surgical aids, but these do not address the fundamental shortcomings of autologous repair that have manifested themselves in variable and sometimes disappointing clinical results. Likewise, the vagaries of healing in the synovial environment and other factors have thwarted attempts to regenerate human cruciates with degradable implants.[19]

We agree that the ideal solution to the problem would be to stimulate the regrowth of a cruciate ligament so that the regenerated tissue duplicates the strength, stiffness, and functional architecture of the original structure. Further, this should be done in conjunction with some means of providing immediate reconstruction strength so that the patient can be spared the degenerative sequelae of immobilization. In our opinion, this goal is not met by any device or reconstructive method now in use in humans, nor is it likely to be attained through technologies available in the near future.

We chose to pursue the development of a true prosthesis rather than rely on the inconsistencies of intraarticular healing for reconstruction strength. Early attempts at prosthetic replacement of the anterior and posterior cruciate ligaments (ACL and PCL) met with very limited clinical success because the devices had inadequate resistance to tensile loads or flexural fatigue.[1,9,12,20] This experience stimulated research leading to a clearer definition of the mechanical properties of the human cruciates and, therefore, the mechanical requirements for a successful polymer prosthesis.[7,9] With this knowledge of requisite properties, we developed mechanical tests that assess the longevity of cruciate prostheses under simulated in vivo conditions.[2]

MATERIAL AND DESIGN CRITERIA

Throughout our development work our goals were to provide a prosthesis that would:

Allow a relatively simple and atraumatic method of insertion.

Provide immediate strength similar to that of the natural cruciate. Strength of this degree allows immediate mobility and weightbearing, avoiding the atrophy, adhesions, and other undesirable effects of cast immobilization.

Be compatible with the tissues of the knee, particularly the sensitive yet hostile synovial environment.

Have sufficient porosity along the intraosseous segments to allow eventual fixation through the growth of bone and other tissues into the device, freeing the system from long-term reliance on sutures, metallic fixtures, or other artificial attachments that might elongate, loosen, or break.

Possess the mechanical properties necessary to provide an acceptable lifetime under the repetitive tensile and flexural loads imposed during normal activity.

POLYTETRAFLUOROETHYLENE AS A BIOMATERIAL

We chose to construct our cruciate prostheses from polytetrafluoroethylene (PTFE) because of its compatibility with the hard and soft tissues of the knee. This polymer is essentially inert to chemical reaction. The inertness results from its molecular configuration of repeating units of $-CF_2$. Molecular weights range as high as 1×10^7. Carbon atoms form the "backbone" of the molecule, with a protective, strongly bonded outer sheath of fluorine atoms. The strong covalent bonds that result from affinity of the highly electronegative fluorine atoms for the carbon atoms create a material that resists chemical reaction under physiologic conditions. Numerous investigations[3,11] have illustrated the compatibility of this polymer with mammalian tissues.

The chemical and physical stability of PTFE has led to its wide use as an implant in many surgical disciplines, but orthopaedic applications have been limited. Reluctance to implant PTFE in the musculoskeletal system stems largely from tragic early experiences with fluoropolymers in hip and knee arthroplasties. The late Sir John Charnley, a pioneer in low-friction arthroplasty, constructed the acetabular component of his early total hips from PTFE. The primary reason for this choice was the low coefficient of friction of the polymer. Between 1958 and 1961, approximately 300 patients received acetabular prostheses made of PTFE or composites of PTFE and other materials.[5]

Early results were promising, but compression and shear of the stainless steel femoral component against the PTFE socket in this weight-bearing application soon caused the liberation of massive quantities of large ($>100 \mu m$) PTFE particles into the joint. The consequence of this massive infusion was a severe foreign body response with extensive tissue necrosis.[6] The functional results were disappointing, and the revision rate was high.[5]

Similar results were obtained by other investigators in the knee and hip in humans[16,21] and experimental animals.[14]

In retrospect, the use of PTFE in these applications was clearly inappropriate. In weight-bearing prostheses, such as knee and hip arthroplasties, the material has a poor resistance to repetitive shear under compression. The resultant large sizes and quantities of wear particles overwhelmed the body's defenses against intrasynovial particles, resulting in painful, persistent synovitis characterized by a widespread caseating necrosis of the synovial surfaces. Although the chemical inertness of this polymer is well established, massive intrasynovial infusions of particles can cause a morphologically mediated histiocytic/giant cell granulation. In the present cruciate application the material is not placed under compressive loads such as those responsible for generating the massive doses of wear particles observed in the early arthroplasty experiences.

We have determined that small amounts of particles can be generated if the device is inadvertently placed so that it passes over a sharp edge of bone or impingement occurs in the femoral intercondylar notch in ACL replacement. These conditions promote failure of the device. Even if all strands of the device rupture, the total mass of particles liberated is small, no more than a few milligrams.

We have now had the opportunity to examine several devices that went to partial or complete failure (discussed further under Clinical Results) and associated synovial biopsies. Typically, these small particles ($<30\ \mu$m) are found in the synovial tissue immediately adjacent to broken strands. Histologic examination shows microscopic foci of chronic histiocytic inflammation associated with embedded particles, characterized by macrophage accumulation, giant cell formation, and focal fibrosis. No necrosis has been observed nor have patients presented with synovitis caused by particles.

EXPANDED PTFE

The Gore-Tex (Gore-Tex is a trademark of W. L. Gore & Associates, Inc.) cruciate ligament prosthesis is constructed from a unique porous form of PTFE produced through a mechanical stretching process. This material has been used as a vascular graft in nearly one million patients since 1975. Other medical applications of this material include tissue repair patches and sutures. Previous studies have documented the biocompatibility and potential for healthy interstitial growth of host tissue into the pores of the material.[2]

The stretching process used to produce the prosthetic ligament material provides a unique combination of properties: high strength and a porous microstructure allowing direct attachment and ingrowth of connective tissue, including bone. Conventional, full-density forms of PTFE normally exhibit an ultimate strength less than 24 MPa. The expanded PTFE from which the cruciate prosthesis is constructed has a tensile strength more than 20 times as great, owing to a highly oriented molecular configuration.

The microstructure produced through this pro-

Fig. 30-1. Scanning electron micrograph of the expanded PTFE material. In this view, solid "nodes" of PTFE appear black, and the "fibrils" appear white (original magnification $\times$ 1,000).

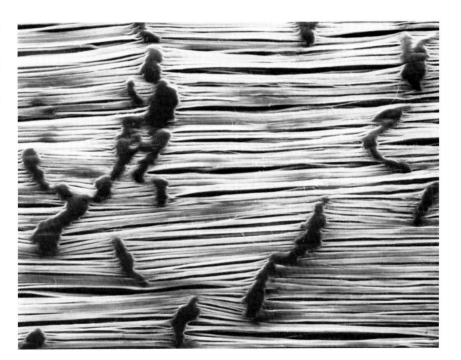

cess (Fig. 30-1) consists of solid PTFE segments (termed "nodes") connected by thin, flexible filaments several molecules in diameter (termed "fibrils"). The distance between nodes averages 60 μm or more. The three-dimensional, radially oriented pathways between nodes form the interstitial spaces into which host tissue can grow. These void spaces constitute more than 75 percent of the volume of the strand.

A critical requirement for materials intended to replace the cruciate ligaments is resistance to fatigue. Expanded PTFE is unique in its absence of internal stresses induced during bending that can lead to fatigue-related material changes in other polymers. In most polymers, bending induces compressive stresses on one side of the structure being bent and tensile stresses on the other. The arrangement of longitudinally oriented, parallel fibrils in expanded PTFE, however, produces slack in one side of the expanded PTFE strand while the other side remains under tension. Under pure bending conditions this characteristic provides an essentially unlimited fatigue life.

STRUCTURAL PROPERTIES OF THE DEVICE

The Gore-Tex cruciate ligament prosthesis is constructed from a single long strand of the expanded PTFE material described above. The strand is nominally 0.6 mm in diameter. It is wound into loops, with eyelets formed at each end of the looped bundle of strands. The air is removed from the strand segments that compose the eyelets through compression and heat. The finished device comprises some 190 strands connecting the two eyelets that provide the means of initial fixation (Fig. 30-2). The 190-odd strands are braided in three bundles to provide a more uniform loading during bending.

During manufacture each device is tested to ensure a minimum ultimate tensile strength of 4448 N. This specification for strength was derived from accelerated mechanical testing. As previously reported, we developed a cyclic creep test that simulates the tensile loads imposed on the human ACL.[2] Previous authors have estimated these in vivo loads.[7,10,15,17,18] For the purposes of these tests, we

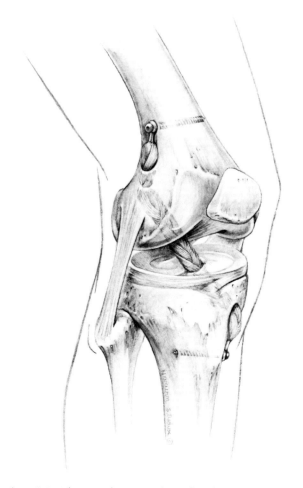

Fig. 30-2. The prosthesis implanted in the ACL position, routed "over-the-top" of the posterior intercondylar fossa of the femur. (Copyright 1985 by Harwin Studios, Portland, Oregon, used with permission.)

assumed 285 N and 405 N to be representative mean physiologic loads. After the equivalent of 8.5 years of testing (3.4×10^7 cycles), elongation of the prosthesis was less than 4 percent under either condition. By using test loads much greater than physiologic, we were able to derive relationships predicting the elongation that occurs over longer periods as well. Perhaps the best illustration of the creep properties of the prosthesis is the observation that the ACL in most young humans would fail with a single application of a load of 2,000 N.[18] The prosthesis, however, requires almost 1,000 of these loads to produce a 10 percent elongation. This degree of strength is necessary to prevent unacceptable elongation of the prostheses through creep.

During a flexion cycle from 0° to 90°, the prosthesis must bend approximately 30° at the tibial entry site. Since this occurs on the order of 4.2×10^6 times per year for the active individual,[7] it was necessary to test the device under these conditions. Using an apparatus that simulates this bending under load,[2] testing was conducted to the equivalent of 20 years (8.4×10^7 cycles). This test essentially confirmed the resistance of the material to bending fatigue. A 25 percent reduction in tensile strength was noted at the conclusion of testing. This was related to a localized creep of the material around the 1.5 mm radius used to simulate the tibial entry tunnel edge, and not to fatigue per se.

DEVICE FIXATION

We believe that one of the principal advantages afforded by the use of a true prosthesis is the elimination of the need for rigid postoperative immobilization. To achieve this goal a prosthesis must have an initial fixation strength similar to that of the original cruciate. Thus, the device was designed to provide integral eyelets at each end. These provide for initial fixation through bicortical bone screws (Fig. 30-2). Animal testing[2] has shown that this means of fixation provides an initial strength similar to that of the natural ACL.

Permanent fixation of the device is achieved through tissue healing in the bone tunnels around and into the microstructure of the individual strands. Testing in sheep[2] has shown that this healing provides a fixation strength (with the tibial fixation screw removed) of approximately 1380 N at 10 mm total system elongation 7 months postoperatively. Since the bone tunnels can be substantially longer in humans, we believe that greater attachment strengths are possible in humans.

CLINICAL TRIALS AND RESULTS

The data considered here were provided by 35 surgeons from 21 institutions. Clinical use of the prosthesis for anterior cruciate replacement was initi-

ated in October 1982. This was extended to use in the PCL position in July 1984. As of August, 1985, 963 patients have received the prosthesis in the United States:

ACL only	921
PCL only	32
combined ACL and PCL	10

Prior to the use of the prosthesis, these patients had undergone an average of 1.2 previous surgical procedures. The mean time from onset of ACL insufficiency to prosthetic reconstruction was 5 years; 6.5 percent had been injured 1 month or less prior to surgery. Most of the original injuries (75 percent) occurred during sports activity (primarily football, basketball, and skiing). The mean patient age was 27 years, and 70 percent of the patients were male.

Concomitant extraarticular reconstructions were performed in 25 percent of the patients. Forty percent of the ACL grafts were inserted under arthroscopic control. Only 5 percent of the patients required rigid immobilization. By the third postoperative month, 97 percent reported that they were able to engage to some degree in their desired daily activities, and 91 percent considered the knee to be improved compared to the preoperative condition. At 1 year after surgery 84 percent were engaged in unrestricted activities. No reduction in mean thigh girth measurements or range of motion was present at intervals greater than 3 months postoperatively.

Follow-up of 1 year or more was available for 326 patients with ACL grafts (mean follow-up of 15 months). Objective stability results for these patients are illustrated in Figure 30-3. At the longest follow-up examination on record, 96 percent of these patients maintained a "0" or "1" score on the pivot shift test, and 88 percent maintained a similar score on the Lachman test.

Twenty-four of the 963 total grafts (2.5%) have been removed:

6 due to infection
2 due to persistent inflammatory effusion
10 due to partial or complete mechanical failure
6 due to surgical misplacement resulting in laxity

Removal rates were evaluated with actuarial methods that account for loss to follow-up.[8] Life

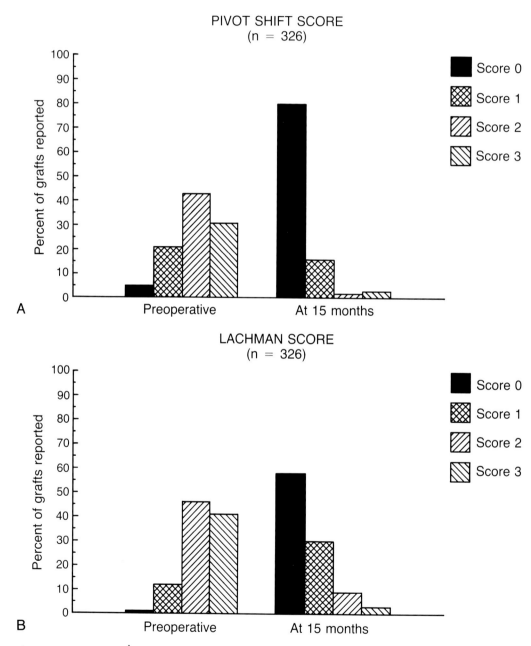

Fig. 30-3. Preoperative and postoperative pivot shift test **(A)** and Lachman test **(B)** scores in a selected group of 326 ACL patients with follow-up of 1 year or more.

table analysis predicts that 94.9 percent of grafts will remain in situ at 28.5 months after surgery (Fig. 30-4).

In the 10 grafts that failed, rupture was associated with notch impingement or a sharp edge in the graft course such as osteophytes or inadequately chamfered drill hole edges. The remaining 14 grafts were removed intact. Of the 16 patients who had devices removed for failure or instability, 12 received a replacement Gore-Tex ligament.

Other complications have not required graft removal:

Inflammatory effusion	34
Instability	15
Screw tightening/removal	13
Infection	2
Femoral supracondylar fracture	2
Intraoperative vein laceration	1

The major source of complications in this category is inflammatory effusions. This condition is characterized by a swollen knee with a cloudy aspirate. Elevated leukocyte counts are often present, and cultures of the aspirate are negative. In some cases the effusion can be clearly ascribed to repeated trauma or overexertion early in the postoperative period. In other cases, however, the cause is obscure. The biologic inertness of PTFE makes it highly unlikely that these effusions represent an immunologic or allergic reaction to the material. No clear correlation is present between the occurrence of effusions and particles that are potentially generated by strand breakage. Most patients have been successfully treated with aspiration, rest, and nonsteroidal anti-inflammatory drugs.

Removal of the devices described above afforded the opportunity for histologic examination of human specimens. We were particularly interested in the condition of the intraosseous segments and whether the healing rate along these segments in humans is similar to that seen in experimental animals.[2]

Ingrowth along the bone tunnels was demonstrated by the tenacity with which the prosthesis adhered to the host tissues in most cases in which revision or removal was attempted. Microscopic examination of these specimens revealed osseous tis-

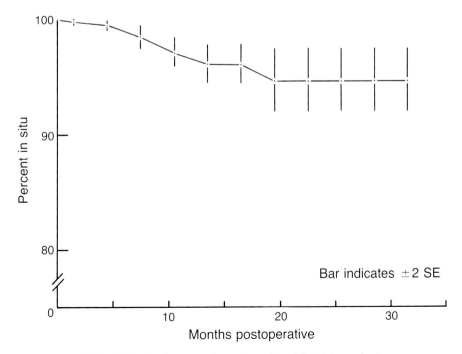

Fig. 30-4. Graft removal rate based on life table analysis.

sue between the strands and within the interstices of the individual strands.

Several specific observations are noteworthy. First, the individual variation in the rate at which tissue invades the graft appears to be greater in humans than in sheep. Second, our observations suggest that the mean rate of bone growth into the device is somewhat slower in humans than in sheep. These are tentative conclusions, since factors other than species differences could account for these observations. Furthermore, these general statements are based on a limited number of human samples, which are often mutilated during removal. *We have noted that thermal necrosis of the bone tunnels through the use of inappropriate drill speeds or dull bits can significantly retard the quality and rate of healing.* In view of these observations, we now recommend that the bone screws used for initial fixation not be removed before 1 year. In those knees in which screws have required removal, no loosening of the device has been noted. With the exceptions noted above, the histologic findings in humans have resembled those in experimental animals.

CONCLUSIONS

The results obtained using this prosthesis in humans generally confirm the predictions of performance based on preclinical studies in laboratory animals and mechanical simulators. In the absence of technical problems, stability has been maintained in patients now in their third postoperative year. The major advantage of the use of this prosthesis is immediate stability, allowing early mobilization and early return to the activities of daily living. This reduces or eliminates the muscular atrophy, articular surface degeneration, and adhesion formation that result from rigid immobilization. Further advantages are its compatibility with the tissues of the knee and its potential for long-term fixation through tissue ingrowth.

The 10 failed grafts illustrate the sensitivity of the prosthesis to implant technique. In ACL implants, generous "notchplasties" are often required to prevent bony impingement on the prosthesis. The eventual resorption of soft tissue trapped beneath the device by improper routing through the poste-

rior capsule can result in increased laxity. All sharp edges must be thoroughly smoothed. Meticulous attention must also be directed toward bone tunnel orientation to minimize stress concentrations. If technical problems such as these arise, the resulting complications generally appear in the first postoperative year.

The early results of the clinical trial of this ligament prosthesis are encouraging. Longevity of the device under the wide variety of loading conditions in the patient population remains to be determined by continuing clinical study.

REFERENCES

1. Beauchamp P, Laurin CA, Bailon J-P: Étude des propriétés méchaniques des ligaments croisés en vue de leur remplacement prothétique. Rev Chirurg Orthop 65:197–207, 1979

2. Bolton CW, Bruchman WC: The GORE-TEX™ expanded polytetrafluoroethylene prosthetic ligament: an *in vitro* and *in vivo* evaluation. Clin Orthop 196:202–213, 1985

3. Boyce B: Physical characteristics of expanded polytetrafluoroethylene grafts. pp. 553–561 In Stanley JC (ed); Biologic and Synthetic Vascular Prostheses. Grune and Stratton, New York, 1982

4. Butler DL, Noyes FR, Grood ES et al: The effects of vascularity on the mechanical properties of primate anterior cruciate ligament replacements. Transactions 29th Annual Meeting Orthopaedic Research Society 8:93, 1983

5. Charnley J: Low-Friction Arthroplasty of the Hip: Theory and Practice. Springer-Verlag, New York, 1979

6. Charnley J, Cupic Z: The nine and ten year results of the low-friction arthroplasty of the hip. Clin Orthop 95:9–25, 1973

7. Chen EH, Black J: Materials design analysis of the prosthetic anterior cruciate ligament. J Biomed Materials Res 14:567–586, 1980

8. Colton T: Statistics in Medicine. Little, Brown, Boston, 1974

9. Grood ES, Noyes FR: Cruciate ligament prosthesis: strength, creep and fatigue properties. J Bone Joint Surg 58A:1083–1088, 1976

10. Henning CE, Lynch MA, Glick KR: An in vivo strain gage study of elongation of the anterior cruciate ligament. Am J Sports Med 13:22–26, 1985

11. Homsy CA: Biocompatibility of perfluorinated poly-

mers and composites of these polymers. p. 59. In Williams DF (ed); Biocompatibility of Clinical Implant Materials, Vol II. CRC Press, Boca Raton, FL, 1981

12. James SL, Woods GW, Homsy CA et al: Cruciate ligament stents in reconstruction of the unstable knee: a preliminary report. Clin Orthop 143:90–96, 1979

13. Kennedy JC, Roth JH, Mendenhall HV, Sanford JB: Presidential address: intraarticular replacement in the anterior cruciate ligament-deficient knee. Am J Sports Med 8:1–8, 1980

14. Leidholt JD, Gorman HA: Teflon hip prostheses in dogs. J Bone Joint Surg 47A:1414–1420, 1965

15. McLeod PC, Kettelcamp DB, Srinivasan V, Henderson OL: Measurement of repetitive activities of the knee. J Biomech 8:369–373, 1975

16. Meachim G, Pedley RB: The tissue response at implant sites. p. 107. In Williams DF (ed); Fundamental Aspects of Biocompatibility, Vol I. CRC Press, Boca Raton, FL, 1981

17. Noyes FR, Butler DL, Grood ES et al: Biomechanical analysis of human ligament grafts used in knee-ligament repairs and reconstructions. J Bone Joint Surg 66A:344–352, 1984

18. Noyes FR, Grood ES: The strength of the anterior cruciate ligament in humans and in rhesus monkeys: age-related and species-related changes. J Bone Joint Surg 58A:1074–1082, 1976

19. Rushton N, Dandy DJ, Naylor CPE: The clinical arthroscopic and histological findings after replacement of the anterior cruciate ligament with carbon-fibre. J Bone Joint Surg 65B:308–309, 1983

20. Scharling M: Replacement of the anterior cruciate ligament with a polyethylene prosthetic ligament. Acta Orthop Scand 52:575–578, 1981

21. Weber BG: Die Rotations-Totalendoprothese des Hüftgelenkes. Z Orthop 107:304–315, 1970

31

Ligament Repair and Reconstruction with an Absorbable Polymer-Coated Carbon Fiber Stent

HAROLD ALEXANDER
ANDREW B. WEISS
JOHN R. PARSONS

Two avenues of research have dominated ligament replacement. The first is a search for an adequately designed permanent prosthetic replacement. Such a replacement must be constructed of a biocompatible material. It must have sufficient mechanical strength with some promise of surviving the millions of fatigue cycles associated with normal ligament use. The second is an avenue of research that utilizes a scaffold replacement approach that allows the ingrowth of new collagenous tissue. This latter technique provides only temporary mechanical integrity until the new tissue can assume the mechanical function. Working along these lines, we found composites of filamentous carbon fiber and absorbable polymers to be a new and useful class of orthopaedic biomaterials. Ribbonlike composite structures have been utilized in the repair and replacement of ligaments.

Perhaps no other material in the history of orthopaedic implants has been surrounded with such controversy as carbon fiber. The earliest use of carbon fiber for ligament repair dates to the work of Jenkins et al.[20,21] in Wales and Wolter et al.[46] in West Germany. Since that time, more than 112 papers have been published on this subject. Of those, 87 have reported positively on its use, 13 have pub-

lished negative reports, and 12 have reported both positive and negative findings.

There are many explanations for the seemingly obvious contradiction in the literature on this subject. However, the overriding explanation is the differences in the materials and devices used by the various investigators. The original work of Jenkins and that of other investigators in the United Kingdom was performed with an extremely brittle fiber that had been coated with a toxic epoxy. Although every effort was made to remove the epoxy, complete removal is impossible. Therefore, the negative reports of Dandy et al.,[14] Amis et al.,[5] and Forster and Shuttleworth[17] are directly attributable to the use of this uncovered, brittle, potentially toxic implant material within the synovial joint. Investigators in West Germany[12,27-29] have used a woven structure of a different carbon fiber that also had been coated with epoxy. They also tried pyrolytic carbon coating to improve the tissue response.[46] The fragmentation of the coating resulted in a worse response. They then obtained fiber that had never been epoxy-coated and coated their implant with collagen. This produced a transient foreign body response, but superior long-term results.

Investigators in South Africa have used yet a different carbon fiber in a twisted form coated with animal collagen.[39,40] This material has also been shown to elicit a foreign body response but provides for adequate tissue ingrowth. Recently, a French group has developed yet another implant of carbon fibers covered with a polyglycolic acid–polylactic acid polymer film.[8] We have drawn upon the successes and the failures of many of these other investigators. We produced a carbon-fiber-based ligament repair and reconstruction material that clinical trials have shown is a useful addition to the armamentarium of the knee surgeon.

Even though these various carbon fiber-based implants have some significant differences, a common feature of all the materials is that filamentous carbon implants act as scaffolds for the development of new fibrous tissue. Carbon fiber succeeds as a scaffolding material for a number of reasons. It provides mechanical strength upon implantation, allowing early return of function. The material is extremely compatible, permitting the ingrowth of new aligned fibrous tissue. Also, the carbon fiber may degrade mechanically as the new tissue matures, allowing for the gradual transfer of load to the regrown tissue structure.

Forster et al.[16] and Jenkins et al.[20,21] used spun carbon fiber tows as replacements for the anterior cruciate ligament (ACL) and medial collateral ligament (MCL) in sheep. They have since used this raw uncoated carbon in humans for various ligament reconstructions[22] including the cruciate ligaments of the knee. Similarly, Wolter et al.,[46] Claes et al.,[12] and Kinzl et al.,[24] used thick braided tows of carbon to replace MCLs in sheep and extraarticular knee and ankle ligaments in humans.[10] In the work of these groups,[10,12,16,20–22,24,46] as well as that reported by Dandy et al.[14] and Rushton et al.[37] replacing ACLs, raw carbon fiber partially fragmented during and immediately after the operative procedure. This permitted carbon to migrate from the implant site before the new fibrous tissue could encapsulate it. Carbon fragments were found in the lymph nodes of the animals and are most likely in the nodes of the humans into whom the uncoated carbon was implanted. Although not shown to be detrimental in any way, spread of carbon fiber fragments to nearby lymph nodes is clearly undesirable.

In this chapter we describe our program of re-search in which we addressed the problem of the mechanical degradation of the brittle filamentous carbon during its implantation and the early phases of tissue growth. This premature mechanical degradation, and the resulting migration of carbon fragments from the implant site, was largely eliminated by using a coating of polylactic acid polymer (PLA) or a copolymer of PLA and poly-ϵ-caprolactone (copolymer). The coated implant has greatly improved handling characteristics compared to raw carbon fiber. After implantation, the polymer slowly degrades, exposing the fibers to the fibroblast cells. The implant, in a ribbonlike configuration, was used in a variety of animal models. In these studies, the implant material was successful as a scaffold for the development of new soft tissue. The implants allowed early resumption of activity and eventual growth of new structures that were histologically and mechanically similar to the natural structures.

The high initial strength, rapid ingrowth, and benign tissue reaction of the composite suggested that this new material might be useful in the treatment of ligament injuries in humans. Consequently, human clinical trials were initiated. As part of a multicenter trial sanctioned by the Food and Drug Administration (FDA), over 800 patients have had implant surgery for the repair of knee ligaments, as well as extensor mechanisms, Achilles tendons, shoulder rotator cuffs, and other soft tissue problems. By 1986, some patients had been evaluated for up to 3 years, and more than 200 patients have been followed up for 2 years. These results have been encouraging. Consequently, FDA approval has been sought and investigators in France, West Germany, Japan, Australia, and the United Kingdom are now using this implant.

LIGAMENT REPLACEMENT MATERIAL

Absorbable polymer–filamentous carbon tissue scaffolding ribbons are produced by coating uniaxial filamentous carbon with either PLA or copolymer. The individual carbon fiber tows typically contain 10,000 fibers, 6 to 10 μm in diameter. The fibers are prepared by pyrolizing a polyacrylonitrile (PAN) fiber tow in an inert atmosphere at approximately 3,000°C. The resulting material is almost pure elemental carbon with mechanical strength and rigidity greater than steel. It has a modulus of over 200 GPa and an ultimate tensile strength of approximately 2.5 GPa.

The polylactic acid polymer is produced from L(−)lactide. This cyclic diester, the lactide of lactic acid, polymerizes by an ionic ring-opening addition mechanism to a high polymer that can be cast into films, spun into fibers, or extruded into rods similarly to the industrial polyesters, such as Dacron. It is a thermoplastic and can be dissolved readily in a number of solvents. Poly-ε-caprolactone alone is similar in character. However, the copolymer of PLA and poly-ε-caprolactone is elastomeric. As such, it is tough and flexible.

Fabrication of coated fiber tows is accomplished by first preparing PLA or copolymer solution. The fibers are coated with the polymer by solution dipping or spraying. For attachment to soft tissues, suture needles are attached to the ends of the fiber tows. The device is then sterilized by gamma irradiation.

The biocompatibility of carbon fiber, polylactic acid, and polycaprolactone has previously been demonstrated. Finely divided carbon particles have been shown to be well tolerated; they do not cause formation of foreign body giant cells in the synovial lining of joints, nor do they produce cytotoxic effects.[19] Studies of tissue tolerance of carbon materials by Christel et al.[11] indicated that carbon materials are well accepted by connective tissues. Filamentous carbon has been used as a component of implants in humans. Studies in rabbits and mice indicated good short- and long-term biocompatibility of this material. The question of foreign body or physically induced carcinogenicity was addressed in carbon fiber connective tissue implant studies conducted by Tayton et al.[42] and Claes (L. Claes, personal communication, 1982). We studied 205 Sprague-Dawley rats and ascertained the long-term effects of carbon fiber resident in the bone, soft tissue, and vital organs. The study lasted 2 years, the approximate life span of a rat. Gross examination at autopsy and microhistologic study of organs revealed tumors in both control and experimental animals with similar occurrence rates. The various lesions observed were consistent with the tumor types seen commonly in aging rats. To date, all these research groups have found no abnormal tumor formation attributable to carbon fiber.

The short and long-term response to polylactic acid was studied by Cutright and Hunsuck,[13] Brady et al.,[9] and Kulkarni et al.[25] Polylactic acid is a biocompatible material that elicits little immunologic response, probably due to the absence of peptide linkages. It biodegrades by undergoing hydrolytic deesterification to lactic acid, a normal metabolic intermediate. The compatibility of poly-ε-caprolactone has been studied by a number of researchers.[33,36] The polymer and its degradation product, hydroxycaporic acid, are compatible. Biologic response to and degradation of PLA/polycaprolactone copolymers were investigated by Schindler et al.[38]

PRECLINICAL TESTING

Because this is a new device produced from new materials without extensive clinical experience, extensive in vitro and in vivo biocompatibility and bench testing were necessary. The laboratory testing performed over the 8 years during which the device was developed are presented in Table 31-1.

The details of much of the in vitro evaluation are beyond the scope of this paper. However, the cell culture, cell–fiber interactions results are presented to provide an understanding of the basis of the scaffold nature of the device.

Table 31-1. Laboratory Testing

Implant mechanical properties
Cell culture, cell–fiber interactions
Carbon fiber ash weight analysis
Polymer ash weight analysis
Trace element analysis
Sterilization polymer degradation
Needle attachment strength
Pyrogenicity
Tissue culture cytotoxicity
Quantitative Ames test
Extract cell transformation
Direct contact cell transformation

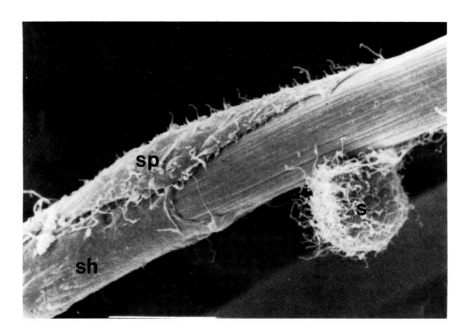

Fig. 31-1. Scanning electron micrograph of a neonatal rat tendon fibroblast cell culture on carbon filaments showing a spherical cell *(s)*, a spindle cell *(sp)*, and a sheath cell *(sh)* (bar = 10 μm).

Ricci et al.[35] isolated rat tendon fibroblasts from the hind feet of 14-day old Sprague–Dawley rats. The tendon explants were placed on carbon, Dacron, polyethylene, and nylon fibers in Dulbecco's modified Eagle's medium containing 10 percent fetal calf serum and 1 percent penicillin–streptomycin. After 5 to 7 days in culture, the cells were fixed and examined by scanning electron microscopy. The orientation of the cells grown on different substrates was controlled by the surface characteristics of the substrate. On smooth substrates, such as the polymer fibers, the cells oriented randomly. On small (7 to 15 μm) striated fibers, such as the carbon fibers used in the ligament implant, the cells aligned parallel to the longitudinal surface striations. Also, cells grown on the striated surfaces lacked the ruffling membrane common to cells grown on smooth surfaces. Figure 31-1 is a scanning electron micrograph demonstrating the types of cells commonly seen on carbon filaments in this study. Spherical cells are those undergoing cell division. Spindle and sheath cells were those most often seen. These cells migrated along the fibers, orienting themselves parallel to the fibers. They appeared to be aggressively attached to the fibers by filopodia-like structures. In vivo, after attaching to the fibers, the cells appear to extrude new collagen parallel to the fibers, producing a new fibrous tissue. This has been demonstrated in numerous animal[1,6] and human[43] specimens.

The device has also been subjected to extensive animal testing before its clinical use. It has been preclinically tested for biocompatibility and in-use simulation studies in animals. Since the function of ligaments and tendons is to transfer mechanical load, a major evaluation method is to measure the mechanical properties of the replaced structure and compare them with those of the original struc-

Table 31-2. Animal Testing

Systemic injection toxicity
Intracutaneous reactivity
Acute intramuscular tissue toxicity
Long-term rat biocompatibility
C-fiber debris in the synovial joint[31]
Rabbit patella tendon
Canine patella tendon[1]
Rabbit Achilles tendon[5,30]
Canine medial collateral ligament[6]
Canine anterior cruciate ligament[2]
Sheep anterior cruciate ligament

ture. The implant must also be compatible with the host tissue and not cause excessive adverse tissue response. Therefore, histologic evaluation is also of extreme importance. The animal testing performed with this device is listed in Table 31-2.

CLINICAL TESTING

After extensive preclinical testing, the implant system was placed in phase I clinical trials with one of the authors (ABW) as sole investigator for a 1-year period. In April, 1982, it was approved for phase II multicenter clinical trials. The trials are now in progress at 25 centers around the United States and Europe. The implant in clinical use is a double-armed uniaxial tow of 10,000 fibers coated with a copolymer of PLA and poly-ϵ-caprolactone. It is 1 m long, 0.5 cm wide, and has an ultimate tensile strength of approximately 425 N. The system had been used initially with soft tissue attachment only, using the locking-weave anastomosis shown in the animal studies. More recently, bone attachment has been accomplished through the use of a newly designed composite material attachment device (expandable fastener).

In an early report of the clinical results, Alexander et al.[4] discussed 30 surgical repairs of ligament and tendon injuries. These repairs included lateral and medial knee instability, Achilles tendon ruptures, extensor mechanism ruptures, and rotator cuffs. Seven months follow-up indicated that no complications associated with the implant had been noted. All patients showed improvement, with many demonstrating good to excellent stability and/or function.

In a later report[43] the results from 82 patients treated over a 27-month period for both acute (8 percent) and chronic (92 percent) knee ligament instabilities were presented. Preoperative and postoperative evaluation, consisting of questionnaires, physical examination, and isokinetic testing, revealed significant improvements in categories of stability, pain, function, and strength. Arthroscopic examination and histologic studies of retrieved specimens demonstrated well-vascularized reconstructions of the ACL with collagenous tissue ingrowth into the carbon–copolymer implants. Par-

sons et al.[32] reported results from 27 patients surgically treated for Achilles tendon rupture. Fourteen patients had at least 9 months of follow-up (average follow-up, 14.4 months) and had been objectively and subjectively evaluated on a temporal basis for return of function. Results were encouraging, with 90 percent return of function at 18 months.

Reports from the other clinical centers indicated early results either as good[34,41,45] or better[23] than previously used repairs. King and Bulstrode[23] reported that free carbon fibers had been spread in the joint as a result of using a technically incorrect implantation procedure. However, there did not appear to be any clinically deleterious consequences of this fiber spread, which corroborated the results of the animal study reported by Parsons et al.[31] Witvoet and Christel,[45] performing a combined reconstruction of the ACL and collateral structures, reported that the use of the implant allowed an earlier return to normal activity than would have been possible with a standard autogenous tissue repair.

Materials and Methods

The total patient population from the 25 clinical centers around the United States is 848 patients with up to 3 years of follow-up available. A recent compilation of the data from cases at the author's institu-

**Table 31-3. Surgical Cases
(At Least 12 Months Postoperative)**

Surgical Site	Number of Cases
Combined knees	87
Intraarticular knees	7
Extraarticular knees	12
Extensor mechanism	10
Total knees	5
Achilles tendons	9
Shoulder rotator cuffs	8
Ankle ligaments	2
Total shoulders	1
Shoulder separations	1
Triceps tendons	2
Elbow ligaments	1
Biceps tendons	1
Hand ligaments	4
Total	150

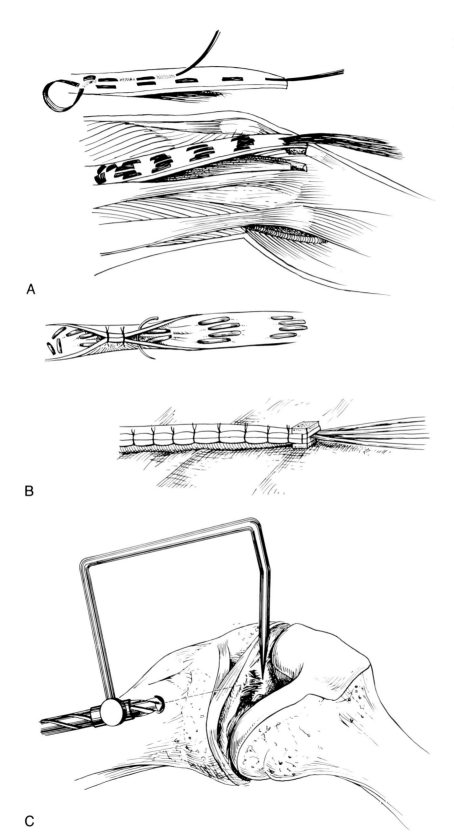

Fig. 31-2. (A) Carbon tow is woven into fascial strip from proximal to distal direction. **(B)** Fascial tube is formed with exposed carbon tows on the inside of the tube. **(C)** Tibial hole is made using the 3/8-inch drill bit and tibial guide. *(Figure continues.)*

B

C

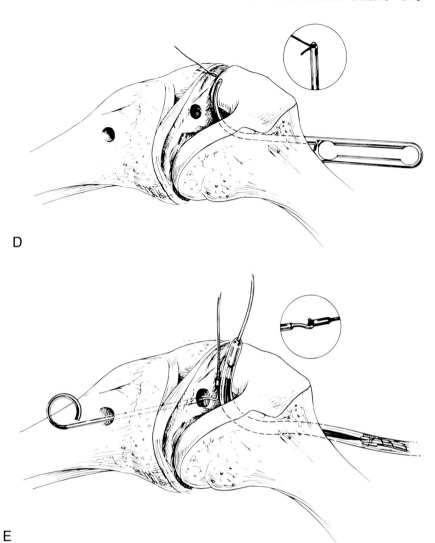

Fig. 31-2 *(Continued).* **(D)** Strover hook is placed into the knee joint from lateral aspect. Guidewire is then connected to the hook. **(E)** Shrink tubing. Tendon passer and carbon tows are pulled into the knee joint by hand and then through the tibial hole using the tibial hook. (Weiss AB, Hatam M, Alexander H: Surgical protocols for PLA-carbon ligament implants. Contemp Orthop 7:39–48, 1983.)

D

E

Fig. 31-3. Side-to-side difference in anterior Drawer of the knee evaluated preoperatively and postoperatively. (Data for combined knees; measured on a KT-1000.)

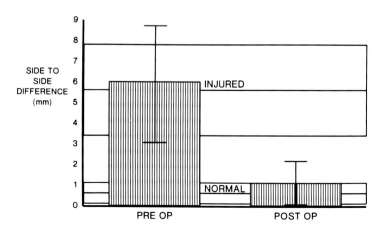

tion indicated that 150 surgical cases had been done at least 12 months previously. A list of these surgical cases is in Table 31-3. They include a great variety of surgical procedures. However, the largest group is the combined knees (cruciate ligament repair combined with lateral and/or medial collateral ligament repair). In the combined knees' group, 17 have been lost to follow-up. Consequently, data on 70 patients with 12 months of follow-up and 30 patients with 24 months of follow-up are available. The 70-patient group includes 54 male and 16 female patients with a median age of 26 years and an average of one previous surgical attempt at repair. Therefore, on average, they were someone else's failures. Fifty percent of them were injured in sporting activities, 17 percent in vehicular accidents, 10 percent at work, and 3 percent by miscellaneous other modes.

The procedures for surgical repair were described by Weiss et al.[43,44] They involve augmenting iliotibial band tissue for anterior cruciate ligament repair (Fig. 31-2) and using the implant directly for collateral ligament repair. Postoperative care procedures are outlined in detail by Weiss et al.[43]

Results

The patients were evaluated for stability, function, and isokinetic muscle strength at regular intervals. Using a KT-1000 arthrometer,[15,26] side-to-side differences in anterior Drawer of the knee were evaluated preoperatively and postoperatively. Figure 31-3 shows that the preoperative results were in the expected injured range and the postoperative results were at the upper edge of the expected normal range. Four patients failed to maintain stability. Out of a possible total stability score of 20, the preoperative average was 7 and rose to a significantly more stable value of 15 by 6 months. Following both the 12 and 24-month groups, they parallel each other, maintaining stability out to 2 years (Fig. 31-4).

Initial average scores for function were 11 and 12 for the 12- and 24-month groups, respectively. They reached 19 out of a possible 25 points by 12 months and stabilized at 20 until 24 months into the study (Fig. 31-5).

Low-speed isokinetic testing (30°/sec) results were expressed as percent deficit of maximum torque generated as compared to the uninjured leg

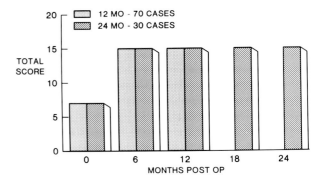

Fig. 31-4. Stability score for combined knee ligament reconstructions. Maximum score possible is 20.

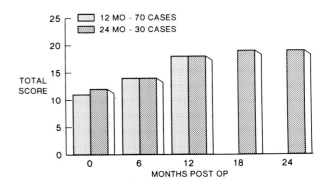

Fig. 31-5. Function score for combined knee ligament reconstructions. Maximum score possible is 25.

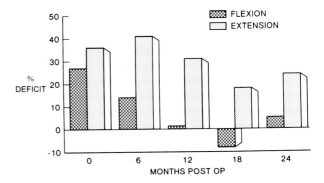

Fig. 31-6. Isokinetic knee testing at 30°/sec. Results expressed as percent deficit of maximum torque generated as compared to the uninjured leg preoperation. (Data for combined knees.)

Fig. 31-7. (A) Light and **(B)** scanning electron micrographs showing collagenous ingrowth around the carbon fibers in a reconstructed ACL at 18 months post-operatively. (**A** × 100;   **B** × 1,000;   bar = 10 μm.) (Weiss A, Blazina ME, Goldstein AR, Alexander H: Ligament replacement with an absorbable copolymer carbon fiber scaffold—early clinical experience. Clin Orthop 196:77–85, 1985.)

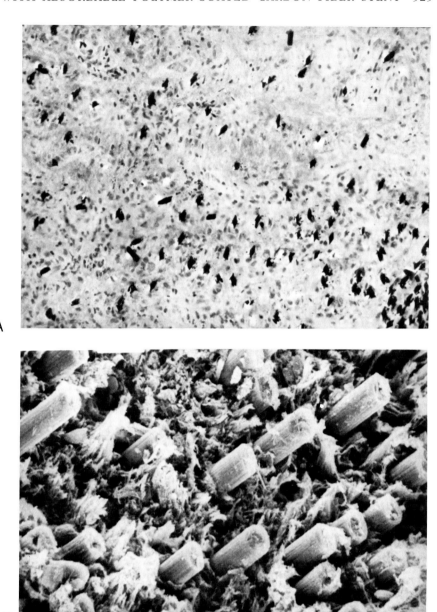

A

B

before operation. By 1 year, strength in flexion reached preoperative values. However, extension strength continued to register a deficit even after 2 years (Fig. 31-6). This may be a result of the considerable quadriceps damage caused in performing the arthrotomy.

The histologic appearance of the regrown tissue was previously presented by Weiss et al.[43] Both light and electron microscopy demonstrated collagenous ingrowth surrounding the carbon fibers used to reconstruct the anterior cruciate ligament (Fig. 31-7). Various samples were enzymatically degraded with pepsin and interrupted gel electrophoresis was performed to characterize the types of collagen present (Table 31-4). The collagenous ingrowth was composed of types I and III collagen

Table 31-4. Percentage of Type III Collagen in Various Tissues

Tissue	Percentage
Skin	24
Joint capsule	51
Healing ACL	44
Joint capsule with carbon	40
Carbon fiber ACL repair	42
Normal ACL	25
Carbon fiber MCL repair	52
Normal MCL	11

in similar proportions to that found in normal healing ligamentous tissue.

Complications are best described in terms of the entire study group from all 25 centers, where the large number of patients makes the complication percentages significant. The deep infection rate was 1.2 percent, the resurgery rate was 5.1 percent, and the instability–failure rate was 6.1 percent. The rate of the development of limited range of motion or adhesions was 4.4 percent and the joint effusion rate was 4.4 percent. All of the complication rates are within expected limits for implant surgery of this type.

Comments

This series of animal experiments and clinical trials suggests that carbon fiber–absorbable polymer composites are useful in soft tissue repair. Fibrous tissue ingrowth appears to be consistent with some organization of the tissue evident as early as 4 weeks. Complete envelopment of the implant by aligned collagen fibers has been noted at 8 weeks in the animal studies. Bone ingrowth around the carbon fibers in the drill holes in beagle tibias (patellar tendon study) was also evident. However, this process is clearly much slower than soft tissue ingrowth: it requires upward of 1 year. Within the synovial joint, protection of the carbon fiber with autogenous tissue appears to be necessary to counteract the slower growth rates in this environment.

Carbon fiber composite clinical implants have, to date, demonstrated ingrowth potential similar to that seen in the animal studies. Two-year evaluation results have been encouraging. Most patients have shown significant improvement, with many demonstrating good to excellent stability and function.

The carbon composite has high strength and reasonable flexibility when woven into soft tissue. It is highly biocompatible and encourages rapid tissue ingrowth. The absorbable polymer coating appears to delay the fragmentation of the fibers, thereby preventing migration. It is anticipated that this new material will soon be a useful addition to the surgeon's armamentarium for the treatment of unstable joints and tendon injuries.

ACKNOWLEDGMENTS

This work has spanned an 8-year period and has benefited from the contributions of many individuals. Amos Gona, Ophelia Gona, and Irving Strauchler contributed to much of the early planning of these experiments. Research residents Stephen Corcoran, James Aragona, Richard Fong, Albert Mylod, Richard Rosa, Leigh Ende, Anthony Rosario, Marie Hatam, Teresa Vega, and Andrew Goldstein attended to much of the day-to-day experimental details. Helen Chen and Irene Collins did all of the tissue histologic study. Robert Ainsworth and Kenneth St. John of the Hexcel Corporation prepared the implants and Linda Wilson and Brenda Hershey-Fell monitored the clinical trials. The care and thoughtfulness with which they approached this project contributed to the FDA's approval of early clinical trials and their recent acceptance of a premarket approval application. Martin Blazina, Vert Mooney, Melvin Post, Robert Larson, and John King provided many of the early clinical cases and helped in planning the various surgical procedures. The many other clinical investigators, too numerous to mention here, contributed much to the study. The authors owe all of these individuals a debt of gratitude.

This project has been funded by the generous support of the William Lightfoot Schultz Foundation through the Foundation of the University of Medicine and Dentistry of New Jersey and the Hexcel Corporation.

REFERENCES

1. Alexander H, Parsons JR, Strauchler ID et al: Canine patellar tendon replacement with a polylactic acid polymer-filamentous carbon tissue scaffold. Orthop Rev 10:41–51, 1981

2. Alexander H, Parsons JR, Smith G et al: Anterior cruciate ligament replacement with filamentous carbon. Orthop Res Soc 7:45, 1982 [abstr]

3. Alexander H, Weiss AB, Parsons JR, Strauchler ID, Gona O: Ligament and tendon replacement with absorbable polymer-filamentous carbon tissue scaffolds. 25th Annual Meeting of the Orthopaedic Research Society, February 1979 [abstr.]

4. Alexander H, Weiss AB, Parsons JR: Absorbable polymer filamentous carbon composites. A new class of tissue scaffolding materials. p. 83. In Burri C, Claes L (eds): Aktuelle Probleme in Chirurgie und Orthopaedie. Hans Huber, Bern, 1983

5. Amis AA, Campbell JR, Kempson SA, Miller JH: Comparison of the structure of neotendons induced by implantation of carbon or polyester fibres. J Bone Joint Surg 66B:131–139, 1984

6. Aragona J, Parsons JR, Alexander H, Weiss AB: Soft tissue attachement of a filamentous carbon-absorbable polymer tendon and ligament replacement. Clin Orthop 160:268–278, 1981

7. Aragona J, Parsons JR, Alexander H, Weiss AB: Medial collateral ligament replacement with a partially absorbable tissue scaffold. Am J Sports Med 11:228–233, 1983

8. Bercovy M, Goutallier D, Voisin MC et al: Carbon-PGLA prostheses for ligament reconstruction. Clin Orthop 196:159–168, 1985

9. Brady JM, Cutright DE, Miller RA et al: Resorption rate route elimination and ultrastructure of the implant site of polylactic acid in the abdominal wall of the rat. J Biomed Materials Res 7:155–166, 1973

10. Burri C, Henkemeyer H, Neugebauer R: Techniques and results of alloplastic carbon fiber ligament substitution. p. 146. In Burri C, Claes L (eds): Aktuelle Probleme in Chirurgie und Orthopaedie. Hans Huber, Bern, 1983

11. Christel P, Buttazzoni B, Leray JL, Morin C: Tissue tolerance of carbon materials. Trans World Biomaterials Congress 1:4,7,9, 1980

12. Claes L, Wolter D, Gistinger G et al: Physical and biological aspects of carbon fibres in the ligament prosthesis. In presentation, 3rd Congress on Mechanical Properties of Biomaterials, Keele University, 1978

13. Cutright DE, Hunsuck EE: Tissue reactions to the biodegradable polylactic acid suture. Oral Surg 31:134–139, 1971

14. Dandy DJ, Flanagan JP, Steenmeyer V: Arthroscopy and the management of the ruptured anterior cruciate ligament. Clin Orthop 167:43–49, 1982

15. Daniel DM, Malcom LL, Losse G et al: Instrumented measurement of anterior laxity of the knee. J Bone Joint Surg 67A:720–725, 1985

16. Forster IW, Ralis ZA, McKibbin B, Jenkins DHR: Biological reaction to carbon fiber implants. The formation and structure of a carbon-induced "neotendon." Clin Orthop 131:299–307, 1978

17. Forster IW, Shuttleworth A: Tissue reaction to intraarticular carbon fibre implants in the knee. J Bone Joint Surg 66B:282, 1984 [abstr]

18. Goldstein AR, Alexander H, Collins I, Poandl T, Weiss AB: Sheep anterior cruciate ligament reconstruction using a collagen-coated absorbable copolymer carbon ligament prosthesis. Proceedings Society for Biomaterials, 1986.

19. Haubold A: Carbon in prosthetics. Ann NY Acad Sci 283:383–395, 1977

20. Jenkins DHR: The repair of cruciate ligaments with flexible carbon fibre. J Bone Joint Surg 60B:520–522, 1978

21. Jenkins DHR, Forster IW, McKibbin B, Ralis ZA: Induction of tendon and ligament formation by carbon implants. J Bone Joint Surg 59B:53–57, 1977

22. Jenkins DHR, McKibbin B: The role of flexible carbon-fibre implants as tendon and ligament substitutes in clinical practice. A preliminary report. J Bone Joint Surg 62B:497–499, 1980

23. King JB, Bulstrode C: Polylactate-coated fiber in extra articular reconstruction of the unstable knee. Clin Orthop 196:139–142, 1985

24. Kinzl L, Wolter D, Claes L: Aspects of coated carbon fibres in the ligament prosthesis. Trans Soc Biomater 3:71, 1979 [abstr]

25. Kulkarni RK, Moore EG, Hegyeli AF, Leonard F: Polylactic acid for surgical implants. Arch Surg 93:839–843, 1966

26. Malcom LL, Daniel DM, Stone ML, Sachs R: The measurement of anterior knee laxity after ACL reconstructive surgery. Clin Orthop 196:35–41, 1985

27. Neugebauer R, Burri C, Claes L et al: The anchorage of carbon fibre strands into bone. A biomechanical and biological evaluation on knee joints. Trans Europ Soc Biomater 2:64, 1979 [abstr]

28. Neugebauer R, Burri C, Claes L et al: The replacement of the abdominal wall by a carbon-cloth in rabbits. Trans Soc Biomater 3:135, 1979 [abstr]

29. Neugebauer R, Burri C, Claes L, Helbing G: The trap door. A possibility of fixation of carbon fibre strands into cancellous bone. Trans World Biomater Congress 1:4,5,7, 1980

30. Parsons JR, Alexander H, Ende LS, Weiss A: Fiber reinforced absorbable polymer tissue scaffolds. A comparison of carbon fiber and dacron fiber systems. Trans Orthop Res Soc 8:86, 1983 [abstr]

30a. Parsons JR, Alexander H, Weiss AB: Soft tissue repair and replacement with carbon fiber. Absorbable polymer composites. pp. 417–452. In Heppenstall RB, Pines E, Rovee D (eds): Soft and Hard Tissue Repair: Biological and Clinical Aspects of Soft and Hard Tissue Repair. Praeger Publishing, Westport, CT, 1984

31. Parsons JR, Bhayani S, Alexander H, Weiss AB: Carbon fiber debris within the synovial joint. A time-dependent mechanical and histologic study. Clin Orthop 196:69–76, 1985

32. Parsons JR, Rosario A, Weiss AB, Alexander H: Achilles tendon repair with an absorbable polymer-carbon fiber composite. Foot Ankle 5:49–53, 1984

33. Pitt CG, Gratzlk MM, Kimmel GL et al: The degradation of poly (DL-lactide) poly (E-caprapectone) and their copolymers M-V in vivo. Biomaterials 2:215, 1981 [abstr]

34. Post M: Rotator cuff repair with carbon filament. A preliminary report of five cases. Clin Orthop 196:154–158, 1985

35. Ricci JL, Gona AG, Alexander H, Parson JR: Morphological characteristics of tendon cells cultured on synthetic fibers. J Biomed Mater Res 18:1073–1087, 1984

36. Rice RM, Hegyeli AF, Gourlay SK et al: In vitro studies with in vitro correlation. J Biomed Mater Res 12:43–54, 1978

37. Rushton N, Dandy DJ, Naylor CPE: The clinical arthroscopi and histological findings after replacement of the anterior cruciate ligament with carbon-fibre. J Bone Joint Surg 65B:308–309, 1983

38. Schindler A, Jeffcoat R, Kimmel GL et al: Biodegradable polymers for sustained drug delivery. p. 251. In Pearce E, Schaefgen J (eds): Contemporary Topics in Polymer Science, Volume II. Plenum Press, New York, 1977

39. Strover AE: Technical advances in the reconstruction of knee ligaments using carbon fiber. p. 127. In Burri C, Claes L (eds): Aktuelle Probleme in Chirurgie und Orthopaedie. Hans Huber, Bern, 1983

40. Strover AE, Firer P: The use of carbon fiber implants in anterior cruciate ligament surgery. Clin Orthop 196:88–98, 1985

41. Strum GM, Larson RL: Clinical experience and early results of carbon fiber augmentation of anterior cruciate reconstruction of the knee. Clin Orthop 196:124–139, 1985

42. Tayton K, Phillips G, Ralis ZA: Long term effects of carbon fibre on soft tissue. J Bone Joint Surg 64B:112–114, 1982

43. Weiss AB, Blazina ME, Goldstein AR, Alexander H: Ligament replacement with an absorbable copolymer carbon fiber scaffold. Early clinical experience. Clin Orthop 196:77–85, 1985

44. Weiss AB, Hatam M, Alexander H: Surgical protocols for PLA-carbon ligament implants. Contemp Orthop 7:39–48, 1983

45. Witvoet J, Christel P: Treatment of chronic anterior knee instabilities with combined intra and extra-articular transfer augmented with carbone-PLA fibers. Clin Orthop 196:143–153, 1985

46. Wolter D, Fitzer E, Helbine G, Goldaway J: Ligament replacement in the knee joints with carbon fibers coated with pyrolitic carbon. Trans Soc Biomater 1:126, 197 [abstr]

32

Bovine Xenograft Reconstruction of the ACL

ROBERT A. TEITGE

Replacement of the anterior cruciate ligament (ACL) has not been reliably mastered. Approaches include autografts, allografts, xenografts, prosthetic stents, and total prosthetic replacement.

Xenograft (the old term was "heterograft") is the transplantation of a graft between different species. Historically this has not been successful because the species-specific antigens evoke a host-vs.-graft response in the recipient. Ultimately the graft is destroyed. The use of a collagen structure to replace an absent collagen structure is an extremely attractive goal. Species-to-species collagen chemical differences are relatively small. Blockage of the immunologic reaction might be easier with relatively solid collagen structures than with other tissues. Peacock and Petty,[16] Potenza,[17] and Potenza and Melone[18] all failed to demonstrate significant rejection-type reactions in their animal studies of tendon allografts.

A tendon or ligament graft made of collagen that did not provoke an immunologic or other host reaction, was resistant to degradation, maintained desirable mechanical properties, and was easy to handle would advance our potential for replacing the crucial ligaments in the knee with a reliable material.

CHEMISTRY

Tanning is the process of chemically stabilizing tissues. Although many agents stabilize structures, perhaps the best known is chromium, which is used in the manufacture of "chromic catgut" suture. Cross-linkage is an effective means of controlling the biodegradation rate of collagen-based materials, preventing elution of the material into wound fluids, and increasing the tensile properties of the material to the level at which they can be handled conveniently. Cross-linked collagen has a greater modulus of elasticity, greater resistance to proteases, and lower degree of swelling than un-cross-linked collagen. The latter property is used as a measure of the degree of cross-linking. A variety of chemical and physical agents are used to cross-link collagen: aldehydes, isocyanates, alkyl and aryl halides, imidoesters, carboiimides, N-substituted maleimides, and acylating compounds. Collagen intermolecular cross-links are covalent and they can support high stresses. The cross-linking efficiency of any reagent is a function of the pH, temperature, the number of available amino acid residues that can react with the reagent, the bond energy associated with each cross-link, and the stability of that cross-link.[23] Of the various aldehydes commonly used for tanning, a greater number of more stable cross-linkages are formed with glutaraldehyde than with formaldehyde. Glutaraldehyde is an effective sterilization agent; it has been used successfully as a disinfectant and sterilizer of surgical equipment for over 20 years. Toxic effects of glutaraldehyde on cells of any type are apparent at very low concentrations and thus adequate rinsing is a prerequisite for its use. Glutaraldehyde has a molecular size that appears to be particularly suitable for bridging the gap between amino groups of the polypeptide chains of collagen and introduces more cross-linkages into collagen than other aldehydes. The glutaraldehyde cross-linkages are more stable than the other cross-linkages.[24]

HISTORICAL PERSPECTIVES

The current use of xenograft to replace the ACL really had its genesis in an extrapolated use of the successful xenograft heart valve. Alain Carpentier, Professor of Cardiac Surgery at the University of Paris, began using xenograft heart valves in 1964. A French law forbade removal of tissue from a cadaver within the first 48 hours of death. The possibility of using an allograft was blocked; the choice of xenografts was second best. He hoped that the xenograft would serve as a frame into which host cells would grow by creeping substitution. Buffered mercurial solution was used initially to guarantee sterilization and histologic preservation. A series of patients had these mercurial-fixed xenografts implanted. Within 5 years, because of collagen degeneration and an inflammatory (immune) reaction, the xenografts failed in all patients. Consequently, the fixation agent was changed from the mercurial solution to formalin. Within 4 years, all the xenografts failed due to inflammatory (immune) reaction.

At this point, according to Carpentier,[4] he realized that the theoretical possibility of graft regeneration by host fibroblast infiltration had failed to materialize. When the graft did show cellular ingrowth, it was invaded by inflammatory cells not fibroblasts. Research concepts were changed and directed toward using the xenograft as a biomaterial to construct a prosthetic valve. The term "bioprosthesis" was coined to indicate a prosthesis manufactured from biologic tissues, as opposed to a graft that would be replaced by host tissue. Various chemicals were investigated in an attempt to reduce the antigenicity of the tissue and increase its long-term stability. After several fixation methods were tested, a series of patients had xenografts inserted that had been processed in glutaraldehyde and an oxidant. Although these appeared mechanically sound in vitro, in vivo calcification of the valves developed within 7 years. Subsequently, buffered glutaraldehyde proved to yield biologically acceptable xenografts and a large industry developed for their production.[2,4]

The success of the porcine valvular xenobioprosthesis led directly to the current trials of xenograft ligament replacement. McMaster et al.[13,14] recognized the potential for similar bioprostheses in orthopaedics and initiated animal investigations.

ANIMAL STUDIES

In 1975, McMaster et al.[13] reported on a series of five rabbits in which the medial collateral ligament (MCL) was replaced by a glutaraldehyde-treated allograft. One knee was unstable because of loss of internal fixation but none of the five showed evidence of granuloma, exudate, or hypertrophic scarring. Microscopic evaluation was interpreted to show changes within the ligament consistent with host invasion by capillaries and viable-appearing fibroblasts. They also noted material between strands of implant tendon that appeared to have the most fibroblasts, with occasional round cells and giant cells but no granuloma or abscess formation.

In 1976, McMaster et al.[14] published the results of three experiments involving the use of glutaraldehyde-treated tendons. In the first experiment, 2 cm pieces of glutaradehyde-fixed homogeneous grafts were implanted into the subcutaneous space on the backs of 14 rabbits. Examination at 3 days to 15 weeks showed no alteration of the implant, which was surrounded by a thin scar of fibrous tissue without granuloma or leukocyte collections.

In the second experiment, 40 rabbits had a 2 cm segment of glutaraldehyde-fixed Achilles tendon homograft inserted as an interposition graft. Histologic evaluation at 5 weeks to 1 year was interpreted as showing areas of replacement of the graft by host collagen. Granulation buds appeared as well as scattered macrophages, plasma cells, mast cells, lymphocytes, polymorphonuclear leukocytes, and occasional giant cells but no evidence of an acute inflammatory response or granuloma formation.

In the third experiment, 10 chickens had a segment of profundus tendon replaced with a 2 cm fixed homograft on one claw. A reversed autogenous tendon graft was used as a control. The anastomosis and its investing scar was subjected to tensional pull-to-failure and the mean tensile strength at failure was nearly identical (4.3 lb vs. 4.6 lb), al-

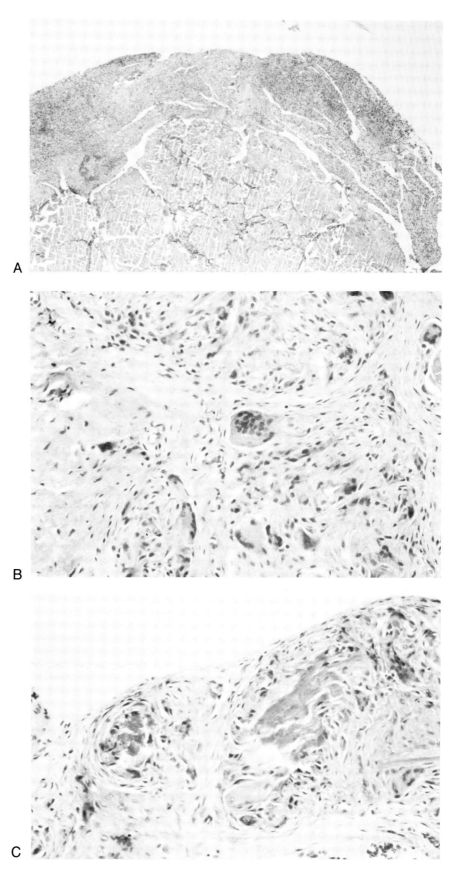

Fig. 32-1. **(A)** Low-power view of inert graft material surrounded by fibrous tissue and an inflammatory cell infiltrate. **(B)** High-power view of subjacent area showing granuloma response to "inert" graft material. **(C)** Surface of granuloma showing apparent engulfing of graft particulate material.

A

B

C

though nearly half of the autogenous grafts failed at their middle and all the homogenous grafts failed at the suture line.

In 1984, Gambardella et al.[6] reported the results of implantation of glutaradehyde-fixed bovine tendons used to replace the anterior cruciate ligaments in 14 rabbits. All of the fixed tendon grafts were covered with a Dacron sleeve. At sacrifice between 4 and 52 weeks all implants except one were intact. At 52 weeks, there was fibrocartilage between the tendon implant and the adjacent bone tunnels and also ingrowing fibroblasts and cartilage cells between filaments of implanted ligament. The intraarticular graft was surrounded by a connective tissue.[6]

In 1985, McMaster[12] reported on the anterior cruciate ligament replacement with a bovine xenograft in eight dogs sacrificed at 3 to 12 months. The knees were examined grossly and microscopically. Grossly there was minimal osteophyte formation in several knees and all xenografts were intact and covered with synovial tissue. Microscopically, there was no evidence of resorption of graft material. There was evidence of granulation buds in the interstices of the graft but no evidence of granulomas, eosinophils, round cell aggregations, or foreign body giant cells.

HUMAN STUDIES

The first series of human patients receiving bovine xenograft ACLs was reported at the 1982 Eastern Orthopaedic Association Meeting by Abbink and Kramer.[1] In their series,[1] 78 patients had received 72 ACL, 20 PCL, and 13 MCL implants; 73 patients (95 percent) were functioning well. Five patients had problems with pain, effusion, or restricted range of motion and three of these had synovectomies, which resulted in resolution of symptoms.

In North America, the first series was reported by Teitge and Rojas.[21] They evaluated 18 patients over an average of 18.1 months. This report contrasted sharply with that of Abbink and Kramer[1] and was criticized by the manufacturer.[11] In these 18 patients, 9 grafts had been removed by the time of the report. Ten patients complained of large recurrent effusions at 6 months postoperatively or later with cell counts up to 150,000/mm[2] and negative cultures. At follow-up evaluations, only one patient was

stable by KT-1000 measurement and this patient had a documented broken graft in the femoral tunnel. Two patients had relatively improved stability with only a 3 mm increase by KT-1000 value and four other patients were subjectively improved but remained unstable by KT-1000 testing. Histologically, six pathology reports described chronic inflammation with foreign body giant cell granulomatous reaction of the removed graft, while three other reports were only of chronic inflammation (Fig. 32-1).

PHYSICAL PROPERTIES

Mechanical studies of the bovine xenograft began after human studies were underway. Few studies are available; also, the different mechanical variables and testing conditions make comparisons difficult. The published reports[3,15,23,24] and one set of data presented in 1985 are summarized in Table 32-1. In general, increasing the cross-linkages in collagen results in a larger slope of the stress–strain curve, a decrease in gliding, and a decrease of stretching of the collagen fibers. The maximum load, ultimate strength, stiffness, and elastic modulus are all higher than the natural human ACL.

IMMUNOLOGIC AND TOXIC REACTIONS

Salgaller and Bajpai[19] compared the immunogenicity of glutaraldehyde-treated bovine pericardial tissue with untreated bovine pericardial tissue implanted in rabbits and concluded that treating the tissue with glutaraldehyde reduced the reaction but did not render the tissue immunogenic. Magilligan et al.[10] and Heinzerling et al.[9] have shown the presence of antibodies against glutaradehyde-treated porcine heart valve leaflets in patients implanted with these valves. Also, they discovered circulating antibodies against bovine collagen in patients receiving the glutaradehyde-treated cruciate ligament grafts but the histologic appearance of the reactive synovium around the removed grafts was not characteristic of an immune or rejection reaction.

Toxic chemical reactions could be a concern with the use of glutaraldehyde-treated tissue implants. On the basis of a morphologic study of gluteralde-

Table 32-1. Summary of Studies

Factors Measured	Noyes and Grood[15]	An[1a]	Berg et al.[3]	Xenotech[25]	Weadock et al.[23]
Maximum load	—	2180 N	855–1027 N	855–1027 N	—
Linear force	0.622–1.17 kN	—	—	—	—
Maximum force	0.73–1.73 kN	—	—	—	—
Linear stress	11–25 MPa	—	—	—	—
Maximum stress	13–38 MPa	—	—	—	—
Ultimate tensile strength	—	70 MPa	—	—	—
Maximum tensile strength	—	—	27–33 MPa	27–33 MPa	—
Stiffness	129–182 kN/m	53 kN/strain	—	—	—
Elastic modulus	65–111 MPa	1696 MPa	2363–2924 MPa	2363–2924 MPa	—
Low strain modulus	—	—	—	—	167–233 g/mm^2
High strain modulus	—	—	—	—	1611–2148 g/mm^2
Initial strain @ toe	—	2.2%	—	—	—
Strain @ linear stress	22–25%	—	—	—	—
Strain @ maximum stress	30–44%	—	—	—	—
Strain @ failure	48–60%	—	—	—	—
Final strain	—	—	—	1.71–2.38%	—
Maximum strain	—	—	—	—	0.16–0.23 [sic]
Strain energy	—	—	—	0.186–0.199 Nm/cm^3	—
Strain energy to failure	3–10.3 Nm/ml	—	—	—	—
Energy to failure	4.9–12.8 Nm	—	—	—	—
Strain rate	100%/sec	—	—	0.33–33%/sec	10%/min
Loading rate	—	—	0.5–50.8 cm/min	0.5–50.8 cm/min	—

hyde-treated sponges, Chvapil et al.[5] proposed that leaching of glutaraldehyde exerts a cytotoxic effect that prevents the ingrowth of cells into the central core of the matrix. They also showed that the glutaraldehyde may be detected as residual effects for up to 6 months after implantation.[5] In another study, the group[20] showed some enhancement of healing of osteochondral defects by collagen sponge but believed that collagen without residual glutaraldehyde would be preferable for ingrowing cells. Gendler et al.[7] suggested that glutaraldehyde-fixed tissues washed for as long as 4 hours before implant still showed slight inflammatory reaction potential.

COMMENTS

The concept of using a collagen-based prosthesis as a ligament replacement remains attractive. Tanning of a graft may make it sufficiently inert that it may not be replaced by host fibroblasts and collagen of liga-ment capability and, in fact, it may remain a bio-prosthesis. The difference in natural human history between a biologic ligament xenograft and a ligament bioprosthesis has not been defined. Tanning of the graft significantly alters its mechanical properties and the resultant fixed graft may then be mechanically unsuited for its new function. Rates of fatigue failure for the xenograft as a prosthesis remain to be published. Grood and Noyes[8] evaluated the failure of the polyethylene prosthesis and concluded that it was mechanically unsound. The normal ACL has a strain of 15 percent without failure and the bone–ligament–bone complex may elongate over 50 percent before failure.[15] Trembley et al.[22] have suggested that the normal knee may require the ACL to elongate 14 percent through a normal range of motion. If this is the case, the 1.7 percent elongation reported for the bovine CLR xenograft may be too little to avoid overloading of the prosthesis, even when placed in the most exact "isometric" location. Other reasons for mechanical failure might include chafing from bone tunnels, turning angle being too acute between the intercondylar notch and the bone tunnels, or preload placement being too great or too little and therefore requiring too much strain before failure (not at the so-called isometric points). The possibilities of immunologic or chemical contributions to failure of the xenograft have been shown in studies involving porcine cardiac valves and pericardium. When control of these variables is mastered, the xenograft bioprosthesis may prove a valuable adjunct to the reconstruction of ligaments.

REFERENCES

1. Abbink EP, Kramer FJK: Preliminary report on the use of xenografts in knee instability problems. Orthop Trans 7:84, 1983 [abstr]

1a. An K-N: Biomechanical evaluation of xenograft CLR. Paper presented at the Symposium on Prosthetic Ligament Reconstuction of the Knee, Palm Springs, CA March 21–24, 1985

2. Barratt-Boyes BG: Cardiothoracic surgery in the antipodes. J Thorac Cardiovasc Surg 78:804–822, 1979

3. Berg WS, Stahurshi TM, Moran JM, Greenwald AS: Mechanical properties of bovine xenografts. Orthop Trans 7:279, 1983 [abstr]

4. Carpentier A: From valvular xenograft to valvular bioprosthesis (1965–1977). Med Instrument 11:98–101, 1977

5. Chvapil M, Speer DE, Mora W, Eskelson C: Effect of tanning agent on tissue reaction to tissue implanted collagen sponge. J Surg Res 35:402–409, 1983

6. Gambardella RA, Jurgutis JA, Gendler E et al: The replacement of anterior cruciate ligaments with glutaraldehyde (GTA) fixed bovine implants. Orthop Trans 8:248, 1984 [abstr]

7. Gendler E, Gendler SK, Nimni ME: Toxic reactions evoked by glutaraldehyde-fixed pericardium and cardiac valve tissue bioprosthesis. J Biomed Materials Res 8:727–736, 1984

8. Grood ES, Noyes FR: Cruciate ligament prosthesis. Strength, creep, and fatigue properties. J Bone Joint Surg 58A:1083–1088, 1976

9. Heinzerling RH, Stein PD, Riddle JM et al: Immunological involvement in porcine bioprosthetic valve

degeneration. Preliminary studies. Henry Ford Hosp Med J 30:146–151, 1982

10. Magilligan DJ, Jr., Lewis JW, Heinzerling RH, Smith D: Fate of a second porcine bioprosthetic valve. J Thorac Cardiovasc Surg 85:362–370, 1983

11. Martin C: Letter to the Editor. Orthop Today 4:3–4, 1984

12. McMaster WC: A histological assessment of canine anterior cruciate substitution with bovine xenograft. Clin Orthop 196:196–201, 1985

13. McMaster WC, Liddle S, Anzel SH, Waugh TR: Medial collateral ligament replacement in the rabbit model. A preliminary report. Am J Sports Med 3:271–276, 1975

14. McMaster WC, Kouzelos J, Liddle S, Waugh TR: Tendon grafting with glutaraldehyde fixed material. J Biomed Materials Res 10:259–271, 1976

15. Noyes FR, Grood ES: The strength of the anterior cruciate ligament in humans and rhesus monkeys. J Bone Joint Surg 58A:1074–1082, 1976

16. Peacock EE, Petty J: Antigenicity of tendon. Surg Gynecol Obstet 110:187–192, 1960

17. Potenza AD: Concepts of tendon healing and repair. pp. 18–47. American Academy of Orthopaedic Surgeons, Symposium of Tendon Surgery. CV Mosby, St. Louis 1975

18. Potenza AD, Melone C: Evaluation of freeze-dried flexor tendon grafts in the dog. J Hand Surg 3:157–162, 1975

19. Salgaller ML, Bajpai PK: Immunogenicity of glutaradehyde treated bovine pericardial tissue xenografts in rabbits. J Biomed Materials Res 19:1–11, 1985

20. Speer DP, Chvapil M, Volz R, Holmes M: Enhancement of healing of osteochondral defects by collagen sponge. Clin Orthop 144:326–335, 1979

21. Teitge RA, Rojas F: Anterior cruciate ligament reconstruction using a bovine xenograft prosthesis. Paper presented at the AOSSM interim meeting, Feb. 8, 1984, Atlanta, Georgia

22. Tremblay G, Laurin C, Drovin G: The challenge of prosthetic cruciate ligament replacement. Clin Orthop 147:88–92, 1980

23. Weadock K, Olson RM, Silver FH: Evaluation of collagen crosslinking techniques. Biomater Med Devices Artif Organs 11:293–318, 1984

24. Woodroof EA: Use of glutaraldehyde and formaldehyde to process tissue heart valves. Processed Tissue Valves—Mini review. J Bioenerg 2:1–9, 1978

25. Xenotech Laboratories Inc: Ligament and Tendon Bioprosthesis Investigational Plan IDE No. G810163, May 1963

33

Laboratory Studies of Biodegradable Materials for Cruciate Ligament Reconstruction*

WILLIAM G. RODKEY

Management of moderate to severe knee injuries has frustrated surgeons throughout medical history. Specifically, injuries and deficiencies of the anterior cruciate ligament (ACL) frequently result in disabilities that are permanent and devastating.

In 1977 Dr. Edward Cabaud and I realized that we shared a common frustration: we recognized the ACL as a highly unique anatomic structure on which all mammals depend for knee joint stability, and yet we could not adequately repair and restore the ACL following severe injury. His patients were predominantly athletes and young soldiers. My patients were primarily young and athletic but of the canine species. Rarely did any of our patients return to their original level of activity and ability following the

traumatic disruption of the ACL. Consequently, we decided to approach this problem of repairing or reconstructing the ACL in the laboratory. We began performing well-conceived studies in a controlled environment.

Our laboratory at the Letterman Army Institute of Research, like many others, has actively pursued a solution to the optimal management of ACL injuries. We began with the basic philosophy that acute ACL injuries should be treated as early as possible. We considered that repair or reconstruction of the acutely injured ACL would provide the patient with a better long-term result and minimize secondary degenerative changes. Our initial long-term plans called for studies in four general areas: primary repairs of the disrupted ACLs, augmentation of the repaired ACL with autogenous tissue, the use of permanent materials to repair or reconstruct the ACL, and the use of absorbable or biodegradable materials for the ACL repairs. This chapter describes the findings of our laboratory studies in those four areas. Based on these efforts and the philosophies that developed in our laboratory, a discussion follows on the current (1980s) status of biodegradable materials and the future application of 100 percent biodegradable prosthetic ligaments.

---

* The opinions and assertions contained herein are the private views of the author and are not to be construed as official or as reflecting the views of the Department of the Army or the Department of Defense. In conducting the research described in this report the investigators adhered to the *Guide for Laboratory Animal Facilities and Care* as promulgated by the Committee on the Guide for Laboratory Animal Resources, National Academy of Sciences, National Research Council.

DEVELOPMENTAL AND EXPERIMENTAL LABORATORY STUDIES

Acute Primary Repairs

Through our studies we hoped to provide some definitive answers to the questions of whether a ruptured ACL should be repaired, removed, replaced, or ignored. Our first study[4] was designed with four objectives: to determine if there was any difference in the potential for the ACL to heal if it was lacerated at the femoral vs. the tibial end; to identify the factors responsible for healing of the ligament or for failure to heal and consequent resorption of the repaired ligaments; to detect the healing characteristics of the ACL following repair with absorbable suture materials; and to evaluate the physical properties of repaired and normal ACLs based on biomechanical testing.

In that initial study[4] of acute primary repairs of the ACL, 10 dogs and 6 monkeys underwent transection and repair of the ACL in one knee. Half of the procedures involved transection of the ACL at the femoral end and the remainder were transected at the tibial end. The ligaments were repaired with size 0 polyglycolic acid suture (Dexon, Davis & Geck, Danbury, CT) in a figure-eight pattern with parallel drill holes in the lateral femoral condyle or the medial proximal tibia, depending on whether the ligament was severed at the femoral or tibial end. The insertion sites were decorticated so that the lacerated surface of the ligament was placed in approximation with bleeding bone in the hopes of stimulating healing and bony ingrowth into the repaired ligament. The operated legs were immobilized for 6 weeks in casts, and following cast removal, the animals were allowed unrestricted activity until final evaluation 4 months postoperatively.

Seven of the canine and all of the primate ACLs that had been transected and repaired healed. However, two of the healed canine ligaments were so weak that they ruptured during light exercise just before the animal was sacrificed. All of the canine knee joints showed moderate to severe instability and degenerative changes while the primate knees had fewer degenerative changes but still had gross instability. When the unoperated control ACLs were tested biomechanically, the predominant disrup-

tion pattern in both the dogs and monkeys was failure of the anteromedial band at the tibial insertion and interstitial failure of the posterolateral part. The canine ACL failed at a maximum strength of about 123 kg$_f$ and the primate ACL failed at about 48 kg$_f$.

All of the repaired ligaments suitable for biomechanical testing failed at or near their repair sites. For the canine ACLs the maximum strength for those repaired at the femoral end was 10 percent of the control ligaments, and it was 2 percent of control for those repaired at the tibial end. For the primates, maximum strength was about 47 percent for the femoral end and 63 percent of the control values for tibial end repairs.

We believed that inadequate immobilization and too early stress were the primary causes of the poor results obtained in this study, especially in the dogs. We demonstrated that under appropriate conditions, transected and repaired ACLs will undergo some degree of healing. Certainly, anatomic repair under appropriate tension and effective immobilization are essential if healing is to occur. Other than these factors we were unable to identify causes for failure to heal and ACL resorption. While we were unable to predict which acutely injured and repaired ACLs would heal, we did conclude that supplemental dynamic and static supporting procedures should be used to augment the acute ACL repair.

ACL Repairs Augmented with Autogenous Tissue

If an injury is sufficient to rupture the ACL completely, then the ligament has been stretched and lengthened about 30 percent before ultimate failure occurs.[1,8] Once stretched and disrupted with complete interruption of the blood supply, as in so called "mop-end" injuries, it is little wonder that primary repairs hold questionable promise. A 5-year follow-up study by Feagin and Curl[7] in patients who had surgical repair of isolated ACL injuries revealed the following discouraging facts: On a subjective basis, 12 of 34 patients questioned indicated impairment even in ordinary activities, and 24 of the total of 34 considered themselves athletically handicapped. Furthermore, eight of the total were frankly dissatisfied with their surgical results.

The reasons for failure of primary repair might be attributed to (1) initial stretching of the ligament at the time of the original injury; (2) decreased blood supply following injury; (3) inadequate immobilization of the leg following surgical repair of the ACL; and (4) perhaps excessive stress too early during the rehabilitation period. Based on both the 5-year clinical follow-up and our acute experimental studies, we believed that a technique for primary repair of the ACL and augmentation with autogenous tissue was needed to restore predictably the biomechanical capability of the acutely injured ACL. Therefore, we developed a technique to augment primary repairs in order to supply an additional source of blood, to act as an internal splint to protect the ACL during healing, and perhaps to provide additional strength to the repair complex.[2]

The technique was modeled after that of Eriksson.[6] In our study the acutely lacerated ACL was repaired in its anatomic position in a manner similar to that described for our first study. Additionally the medial one-third of the patellar tendon was elevated with a fragment of patella bone in a groove prepared from the tibial tubercle to the base of the anterior tibial spine. The medial third of the patellar tendon was then transferred and stabilized with nonabsorbable sutures that were carried through the same parallel drill holes used for the ACL repair. The cut end of the repaired ACL as well as the cut end of the patellar tendon was held firmly against the decorticated repair site in the lateral femoral condyle.

Following 6 weeks of cast immobilization of the operated leg, the dogs in this study were allowed unrestricted activities. Four months after the surgical procedure six dogs were evaluated and after 8 months five other dogs were evaluated. All 11 repaired and augmented ACLs healed sufficiently to provide clinical and functional stability to the knee joints. Although there were minimal degenerative changes, there were no articular erosions, as had been noted in the study with primary repair alone. Biomechanical testing revealed a maturation phenomenon between the 4- and 8-month groups with bony ingrowth of the femoral insertion site producing increased strength and, ultimately, interstitial failure of the repaired ACL occurred. This maturation is reflected in the physical properties (Table 33-1). Although the augmented ACLs were not as strong or as stiff as the normal control ACLs, the 8-month group had physical properties in a functional range and all animals in that group displayed clinical joint stability. In fact, one repaired and augmented ACL was stronger than the contralateral control. Furthermore, histologic studies confirmed the bony ingrowth at the repair site that had been noted on gross examination. This bony ingrowth was largely responsible for the fact that ACL failure occurred interstitially during biomechanical testing.

We were extremely encouraged by the results of these augmented ACL repairs in dogs. However, in our continuing long-term plan our next investiga-

Table 33-1. Physical Properties of Repaired Anterior Cruciate Ligaments[2,3]

	Control (N=11)	4 Months (N=6) Patellar Tendon Augmented[2]	8 Months (N=5) Patellar Tendon Augmented[2]	4 Months (N=10) PGA Splint[3]
Maximum linear load (kg$_f$)	101.6 ± 11.6[a]	33.8 ± 9.9	57.5 + 15.5	46.0 ± 5.0
Maximum load (kg$_f$)	122.7 ± 11.6	46.2 ± 10.9	64.3 ± 14.3	54.2 ± 6.3
Slope of linear load (kg$_f$/mm)	20.0 ± 1.8	9.8 ± 2.8	11.5 ± 1.7	13.4 ± 1.1
Ultimate stress (kg$_f$/mm^2)	7.6 ± 0.8	1.3 ± 0.2	2.0 ± 0.3	3.5 ± 0.5
Modulus of elasticity (kg$_f$/mm^2)	23.3 ± 3.0	6.0 ± 1.2	8.1 ± 0.4	18.1 ± 2.7
Strain at maximum linear load (%)	27.9 ± 3.1	20.5 ± 7.2	22.5 ± 5.2	16.8 ± 0.9
Strain at maximum load (%)	35.5 ± 4.2	29.9 ± 10.3	29.1 ± 3.4	22.6 ± 2.6
Strain at failure (%)	58.6 ± 3.8	67.0 ± 10.4	64.4 ± 10.0	61.6 ± 8.2
Energy absorbed to failure (kg$_f$ · mm)	733.2 ± 69.8	298.7 ± 76.1	382.0 ± 51.0	268.4 ± 41.1

[a] Values are mean ± SEM.

tive effort was to find a method of supporting the repaired ACL without the use of an autogenous tissue graft.

Reinforcement with a Completely Biodegradable Intraarticular Ligament

In our third research study in this series,[3] we attempted to develop a biodegradable intraarticular ligament that would provide the same function as the patellar tendon grafts while functioning as an intraarticular splint. While this splint would allow us to avoid the use of autogenous tissue, we also hoped to minimize or preclude postoperative immobilization and allow normal motion of the joint during healing.

Our team selected braided polyglycolic acid (PGA) as the material from which to construct the biodegradable ligament. This 100 percent biodegradable material is strong, easy to handle, produces little tissue reaction, was readily resorbed, and was well tolerated intraarticularly. We evaluated several hand-braided patterns of this material before we selected a Y-shaped design with physical properties that approximated those of the normal canine ACL. The prosthesis used three strands with 10 size 2-0 Dexon sutures in each strand. The tails of the "Y" were braided contiguously with the main portion of the ligament (Fig. 33-1). The PGA ligament was more than 80 percent as strong as the normal canine ACL but it was slightly more compliant. We again used our canine ACL model as we had done in our previous studies to evaluate this biodegradable intraarticular splint. As before, the ACL of one leg was transected at the femoral condyle and a primary repair was performed. We then reinforced the primary repair with the PGA ligament, allowing it to act as an internal splint. The Y-shaped prosthesis was applied by passing the tails through the two parallel drill holes in the lateral femoral condyle that were placed as part of the repair of the ACL. As the tibia was held in a completely reduced position, the suture in the ACL was tied and then the two tails of the PGA ligament were similarly tied over the femoral condyle. The portion of the PGA ligament that composed the base of the Y was secured to the tibia through three drill holes in the tibial tubercle.

The vertical hole was passed anterior and slightly medial to the tibial insertion of the ACL. The remaining two holes were transverse across the prominent tibial tubercle. The biodegradable ligament finally was passed through these three holes and sutured to itself, after the tension was adjusted to be slightly greater than that on the repaired ACL. This procedure was performed on a total of 12 dogs.

Two of the dogs had no immobilization of their operated leg so that we could assess the intrinsic ability of the PGA prosthesis to protect the joint. The operated legs of the remaining 10 dogs were immobilized in a manner similar to that described in our previous studies. One dog was sacrificed and evaluated at 2 weeks after surgery, one dog at 5 weeks, and the remaining 10 dogs at 16 weeks. In the 2-week specimen the PGA ligament was intact and there was no evidence of degenerative changes and no synovitis. The repaired ACL and PGA intraarticular splint together required over 40 kg$_f$ to rupture when tested biomechanically, which is about one-third of the maximum strength of the contralateral control ACL. The intraarticular portion of the PGA ligament was nearly completely resorbed in the 5-week specimen, but the extraarticular portions of the prosthesis remained intact and showed no gross change compared to the original appearance. In that 5-week specimen again there was no synovitis or degenerative changes, but a thick synovial envelope surrounded the complex of the repaired ACL and the PGA prosthesis. Biomechanical testing required only 16 kg$_f$ to disrupt this complex. When the remaining 10 dogs were evaluated 4 months postoperatively, all repaired and reinforced ACLs had healed. There were no or only minimal inflammatory or degenerative changes, but the repaired complex uniformly was enveloped in a thick synovium. Clinically, all of the operated joints remained stable. Biomechanical testing revealed that the strength of the repaired ligaments was about one-half of the maximum strength of the normal control ACL. Furthermore, in addition to being weaker the repaired ligaments also were more compliant (Table 33-1). It also was interesting to note that there was essentially no difference observed in the two joints that had not been immobilized compared to those that did remain in a cast for 6 weeks following surgery.

Figure 33-2 summarizes schematically the load

Fig. 33-1. (A) Hand-braided PGA ligament consisting of 30 size 2-0 Dexon sutures. **(B)** Close-up view of interface between tails and main portion of ligament. (Cabaud HE, Feagin JA, Rodkey WG: Acute anterior cruciate ligament injury and repair reinforced with a biodegradable intraarticular ligament. Am J Sports Med 10:259–265, 1982. © 1982 American Orthopaedic Society for Sports Medicine.)

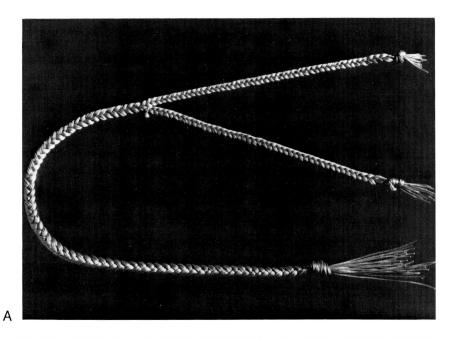

A

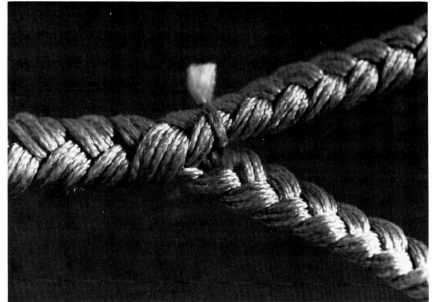

B

deformation curves obtained from the biomechanical testing in our first three studies.[2–4]

Based on the results of this study[3] we concluded that the 100 percent biodegradable PGA ligament was safe, strong, well-tolerated, and provided adequate early splinting function to provide stability to the repaired ACL in our canine model. However, the intraarticular portion of the material was almost completely resorbed by 5 weeks, and an intraarticular splint or prosthetic ligament intended for human

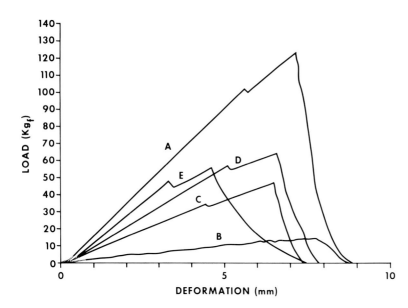

Fig. 33-2. Schematic load deformation curves of *(A)* normal canine ACL compared with *(B)* simple primary repair at 4 months, *(C)* patellar-tendon-augmented repair at 4 months, *(D)* patellar-tendon-augmented repair at 8 months, and *(E)* ACL repair reinforced with a PGA intraarticular splint at 4 months.

clinical use must provide support over a much longer period of time. Hence, it was obvious that any such prosthesis needed greater staying power.

Partially Biodegradable Materials

Although we were encouraged by the results of our study using the 100 percent biodegradable intraarticular splint, we believed that it was necessary to identify a material device that would remain permanently in the knee joint as a replacement or augmentation to the repaired ACL. We realized that such a device must have the functional, physiologic, and biomechanical characteristics of the normal ACL, and that it must be capable of enduring the hostile environment of the knee joint. As we reviewed the work of others, it became apparent that numerous materials, both biologic and nonbiologic, have been used in the construction of prosthetic ACLs, and all have produced varying degrees of limited success and disappointment.[5] These various materials can be placed into two broad categories: (1) permanent materials that must accept complete biomechanical load with little or no initial reliance on host tissues, and (2) completely or partially biodegradable materials that provide immediate stabilization to the repaired ligament and act as a "scaffold" for ingrowth and/or replacement by host

tissues. Regardless of the classification of the prosthesis, the demands placed upon it are numerous and rigorous. Certainly it must be durable with adequate strength to withstand the extreme forces placed upon it, yet compliant enough to allow for repetitive motion without failure or excessive creep elongation. It must be tolerated by the host with no antigenic or carcinogenic reaction and, if partially or completely biodegradable, the size of the individual fibers and the construction pattern must be appropriate to support and allow eventual reconstitution of the repaired structure with ingrowth of fibrous tissue that matures to normal or near normal collagen. The device must tolerate sterilization and storage and it should be easily implanted using surgical and potentially arthroscopic techniques.[9]

With these factors in mind and with consideration of the results of our earlier studies, we identified a combination of materials that was partially biodegradable and met many of our criteria. This material was a combination of polyglycolic acid and Dacron. We chose this machine-woven material that was 80 percent PGA and 20 percent Dacron because its strength and compliance were comparable to a normal canine ACL. We theorized that as the PGA was resorbed, a porous matrix or scaffold of Dacron would be left behind into which would grow fibrous tissue. It was hoped that this collagenous tissue then would remodel in response to mechanical demands placed upon it to become organized and function as a normal ligament.

In that study,[10] we found the strength of this PGA–Dacron material was greater than the normal canine ACL (145 kg_f vs. 125 kg_f), but it was more compliant (Fig. 33-3). When we used this material in our canine ACL repair model, we found that the material had excellent handling characteristics and its simple design made it easy to use. The overall success in this study was limited despite the excellent initial and residual strength of the PGA–Dacron material. The most significant problem was that the open woven pattern was not satisfactory because the weave opened excessively as the PGA was resorbed. This change led to markedly increased compliance of the prosthesis. As a result there was significant clinical instability of the repaired joints within 2 to 4 months after implantation of the material.

The next phase of this study involving partially biodegradable materials led us to evaluate a PGA–Dacron material of a bicomposite design. This device had a distinct central core of polyglycolic acid and Dacron and a separate outer sleeve woven from polyglycolic acid and Dacron of a different percentage of composition. This biocomposite device was 3.2 mm in diameter and constructed to exceed the

strength and stiffness of a normal ACL (Fig. 33-3). It avoided the problem of brittleness as seen in various other materials and the design minimized the problem of increased compliance as observed in our initial work with the PGA–Dacron combination. We believed that this device would provide a scaffold for fibrous tissue and/or bony ingrowth while the prosthesis remained intact. We also believed that the modification of the design and composition of the PGA and Dacron would provide better mechanical properties and would better tolerate the intraarticular environment of the knee joint.

In this phase of the study (Rodkey and Cabaud, unpublished data) we again used our canine ACL model. There were two experimental groups. One group had transection of the ACL at the femoral condyle followed by repair of the ACL with a single size 0 PGA suture in a Kessler pattern. The repaired ACL was then reinforced with the PGA–Dacron prosthesis, which was placed anterior to the ACL through drill holes in the lateral femoral condyle and the anterior tibia. Laterally the prosthesis was placed beneath the fibular collateral ligament, then through a drill hole in the tibial tubercle. The ends of the prosthesis were secured under a bone staple along the medial flare of the tibial tubercle. The other experimental group had transection of one ACL and reconstruction using a strip of tensor fascia

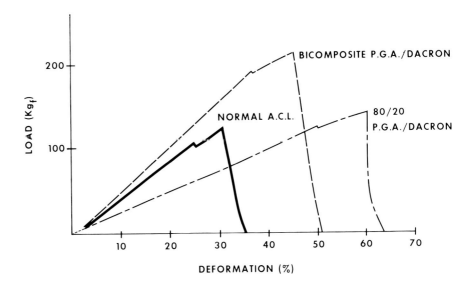

Fig. 33-3. Schematic load deformation curves comparing a normal canine ACL, the machine-woven combination of 80 percent PGA and 20 percent Dacron, and the biocomposite PGA–Dacron device.

lata and the PGA–Dacron prosthesis as an augmentation device. A strip of the tensor fascia lata was dissected free and left attached distally. This strip of tissue was wrapped around the PGA–Dacron prosthesis and sutured to it with a size 2-0 PGA suture. This complex then was carried over the top of the lateral femoral condyle and through a drill hole in the tibia. The ends of the prosthesis were secured by a bone staple in the medial aspect of the tibial tubercle. After 6 weeks of immobilization, the long leg casts were removed and the dogs were permitted unrestricted activity and exercise. Evaluations were carried out at varying intervals up to 9 months postoperatively and included functional and clinical testing, grading of intraarticular changes, biomechanical testing of the repaired complex, and selected histologic study.

We found that all dogs in both experimental groups had competent ACLs at the time of their evaluation, although the amount of degenerative changes and the degree of instability varied. Joints evaluated at 3 months postoperatively demonstrated slightly increased laxity in both groups with equivalent mild degenerative changes. The maximum strength at failure for both groups was about 40 kg_f, or about one-third the strength of the normal control ACL. All of the 3-month specimens failed by bony pullout. The repaired ACLs appeared healthy grossly and viable histologically. One ACL had established solid bony healing and thus failed interstitially during biomechanical testing. In the reconstructed group it was noted that the PGA–Dacron prosthesis could be readily exposed by gentle dissection of the tensor fascia lata. There was no gross or microscopic evidence of tissue ingrowth into the residual Dacron in the intraarticular portion of the device. However, the appearance of the tensor fascia lata and the PGA–Dacron prosthesis extraarticularly was quite different. There was healthy, vigorous fibrous tissue encapsulating and protecting the extraarticular portions of the prosthesis. Histologically there was superficial ingrowth with some orientation of the fibrous tissue.

In the joints that were evaluated 6 months postoperatively there appeared to be some maturation of both the repaired ACLs and the transferred tensor fascia lata. Laxity of the joints and degenerative changes were comparable in both experimental groups. In the reinforced group the average maximum strength of the repaired complex was 60 kg_f. All of the repaired ACLs had achieved bony healing and failed interstitially during testing. Although some fraying of the residual Dacron intraarticularly was a consistent finding, there was no apparent inflammatory reaction or mechanical interference noted. In the group reconstructed with the tensor fascia lata, the average maximum strength also was about 60 kg_f, but bony ingrowth had not stabilized the prosthesis in the bone canals where the tensor fascia lata had surrounded it. Biomechanical testing failure occurred uniformly by pullout of the prosthesis from the bony tunnels. Once again there was no histologic evidence of fibrous ingrowth intraarticularly, but excellent fibrous tissue encapsulation and ingrowth protected the PGA–Dacron prosthesis extraarticularly with definite orientation in a load-bearing direction of the fibrous tissue. Histologically there was also a difference between the intra- and extraarticular portions of the transferred tensor fascia lata. The extraarticular portion appeared healthy and normal, but the intraarticular portion had focal areas of degenerative change compatible with hypovascularity.

By 9 months postoperatively there was fair clinical stability in both experimental groups. In the group with the repaired and reinforced ACL, the healed ACL required 47 kg_f to rupture. The PGA–Dacron prosthesis was contributing little if any support for the healed ACL and it had become markedly frayed. In the group reconstructed with the tensor fascia lata, fair to moderate clinical stability was observed. When the joint was opened, the tensor fascia lata appeared healthy but the residual Dacron was readily exposed and once again showed no evidence of fibrous tissue ingrowth. The extraarticular portions of the prosthesis and the tensor fascia lata appeared healthy and compatible.

In every operated animal, internal rotation of the joint remained reduced compared to the control values, thus indicating that the extraarticular portions of the PGA–Dacron prosthesis continued to provide exceptional lateral support. *No animal in the entire study had exposure, fraying, wear, or abrasion of any extraarticular portion of the prosthesis.*

We drew several conclusions based on the results

of this study. Extraarticularly, this material may ultimately prove to have advantages over any other prosthetic material currently available. Certainly it was extremely safe since the prosthesis was constructed of materials that have been shown to be well tolerated and produce little tissue reaction over many years of use. The prosthesis was designed to be adequately strong with appropriate compliance and to retain reasonable strength even after the PGA was hydrolyzed. It was easy to use, versatile, and adaptable for a variety of clinical situations. Potentially it had use in reconstructive procedures in multiple anatomic areas. Unfortunately, the intraarticular results remain speculative, much as they have with all other prosthetic materials thus far evaluated. We acknowledge that if used alone this device ultimately would fail. Only as a splint for reinforcement or as an augmentation device in conjunction with appropriate biologic or autogenous tissue might this material hold significant promise for intraarticular use. Even under ideal conditions the hostile intraarticular environment seemed virtually to preclude fibrous tissue ingrowth.

Although we were disappointed with the overall results of the intraarticular use of the PGA–Dacron device, we still believed that further investigation of this material was warranted, especially in the surgical management of disrupted extraarticular soft tissues. We therefore designed a study to assess the applicability and in vivo characteristics of this partially biodegradable PGA–Dacron material to repair or replace severely injured extraarticular soft tissue structures of the extremities. We determined the strength and physical properties of the repaired tissue and the residual material complex. Finally, we examined the quantity and quality of fibrous tissue ingrowth into this material and its degree of remodeling when placed under a functional load. For our extraarticular experimental model we chose the rabbit Achilles tendon. In this extraarticular study[11] our research team found that the PGA–Dacron material had adequate strength and physical properties to use both for primary tenorrhaphy and to bridge tendon defects. However, we were unable to identify any significant advantage of this device over other materials available or known to be under evaluation.

Forty adult rabbits were placed randomly into one of three experimental groups. All animals were subjected to complete laceration and repair of one Achilles tendon. Eight animals had end-to-end tenorrhaphy with size 0 braided polyester suture, and 16 animals had their tendons primarily repaired with the biocomposite designed PGA–Dacron device similar to that described above and used intraarticularly in dogs. The only difference was that for the rabbit study the PGA–Dacron device was only 1.55 mm in diameter as opposed to 3.2 mm diameter when used in the dogs. An additional 16 rabbits received laceration and removal of 1 cm of tissue from their Achilles tendon, and the defect then was bridged with this same PGA–Dacron material. No postoperative immobilization was applied to any of the operated legs. Evaluation was carried out at 4 or 8 weeks after tenorrhaphy and consisted of biomechanical testing or histologic inspection. We found that all tendons healed, and at 8 weeks the maximum load at failure of tendons repaired with the braided polyester suture was 32 kg_f, 40 kg_f for the end-to-end tenorrhaphy with the PGA–Dacron device, and 32 kg_f for those tendons in which a 1 cm defect was bridged. Even though we found that these values for load at failure between the groups were not significant in their difference, all were significantly less than the strength of the unoperated control tendons, which averaged 56 kg_f. *Our most noteworthy observation was that lengthening of the repaired tendons, due to scar elongation at the tenorrhaphy site, occurred during healing in all three groups.* This lengthening, however, was significantly less in the two groups in which the PGA–Dacron device was used, perhaps due to some fibrous tissue ingrowth into the device that provided additional anchorage and stabilization after some early displacement.

Although this PGA–Dacron device had excellent strength and handling properties similar to those we had observed in our previous studies, we again were disappointed with the inadequate fibrous tissue that grew into the Dacron scaffold that remained after the PGA was hydrolyzed. Indeed, the fibrous tissue present did not mature or align in response to load to form a neotendon; instead it remained disorganized and of inadequate quantity and quality (Fig. 33-4). Eight weeks may have been an insufficient

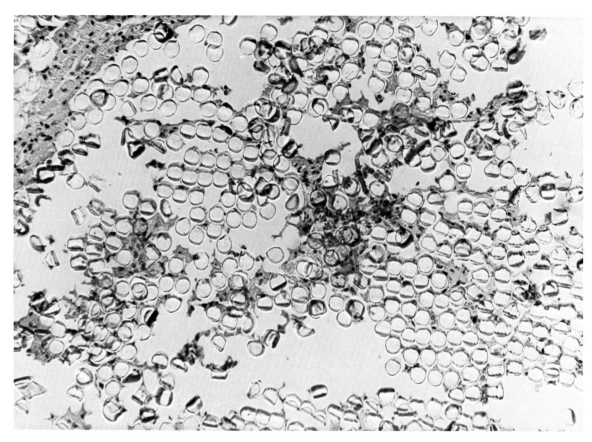

Fig. 33-4. Histologic section of an 8-week extraarticular PGA–Dacron specimen showing poor quality and quantity fibrous tissue ingrowth.

period of time to expect adequate mature collagen, and longer-term evaluation should be considered. Regardless of these shortcomings, this PGA–Dacron device did meet several critical requirements: (1) it was biologically compatible and no adverse reactions were observed; (2) it had adequate strength to support the repaired tendon during the healing process; (3) it was relatively easy to implant surgically; and (4) biomechanically it accepted the load of the normal tendon. Consequently, a device of this type might be appropriate for primary repairs of injured tendons with minimal postoperative immobilization.

The lack of more positive findings with this PGA–Dacron bicomposite device both intra- and extraarticularly has prevented any consideration of human clinical trials with the material in its present composition and configuration. Our efforts continue with modification of the structural design of the device and with substitution for the PGA by different completely biodegradable synthetic materials that maintain in vivo strength for longer periods of time.

STATUS OF BIODEGRADABLE MATERIALS FOR ACL REPAIR

Prosthetic ACLs biologically could be considered biodegradable, biodegradable and replaced, partially biodegradable, or permanent. While many materials have been evaluated for prosthetic ACLs,[5,9] the only truly biodegradable substance critically evaluated and reported is polyglycolic acid.[3] Our research team is unaware of any other similar published reports.

Although descriptions of various autogenous tissues have been promising, we share a strong belief that there is an overwhelming need for a prosthetic material for both intra- and extraarticular uses. Based on the results of our own studies[2–4,10,11] and the literature we cited, we believe that a completely biodegradable material device holds the greatest potential value for development. We base this opinion on several factors: (1) a better understanding of the mechanics of the knee joint and the specific biomechanical requirements of a prosthetic ACL; (2) appreciation of the biology and physiology of the knee joint and particularly the hostile nature of the intraarticular environment; and (3) the development of new or improved biodegradable synthetic materials for in vivo use.

The biodegradable prosthesis should adhere to the scaffold principal. During the period of controlled biodegradation there would be ingrowth of fibrous tissue into the device. The prosthesis would be required to provide sufficient strength to permit adequate amounts of collagen formation that then would accept slowly the mechanical load from the degrading device. The quality of the collagen must be such that it would mature and become near-normal by aligning itself in response to the ever-increasing biomechanical load.

Unfortunately, we are faced with the dilemma of designing a device that provides adequate stability to the joint to preclude motion-induced degenerative changes yet must be elastic enough to permit some load to be placed on the new collagen. If the collagen remains unloaded due to the stiffness of the prosthesis, we would expect the new collagen to be stress-shielded or stress-protected, hence there would be no stimulation for functional alignment or maturation. Furthermore, at this time we do not

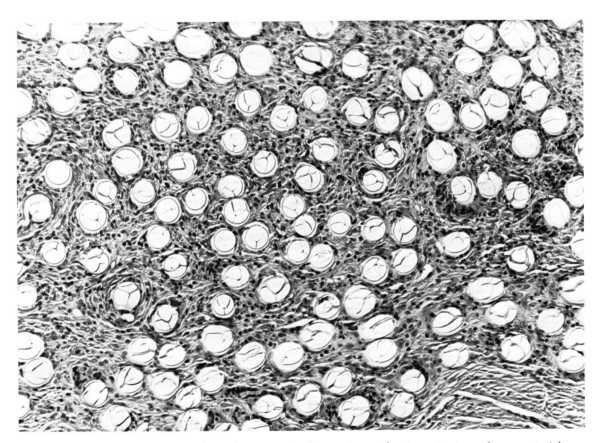

Fig. 33-5. Histologic section of a 90-day extraarticular specimen of an investigative polymer material that is longer lasting but completely biodegradable.

know if the new collagen would be of an appropriate type, and it may be necessary to influence the collagen type by some biochemical manipulation.

At present, we do not have a material that satisfies all of our demands. However, we have identified several completely biodegradable synthetic polymer materials that have significant residual strength in vivo for up to 200 days. If the construction and geometric design of devices made from such materials will permit us to match the physical properties of the normal ACL, we believe that these materials may provide adequate residual strength and hold significant promise for the repair or reconstruction of the ACL.

One such candidate material has undergone preliminary evaluation in vitro and in vivo in our laboratory (December, 1985). When placed extraarticularly in experimental animals, the material retains about 80 percent of its strength after 90 days. This material also supports abundant fibrous tissue ingrowth with early evidence of load-bearing orientation (Fig. 33-5). Further positive findings in the evaluation of this or a similar material likely will lead to studies in which the material is used to repair or reconstruct acutely injured ACLs.

THE FUTURE OF 100 PERCENT BIODEGRADABLE PROSTHETIC LIGAMENTS

Other authors in this book have described the anterior cruciate ligament as a unique, dynamic, and biomechanically complex structure. Consequently, ACL injuries present a very difficult management problem to knee surgeons. Our own philosophy is that such injuries should be treated surgically as soon as possible following injury. We believe that there is a definite need for a reliable prosthetic material device for both intra- and extraarticular use to repair surgically acute ACL injuries. Numerous laboratories, including our own, have made concentrated efforts to identify such a solution. While other investigators have focused primarily on permanent materials or materials that are mechanically degradable, we have developed a strong philosophy that the most appropriate prosthesis would be one that is 100 percent biodegradable and thus, over a period

of time, would be removed completely from the body. We believe that the technology now exists to modify and manipulate biodegradable synthetic polymers to such an extent that all of our critical elements for a prosthesis can be met. Certainly other investigators in this text have described materials that also hold great promise. Nonetheless, our team will continue to pursue the goal of identifying a 100 percent biodegradable material device that can be used routinely to repair or reconstruct the acutely injured ACL.

REFERENCES

1. Cabaud HE: Biomechanics of the anterior cruciate ligament. Clin Orthop 172:26–31, 1983
2. Cabaud HE, Feagin JA, Rodkey WG: Acute anterior cruciate ligament injury and augmented repair: experimental studies. Am J Sports Med 8:395–401, 1980
3. Cabaud HE, Feagin JA, Rodkey WG: Acute anterior cruciate ligament injury and repair reinforced with a biodegradable intraarticular ligament. Am J Sports Med 10:259–265, 1982
4. Cabaud HE, Rodkey WG, Feagin JA: Experimental studies of acute anterior cruciate ligament injury and repair. Am J Sports Med 7:18–22, 1979
5. Cabaud HE, Rodkey WG, Feagin JA: Prosthetic anterior cruciate ligament repairs: current status. p. 230. In Finerman G (ed): AAOS Symposium on Sports Medicine. The Knee. CV Mosby, St. Louis, 1984
6. Eriksson E: Sports injuries of the knee ligaments: their diagnosis, treatment, rehabilitation, and prevention. Med Sci Sports 8:133–144, 1976
7. Feagin JA, Curl WW: Isolated tear of the anterior cruciate ligament: 5-year follow-up study. Am J Sports Med 4:95–100, 1976
8. Noyes FR, Grood ES: The strength of the anterior cruciate ligament in humans and rhesus monkeys. Age-related and species-related changes. J Bone Joint Surg 58A:1074–1082, 1976
9. Rodkey WG: Prosthetic materials for repair and reconstruction of the anterior cruciate ligament. Orthop Surg Update Series, Vol. 4, No. 15, 1986
10. Rodkey WG, Cabaud HE, Feagin JA, Bradley MA: Preliminary evaluation of a partially biodegradable ligament substitute. Orthop Trans 7:174–175, 1983
11. Rodkey WG, Cabaud HE, Feagin JA, Perlik PC: A partially biodegradable material device for repair and reconstruction of injured tendons. Experimental studies. Am J Sports Med 13:242–247, 1985

H. Edward Cabaud, M.D. (1944–1985)

You influenced our scientific thinking; you established standards of excellence; and through your research and eagerness you quickened our pace.

Resident, friend, mentor, respected physician, scientist—we are the richer for your contributions.

May this book embrace the quality of your work and reflect the respect of your colleagues.

Glossary

A

ACL Anterior cruciate ligament. (*See under* Ligament.)

ACL augmentation Reinforcement of the ACL by stenting, whether with autogenous graft, allograft, or prosthetic material. Augmentation may be performed for acute or chronic ACL insufficiency.

Activities of daily living (ADL) Those tasks deemed necessary to maintain one's daily lifestyle, but not including sport participation.

ADL *See* Activities of daily living.

Adhesions *See* Stiffness.

Age, sex A patient's age and sex may be critical determinants of the activity level, which in turn dictates the rate of deterioration of the unstable knee. Age and sex are specified in the Case Studies of *The Crucial Ligaments* to emphasize how they may affect the choice of treatment.

American football The most pernicious of the contact sports in terms of knee injuries because the helmet and padding allow vicious tackling below the waist, resulting in a high incidence of knee injuries.

Ankylosis *See* Stiffness.

AP Anteroposterior.

Antalgic gait A gait characterized by shifting of the shoulders to unload the painful knee. An excellent diagnostic sign.

Anthropometric evaluation Athletes cannot be categorized as mesomorphs, endomorphs, or ectomorphs in a classic fashion, but some athletes are

more "at risk" because of a body habitus that is disadvantageous in their sport.

Arthritis, degenerative No absolutely satisfactory term exists to describe the deterioration of a joint the kinematics of which have been violated. *Degenerative arthritis* adequately reflects the osteophytosis and joint space narrowing and flattening visible on radiography. *Degenerative arthritis* in the knee is used synonymously with "traumatic arthritis" and "gonarthrosis."

Arthrometer An instrument that measures relative laxity. Although still in the development phases, laxity arthrometers are a useful clinical adjunct. Current examples are KT-100, Stryker Knee Ligament Test, and Genucom.

Anterior cruciate ligament *See under* Ligament.

Athlete A player in organized sport(s), team or individual, or a participant in recreational sports activities.

  Elite athlete One who has been tested in competition and ranks persistently among the top finishers. The term is not age-dependent.

  College athlete College athletes are usually 19 to 23 years old. Their epiphyses are closed, and they are nearly skeletally mature.

  High school athlete High school athletes are usually 16 to 19 years old; they frequently have open epiphyses, and are skeletally immature.

Athlete-at-risk The athlete who, whether by sport, physical ability, body habitus, or fatigue, is at greater risk for injury or reinjury.

Avalement A term coined by Joubert to mean upward unweighting. This maneuver is used in skiing to achieve a brisk turn of the skis. When improperly performed, the maneuver may place the ACL at risk.

Avulsion The ligament may tear partially or completely within its collagenous portion or may "avulse" from the bone, with or without a bony or chondral attachment.

B

Bicycle/stationary bicycle A useful adjunct in knee rehabilitation, since range of motion can be emphasized without significant impact or torque. The patellofemoral joint is minimally loaded. Minimum quadriceps stress is imparted to the ACL. The stationary bicycle usually gives the advantage of controlling the resistance, which may be advantageous.

Bracing/braces, knee Braces (orthotics) are still relatively unscientific. Most knee braces have hinged joints, and some have proved efficacious; however, reinjury may occur in spite of bracing. Neither preventive nor prophylactic bracing is of proven worth.

Bumper model* A model of the knee where the motion of the tibia is represented as being limited by bumper stops. The bumpers simulate the tethering action of the ligaments and are placed so the tibia cannot move past the position where the ligaments become taut. (See Chapters 9 and 10.)

Burmester curve A mathematical construct to explain the form and function of the MCL.

C

Chamfering The technique of smoothing the bony tunnel and decompressing its outlet so there is less likelihood of abrasion where the implanted ligaments or prosthetic stents are placed.

Chondromalacia An objective term meaning softening of cartilage. In common usage, it connotes the parapatellar pain that is a frequently concomitant of internal derangement of the knee.

Clancy operation (procedure) Variation of the Jones procedure (*See* Jones procedure.)

Conservative care *See* Nonoperative care.

Course of action The therapeutic course that the surgeon chooses on the basis of the given facts, the patient's desires, and the surgeon's best judgment.

CPM Continuous passive motion.

Crossed four-bar linkage A graphic model, popularized by Müller, that interprets the role of the cruciate ligaments. It is an excellent analogy which serves the knee surgeon well in the quest for anatomic restoration of the patient's knee function.

Cutting An abrupt change of direction in sport.

Cutting sports Sports such as soccer, football, and tennis, which require abrupt changes of direction that impose rotational torque on the knee. It is more difficult for patients with ACL insufficiency to regain elite status in the cutting sports.

D

Dashboard injury Injury caused by impact with the dashboard of a car. The term implies that the injury occurs by abrupt deceleration with the knee and hip flexed 90 degrees, making the posterior cruciate, posterior capsule, popliteal artery, femur, and femoral neck vulnerable to injury.

Degenerative arthritis *See* Arthritis.

Degrees of freedom* A term used to refer to the types of distinct and independent motions that are possible. Each separate, independent motion is one degree of freedom. In three dimensions there are six independent motions or degrees of freedom. Three of the six degrees of freedom are translations, and three are rotations. The three rotational degrees of freedom in the knee are (1) flexion–extension rotation, (2) adduction–abduction rotation, and (3) internal–external tibial rotation. The three translational degrees of freedom are (1) anterior–posterior translation, (2) caudad–cephalad translation (which produces joint distraction and compression), and (3) medial–lateral translation.

Dislocation* A malposition of the bones forming a joint. In common usage, a dislocation involves a malposition so large that the normally opposed articulating surfaces can no longer come in contact with each other.

Displacement* The net change in position that results from a motion; the difference between the initial and final positions.

Drawer test *See under* Test.

Drill guide   A device to channel the surgical drill. It is essential for accuracy in restorative ligament surgery. Many drill guides are available, and there is no single universally accepted guide.

E

Effusion   The escape of fluid from the blood vessels or lymphatics into tissues or a cavity. Often it is not known whether effusion in the knee is grossly hemorrhagic or not. *Mild, moderate,* and *tense* are subjective terms related to the pressure and distention caused by the effusion. An acute tear of the ACL usually results in a moderate effusion, whereas an intraarticular fracture will result in tense effusion. If the capsule is compromised, neither of the above holds true.

Elastic limit   The elastic limit of the normal ACL—the amount by which it can be stretched without causing permanent deformation—is approximately 10 percent of its resting length. Deformation beyond this point may cause rupture.

Elite athlete   *See under* Athlete.

End points (soft, hard)   The normal ACL and PCL firmly limit the anteroposterior (AP) glide of the knee and provide a hard end point for the examiner. In contrast, when these ligaments are disrupted, the secondary restraints oppose the examiner, and their resiliency provides the examiner with a "softer" (less abrupt) end point.

Eriksson operation (procedure)   Variation of the Jones procedure. (*See* Jones procedure.)

EUA   *See* Examination under anesthesia.

Examination under anesthesia (EUA)   EUA is more revealing than ordinary examination because the state of the knee is not masked by muscle tension. It should be performed before inflation of the tourniquet. As always, the well leg should be examined first.

Extension   The leg in extension is straight at its neutral position (zero degrees of flexion). In hyperextension, the knee is at its maximum bend past the neutral position.

F

Finochietto's sign   The tibia subluxes so far anteriorly on the femur that the meniscus becomes trapped anterior to the femoral condyle.

Flexion (of the knee)   A decrease in the distance between the heel and hip. Ninety degrees flexion means the leg is bent at a right angle.

Functional rehabilitation program   A rehabilitation program that involves agility training and purposeful adaptation in addition to the standard techniques. Such a program includes activities that promote endurance and strength through a range of motion.

G

Gonarthrosis   A term synonymous with *degenerative arthritis* and *traumatic arthritis.* (*See under* Arthritis.)

H

Hemarthrosis   Blood in a joint. (*See* Effusion.)

Hyperextensile joints   This condition is not precisely defined, but it is known that people whose joints are inherently lax seem to have a less than satisfactory result after ligament repair. People who are "loose jointed" may sustain more injuries at sport. The work of Nicholas addressed this point, but subsequent work was unable to verify this trend. Nevertheless, the tests described by Nicholas are useful to standardize loose versus tight jointedness.

Hyperextension   The position of the knee at its maximum bend past the neutral (zero degrees), straight-leg position.

I

Iliotibial tract   A coalescence of fibers of the iliotibial band which serves as a lateral stabilizing structure.

Induration   A feeling of hardness. The sensation the examiner can appreciate with the fingertips when there is fluid within the tissue elements and planes, which connotes injury or inflammation.

Instability* 1. A clinical sign, a condition of increased joint motion or mobility due to ligament injury. 2. A symptom, a giving-way event during activity. It is preferable to say *giving way* when this meaning is intended. (*See also* Laxity.)

Intercondylar notch The anatomic indentation between the femoral condyles. It is variable in size and shape. The posterior outlet, in particular, is responsible for amputating the ACL when the knee is suddenly hyperextended and internally rotated.

Interference fit fixation This term was introduced by Lambert and Cunningham to describe a technique of wedging the patella tendon bone graft into the recipient bone tunnels. The enhanced fixation provided by this technique allows earlier motion, earlier weightbearing, and more rapid rehabilitation. The bone plugs are believed to be healed by 6 weeks when held in this manner. The technique represents an application of the Charnley compression principle.

Isokinetic (knee rehabilitation) Exercise and activities to restore endurance and agility. This is stage III in knee rehabilitation—gaining strength through range of motion. (*See also* Isometric, Isotonic knee rehabilitation.)

Isolated ACL This term is a misnomer. No ligament "lives" alone. One of the most fascinating aspects of knee care is the interrelationship and interdependency of the anatomic parts.

Isometric (surgical reconstruction of the ACL) The term *isometric* implies that the distance between two points remains constant (through an arc of motion). If the ACL is replaced to its anatomic origin and insertion, the reconstruction is said to be isometric.

Isometric (knee rehabilitation) The first phase (stage I) of knee rehabilitation in which muscles are strengthened without joint motion (concentric tightening of the quadriceps and hamstrings so as not to impart quadriceps thrust, which might jeopardize the ACL). (*See also* Isokinetic, Isotonic knee rehabilitation.)

Isotonic (knee rehabilitation) Muscle contraction through a range of motion, progressively increasing the resistance or weight load. This constitutes stage II in knee rehabilitation. (*See also* Isokinetic, Isometric knee rehabilitation.)

J

Jakob test *See under* Test.

Jerk test *See under* Test.

Joint motion *See* Motion *and* Limits of motion.

Jones operation (procedure) The original procedure for using the middle third of the patella tendon as a graft to replace the ACL. Described by Dr. Kenneth Jones (See Ch. 20.)

Jones compression dressing Named after Sir Robert Jones, who described a compression dressing of alternate layers of wool and flannel, seldom seen in the operating room today. Nevertheless, most surgeons who apply compression dressings about the knee pay homage to Sir Robert Jones and his contributions to orthopaedic surgery.

K

Kessler suture A suture which does not constrict but has superior grasping qualities.

Knee bracing *See* Bracing.

Knee reconstruction The attempt to restore stability to the knee through ligamentous replacement, augmentation, or redirection.

Knee rehabilitation *See* Isometric, Isotonic, Isokinetic knee rehabilitation.

Knee surgeon In an international context, many of the surgeons who specialize in knee surgery are not orthopaedic surgeons. *The Crucial Ligaments* is intended for all surgeons who are dedicated to improvement in diagnosis and care of knee ligament injuries. The surgical skills are a logical extension of this care.

L

Lachman test *See under* Test.

Lateral collateral ligament *See under* Ligament.

Lateral meniscocapsular ligaments *See under* Ligament.

Lateral tenodesis The MacIntosh, Losee, Andrews, and Ellison operations are examples of lateral tenodeses of the iliotibial band, meant to restrain subluxation of the lateral compartment and thus complement the function of the ACL.

Laxity A general term meaning looseness. Laxity may be normal — the "normal physiological laxity of the knee," or abnormal, such as the increased laxity following rupture of knee ligaments. We have excluded from this definition the common use of the term *laxity* to describe only abnormal looseness. Laxity in the knee may be normal or abnormal; it must be made clear which is meant when the term is used. The amount of laxity is a clinical sign — a descriptive term — used in differential diagnosis. Diagnosis is described ultimately in anatomic terms. (*See under* Instability.)

    Global laxity Pathologic laxity in all planes of motion. It is a result of disruption and/or attritional tearing of both primary and secondary restraints about the knee.

    Multiplanar laxity *Multiplanar laxity* connotes that there is a varus or valgus opening with a rotatory component.

    Uniplanar laxity *Uniplanar laxity*, such as results from a tear of the MCL, allows pathologic opening (laxity) in only one plane, i.e., valgus opening without rotation.

    Rotatory laxity Laxity in which there is a rotatory component, in addition to simple translation of the tibia on the femur. The combination of translation and rotation is one that should be appreciated by the examiner.

LCL Lateral collateral ligament. (*See under* Ligament.)

Ligament

    ACL — Anterior cruciate ligament This ligament is frequently described as consisting of two bands, anteromedial and posterolateral. In reality, it is a mutistranded helicoid structure which limits anterior glide of the tibia on the femur.

    LCL — Lateral collateral ligament

    MCL — Medial collateral ligament This ligament consists of superficial and deep portions

and also meniscotibial and meniscofemoral portions.

    Medial and lateral meniscocapsular ligaments The secondary restraints for the ACL consists of the lateral meniscus and the capsular portion of the arcuate complex, as well as the medial meniscus and the meniscotibial and meniscofemoral ligaments. These ligaments are the lateral secondary restraints when the ACL fails.

    Medial patellofemoral ligament This ligament inserts on the medial intermuscular septum beneath the vastus medialis obliquus and is frequently torn with patella luxation.

    PCL — Posterior cruciate ligament The PCL is often described as two bands in association with the ligaments of Humphry and Wrisberg. In reality, like the ACL, it is a continuum of fibers. More vertically oriented than the ACL and also thicker and stronger, it resists posterior glide of the tibia on the femur. Like the ACL it is a primary restraint.

    POL — Posterior oblique capsular ligament The POL is a separate ligament. It is an important medial knee stabilizer.

    Primary and secondary ligamentous restraints A concept emphasizing that for any displacement about the knee, there is a primary stabilizer backed by secondary ligamentous restraints. The ACL and PCL are usually considered the primary stabilizers of AP translation.

Ligamentous restraints *See* Primary and secondary ligamentous restraints *under* Ligament.

Ligament tensioning Ligaments have a proprioceptive function. They can be overtightened, and this is damaging to the joint surfaces. The tension on ligaments should be adjusted using tensioning devices during ligament reconstruction procedures.

Limits of motion *See* motion.

Losee test *See under* Test.

M

MacIntosh test *See under* Test.

MCL Medical collateral ligament. (*See under* Ligament.)

Medial capsuloligamentous structures A term designed to imply that the meniscus and adjoining ligamentous structures are interrelated/and along with the lateral capsuloligamentous structures are the secondary restraints after loss of the ACL or PCL. The medial capsuloligamentous structure consists of the medial meniscus, the meniscotibial and meniscofemoral ligaments, and the posterior oblique capsular ligament.

Medial collateral ligament *See under* Ligament.

Medial meniscocapsular ligament *See under* Ligament.

Medial patellofemoral ligament *See under* Ligament.

Merchant view One of the many tangential patella views, but the one most often used for reproducibility

Motion* The act or process of changing position or orientation. Motion is described by specifying the path of motion or the sequential positions and orientations that occur during the motion. Motion is a general term. There are two types of motion—translation and rotation. (*See also* Degrees of freedom.)

Limits of motion* The positions of the knee at its extremes of motion. The limits or extreme positions are determined by the ligaments and joint geometry. Because the ligaments can stretch, the limits depend to some extent on how much load is applied. Each degree of freedom has two limits of motion, one for each direction (sense). For example, for anterior–posterior translation there is an anterior limit and a posterior limit. There are a total of twelve limits. (*See* Degrees of freedom.) The normal limit is usually considered to be that shown by the uninjured knee. The limits of motion depend on the position of the knee. An example is the limit to adduction rotation. This limit increases as the knee is flexed due to increasing slack in the lateral collateral ligament.

Range of Motion* The maximum amount of motion, between two limits or extreme positions, that a joint can move.

N

Neutral position The position of the knee in which the leg is extended straight, with zero degrees of flexion at the knee.

Nonoperative care Often synonymous with "conservative care." Nonoperative care can be equally demanding and rewarding as operative care.

Noyes' test *See under* Test.

O

Objective Viewing events or phenomena as they exist impersonally or in an unprejudiced way; open to observation by oneself and others; opposite of subjective. The Lachman test should be objective. Arthrometers provide more objectivity than a manual test because the clinical measurements can be reliably reproduced. (*See also* Subjective.)

O'Donoghue' triad The "unhappy" triad. The classic injury of American football, consisting of disruption of the ACL, MCL, and medial meniscus. The term was coined in the early 1950s by the father of American sports medicine, Dr. Don O'Donoghue.

Olecranization of the patella A procedure described by Müller that prevents tibial translation immediately subsequent to repair or reconstruction of the knee for posterior or posterolateral instability.

On-field examination Examination of an injured athlete by the physician, therapist, or trainer who comes on to the playing field to see the athlete before he or she is removed or resumes play. The on-field examination is clearly a manual examination.

Orthotics *See* Bracing.

Over-the-top procedure The direction of ACL graft material over the lateral femoral condyle. The isometricity of this placement has been questioned.

P

Patel arthroscopic portal Superomedial and superolateral arthroscopic approaches that give excellent visualization into the anterior compartment and intercondylar notch of the femur. An essential adjunct to arthroscopic diagnosis and treatment.

Patella apprehension test *See under* Test.

Patella compressive syndrome Postsurgical contracture of the periarticular soft tissues in the knee; a frequent concomitant of degenerative arthritis. Described by Ficat and Hungerford.

Pathologic laxity The adjective *pathologic* signifies abnormal excursion of the tibia on the femur in the injured knee compared to the well knee. Thus, a 1+ Lachman test signifies approximately 5 mm of increased excursion of the injured leg over the well leg, and implies an injury to the ACL. (*See also* Laxity.)

Patient selection The choice of which patients are candidates for ACL surgery, and of the appropriate surgical procedure. The patient's activity level is one of the key variables in the equation, and sometimes the most difficult to determine (or modify).

PCL Posterior cruciate ligament. (*See under* Ligament.)

Pivot shift test *See under* Test.

Plan of action As used in this test, the plan of action is the response to the hypothetical case study as it is presented, which implies the judgment involved with the facts and circumstances.

POL Posterior oblique ligament. (*See under* Ligament.)

"Pop" The "pop" is the characteristic sound or feeling that the patient experiences when the ACL is torn. The pop is characteristic of ACL injury and is not associated with tears of other ligamentous or periarticular structures in the knee.

Position* The relative location and orientation of two objects. The position of the knee is described by the three rotational positions and three translational positions, which make up the six degrees of freedom. (*See also* Degrees of freedom.)

Posterior cruciate ligament *See under* Ligament.

Posterior oblique ligament *See under* Ligament.

Primary ligamentous restraint *See* Primary and secondary ligamentous restraints, *under* Ligament.

Prone Lachman test *See* Lachman test, *under* Test.

Protective weightbearing The use of crutches for external support to unload the injured knee.

Q

Q-angle An anthropometric term coined by Duchenne and popularized by James and others. The Q-angle relates to the alignment of the patella with the femur and tibia. The significance of the Q-angle has never been fully established.

R

Rehabilitation Those treatment modalities, exercises, and activities that we owe our patients after knee ligament surgery. Rehabilitation is that discipline which enhances return to function, which is the goal of the athlete and surgeon.

Reverse Lachman test *See* Lachman test, *under* Test.

Rolling/gliding principle The motion of the femur on the tibia; an explanation of the geometry of the femoral condyles.

Rosenberg view The weightbearing tunnel view that best visualizes weightbearing surface of the knee joint. This view is useful in evaluating degenerative arthritic conditions of the knee.

Rotation* A type of motion or displacement in which all points on a body move in circular paths about a fixed axis.

S

SAID principle "Specific adaptation to imposed demands." The secret to returning an athlete to high-level performance within a sport.

Secondary ligamentous restraints *See* Primary and secondary ligamentous restraints, *under* Ligament.

Segond's sign A fracture of the lateral tibial metaphysis at the joint line, probably secondary to avulsion of the mid-third lateral capsular ligament and usually associated with a tear of the ACL.

Shoe–turf fixation One of the reasons that ACL injuries are on the increase is increased efficiency of shoe–turf fixation, which allows more torque to be transmitted to the knee. The swivel heel introduced by Hanley was an attempt to negate this factor; perhaps we should return to this line of investigation.

Slocum test *See under* Test.

Sports medicine The medical care of those who participate in sport. The specific sport or the level of participation is unimportant. The patient defines the discipline by his or her intense desire to "return to play."

Sprain A tear of the ligament. The severity of a sprain may be rated as grade I, II, or III.

Grade I: Mild, interstitial tear without disruption. Usually calls for symptomatic care.

Grade II: Moderate, some disruption of the ligament form. Usually requires some support for immobilization and attendant rehabilitation.

Grade III: Severe, complete ligamentous disruption. May require surgical restoration. "Ligament disruption" is synonymous with grade III sprain.

Stability As it relates to the knee, *stability* signifies the lack of pathologic motion.

Stable hinge A jargon term describing the residual untorn knee ligaments. Even in dislocation some ligaments usually remain intact, and these are the foundation about which the repair or reconstruction is accomplished.

Steadman modification Implies AO screw fixation of the lateral tenodesis.

Stiffness (ankylosis) Intraarticular surgery invites the formation of intraarticular adhesions and the contracture of the periarticular structures. These adhesions and contractures affect patella mobility. Contractures are particularly likely to form in the suprapatellar pouch and along the medial and lateral plicae, resulting in a relative patella baja. Adhesions must be guarded against, as they result in stiffness, ankylosis, and loss of mobility in the joint.

"Stretching out" When ligaments are replaced away from their anatomic origin or insertion, they are not isometric and may "stretch out" with range of motion.

Subjective Perceived by the individual. The patient's history is subjective. (*See also* Objective.)

Subluxation* Partial dislocation. A malposition in which the articulating surfaces can still contact each other, but the location of the contact on at least one bone is abnormal. In the knee, the direction of subluxation (anterior or posterior) and the tibiofemoral compartment involved (lateral or medial) should be specified.

Synovial steal Procedure involving transfer of synovium from the PCL to the ACL to enhance revascularization subsequent to autogenous augmentation. Described by Hewson.

T

Tear, interstitial *See* Avulsion.

Tenderness Pain upon touch or contact. Tenderness is elicited by a lighter touch than is used to detect induration. Tenderness may be used to outline the injured parts of the anatomic structures. The examiner should palpate each anatomic structure for tenderness.

Test

Drawer test The origin of this test is obscure, but it is generally performed with the knee flexed 90° and the examiner sitting on the patient's foot and demonstrating AP glide of the tibia on the femur. The test is best accomplished with the knee flexed 90°, the leg dangling so that gravity assists the examiner, and the foot free so that the internal and external rotation of the compartments may be measured as the anterior Drawer is accomplished. The position of the hands is also important; the thumb should be able to measure the amount of tibial excursion on the femur.

Jakob test A reverse pivot shift test for posterolateral laxity.

Jerk test A palpable "jerk" occurs during translation and rotation of the tibia on the femur. Described by Hughston.

Lachman test Measures the anteroposterior excursion of the tibia on the femur at 30° knee flexion. The end point should be graded as hard or soft. Increased excursion and a soft end point are pathognomonic of ACL incompetence. The standard Lachman test may be difficult to perform for an examiner with small hands, in which case the reverse or prone Lachman test may be used.

Prone/reverse Lachman test The patient is placed prone. The knee is flexed 30°, and the tibia is translated on the femur. Gravity assists the examiner in this test, and the fingers may be placed at the joint line. Thus, posterolateral instability as well as AP excursion can be palpated.

Losee test A version of the pivot shift test. Losee's appreciation of knee ligament pathophysiology is apparent in Chapter 12. A positive Losee test is usually pathognomonic of ACL insufficiency. A false positive result is rare; a false negative result can be caused by muscle spasm or an incompetent medial collateral ligament.

MacIntosh test A pivot shift test similar to the Losee test. It was described before the Losee test.

Noyes test The Noyes test is a flexion external rotation Drawer test. Since it is done with the hip and knee flexed, the patient is usually well relaxed and gravity is on the side of the examiner. This test should be used to complement the other lateral compartment tests.

Slocum test A position that advantageously demonstrates lateral compartment subluxation in cases where the patient's size or muscle guarding prohibits the free manipulation of the lower leg. The foot is fixed in this test, which may limit the subtleties available in the Losee test.

Patella apprehension test Lateral excursion of the patella causes evident discomfort usually associated with recent patellar subluxation.

Test results Positive test results may be classified as trace positive, 1+, 2+, or 3+.

Trace positive A perceptible but nonmeasureable pathologic difference between the injured leg and the well leg. It may not be specific for a particular ligament, but indicates some pathologic laxity of either the primary or the secondary ligamentous restraints.

1+ A 0 to 5 mm pathologic excursion of the tibia on the femur.

2+ A 6 to 10 mm pathologic excursion of the tibia on the femur.

3+ An 11 mm or more pathologic excursion of the tibia on the femur.

Teton sign Spurring of the tibial intercondylar eminences—an early sign of rotatory laxity.

Timeline An adjunct used at the end of each case study in this book to bring the critical events of the care of that patient into focus and stress the sequence of rehabilitation.

Toe rises Toe rises (lifting the heels off the floor and transferring the body weight to the balls of the feet) is a useful exercise in the immediate postoperative period to stimulate gastrosoleus function. Toe rises can be done with or without crutch support, and may involve active plantar flexion with the weight distributed as comfort dictates.

Translation* A type of motion or displacement where all points of a body move parallel to a fixed line. When an object undergoes complex motions involving combined translations and rotations, *translation* refers to the motion of a single point. The location of the point on the object must be specified for the translation motion to be meaningful. In the knee, it has been customary to describe translation by the motion of a point on the tibia located midway between the medial and lateral margins (edges) of the joint.

Compartmental translation The motion of a point located on the medial or lateral tibial plateau. The location of the point must be described for the translation to be meaningful. It can be shown that the translation of a central point located on the medial–lateral midline (knee center) is always the average value of the medial and lateral.

V

Vastus medialis obliquus (VMO) A portion of the quadriceps muscle.

W

Weightbearing The portion of the body weight applied through the limb. It can be influenced by an antalgic gait or crutches. "Weightbearing to comfort" implies that the patient selects the amount of weight borne by the leg, and thereby the floor reaction force is imparted to the injured knee.

W

Well leg   The uninjured leg. Sometimes the athlete does not have a normal knee with which to compare the injured knee. In this case, the examiner must rely on clinical acumen. In the Case Studies, the injured leg is compared to the other, "well," leg for purposes of uniformity.

Wittek procedure   The suturing of the ACL to the PCL, which lessens anterior glide but does not restore the four-bar linkage described by Müller. The procedure is useful as a compromise when open epiphyses are involved. It sometimes happens naturally, explaining the occasional excellent natural history of an untreated or conservatively treated torn ACL.

Index

Page numbers followed by *f* represent figures; those followed by *t* represent tables.